ENCYCLOPEDIA OF

FOODS
AND THEIR HEALING POWER

A Guide to Food Science and Diet Therapy

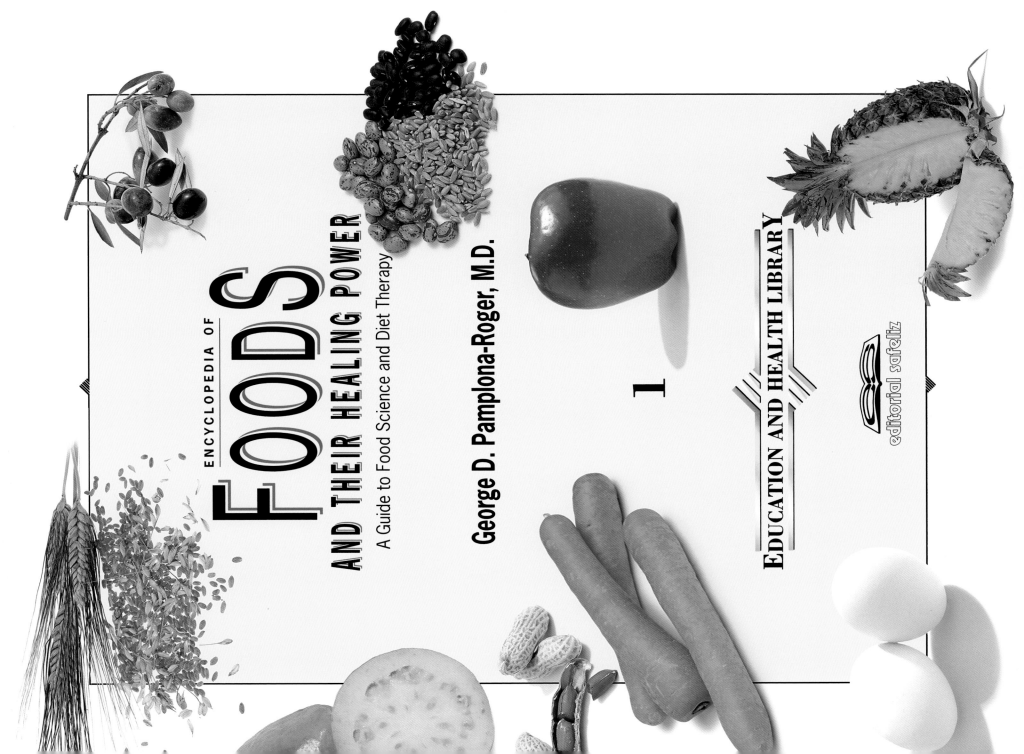

ENCYCLOPEDIA OF

FOODS

AND THEIR HEALING POWER

A Guide to Food Science and Diet Therapy

George D. Pamplona-Roger, M.D.

1

EDUCATION AND HEALTH LIBRARY

editorial safeliz

Education and Health Library
Encyclopedia of Foods and Their Healing Power

EDITORIAL TEAM

General Manager	César Maya Montes
Administration	Sergio Mato Rhiner
Research & Development	George D. Pamplona-Roger
International Marketing	Elisabeth Sangüesa Abenia
Publishing Manager	Leonardo Esteban Ravier
Production & Logistics	Martín González Huelmo

Edition	Raquel Carmona
	Mónica Díaz
	Luis González Soriano
	Juan F. Sánchez Peñas
Layout, Design & Photography	Isaac Chía Mayolas,
	José Mª Weindl,
	Javier Zanuy Pascual

Translation   Annette Melgosa

Copyright by © **EDITORIAL SAFELIZ, S.L.**
Pradillo, 6 – Polígono Industrial La Mina
E-28770 Colmenar Viejo, Madrid, Spain
tel. [+34] 918 459 877 – fax [+34] 918 459 865
admin@safeliz.com – www.safeliz.com

Legal Deposit: V-4966-2006
ISBN: 978-84-7208-345-5 (Complete work)
                 978-84-7208-346-2 (Volume 1)

This Encyclopedia is distributed in USA and Canada by
Review and Herald Publishing Association
55 W. Oak Ridge Drive, Hagerstown, Maryland 21701, USA
tel. [+1] 301-393-3000
email: hhes@rhpa.org

PRINTED IN THE UNITED STATES OF AMERICA

Disclaimer: it is the wish of the author and the publisher that the contents of this work be of value in orienting and in-forming our readers concerning the nutritional, preventive, curative and culinary value of foods and recipes. Although the recommendations and information given are appropriate in most cases, they are of a general nature and cannot take in-to account the specific circumstances of individual situations. The information given in this book is not intended to take the place of professional medical care either in diagnosing or treating medical conditions. Do not attempt self-diagnosis or self-treatment without consulting a qualified medical professional. Some foods and products may cause allergic re-actions in sensitive persons. Neither the publisher nor the author can assume responsibility for problems arising from the inappropriate use of foods or recipes by readers.

TO THE READER

An object of pleasure for some, an effective remedy for others, and an issue of simple survival for the least fortunate among us, foods are an inevitable accompaniment throughout our lives. What is even more, they, along with the air we breathe, come to form the chemical constituents of our bodies.

We each eat between ten and twenty metric tons of food over our lifetime. From this we gain the energy needed to move muscles, for the brain to process thought and for the organs to function properly.

From the foods we eat and the air we breathe, humans gain the materials needed to build and maintain the body.

In addition to these two benefits, that all animals share, human beings should also gain health and happiness from what is taken into the digestive system.

Foods, in addition to providing energy and nutrients, have outstanding healing and preventive power. Scientists are becoming inclined to recognize this and to dissociate the healing power of foods with charlatanism. Unfortunately, the unbridled euphoria that resulted from advances in medical and pharmaceutical technologies during recent decades led to a considerable degree of skepticism concerning the healing properties of natural resources.

Those that once believed that nature would be incapable of compete with what man created in laboratories or accomplished in surgery suites were mistaken. In recent years there has been and ever increasing number of scientific studies demonstrating the healing power of many vegetable foods prepared in their simplest form. Among these we find genuine natural medicines capable of neutralizing and eliminating toxins, regulating vital functions, curbing arteriosclerosis, avoiding cancer, and generally maintaining our health.

No medication can do as much for our health as the healthful foods we eat every day. By the same token, no medication is capable of completely compensating for the harmful effects of the unhealthful foods we eat in an unbalanced diet.

The goal of this ENCYCLOPEDIA OF FOODS AND THEIR HEALING POWER, which forms part of the EDUCATION AND HEALTH LIBRARY, is to provide us with sufficient understanding of food products to enable us to make effective decisions relative to our health.

Editorial Safeliz has provided the best technical resources available in order to make this ENCYCLOPEDIA as current, attractive and easy to use as possible, and thus facilitate a better understanding of the foods that must form part of our diet and our lives.

Doctors Ramón C. Gelabert and Miguel Gracia have contributed their best knowledge to the clarity and accuracy of the text.

My sincere desire is that this ENCYCLOPEDIA assists you in your, often difficult, task of choosing the appropriate foods for your health and well being.

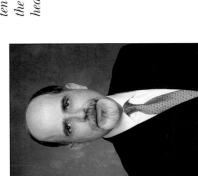

DR. GEORGE D. PAMPLONA-ROGER

General Plan

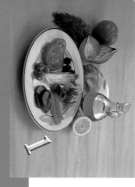

VOLUME ONE

Part One: The Science of Foods

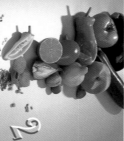

VOLUME TWO

Part Two: The Healing Power of Foods

of the Work

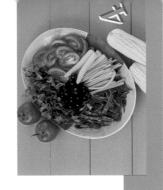

Part Three: The Healthy Kitchen

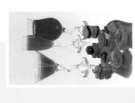

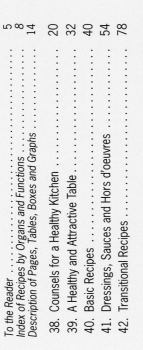

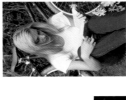

Dressings, Sauces and
Hors d'oeuvres, Ch. 41

Part Four: Recipes that Prevent and Heal

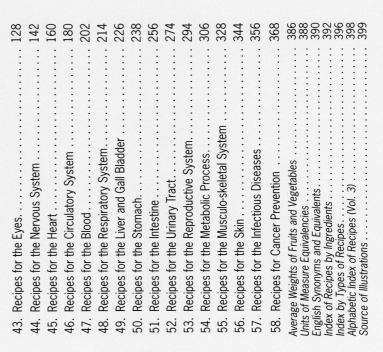

Recipes for the Eyes,
Ch. 43

Recipes for the Skin,
Ch. 56

Recipes for the Musculo-skeletal
System, Ch. 55

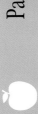

Index of Diseases

This index includes several non-pathological conditions such as pregnancy in addition to diseases.

Those diseases in bold are those that serve as headers in the Tables of Diseases.

Foods Index

Foods Index (Continued)

Besides foods, this index includes nutrients and other products.

See also the Index of Food Names in Other Languages (2/419) and the General Alphabetical Index (2/425).

How To Use This ENCYCLOPEDIA

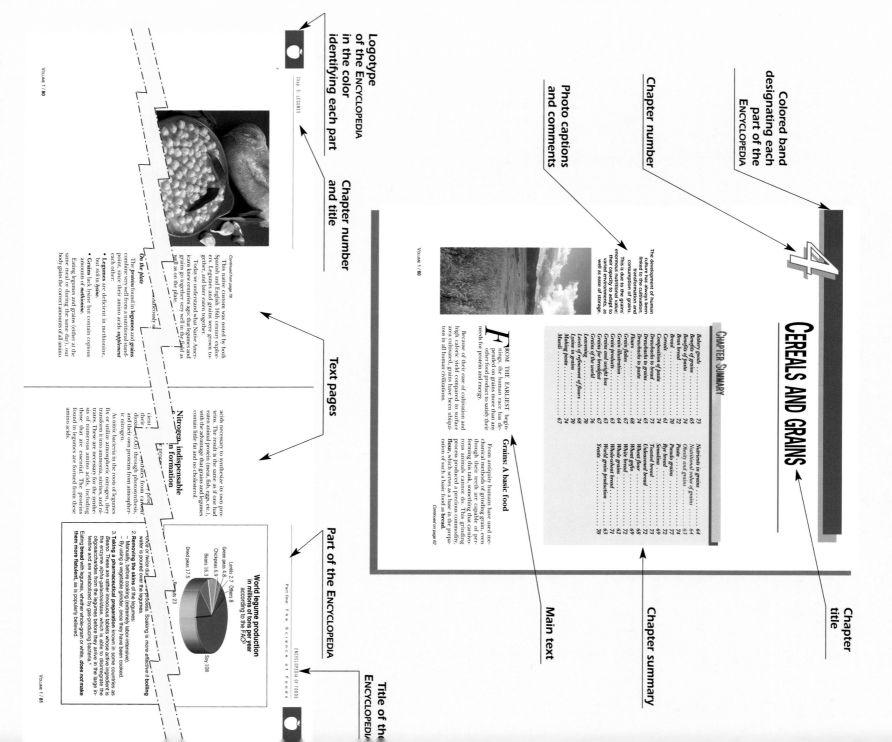

Colored band designating each part of the ENCYCLOPEDIA

Chapter number

Photo captions and comments

Logotype of the ENCYCLOPEDIA in the color identifying each part

Chapter number and title

Text pages

Part of the ENCYCLOPEDIA

Chapter title

Main text

Chapter summary

Title of the ENCYCLOPEDIA

Benefits of Honey

- **Provides energy** (304 kcal/100 g=1,270kj/100g) *very rapidly*. Its **sugars** (glucose and fructose) *do not need to be processed* in the digestive tract; thus, they are quickly absorbed into the bloodstream distributing energy to all the cells of the body.
- It **contains** small quantities of **B** group *vitamins* and *minerals* (calcium and phosphorous) that aid in the metabolism of sugars in the cells.
- **Antiseptic:** When applied to the skin or mucosa (interior of the nose, mouth, pharynx) it destroys pathogens due to its:
  - *elevated sugar concentration*, which inhibits bacterial development;

Chart showing benefits of a food
Identified by a + symbol.

Drawbacks to Honey

- **Botulism:** Although honey does not contain bacterial pathogens, it may contain spores of certain microorganisms such as *Clostridium botulinum*.[29] In the favorable conditions found in the human intestine, these spores transform into the pathogens causing botulism. This *generally* occurs in **infants**, due to their lower resistance level. It is for this reason giving honey to **infants** less than *one year* of age is **not** advised (see caution on the preceding page).
- **Allergies:** These may manifest themselves in a variety of ways: itching in the mouth, digestive disorders, or even severe anaphylactic shock. This is due to the proteins secreted by the bee's glands, as well as the pollen grains in the honey.[30]

Chart showing drawbacks of a food
Identified by a – symbol.

Green: favorable

Red: unfavorable

Amber: neutral

Margarine and Butter Compared

	Margarine	Butter
Natural food	No	Yes
Total fat content	70-80%	81%
Percentage of saturated fat	15%	50,5%
Essential polyunsaturated fatty acids	25%	3%
Trans fatty acids	20-30%	4-5%
Cholesterol	0	219 mg/100 g
Vitamin or provitamin A	799 µg RE/100 g	754 µg RE/100 g
Vitamin E	12,8 mg α–TE/100 g	1,58 mg α–TE/100 g
Relation to heart disease	For some, consumption of **trans-fatty acids**, which is present in large quantities in margarine, does not increase coronary risk.[14] According to the American Heart Association, margarine, especially **light margarine** is **preferable** to butter.[15,16]	For other investigators, such as Doctor Willett, of Harvard University, the animal fat in butter is not as harmful as once thought. On the other hand, consumption of foods rich in **trans-fatty acids** (margarine, bakery goods) are, indeed, associated with greater risk of coronary disease[17,22] and breast cancer.[72]

Comparative table
The color of each cell indicates whether the described element is favorable, unfavorable or neutral.

Information box

Presents additional information regarding a topic in the text or of special interest.

"Mad Cow Disease" and Milk

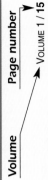

Many ask if milk can transmit the **prions** (infectious proteins) that cause **bovine spongiform encephalopathy**, called "mad cow disease."

Numerous experiments with laboratory animals have shown that milk **does not transmit** mad cow disease.[40]

Inoculation or consumption of infected nerve or bone tissue do transmit it, however, even though physical (heat) or chemical (formol or alcohol) sterilizing techniques have been employed.

Warning box

Presents highlights and advice regarding a food or topic in the text.

Milk and the Heart

*Many studies have shown that milk consumption, **even nonfat milk**, constitutes a risk **factor** for coronary disease (**angina** pectoris and myocardial **infarction**). This is due to negative effects that certain milk components have on cholesterol levels and the cardiovascular system.*

- *Saturated fats: The **predominant** fats in cow's milk are saturated (see Vol. 1, p. 191), which fosters cholesterol production in the body. Using **whole milk** and **butter** increases mortality rates by myocardial **infarction**, since milk fat also promotes **arteriosclerosis** and arterial **thrombosis.**[31] **Replacing** whole milk with **nonfat milk reduces the risk** of coronary disease.[32]*
- **Casein:** *This is the prevalent protein in milk, and gives it its white color. When compared with vegetable proteins, casein **increases** cholesterol level[11,12] (see Vol. 1, p. 191).*
- **Lactose:** *This is the sugar in milk, which also plays a role in the development of coronary disease[8] (see Vol. 1, p. 188).*

Description of the Graphs

Graph of food composition indicating the absolute and relative quantities of **energy** and **nutrients contained.**

Each is represented by a color.

The **numbers** indicate the **absolute energy content** and the mass of each **nutrient** found in 100 grams of a food. This information is provided by the United States Department of Agriculture.[1]

Food

MILK (Whole) composition
per 100g of raw edible portion

Energy	61.4 kcal = 257 kJ
Protein	3.29 g
Carbohydrates	4.66 g
Fiber	
Vitamin A	31.0 µg RE
Vitamin B₁	0.038 mg
Vitamin B₂	0.162 mg
Niacin	0.851 mg NE
Vitamin B₆	0.042 mg
Folates	5.00 µg
Vitamin B₁₂	0.357 µg
Vitamin C	0.940 mg
Vitamin E	0.100 mg α-TE
Calcium	119 mg
Phosphorous	93.4 mg
Magnesium	13.4 mg
Iron	0.050 mg
Potassium	152 mg
Zinc	0.380 mg
Total fat	*3.34 g*
Saturated fat	*2.08 g*
Cholesterol	*13.6 mg*
Sodium	*49.0 mg*

% Daily Value (based on a 2,000 calorie diet) provided by 100 g of this food

Scale: 1% 2% 4% 10% 20% 40% 100%

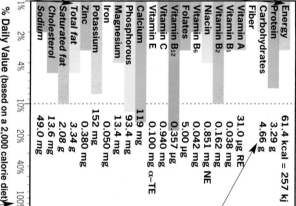

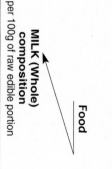

Criteria used in to establish precision of measurement:

- Values less than 1: **3 decimal places**
- Values equal to or greater than 1, but less than 10: **2 decimal places**
- Values equal to or greater than 10 but less than 100: **1 decimal place**
- Values above 100: **no decimal place**

The **length** of the **bars** matches the "**% Daily value**" of each nutrient and food component labeled in food products. The "**% Daily Value**" shows how a food fits into the overall daily diet.

The length of the bars matching the "**% Daily value**" have always been calculated for a male adult taking a 2,000 calorie diet.[2]

Upper bars: Their length show the "**% Daily value**" of each **main nutrient** provided by 100 grams of the analyzed food.

In this case, the "**% Daily value**" represents the percentage of the Reccomended Dietary Allowance (RDA, see Vol. 2, p. 18) for each main nutrient.

Four bottom bars: Their length show the "**% Daily value**" of food components for which there are no RDAs (**total fat, saturated fat, cholesterol** and **sodium**) provided by 100 grams of the analyzed food. Names and figures of these four food components are displayed in italics.

In this case, the "**% Daily value**" represents the percentage of the maximum acceptable daily intake of these food components.

For example, this graph shows that 100 grams of milk provide 0.162 mg of vitamin B₂ (absolute quantity). This represents approximately 10% of the Daily Value (RDA) for vitamin B₂ for an adult male. The RDA of vitamin B₂ is 1.7 mg so 0.162 mg provides approximately 10 % of the RDA (see Vol. 2, p. 18).

If 100 grams of the analyzed product provided the 100% of the Daily Value of a particular nutrient for an adult male, the bar would extend the entire width of the graph.

Nevertheless the **logarithmic scale** for some foods may reach **500%** since some nutrients are present in very high concentrations.

The scale used for the length of the **bars** is **logarithmic**; therefore the length of the bars is not directly proportional to the nutritional content.

---

1 Department of Agriculture, Agricultural Research Service, USDA Nutritional Database for Standard Reference, Nutrient Data Laboratory. http://www.usda.gov/fnic/foodcomp

2 Even though the length of the bars is based on the **RDAs** (Recommended Dietary Allowances) for adult males between 25 and 50 years of age taking a 2,000 calories diet, it may also be used as an orientation for other age groups (see Vol. 2, p. 18);

- **Children:** RDAs are less than for an adult male. Therefore, if 100 grams of milk provides 10% of RDA of vitamin B₂ for an adult male between 25 and 50 years of age, it will provide more than 10% of RDA for women and children, whose needs are less.

- **Women:** The RDAs (Recommended Dietary Allowances) of most nutrients are less for women than for adult males, except of calcium and iron. However, RDAs for pregnant and lactating women are the same or greater than that for adult males.

Used in This Encyclopedia

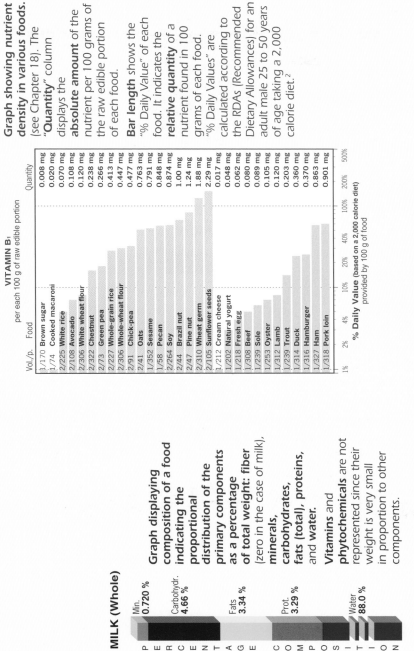

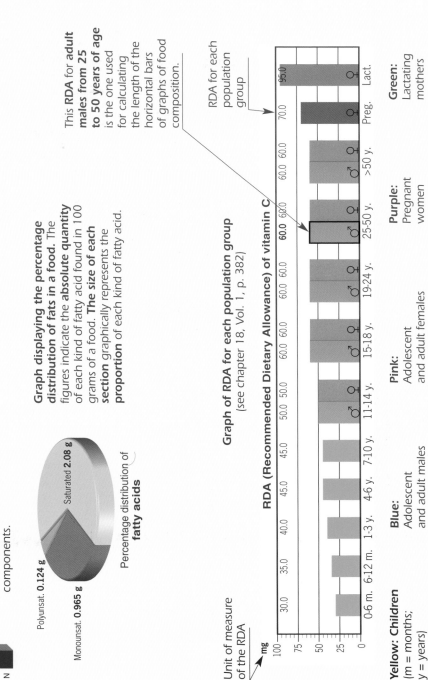

VITAMIN B₁
per each 100 g of raw edible portion

Vol./p.	Food	Quantity
1/170	Brown sugar	0.008 mg
1/74	Cooked macaroni	0.020 mg
2/225	White rice	0.070 mg
2/108	Avocado	0.108 mg
2/306	White wheat flour	0.120 mg
2/322	Chestnut	0.238 mg
2/73	Green pea	0.266 mg
2/227	Whole-grain rice	0.413 mg
2/306	Whole-wheat flour	0.447 mg
2/91	Chick-pea	0.477 mg
2/41	Oats	0.763 mg
1/352	Sesame	0.791 mg
1/58	Pecan	0.848 mg
2/264	Soy	0.874 mg
2/44	Brazil nut	1.00 mg
2/47	Pine nut	1.24 mg
2/310	Wheat germ	1.88 mg
2/105	Sunflower seeds	2.29 mg
1/212	Cream cheese	0.017 mg
1/202	Natural yogurt	0.048 mg
1/218	Fresh egg	0.062 mg
1/308	Beef	0.080 mg
1/239	Sole	0.089 mg
1/253	Oyster	0.105 mg
1/312	Lamb	0.120 mg
1/239	Trout	0.203 mg
1/314	Duck	0.360 mg
1/316	Hamburger	0.370 mg
1/327	Ham	0.863 mg
1/318	Pork loin	0.901 mg

% Daily Value (based on a 2,000 calorie diet) provided by 100 g of food

1% 2% 4% 10% 20% 40% 100% 200% 500%

Graph showing nutrient density in various foods. (see Chapter 18). The "Quantity" column displays the **absolute amount** of the nutrient per 100 grams of the raw edible portion of each food.

Bar length shows the "% Daily Value" of each food. It indicates the **relative quantity** of a nutrient found in 100 grams of each food. "% Daily Values" are calculated according to the RDAs (Recommended Dietary Allowances) for an adult male 25 to 50 years of age taking a 2,000 calorie diet.[2]

MILK (Whole)

Min. **0.720 %**
Carbohydr. **4.66 %**
Fats **3.34 %**
Prot. **3.29 %**
Water **88.0 %**

PERCENTAGE COMPOSITION

Graph displaying composition of a food indicating the **proportional distribution of the primary components as a percentage of total weight:** fiber (zero in the case of milk), minerals, carbohydrates, fats (total), proteins, and water.

Vitamins and phytochemicals are not represented since their weight is very small in proportion to other components.

Polyunsat. **0.124 g**
Monounsat. **0.965 g**
Saturated **2.08 g**

Percentage distribution of **fatty acids**

Graph displaying the percentage distribution of fats in a food. The figures indicate the **absolute quantity** of each kind of fatty acid found in 100 grams of a food. **The size of each section** graphically represents the **proportion** of each kind of fatty acid.

This **RDA for adult males from 25 to 50 years of age** is the one used for calculating the length of the horizontal bars of graphs of food composition.

RDA for each population group

Graph of RDA for each population group
(see chapter 18, Vol. 1, p. 382)

Unit of measure of the RDA: **mg**

RDA (Recommended Dietary Allowance) of vitamin C

100 75 50 25 0

0-6 m. 6-12 m. 1-3 y. 4-6 y. 7-10 y. 11-14 y. 15-18 y. 19-24 y. 25-50 y. >50 y. Preg. Lact.

50.0 45.0 40.0 35.0 30.0 50.0 60.0 60.0 60.0 60.0 60.0 60.0 60.0 70.0 95.0

Yellow: Children (m = months; y = years)

Blue: Adolescent and adult males

Pink: Adolescent and adult females

Purple: Pregnant women

Green: Lactating mothers

PROLOGUE

Whether based on belief or science, certain foods have been credited with healing powers. More than two thousand years ago, the precursor of modern medicine, Hippocrates, coined the aphorism "May your food be your medicine, and may your medicine be your food." The play on words, by this wise Greek demonstrates that our daily food, more than merely sustaining us, may contain curative properties. Although, postulated through the course of medical history, scientific evidence has only recently established the fact that some nutrients in our diet are agents that cause or cure certain diseases.

It was first demonstrated in studies with laboratory animals and later on humans that the lack of certain foods in the diet caused deficiency diseases, such as rickets, and that the inclusion of other foods cured patients with those diseases. Fortunately, deficiency diseases are not a problem for most of the population. However, many do suffer from illnesses and diseases referred to as "diseases of civilization."

Recent years have brought profound changes in the lifestyle of the industrialized world whereas dietary habits, uses and preferences are concerned. Many follow a diet characterized by excessive caloric consumption and frequent nutritional imbalances. The consumption of animal-derived food products continues to increase, with its accompanying increase in saturated fats and cholesterol. The tendency to eat highly refined or processed products reduces the intake of vitamins, certain minerals and other beneficial substances such as fiber contained in foods in their most natural state.

In recent years, nutritional investigation has concentrated on the effect diet has on the prevention and treatment of circulatory disease, diabetes, cancer and obesity, since these are currently the most frequent. Population and clinical studies have demonstrated, for example, that the abundant use of fruits and vegetables prevents the initiation of certain cancers. The eating of whole grain cereals and oil-bearing nuts reduces excess levels of cholesterol in the blood and the risk of myocardial infarction. On the other hand, the consumption of a great deal of meat increases the risk of cardiovascular disease and some types of cancer. Thus we see that the choice, frequency and quantity of the foods that we eat very directly affects our health.

Foods of vegetable origin, rich in fiber, minerals and vitamins, also bring substances to the diet that, although not well understood nor classified as nutrients, display potent anticarcinogenic and curative effects on a variety of diseases and illnesses. These substances, known as phytochemicals, are currently the subject of intense study and represent the new frontier in nutritional investigation. Phytochemical elements are only found in foods of vegetable origin and possess important health and healing properties.

This ENCYCLOPEDIA OF FOODS AND THEIR HEALING POWER provides clear and usable information concerning the composition, nutritional and therapeutic properties of foods. Thus, the reader is led to a prudent selection of the products that form his diet. With this work by Dr. George D. Pamplona-Roger, Editorial Safeliz continues its noteworthy efforts to publish books and materials for an intelligent public interested in maintaining and improving their health by giving preference to natural elements.

DR. JOAN SABATÉ
Professor and Chair
of the Department
of Nutrition,
School of Public Health,
Loma Linda University
(California, USA).

Index of Chapters

VOLUME 1

ENCYCLOPEDIA OF

FOODS

AND THEIR HEALING POWER

PART ONE

The Science of Foods

"I give you every seed-bearing plant on the face of the whole earth and every tree that has fruit with seed in it. They will be yours for food."

THE BOOK OF GENESIS
chapter 1, verse 29

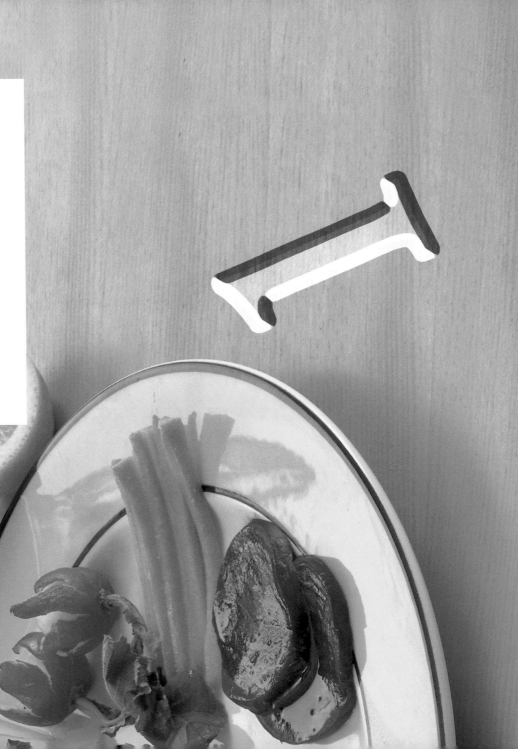

1

FOODS FOR HUMANS

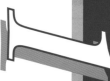

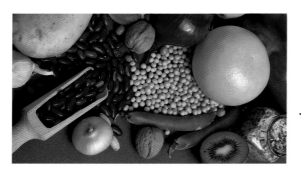

With the exception of mother's milk during infancy, no food by itself provides all of the nutrients needed by humans. Therefore, knowing how to select foods and appropriately combine them is of vital importance.

HUMAN BEINGS can eat just about anything as food, from mammary secretions (milk) to mineral crystals (common salt), including fruits, flowers, seeds, stalks, leaves, roots, seaweed, fungus, eggs of fish and birds or the dead bodies of various animals.

All of these, processed to a greater or lesser degree, provide thousands of different foods to the market.

Does the fact that we can eat this whole variety of foods mean that *all of them are equally fit for human consumption? Is there an ideal diet for humans that, in addition to being nourishing, maintains health and prevents disease?*

Chance or Intelligent Plan

The engineer has finished his work. The shining engine he has built is sitting on the test bench ready to be started for the first time.

"Here is the type of fuel that must be used in this engine", says the engineer to his assistants. "No other will give optimal results. And don't forget the oil. It must be exactly of this type!"

Only the one who has planned and built a engine can knowledgeably prescribe the type of fuel and lubricant the mechanism needs.

Specifically Recommended Foods

And is it not this way with humans? If human presence on planet Earth is just a random and unexpected consequence of evolutionary chance, then there should not be any particularly ideal foods. Man would have simply adapted to whatever foods were available, and whatever those might have been, they would have provided good health and wellbeing.

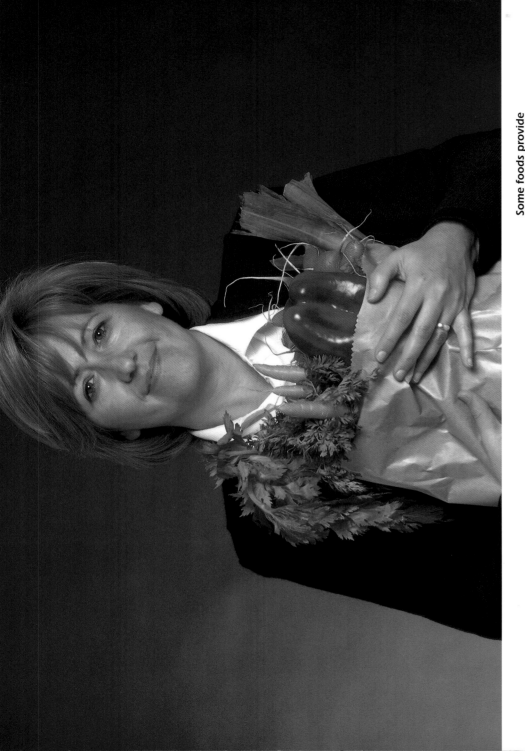

However, if humans were created by a superior Intelligence according to a specific plan and for a particular purpose, there should be, as well, specially created foods to maintain optimal physiological performance. Many believers find answers to these questions in the first chapters of Genesis, where it says that plants that bear seeds, **grains**, and, in a broader sense, **legumes**, **fruit** from trees[1] and **vegetables** that were added later,[2] constitute the *ideal diet* for the human species.

Adaptation, Yes, but Not by Eliminating Necessary Foods

Humans possess great capacity to adapt physiologically to many different types of foods. In spite of this, nutrition science has demonstrated that there are certain foods that ***cannot be eliminated***, such as **fruit** and **fresh vegetables**. Not just any diet can produce good health. No matter how well we adapt to certain foods that are not ideal, such as those of animal ori-

gin, we continue to need vegetables, which are the most healthful and suitable. For example, Alaskan Eskimos have adapted to a diet rich in fish but they suffer a number of chronic diseases due to low consumption of fruit and vegetables.[3]

Some foods provide curative and preventive substances in addition to nutrients. Because of these benefits, foods that are well chosen and carefully used can cure, relieve and prevent many disorders and diseases.

i

Basic Definitions

- ***Food:*** *Natural or manufactured product, solid or liquid, that contains one or more of the nutrients that the human organism requires for the development of vital functions.*

- ***Healing powers of foods:*** *The capacity of certain foods to restore health and to avoid certain disorders and diseases.*

What to expect from foods

	Is this met by foods of vegetable origin?	Is this met by foods of animal origin?
That they will do no harm such as infections, poisoning, or other diseases. *Primum non nocere* (First, do no harm) is the old medical aphorism.	**Yes,** in general.	**Not** always. They contain pathogenic **viruses, bacteria, and parasites at a much higher rate than vegetables.** *Habitual* consumption of some foods is *related* to **cancer** and **cardiovascular disease.**
That they provide the **energy** needed by the organism to function.	**Yes,** basically through carbohydrates (recommended).	**Yes,** primarily through proteins and fats.
That they supply needed **nutrients.**	**Yes,** except in the case of **vitamin B₁₂;** although for reasons that are not well understood, strict vegetarians do not suffer from this lack as might be expected.	**Not completely.** They provide *little* or **no vitamin C, vitamin E, carbohydrates** or cellulose **fiber.**
That they **prevent or cure** disorders and diseases.	**Yes.** They have healing and preventive properties.	**No,** except in **very specific cases.**
That they provide a sense of **pleasure** when eaten.	**Yes.**	**Yes.**

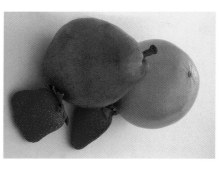

Vegetable Foods, Source of Health and Healing Powers

There has been a rapidly increasing number of scientific discoveries in recent years related to foods of vegetable origin. As methods of chemical analysis have become more precise, it is being proved that fruits, grains, legumes and vegetables contain, in addition to nutrients found in all foods, two types of compounds that are *not found* in foods of **animal** origin:

- *antioxidants* (certain vitamins and minerals), and
- *phytochemicals* with curative properties.

Many scientists are inquisitive about the origin and significance of these beneficial substances found only in vegetables. *Why do humans need them for their health? Why do*

Fruits, grains, legumes as well as vegetables are particularly rich in antioxidants and accompanying substances known as phytochemical elements, that act as true natural pharmaceuticals.

they continue to need them after centuries or millennia of adaptation to a carnivorous diet, such as the traditional diet of the Eskimos? Why is there an ideal diet for the health of humans?

Two Options...

There are those that believe that humans found plants and vegetable foods possessing healing powers by mere chance. These vegetables, according to this reasoning, evolved the capacity to synthesize precisely those nutritional and healing substances that would be needed by humans long before humans existed.[4]

But we may also consider, with no less validity, a rational alternative; that a superior Being created Man and Woman and provided them with an ideal "fuel": vegetable foods.[5]

1

Foods of Animal Origin With Healing Properties

Although foods of vegetable origin hold the most healing powers, some of animal origin stand out because of their preventive and healing properties.

Honey and Other Products of the Hive

Honey is referred to as **sweet medicine** (see Vol. 1, pp. 164-165). Royal jelly, pollen, and propolis (see Vol. 1, pp. 359-361) act as a general tonic.

Yogurt

Yogurt increases immune defenses because of the bacteria it contains, rather than because of its milk content.

Fish

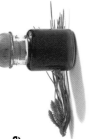

Fish oils are used for their **anti-inflammatory** and **hypolipidemic** *(lowers blood triglyceride levels) effects. Fish liver oil has long been used for the prevention and treatment of rickets because of its high vitamin D content although manufactured preparations of this vitamin are preferred today.*

Beef Liver

Beef liver and that of other mammals has been used in the treatment of different types of **anemia,** because of its high content of iron and vitamin B₁₂. Manufactured products are preferred today, due, among other reasons, to the high level of chemical contamination present in the organs of animals.

Without a doubt many things have happened since then. Therefore in the present state of nature and humanity, **foods of animal origin** can become **necessary** *in some cases;* although *never* **indispensable.** This notwithstanding, the basis of human nutrition as well as the most important source of health-producing materials continue to be fruit, grains, seeds, and vegetables. The exception, of course, is the first phase of life (lactation).

...and the Same Conclusion

In either of these cases, no matter what one may believe about origins, numerous scientific studies demonstrate that vegetable foods prepared simply provide the *best* '**fuel**' for our "engine." They supply the energy necessary to function and the substances to slow the "wear and tear" of the years and helps prevent "breakdown."

And do not forget to provide the *best oil* for this "engine!" (see Vol. 1, p. 112).

Foods and Health

Our health depends on the sum total of the many **"small" decisions** that we take each day, in other words, our **lifestyle.**

Generally speaking, the decisions we make that *most affect* our health have to do with the **foods** we eat. There are so many options available that we must continually decide which foods to select and how they are best prepared.

Information + Correct Choices = Health

The more complete the information we have concerning available foods, the easier it is to make the best choices for health.[6]

Throughout the pages that follow the reader will come to understand that all foods are not of equal value.

Knowing Foods Well

It is vital to understand foods well in order to select those that maintain our health, which is so threatened today, and those that treat various diseases. This ENCYCLOPEDIA OF FOODS AND THEIR HEALING POWERS is designed to provide that understanding.

Harmful Foods, Beneficial Foods

Humans need food throughout their lives. While all foods provide nutrients and energy, some can cause disorders and diseases; while others, bring health and healing. Therefore, there are potentially harmful foods, and, of course, beneficial foods.

Foods can prevent and cure diseases, but they can also cause them. Therefore, the best diet is not one that includes "a little of everything" but one that avoids the harmful and makes moderate use of the beneficial.

Sources of Foods

Humans can adapt to eating almost anything, whether mineral, vegetable or animal. But simply because something can be eaten does not mean that this may be done without risking good health.

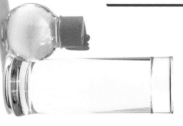

From the Mineral Kingdom

Water and **salt** are two foods (in the broad sense of the word), of mineral origin. Unlike any other food, the water and salt we eat do not originate with any living thing.

From the Vegetable Kingdom

These foods are the *healthiest* and have the *most healing properties*. Various types of vegetables can be used as food:

- **Seaweed:** These are eaten whole, whether they are microscopic single-cell (such as Spirulina, Vol. 1, p. 134) or multicellular such as the rest of the seaweed described in Chapter eight.

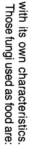

- **Higher plants:** Customarily, these foods are a part of the plant: fruit, seed, bulb, root, etc. (see Vol. 1, pp. 96-97).

- **Fungi:** Although they are grouped with foods of vegetable origin, fungi belong to an independent kingdom with its own characteristics. Those fungi used as food are:

  – certain **microscopic fungi** belonging to the class Ascomycetes, such as brewer's yeast.

  – **mushrooms,** which are, in reality only a part (fruity body) of higher fungi.

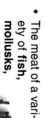 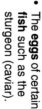 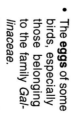

From the Animal Kingdom

Certain secretions, eggs, and meat of various aquatic and land animals can be used for food. However, *not all* of them are **beneficial.**

- The **milk** of various species of mammals and the dairy products that are made from it.

- **Honey** and other **secretions** of certain insects such as **bees.**

- The **eggs** of some birds, especially those belonging to the family *Gallinaceae.*

- The **eggs** of certain **fish** such as the sturgeon (caviar).

- The meat of a variety of **fish, mollusks, amphibians** and **crustaceans.**

- The **meat** and other body tissues of aquatic (whale) or land (lamb) **mammals.**

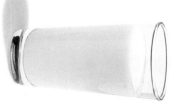

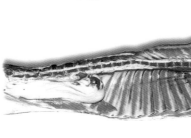

Comparison of Foods of Vegetable and Animal Origin

	Vegetable Origin	Animal Origin
Healing	**Yes.** In addition to their nutritive properties, they act pharmacologically in a manner *similar* to **medicinal plants** (see next page).	Only **very few** and only in very specific cases.
Living	The greater portion can be eaten while their cells are still alive, therefore retaining *all* of their **biochemical and healing potential.**	Their cells are dead when eaten. **Decay** begins in these cells at the moment of the animal's death.
Chemical contamination	Generally speaking, this is *very small and external.* As a result peeling or thorough washing can eliminate it.	**Greater** than with vegetables, since animals **retain and concentrate** contaminants that they consume (see Vol. 1, p. 248).
Harmful components	Generally, they contain *few and of low toxicity.* Any that may be present are normally removed by soaking or cooking (see Vol. 1, p. 84).	May contain very **powerful and dangerous toxins,** particularly seafood and some fish (see Vol. 1, pp. 246-251, 256-261).
Depletion of natural resources	Production requires *few* natural resources. Some crops, such as legumes, do not even require fertilizer (see Vol. 1, p. 80).	**High.** To gain *one* calorie of **animal-based** food, it is necessary to provide *seven* calories of **vegetable-based** feed to livestock or fowl.
Antioxidant action	Fruits, as well as vegetables, are **rich** in **powerful** antioxidants such as vitamins A, C, and E, selenium and flavonoids. They *prevent* **premature aging,** *avoid* cancer and *enhance* the **immune system.**	Contains *only a trace* of antioxidants.
Diuretic	*Promotes* **elimination** of numerous **prejudicial substances** that are the by-products of **metabolism,** such as uric acid and urea. **Purifies** and **detoxifies** the blood and tissues.	**Do not act** as a diuretic. To the contrary, meat, seafood and fish **add** waste material to the organism (see Vol. 1, p. 300).
Na/K quotient (sodium/ potassium)	**Low,** since they contain much more potassium than sodium. This *contributes* to its **diuretic** and **antihypertensive** effects.	**High.** Dairy products, fish, seafood, and meats contain more sodium and less potassium than vegetables. Their *regular* **consumption** may lead to **hypertension.**
Ca/P quotient (calcium/ phosphorous)	**High,** thus *contributing* to the fixation of **minerals** in the **bones.**	**Low.** Since they contain much more phosphorous than calcium fish, seafood, and meat act as **decalcifiers.**
Cholesterol	**No vegetable** food contains cholesterol; not even those rich in fats such as nuts. Additionally they *help* **lower** blood cholesterol levels.	Cholesterol is **only** found in **foods of animal origin. All** animal secretions and animal tissues with the exception of honey and other products of the beehive contain cholesterol.
Heart	**Heart healthy,** help *avoid* **arteriosclerosis** (see Ch. 22 Vol. 2, pp. 82-90).	Milk products, eggs and meat are associated with **coronary disease** (see Vol. 1, pp. 193, 225, 300).
Cancer	Contain substances that **counteract** the effect of **carcinogens** consumed as ingredients of other foods or as a consequence of environmental pollution. Additionally, they stop the **development** of **cancerous cells** (see Vol. 2, pp. 368-373).	Several research studies relate the *liberal use* of milk, eggs and meat with various types of cancer. (see vol. 1, pp. 193, 225, 307). On the other hand, **yogurt** and **fermented milk** products have a **prophylactic** effect.

The Healing Power

Discover the natural pharmacy in your pantry.
This chart presents some of the healing properties of vegetable foods.

Healing Foods

Plant-based foods, like medicinal plants, contain substances that produce pharmacological effects similar to any other medication, but with these **advantages:**

- They **prevent and correct the tendency toward** disease, in addition to having curative properties.

- *Generally speaking, they have no* **side effects.**

Diuretics

Celery: increases urine production, aids kidney function and reduces edema.

Other diuretic foods: eggplant, melon, watermelon, leeks, and asparagus.

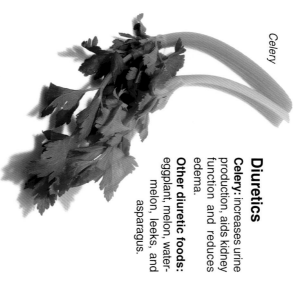

Celery

Persimmon

Astringents

Persimmon: Contains tannins that dry the intestinal mucosa and mucilage that softens it.

Other astringent foods: quince, apple, caimito, pomegranate, and loquat.

Hepatic Tonic

Artichoke: increases bile flow and detoxifies the liver.

Other foods that act as hepatic tonics: loquats, cardoom.

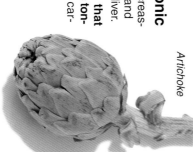

Artichoke

Urinary Antiseptics

Cranberry: Counters the effects of cystitis and other urinary infections without activating bacterial resistance.

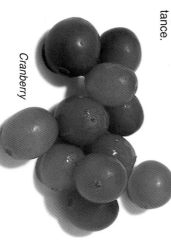

Cranberry

Mineral Restorers

Coconut: very rich in magnesium, calcium and phosphorous.

Other mineral restoring foods: almonds, alfalfa, cabbage, oranges, turnip greens.

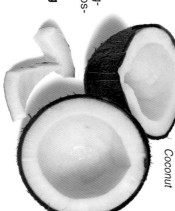

Coconut

# of Vegetables

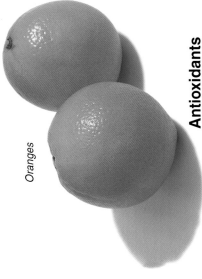

Avocado

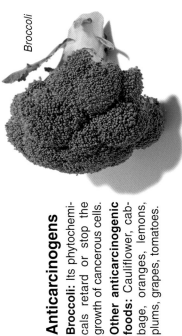

Oranges

Antioxidants

Oranges: contain four potent antioxidants: vitamin C, beta-carotene (provitamin A), flavonoids and folic acid. They help avoid arteriosclerosis and thrombosis.

Other antioxidant foods: strawberries, citrus fruits, and nuts.

Hypolipidemic

Avocado: antianemic, protects the digestive lining and acts as a tonic in addition to lowering blood cholesterol and triglyceride levels.

Other hypolipidemic foods: beans, English walnuts, sunflower seeds, yams.

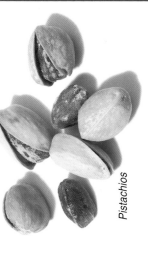

Broccoli

Anticarcinogens

Broccoli: Its phytochemicals retard or stop the growth of cancerous cells.

Other anticarcinogenic foods: Cauliflower, cabbage, oranges, lemons, plums, grapes, tomatoes.

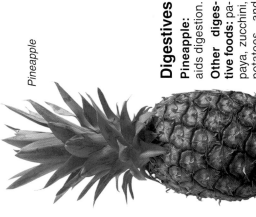

Pineapple

Digestives

Pineapple: aids digestion.

Other digestive foods: papaya, zucchini, potatoes, and okra.

Antianemics

Pistachios: Contain as much or more iron as lentils, in addition to copper and other trace elements that serve to promote blood production.

Other antianemic foods: red beets, apricots, passion fruit, spinach, and lamb's lettuce.

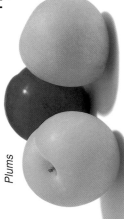

Pistachios

Laxatives

Plums: stimulate intestinal function.

Other laxative foods: eggplant, chard, and whole grain cereals.

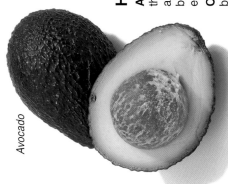

Plums

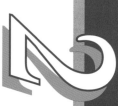

2

FRUITS

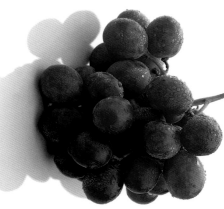

Of the great variety of foods that nature provides none delights the senses or is so healthful as fruit.

THERE IS an old proverb that says: *"Where the sun shines in, the doctor stays away,"* Today, there are so many studies demonstrating the healing powers of fruit that we could say, *"Where fruit is eaten in abundance, there is no need for medicines."*

Characteristics of Fruit

Good To Eat

The first thing we notice about fruits is how appetizing they are. Among all the foods that humans can eat, **none** is so **pleasant and healthful** as fruit.

Fruit produces sensory stimulation that results in a whole series of physiological responses that prepare the system for better digestion: the most obvious is that merely considering a lemon activates salivation.

Mere chance is not enough in itself to explain why fruit attracts us when our sense of taste has not been too dulled by artificial flavors. As with other natural phenomena, there must be some purpose, a design, behind it. The book of Genesis says, *"And the Lord God made all kinds of trees that were pleasing to the eye and good for food."*[1]

Is it unreasonable to believe, then, that fruit has been made to look delicious to our sight because our body cannot live without it?

Continued on page 32

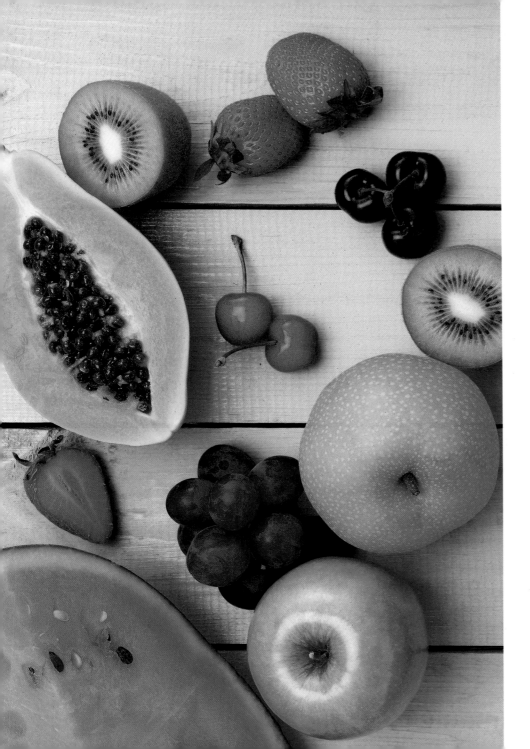

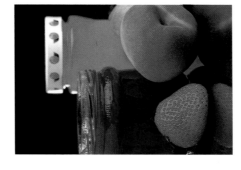

Jams, jellies, and marmalades are prepared by combining sugar, pectin, and citric acid or lemon juice with fruit and then heating the mixture. There are fruits that are high in pectin (a type of vegetable fiber) such as the apple, which can be made into jelly without adding pectin.

Botanical and Dietary Concepts of Fruit

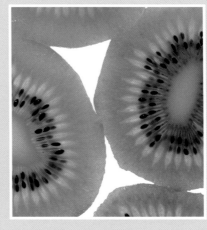

- *Botanical concept: **Fruit** is the edible por-tion of a plant that has developed from a **flower** or **blossom**. It contains internal seeds. The **fruit** is formed from the **mature ovary** of the flower and the **seeds** from its **ovules**.*

- *Dietary concept: The fruit of a plant, sweet and juicy, that is normally eaten fresh and produces particularly pleasant sensations to the five senses.*

*While tomatoes, cucumbers, and eggplants are fruits from a botanical point of view, they are considered **vegetables** from a dietary standpoint. This traditional classification is quite arbitrary. Tomatoes, for example, meet all the requirements to be considered true fruit according to the dietary concept.*

Fruit is the best and most natural source of vitamins, minerals, and fiber, thus the most healthful.

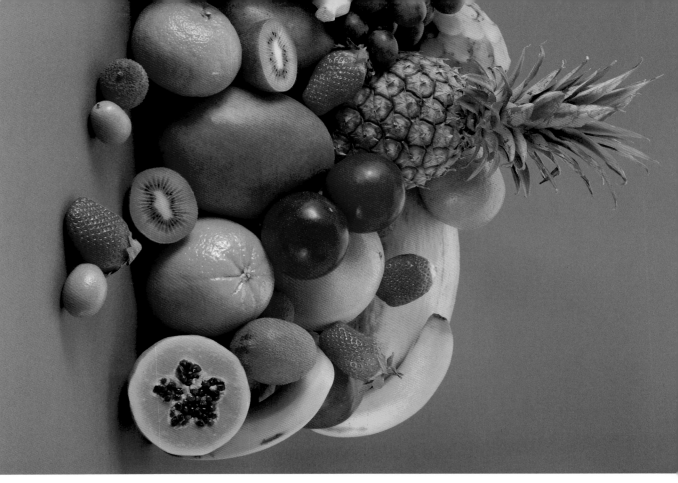

Continued from page 32

Fruit Is Irreplaceable

The majority of living beings synthesize their own vitamin C. Only a few, including humans, must take it in with their food.

The human body's *overwhelming* **need** for *vitamin C* can *only* be *naturally* met by eating *fresh* **fruits.** Although *some* **vegetables** also contain vitamin C, its primary dietary source is fruit.

Neither meat, nor milk, nor eggs, nor grains, nor legumes contain this important vitamin. One can live perfectly well without any of these foods, but without fresh fruits and vegetables it is impossible to remain healthy: the disease of scurvy sets in, followed by death.

Sailors are well aware of this since 1747, when the Scottish physician *James Lind* demonstrated that eating two oranges and a lemon daily prevented and cured scurvy.

Of Little Nutritional Value?

A few decades ago, nutritionists focused their attention on proteins and calories. For many of them fruit was little more than water and sugar. As a result they were relegated to a very secondary dietary role.

Today we are aware that, in addition to vitamins and minerals, fruits contain hundreds of substances known as *phytochemicals* (see Vol. 1, p. 410) that carry out important preventive and healing functions.

When we consider the composition of a fruit, we might be led to believe that it has little food value since the bulk of their nutrients are diluted and, as a result, represent a small proportion of the whole. However, it is possible to consume much greater quantities of fruit than of any other, more concentrated foods, such as meat, eggs, cheese or legumes. This way, eating more fruit partially compensates for its limited content of certain nutrients, thus reducing the differential between fruit and more concentrated foods.

Fruit Stimulates the Five Senses

No other food stimulates the senses as much as a piece of fruit.
Whether hanging from a tree or lying in a fruit bowl, fruit is inviting.

Sight

The mere sight of a piece of fruit attracts and produces an increase in digestive secretions, beginning with saliva.

Smell

The aroma of fruit—all different but all pleasant—depends on thousands of volatile chemical substances (that change easily to a gaseous state) present in the peel and pulp.

Taste

Biting into a fruit produces a sensation of fresh sweetness resulting from the stimulation of thousands of taste, pressure, and temperature sensitive receptors in the mouth and on the tongue.

Touch

Touching fruit as well as placing it to the lips pleasantly stimulates the sense of touch.

Hearing

The crunchy sound of fruits being opened also contributes a pleasant sensation.

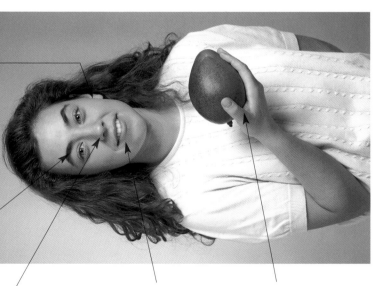

Eating fruit is a pleasant act that contributes to a feeling of physiological and psychological well being; probably because fruit, along with grains, formed the original diet of the human species.

When and How To Eat Fruit?

A person can eat a kilo of oranges or tangerines without any ill effects (quite the contrary; they will prove beneficial). However, one cannot do the same with a kilo of cheese, for example. A kilo of oranges provides 9.4 grams of protein and 400 mg of calcium; approximately the same amounts found in a 50-gram portion of aged cheese.

A pleasure to the senses, a food, and even a medicine, fruit can be eaten anytime. All fruits except citrus, combine well with grains in any form (see Vol. 1, p. 66).

It is wiser to include fruit as a fundamental part of breakfast and/or dinner than as a final complement to a full meal.

Fresh, ripe fruit evidently provides the greatest level of vitamins, flavonoids, and antioxidants. But if fresh fruit is not available, it is always better to eat fruit that has been preserved by some method than not to eat it at all.

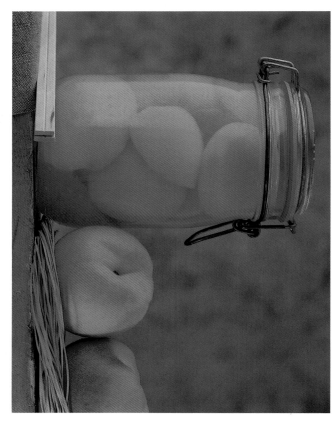

The Processing of Fruit

Fruit can be processed in a variety of ways to make it easier to eat or to preserve it for longer periods. All of these methods result in the *loss* of some portion of *vitamins* and *flavonoids*, which are the most unstable of nutrients. Carbohydrates and minerals are not affected.

Peeling

Discarding the peel represents the **loss** of an important portion of the *vitamins* found in fruit. However, **pesticides and other contaminants** that may be on the surface are also *eliminated.*

Slicing

When fruit is sliced, some cells are broken. As a result, vitamins are released to the air, where they are oxidized, thus made inactive. For this reason it is *best* to slice the fruit *just before* **it is to be eaten.**

Drying

Traditionally fruit has been dried by exposing it to the sun and air. Today, there are devices that generate warm, dry air for this purpose. The drying process destroys a certain amount of provitamin A and vitamin C.

Sodium sulfite is usually added to industrially dried fruits to preserve them and keep them from turning dark. Sulfite helps preserve some of the *vitamins* but completely **destroys** *all* of the *vitamin B.* It can also cause **allergic reactions.**

Freezing

Vitamin loss is *less* in frozen fruits than in canned:[2] 37% of provitamin A; 29% of vitamin B[1]; 17% of vitamin B[2]; 16% of niacin; 18% of vitamin C. When they are unfrozen, these fruits maintain their original appearance and flavor quite well.

Canning

Heating and adding sugar to foods prior or to sealing them is an effort to destroy the ever-present microorganisms that spoil them. The **loss** of *vitamins* through the canning process is *quite significant* according to one study.[2] The losses include 39% of provitamin A; 47% of vitamin B[1]; 57% of B[2]; 42% of niacin; and 56% of vitamin C.

Making of Jams, Jellies, and Marmalades

The **loss** of *vitamins* from making jams, jellies, and marmalades is similar to that of canning because of the cooking of the fruit that is involved. The destruction of flavonoids has not been precisely measured but it is thought to be greater than 50%.

Jams, jellies and marmalades are *not very* **healthful** because of their *high* refined **sugar** content.

Fruit Juices

In recent years, there has been a considerable increase in the consumption of industrially prepared juices with an accompanying decline in the use of fresh fruit. This notwithstanding, juice should not replace fresh fruit, particularly if it is industrially prepared. Neither should juices be used to replace pure water.

Industrially Prepared Juices

The industrial production of fruit juices includes the following processes that alter the composition and properties of natural juice.

1. **Extraction** of the juice by either squeezing or grinding the fruit, which is then filtered to remove peel, pulp, and seed residues.

2. **Enzymatic treatment:** The enzyme **pectidase** is added to clarify the juice by removing its naturally cloudy appearance, thus making it more attractive to many consumers. These enzymes transform pectin (soluble fiber) into carbohydrates and sugars that can cause digestive disorders and diarrhea.[3]

3. **Precipitation with gelatin:** 200 grams of fish or bone gelatin are added to each 1,000 liters of juice to eliminate any remaining dissolved particles.[4] The gelatin combines with the tannins in the juice to form a solid sediment, which is then eliminated by centrifuge. Theoretically, none of the gelatin remains. This process is used primarily with apple, grape, and currant juices.

4. **Concentration:** The bulk of the water is removed from the juice by means of either heat and evaporation or by freezing. This reduction in volume facilitates its storage and transport, although approximate **half** of the **vitamins** are **lost.**

5. **Reconstitution:** The water necessary to reconstitute the juice is added at the bottling plant.

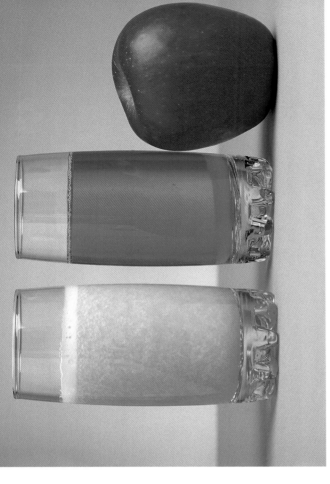

Freshly squeezed natural juices are much preferable to those that are bottled, especially if these have been clarified to eliminate their cloudy appearance.

Clarifying apple or grape juices causes the juice to **lose** their **pectin** (soluble fiber) and **tannin** content. Heating them during the preserving process **destroys** approximately **half** of their **vitamin content.**

Benefits of Juices

Natural juices, more than those that have been processed, are **diuretics** (due to their high potassium and flavonoid content), **alkalizers** (in spite of their own acidity, they reduce the acidity of the blood and tissues), **mineralizers** (because of their high mineral content) and have **invigorating effects** (due to their high levels of sugars and vitamins).

Drawbacks to Juices

- **They are not a substitute for fruit** as they always contain less fiber (pectin) and, if they are not freshly prepared, fewer vitamins.

- Industrial juices, particularly apple juice, may produce **diarrhea** and indigestion (see Vol. 2, p. 231).

- **Preschool-aged children** that drink more than 360 ml (approximately two glasses) a day of industrially prepared juices have a greater tendency toward **obesity** and **slower growth rate,**[5, 6] possibly due to the fact that these juices contain too much sugar, which reduces appetite, and very little protein. It is not healthful to always drink juices in place of water.

- Excessive consumption of acidic juices erodes dental enamel and produces hypersensitivity of the dentine.[7,8] (toothache),

"Nectars" are pureed fruit, to which water, sugar, and fruit acid have been added (see Vol. 1, p. 368).

Continued on page 40

Exotic Fruits:

Fruits considered exotic in countries where they are not produced are just as healthful and nutritious as any other fruit. They do not possess any special properties not found in more common fruits, as was once thought. However, eating them gives a special pleasure that enriches the food experience. This chart displays some of the more attractive.

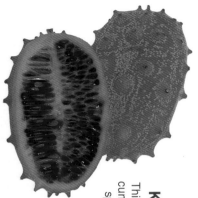

Kiwano

This native of Africa is, in reality, a wild cucumber, very aromatic and flavorful. The spines on its rind are fleshy and its pulp, gelatinous. It has **digestive** and **laxative** properties (see Vol. 1, p. 44).

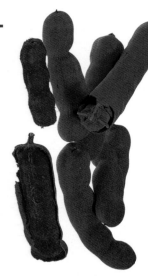

Tamarind

The slightly acid pulp of this legume-like fruit is an effective **laxative** (see Vol. 1, p. 46).

Tamarillo

Also called **tree tomato**, because of its appearance, which is similar to the tomato. They are native to South America. They are eaten fresh and have a slightly acid taste (see Vol. 1, p. 51).

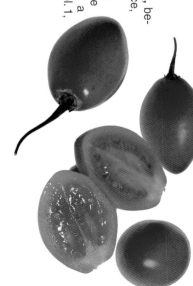

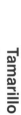

Mangosteen

These are native of Thailand, where they are considered a true delicacy. Its bittersweet taste is reminiscent of plums (see Vol. 1, p. 45).

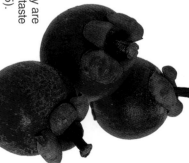

Delights of Paradise

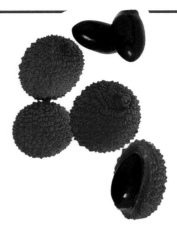

Litchi

This fruit of a tree from China is noted for its **high vitamin C content**, which is greater than that of oranges or lemons. They enhance the **immune system** (see Vol. 2, p. 366).

Rambutan

This native of Malaysia has a pulp similar to the litchi, with a flavor similar to almonds (see Vol. 1, p. 51).

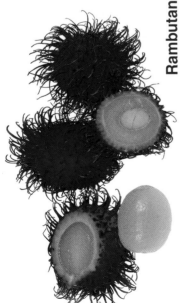

Winter Cherry

Originating in East Asia and China, these are now grown in Colombia. It is like a cherry with a pleasantly tart flavor (see Vol. 1, p. 51).

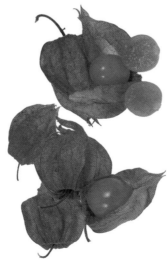

Night-Blooming Cereus

This fruit is covered with spines, like the cactus that it is. Its pulp, however, is very sweet and aromatic (see Vol. 1, p. 43).

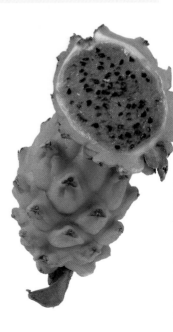

Attracted by the Exotic

In European countries, particularly, **'exotic'** fruits are those coming from faraway, generally tropical, places. Their brilliant colors, unique shapes, and delicate aromas have always attracted travelers and explorers. Today, thanks to better transport, more and more exotic fruits are finding their way to the markets of the world.

Two historic figures stand out as special contributors to our knowledge of tropical fruits:

Christopher Columbus was so taken by the richness of the vegetation in Central America that he thought he had found the earthly Paradise. He and his men brought many American species to Spain, thus making them known for the first time in Europe in the 16th century.

Georg Meister, a German botanist, traveled to Southeast Asia in the 17th century in search of new fruits. Ten years later, never ceasing to marvel at the "magnificent work of the Eternal in these beautiful lands", he returned to his native Saxony. In 1692 he published an illustrated book on exotic fruits that constitutes one of the great classics of universal botany.

Many fruits ceased being exotic when they acclimatized and were cultivated in other places. For example, the orange was considered exotic in 15th century Europe when it was introduced to the West from China. The same has happened with the avocado and cherimoya, which have been successfully grown in southern Spain for many years.

Nutritional Value

Peel

Also known as the **epicarp**. As they receive more solar radiation, the peel and the pulp just beneath it contain the greater portion of **vitamins** as well as **flavonoids** and other **phytochemicals** (see Vol. 1, p. 410). However, since the peel is *most* **contaminated** by **pesticides**, it is best to remove it, if possible, by peeling the fruit. It is *only* safe to eat the peels of **organically grown** fruit.

Pulp

Known, as well, as **mesocarp**. Taken together with the **epicarp**, they form the pericarp, which is the **edible part** of the fruit.

The pulp just below the peel of fruit from the family Rosaceae (see Vol. 1, p. 48) is also rich in vitamins and flavonoids. If they are peeled carefully there is minimal nutritional loss.

Pit

Also called **endocarp**, this contains the **seed**. In general, fruit seeds are not edible. The seeds of some Rosaceae (peaches, apricots, plums and bitter almonds) contain hydrocyanic acid, which is toxic.

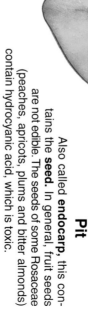

What Fruit Provides

- **Water** constitutes between 80% and 93% of most fruits. This is **"living"**, pure, uncontaminated water that contains numerous biologically active substances.

- **Sugars:** The most abundant are **glucose** and **sucrose**, which are absorbed directly into the bloodstream without need of digestion, thus providing **quick energy**. Some fruits such as oranges, apples, melons, watermelons and mangos also contain **saccharose**.

- **Starch:** Most fruit contains *little or none*, since it is converted to simple sugars (glucose and fructose) during the maturation process. The banana is the fresh fruit richest is starch (1%-2%).

- **Fiber:** For the most part, soluble **(pectin and hemicellulose)**.

- **Organic acids**, such as citric acid, which facilitates the action of **vitamin C**: they are **antiseptics**, and produce an alkalizing effect in the blood and internal organs.

- **Vitamins:** Above all, **vitamin C** and **provitamin A** (beta-carotene), which are *powerful* **antioxidants**.

- **Minerals:** particularly potassium, magnesium, calcium and iron.

- Flavonoids, anthocyanins and other **phytochemicals**, acting as *true* **medicines** avoiding arteriosclerosis, maintaining the fluidity of the blood, and preventing cancer.

What Fruit Does Not Contain

- **cholesterol**
- **purine**, which forms uric acid,
- **antinutritive factors** (factors interfering with the absorption of nutrients. See Ch. 18),
- **toxic substances.**

# of Fruit

Benefits of Fruit

Fruit is a synonym of **good health**. *No other* type of food has *so many* **preventive** and **healing properties.** Some nutrition specialists see each piece of fruit as a *true* **natural medication.** The National Cancer Institute of the United States of America recommends that everyone eat, at least, *five* **servings** of fruit or vegetables a day.[12]

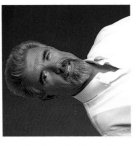

Natural, Healthful Food

- Fruit is attractive, appetizing, easy to eat, and refreshing.
- It can be eaten **naturally** without cooking or other processing.
- Fresh fruit is a **living food** in which the marvelous chemical reactions that constitute life continue.

Detoxifies the Organism

Fruit *does not generate* **toxic residuals** as it is digested and metabolized as does foods of animal origin. *Quite the opposite.* Its **diuretic** effect *facilitates* the **elimination** of wastes and blood impurities such as uric acid.

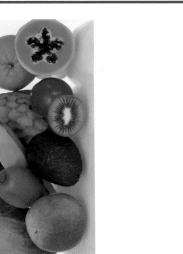

Kidney

Regulates the Intestine

Most fruit is laxative, softening the intestinal mucosa and facilitating evacuation. Others, such as the apple and the quince, regulate the digestive function, and combat diarrhea.

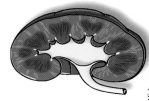

Large intestine

Prevent Cancer

Numerous studies demonstrate that the *more* **fruit consumed**, the *lower* **the risk** of cancer, particularly of the digestive, respiratory, and urinary organs.[11]

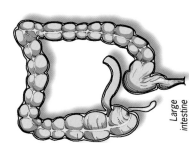

Antioxidant

Fruit is the *primary source* of **antioxidants** in our diet. Thanks to them, we *can avoid* **premature aging, arteriosclerosis, cancer** and other diseases.

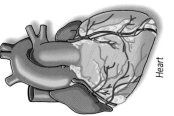

Avoid Cardiovascular Disease

According to a study that took place at Forvie Site University at Cambridge (UK)[9], the consumption of fruit is *very effective* in the prevention of **stroke** (cerebrovascular accidents such as thrombosis and embolism), and *quite effective* against **coronary disease.** A similar study at the Harvard Medical School (USA) reached a similar conclusion.[10]

Heart

Types of Fruits

Drupes

The fruits in this group contain a **single seed** called a pit or stone surrounded by a fleshy, edible portion (pericarp). Drupes, such as the peach, apricot, plum, and cherry, are noted for their *provitamin A* content.

Pomes

Apples and pears belong to this group. Pomes are particularly rich in *pectin* and *maleic acid.*

Berries

These are characterized by a **juicy pulp** containing **small seeds,** such as grapes or blueberries.

Citrus

Botanically known as **hesperidia,** they are a specialized type of berry with a leathery peel: orange, grape-

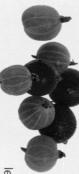

fruit, lemon, etc. They are rich in *citric acid* and *vitamin C.*

Pepol

These **large** fruits contain many *seeds* in their interior. Examples are the melon and the pumpkin.

Aggregate Fruits

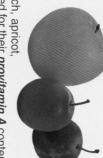

These are **clusters of fruit** coming from individual blossoms. The fig, the blackberry and the pineapple are aggregate fruits.

The **strawberry** is a special case: in reality it is the fleshly receptacle of multiple small, dry, one-seeded fruit of the strawberry are the seed-like grains on its surface.

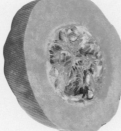

Continued from page 35

Is Fruit Fattening?

This is one of the most widespread fallacies concerning fruit. In fact, abundant use of fruit is not only non-fattening, but is *one of the best ways to lose weight.*

While it is true that fruit contains calorie-bearing *sugars,* when compared with other foods with the same caloric content as fruit:

- produces a *greater* sense of **satiety,**
- contains *virtually* no **fat,**
- acts as a *natural* **diuretic,** thus contributing to weight loss,
- given its high B vitamin content, its sugars are *easily* **metabolized** (burned) thus are not turned into fat as happens with refined bakery products.

A large apple (approximately 200 grams), for example, contains about 120

kcal, the same as a *doughnut;* however it satisfies more, and is virtually non-fattening.

Drawbacks to Fruit

Even though fruit is the most healthful and healing of all foods, there are *some* that require discretion in the following circumstances:

- **Diarrhea:** Certain fruits, such as grapes, melons, and plums, acts as laxatives and should be avoided. Apples, quince, and loquats are astringents and have a beneficial effect under these circumstances.
- **Diabetes:** Avoid fruits with a very high sugar content such as grapes or dates.
- **Dental caries:** If one is predisposed to caries, eat less citrus[8] and drink juices using a straw to minimize contact with the teeth.

LIVING ON FRUIT

Living exclusively on fruit for a period of time is a very healthy habit. There are several ways to carry it out:

- Fruit cure.
- Eating exclusively fruit once a week.
- Having just fruit for supper.

World Fruit Production

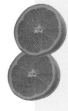

Natural Vitamin C
Plenty for Everyone

The **orange** is, undoubtedly, the most consumed fresh fruit in the world. The 52.2 million tonnes (metric tons or MT) of oranges produced every year provide **27,770 tonnes** of **vitamin C**. Such an enormous amount is equivalent to more than a fifth of the yearly needs of all the inhabitants of the Earth, estimated to be about 131,400 tonnes (60 mg a day x 6 billion inhabitants x 365 days = 131,400,000 kg = 131,400 tonnes of vitamin C).

In other words, just with the oranges produced in our planet, humans can obtain more than a fifth of the **vitamin C** they need. Additionally, taking into account the vitamin C that comes from other cultivated fruits and vegetables, we can be certain that mankind has a guaranteed supply of this important vitamin.

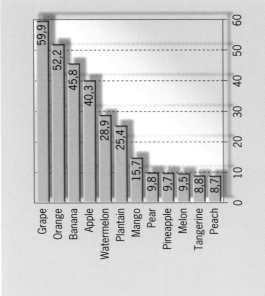

Fruit	Production
Grape	59,9
Orange	52,2
Banana	45,8
Apple	40,3
Watermelon	28,9
Plantain	25,4
Mango	15,7
Pear	9,8
Pineapple	9,7
Melon	9,5
Tangerine	8,8
Peach	8,7

*This graph displays annual world production of the most cultivated fruits in millions of metric tons. (Source, FAO[13]) The **grape**, as can be plainly seen, is the most cultivated fruit in the world. Unfortunately, only a small percentage of this production is destined for the fresh market. The vast bulk is for the production of wine.*

Sources of Common Fruits
Areas where common fruits are grown

❶ Central America
Acerola
Avocado
Pineapple
Passion fruit
Papaya
Sapote

❷ South America
Cashew
Cherimoya and sugar apple
Feijoa
Guava
Tamarillo

❸ Central and Northern Europe
Cherry
Strawberry
Gooseberry
Apple
Raspberry
Elderberry

❹ Mediterranean
Date
Pomegranate

Fig
Grape
Orange

❺ China and Central Asia
Apricot
Chinese date
Persimmon
Carambola
Kiwi
Lemon
Litchi
Peach
Quince
Loquat
Orange

❻ India and Southeast Asia
Durian
Breadfruit
Mango
Mangosteen
Banana
Rambutan
Tamarind

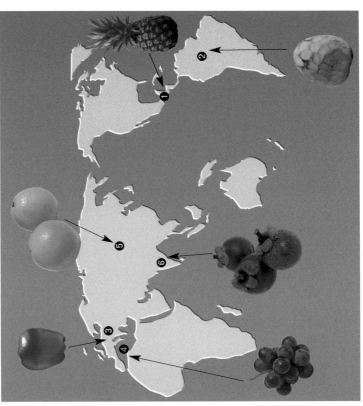

FRUITS OF THE WORLD

Botanical Family	Food	Vol./Page	Description and Use
ACTINIDIACEAE Family of some 300 trees and bushes, many of which are vines and ornamentals from the Southern hemisphere.	**KIWI** *Actinidia chinensis*	2/356	Widely cultivated but primarily in New Zealand. Contains **more vit-amin C** than the orange or lemon.
ANACARDIACEAE Composed of 500 species spread through tropical and sub-tropical Africa, India, America, and the Mediterranean. Their **fruits** are rich in **essential oils**, and many, such as the Mango, contain **resins** that give them a delicious flavor and the aroma of turpentine. This family takes its name from the cashew, which is included in the Table of Nuts (see Vol. 1, p. 58). **Mangifera:** Genus some seven species of large tropical trees with very aromatic fruit **rich in provitamin A.** The *M. indica* provides the most prized fruit. **Spondias:** Genus of trees found in the tropical regions of America and Southeast Asia. All produce a **fruit** similar to the plum but more acid and with a tougher peel. These fruits are eaten raw, in jelly, in jam or as juice. The **leaves** of these trees are eaten as vegetables.	**GANDARIA** *Bouea macrophylla*		Produced in Thailand and Indonesia. Its appearance is similar to the mango, but smaller. It has an aroma of turpentine, as well, but is more acid than the mango. It is used primarily as a **spice** in oriental cuisine.
	MANGO *Mangifera indica*	2/341	**Syn.** *Man-gay, Mangga, Man-kay.* One 300 g mango provides the RDA (Recommended Dietary Allowance) of **provitamin A.**
	AMBARELLA *Spondias cytherea*		**Scientific syn.** *Spondias dulcis.* **Syn.** *Golden apple, Jew plum.* This **fruit** is yellow or orange in color, similar to the mango but smaller (5-10 cm). It is sweet and somewhat resinous, as is the mango. It is grown in Indonesia, Philippines, and Brazil.
	YELLOW MOMBIN *Spondias mombin*		The **fruit** is yellow and measures 3-5 cm. It ripens on the tree after the leaves have fallen. Contains 28 mg/100 g **vitamin C** and is a good **diuretic.**
	RED MOMBIN *Spondias purpurea*		**Syn.** *Spanish plum.* This **fruit** is purple or violet and measures 3-7 cm. Its acidic, aromatic taste makes it more pleasant than the yellow mombin. This **fruit** is the richest of its genus (Spondias) in **vitamin C** (45 mg/100 g, as much as citrus). It is a good **diuretic** (stimulates kidney function). It is recommended in cases of **kidney stones, fluid retention, gout,** and **obesity.**
	IMBU *Spondias tuberosa*		**Syn.** *Umbu, Umbú.* This **fruit** is smaller than others of their genus (Spondias), with very pleasant-tasting pulp. They are grown in northern Brazil and Bolivia.
ANNONACEAE Consists of some 800 tropical tree species with fleshy berries. **Annona:** This genus consists of some 800 species of which about 120 are cultivated for their **fruit** in tropical America and Southern Europe. All Annona are rich in **B vitamins** and **minerals** (particularly calcium and potassium), and are very **low** in **fat** and **sodium.** For these reasons, they are **highly recommended** in cases of **cardiovascular disease.** Its heart shape has given it the ancient reputation of strengthening the heart.	**CHERIMOYA** *Annona cherimola*	2/59	Fortifies the **heart.** Useful in the treatment of congestive heart failure, **stomach disorders and obesity.**
	SOURSOP *Annona muricata*	2/62 EMP 489	The largest and most acid of the Annonaceae.
	CUSTARD APPLE *Annona reticulata*	2/62	Its pulp is valued for drinks and desserts.
	SUGAR APPLE *Annona squamosa*	2/62	The sweetest of the Annona, with a flavor reminiscent of cinnamon.
	PAPAW *Asimina triloba*		**Syn.** *Pawpaw.* This fruit, grown in southeastern United States, is **very rich in pro-tein** (up to 5%). It is eaten as a dessert with other fruit or in juice.

Mango

VOLUME 1 / 42

EMP = *Encyclopedia of Medicinal Plants,* EDUCATION AND HEALTH LIBRARY, Editorial Safeliz.

FRUITS OF THE WORLD – continued

Botanical Family	Food	Vol./Page	Description and Use
APOCYNACEAE This family is composed of more than 1,000 species of herbaceous and woody plants found in tropical and subtropical regions. Some produce **toxic** alkaloids and glucosides. The periwinkle (EMP 244) and rosebay (EMP 717) are part of this family.	**KARANDA** *Carissa carandas*		*Syn. Caraunda.* This small **fruit** comes from a thick-barked, rubber producing, spiny tree found in India. It is red outside with a white interior. Its flavor is very acid and it is used as an **aperitif.**
BERBERIDACEAE This family is made up by some 200 species of plants and shrubs found in warm regions.	**BARBERRY** *Berberis vulgaris*	EMP 384	*Syn. California barberry, Oregon grape, Holly-leave barberry.* This very small **fruit**, rich in **vitamin C** and **organic acids**, grows on a spiny bush. Taken either fresh or in juice, the tiny fruit has a **febrifuge** (fever-reducing) effect as well as acting as a general **tonic.**
BOMBACACEAE Consists of 150 species, almost all tree-like, found in tropical regions. Their fruit is generally very large.	**BAOBAB** *Adansonia digitata*		*Syn. Monkey bread.* A tree found in tropical Africa and South America cultivated for its edible **fruit** and its **seeds**, from which an **oil** is extracted. The **juice,** called **Baobab milk** or **gubdi,** is **richer** in **protein, calcium** and **iron** than human milk. In Africa it is used as **infant food.**[14]
	DURIAN *Durio zibethinus*		*Syn. Civet-cat fruit, Lahong, Tutong.* This fruit looks like a hedgehog and weighs 3 to 10 kg. It is quite rich in **fiber** (1.7%) and **vitamin C** (24 mg/100 g). It is eaten fresh as a **vegetable.** It comes from a tree from Southeast Asia that grows up to 40 meters tall.
	COLUMBIAN SAPOTE *Matisia cordata*	2/220	Brown fruit with orange-colored, sweet, fibrous pulp. It is rich in **provitamin A** and in **vitamins C and E.** Its flavor is reminiscent of the mango. It is generally eaten fresh, although it is used in juice, compote or jam. Colombian sapote comes from a tropical tree grown in South America.
BROMELIACEAE Consists of 1,400 species of mostly herbaceous plants with perennial leaves and very bright flowers. Some of these produce **proteolytic enzymes** (capable of digesting proteins). All of them grow in tropical America.	**PINEAPPLE** *Ananas comosus*	2/189 EMP 425	Aids in the **digestion of proteins.**
CACTACEAE Consists of more than 600 species known as cactus. They produce mucilage and glucosides. Only those of the genus *Opuntia* produce edible fruit.	**PRICKLY PEAR** *Opuntia ficus-indica*	EMP 718	*Syn. Barbary fig, Barbary pear, Cactus pear, Indian fig, Tuna fig, Indian pear, Nopal.* The **prickly pear** is an **astringent** that contains **B group vitamins, vitamin C,** and **calcium.** The juice of the prickly pear is used in Mexico as a cough remedy. The tender, **fleshy leaves** of the prickly pear and another similar species (*Opuntia streptacantha*) are eaten as vegetables, called **nopalitos.** They reduce the blood glucose level. For this reason they greatly benefit **diabetics.**[16]
	NIGHT-BLOOMING CEREUS *Selenicereus grandiflorus*	1/37 EMP 216	*Syn. Night-flowering cactus, Queen of the night.* Its **spiny fruit** is yellow or deep red. Its pulp is sweet, refreshing, and slightly laxative.

Colombian Sapote

Prickly pear

EMP = *Encyclopedia of Medicinal Plants,* EDUCATION AND HEALTH LIBRARY, Editorial Safeliz.

FRUITS OF THE WORLD – *continued*

Botanical Family	Food	Vol./Page	Description and Use
CAPRIFOLIACEAE This family if composed of bushes or small trees found in temperate regions of the Northern Hemisphere. They produce *glucosides*. Their fruits are either **berries** or **drupes**. *Sambucus:* Genus composed of bushes with small berries that are **very rich in potassium** (1,300 mg/100 g), **vitamin C** (36 mg/100 g), **fiber** (7%), **provitamin A**, and **antioxidant flavonoids.**	**AMERICAN ELDERBERRY** *Sambucus canadensis*		**Syn.** *Sweet elder, Eastern elderberry.* Species of elderberry found in Canada. Its juice is **very rich in antioxidant flavonoids.**
	ELDERBERRY *Sambucus nigra*	EMP 767	This fruit possesses **tonic** and **laxative** effects. However it can be **toxic** if eaten in large amounts because it contains sambugrine, a cyanogenetic glucoside.
CARICACEAE Formed by 71 small, branchless trees, such as the papaya, producing large **fruits** and growing in tropical regions of Africa and South America.	**PAPAYA** *Carica papaya*	2/157 EMP 435	Neutralizes excess **gastric acidity** and combats **intestinal infections.**
	PAPAYUELA *Carica goudotiana*		**Syn.** *Wild papaya.* Possesses the same properties as the papaya. The **seeds** cause stomach pain and therefore must be removed.
	BABACO *Carica pentagona*		**Syn.** *Chamburo.* Originally from the Andean valleys of Ecuador, this plant is now also grown in other American and European countries. Its fruit resembles a thick cucumber 20 or 30 cm in length. Its **pulp** is very pleasant, resembling an apple in taste. It is rich in **vitamin C** and in **papain,** which makes it **highly digestible.**
	MOUNTAIN PAPAYA *Carica pubescens*		This fruit grows in cooler, mountainous areas of the tropics. It is smaller and sweeter than the papaya. It acts as a **digestive** and a **laxative.**
CUCURBITACEAE Contains 850 species of mostly herbaceous climbing or low-growing vines that produce generally very large **fruits** that are protected by a thick rind. See Vol. 1, p. 107 for other *Cucurbitaceae* that are used as vegetables.	**WATERMELON** *Citrullus lanatus*	2/251	**Diuretic** and **purifying agent.** Eliminates blood impurities.
	MELON *Cucumis melo*	2/254	**Syn.** *Muskmelon, Sweet melon.* Aptly considered a true **vegetable serum** because of its hydrating and diuretic effects.
	CANTALOUPE MELON *Cucumis melo*	2/255	This is a smaller variety of melons, but it is the richest in **Beta-carotene** (provitamin A).
	KIWANO *Cucumis metuliferus*	1/36	Its cultivation has extended from its African origins to Brazil, Israel, and New Zealand. It can be eaten fresh or as a garnish with other foods. It is **very rich in potassium, aids digestion,** and is **slightly laxative.**
EBENACEAE Covers some 300 species of trees, including those that produce the famous wood, ebony. The only genus that produces edible **fruit** is *Diospyros.*	**PERSIMMON** *Diospyros kaki*	2/222	**Syn.** *Kaki fruit, Sharon fruit.* Combats **diarrhea** and **intestinal inflammation.**
	DATE PLUM *Diospyros lotus*		**Syn.** *Caucasian persimmon.* Similar to the persimmon but smaller (about the size of a cherry). They are grown in China, Korea, and Japan. Its very sour taste is due to its **high tannin content.** Soaking in hot water eliminates some of these tannins. It is **very** astringent.
	AMERICAN PERSIMMON *Diospyros virginiana*	2/224	**Richer in sugars, minerals,** and **vitamin C** than the common persimmon or the Japanese variety.

Papaya

Watermelon

Persimmon

EMP = *Encyclopedia of Medicinal Plants.* EDUCATION AND HEALTH LIBRARY, Editorial Safeliz.

FRUITS OF THE WORLD – continued

Botanical Family	Food	Vol./Page	Description and Use
ERICACEAE Small bushy or woody plants with perennial leaves. **Vaccinium:** Genus formed by a dozen plants that produce dark-colored, blue or red **berries.** They are **rich** in **anthocyanins** (a vegetable pigment flavonoid). They are of value in cases of **cystitis**, loss of **visual acuity**, and, urinary **stones** of calcium phosphate. *Blueberry*	**ARBUTUS BERRY** *Arbutus unedo*	EMP 563	**Syn.** Strawberry tree berry. These are found wild in southwestern Europe. Their pulp is creamy and **astringent.**
	BLUEBERRY *Vaccinium corymbosum*	2/259	**Syn.** Highbush blueberry. Cultivated in North America for its large, juicy fruit.
	CRANBERRY *Vaccinium macrocarpon*	2/259	Cranberry juice is among the **most effective** urinary disinfectants of the genus Vaccinium. It is effective in cases of **cystitis.** The fruit is red in color and slightly larger than the European cranberry.
	BILBERRY *Vaccinium myrtillus*	2/257 EMP 260	**Syn.** Huckleberry, Whortleberry. This species is the **richest** in **anthocyanins,** which are effective against **urinary infections, infectious diarrhea, varicose veins,** and alterations of the **retina.**
	EUROPEAN CRANBERRY *Vaccinium oxycoccus*	2/259	This kind of cranberry is found in Northern Europe and North America. Their reddish fruit is oval-shaped and acidic in taste. It is very effective as a urinary antiseptic.
	COWBERRY *Vaccinium vitis-idaea*	2/259 EMP 261	Red, acid tasting fruit.
EUPHORBIACEAE This family comprises more than 7,000 species spread through all the subtropical regions of the world. Their **fruit** is contained in a capsule The genera **Baccaurea** and **Phyllanthus** originated in Malaysia but their cultivation has extended to India and some tropical regions of America. Manioc or yuca also belongs to this family (Vol. 1, p. 108).	**RAMBAI FRUIT** *Baccaurea motleyana*		These fruits are 2 to 4 cm in length and enclosed in a shell. The pulp is translucent white.
	OTAHEITE GOOSEBERRY *Phyllanthus acidus*		These green or light yellow fruits hang in bunches similar to grapes. They are used as **aperitifs** because of their bittersweet taste.
GUTTIFERAE Family of tropical trees from Asia and America, many of which exude **gums** and **resins.** **Garcinia:** Genus formed of tropical trees native of Southeast Asia. *Mamey*	**GARCINIA** *Garcinia cambogia*	1/36	**Extracts** of this fruit are used for the treatment of **obesity** due to its anorectic (reduction of appetite) properties without toxic side effects. They produce a sensation of satiety and aid the metabolism of sugars, inhibiting their conversion to fat. **Hydroxycitric acid** is the active ingredient in this fruit and is found in its **peel.**
	MANGOSTEEN *Garcinia mangostana*		**Berries** the size of a tomato, but with a tough, purple rind. Its whitish pulp has a pleasant bittersweet taste.
	MAMEY *Mammea americana*		**Syn.** Mamee apple, Mamey apple, Mammey sapote. This tree is found in Indonesia and tropical America. The 15 cm fruit with its leathery brown rind contains a very aromatic, slightly acid yellow pulp similar to the apricot. It contains from one to four **poisonous seeds.** It may be eaten fresh or cooked in a compote or jam.
	MADRONO *Rheedia acuminata*		**Syn.** Madroño, Madrone. This tree grows **wild** in Colombia. Balsam of Maria, which is used throughout South America, is produced from the medicinal **resin** of this tree. The **fruit** is round or oval shaped, up to 9 cm in diameter and has a yellow rind. Its pulp is tart and refreshing.

EMP = Encyclopedia of Medicinal Plants, EDUCATION AND HEALTH LIBRARY, Editorial Safeliz.

Botanical Family	Food	Vol./Page	Description and Use
LEGUMINOSAE This family of herbaceous and woody plants is found throughout the world. Most are grown for their **seeds**, which **are** contained in **pods.** They are considered **legumes** or pulses (see Vol. 1, p. 78) from a dietary standpoint. The four examples listed here are valued for their **pods** themselves, rather than the **seeds.** **Inga:** Botanical genus that includes more than a dozen trees from tropical America. Their seedpods, all edible, can reach a meter in length.	**PURGING CASSIA** *Cassia fistula*	EMP 494	Children in Mexico eat this as a treat because of its sweetness. Its black pulp is mildly **laxative.**
	CAROB *Ceratonia siliqua*	EMP 497	Flour made from these pods is a **restorative** and **antidiarrheal** agent.
	GUAMA *Inga laurina*		*Syn.* Ice-cream bean. The pulp surrounding the seeds is dry but very sweet.
MALPIGHIACEAE This family includes most of the tropical vines found in America and some trees, such as the acerola.	**TAMARIND** *Tamarindus indica*	1/36 EMP 536	Its bittersweet pulp is used as a condiment in various tropical countries. Its properties include **laxative, choleretic, cholagogue,** and **invigorating.** It works well in case of **constipation** and disorders of the **gallbladder** and the **liver.**
	ACEROLA *Malpighia glabra*	2/367	This fruit is the **richest of any** in **vitamin C.**
MELIACEAE Certain valuable hardwoods, such as mahogany, as well as others with edible **fruit,** are members of this family.	**LANGSAT** *Lansium domesticum*		*Syn.* Duku, Lanzone. Exquisite Southeast Asian fruit with a slightly bitter taste. The **DUKU** is a sweeter variety of the langsat.
	SANTOL *Sandoricum koetjape*		A round fruit about 10 to 12 cm in diameter with a very thick rind and an aroma similar to the peach. These are grown in Southeast Asia.
MORACEAE This family consists of more than 1,500 species of latex-producing bushes and trees that grow in tropical regions. **Artocarpus:** Trees originally from Southeast Asia and spread throughout tropical America and Africa as well as Polynesia. They produce very large **fruit** with high **starch** content; thus, they are called the "bread of the tropics." **Morus:** Mulberry trees with origins in the Caucasus. Their leaves are used to feed silkworms.	**JACKFRUIT** *Artocarpus heterophyllus*		*Syn.* Jakfruit, Jack, Nangka. This is the **largest** edible **fruit** known (up to 40 kg). It is rich in **starch, protein, calcium** and **phosphorus.**
	BREADFRUIT *Artocarpus communis*	2/295	Nutritious and energy-producing.
	FIG *Ficus carica*	2/145 EMP 708	These **aid digestion** and soften the **bronchial** and **digestive mucosa.**
	WHITE MULBERRY *Morus alba*		*Syn.* Chinese mulberry. This berry is sweeter and smaller than the black mulberry. They are a good source of **iron** and **vitamin C.**
	BLACK MULBERRY *Morus nigra*		*Syn.* Russian mulberry. Black mulberries are rich in **iron** (3 mg/100 g), **vitamin C** (39 mg/100 g), and **anthocyanins.** During the ripening process these berries go from red to black at maturation.
MUSACEAE This family comprises some 200 species of trees and bushes, primarily tropical, known for their bunches of fleshy **fruit.** The Genus *Musa,* which includes the common banana and all of its variants, is the most abundant of the family consisting of some 60 species.	**BANANA** *Musa paradisiaca*	2/70	**Rich** in **potassium** making it excellent for **cardiac disorders.**
	PLANTAIN *Musa paradisiaca*	2/72	Contains high levels of **starch** and **potassium.** Must be cooked before eating.

Plantain

FRUITS OF THE WORLD – continued

Botanical Family	Food	Vol./Page	Description and Use
	FEIJOA *Feijoa sellowiana*	2/263	**Very rich** in **folates** and **iodine. Particularly beneficial** for pregnant women.
	PARA GUAVA *Psidium acutangulum*	2/115	These are used in the same manner as the **guava** (*P. guajaba*).
	WILD GUAVA *Psidium friedrichsthalianum*	2/115	**Syn.** *Costa Rican guava.* This is the best tasting of the guavas. It is used in the same manner as the **guava** (*P. guajaba*).
	GUAVA *Psidium guajaba*	2/115 EMP 522	All **guavas** (fruit of trees of the botanical genus *Psidium*) are **very rich** in **vitamin C** (more than triple that of oranges) and in soluble **fiber** (pectin and mucilage). They are **highly recommended** for **hypertension** and **high cholesterol**.
	BRAZILIAN GUAVA *Psidium guineense*	2/115	These grow **wild** in Brazil and are similar in use to the **guava** (*P. guajaba*).
	WATER ROSE APPLE *Syzygium aqueum*		Similar to the Java apple, but smaller. Its pulp is similar to the common apple.
	ROSE APPLE *Syzygium jambos*		**Syn.** *Jambos, Jambu, Wax-apple.* Similar to an apple, but smaller and with rose-colored pulp. They are used to make jams and compotes. They are 93% water but contain some sugars (5.7%), **provitamin A** (34 RE), **vitamin C** (22.3 mg/100 g), and **potassium** (123 mg/100 g).
	PITANGA *Syzygium malaccense*		**Scientific syn.** *Eugenia uniflora.* **Syn.** *Petanga, Brazilian cherry, Surinam cherry.* Red **aggregate** fruit the size of a plum, with an acid taste and somewhat sour. It is noted for its **provitamin A, vitamin C,** and **calcium** content. It is usually made into jams and jellies, however it can be eaten fresh.
	JAVA APPLE *Syzygium samarangense*		**Syn.** *Makopa, Wax jambu, Jambos, Wax-apple.* These can be either red or green, and have a refreshing, acid flavor.
	BILIMBI *Averrhoa bilimbi*		This is shaped like a small cucumber. It is generally used in the preparation of other foods in Southeast Asia and Central America, since it is sour when eaten fresh.
	CARAMBOLA *Averrhoa carambola*	2/219	Gentle **laxative** due to its **fiber** content (2.7%).

MYRTACEAE

Includes more than 3,000 species of trees and bushes on the five continents. Many of these are aromatic, such as the eucalyptus and clove.

Psidium: Trees from this genus produce all guavas. They grow in the tropical regions of America, Asia, and Oceania.

Syzygium: These trees are typical of Southeast Asia, particularly Thailand. They are also found in the Caribbean and Brazil. They produce **fruits** that are reminiscent of apples.

Feijoa

Guava

OXALIDACEAE

This family is composed of about 900 species of bushes and small trees, such as the genus *Averrhoa*. **Oxalic acid** is produced in their **leaves** and other green parts.

Carambola

EMP = Encyclopedia of Medicinal Plants, EDUCATION AND HEALTH LIBRARY, Editorial Safeliz.

Strawberry

Botanical Family	Food	Vol./Page	Description and Use
PALMAE Palms constitute one of the families most typical of tropical plants. It includes almost 200 genera and more than 2,000 botanical species found in desert regions of America and Asia. They provide shade, beauty, and exquisite **fruits** such as the **date** and the **coconut**. The **pulp** (mesocarp) of all palm fruit, except the coconut, is used. The case of the coconut is special since it is the seed (endocarp) that is used. The edible part of all palm fruit is the **pulp** (endocarp), except for the coconut, what we eat of this fruit is its seed (endocarp). For this reason the coconut is grouped with nuts and seeds (see Vol. 1, p. 59).	**PEACH PALM** *Bactris gasipaes*	2/296	Pulp **very rich** in carbohydrates (**starch**).
	BEACH PALM *Bactris major*	2/328	Small fruit similar to dates with a bittersweet taste.
	PALMYRA PALM *Borassus flabellifer*	2/328	**Syn.** Borassus palm. Its pulp is used to prepare refreshing **beverages**.
	DATE *Phoenix dactylifera*	2/147	**Very rich** in **B vitamins, minerals,** and **fiber.** Softens the bronchial mucosa.
	SALAK *Salacca edulis*	2/328	Bittersweet pulp with a mildly astringent effect.
PASSIFLORACEAE Encompasses 530 species of climbing plants with bright flowers that grow in hot regions of America and Southern Europe. **Passiflora:** this is the most important genus of this family. Spanish explorers called their fruit **granadillas** or "little pomegranates" because of their similarity to that fruit.	**PASSION FRUIT** *Passiflora edulis*	2/133 EMP 168	Rich in **iron** and in **vitamin C**. Antianemic and mildly **sedative.**
	CURUBA *Passiflora mollissima*		**Syn.** Banana passion fruit. These are cultivated primarily in Colombia. The **fruit** is about 10 cm in length. Its long, ovoid shape slightly resembles the banana. They are yellow and orange. The pulp is used to make milkshakes, cremes, yogurts, and jellies.
	GIANT GRANADILLA *Passiflora quadrangularis*		This is the **largest** (up to 20 cm) of the passion **fruits.**
PUNICACEAE Small family of trees or bushes whose **fruit** has juicy, triangular fruit.	**POMEGRANATE** *Punica granatum*	2/236 EMP 523	**Astringent** and intestinal **anti-inflammatory.** Suggested for **anemia, arteriosclerosis and hypertension.**
RHAMNACEAE Composed of more than 500 species woody plants found in temperate regions. They produce **glycosides** and are **laxative.**	**JUJUBE** *Ziziphus jujuba*	2/149	**Syn.** Chinese date. Rich in **mucilage** that has a **balsamic** effect on the respiratory mucosa. It is also laxative.
ROSACEAE Includes more than 2,000 herbaceous plants, bushes, and trees throughout the temperate regions of the world. They produce **organic acids, vitamin C,** and small amounts of essences. These are the **primary European fruits,** in addition to the rose, belong to this family.	**COCOPLUM** *Chrysobalanus icaco*		**Syn.** *Icaco* (plum). **Fruit** of a tree approximately 8 meters tall that grows in tropical America. It has an **astringent** effect. It is used in making compotes and preserves.
	AZAROLE *Crataegus azarolus*	2/367	This **fruit** is similar to cherries, rich in **vitamin C** although not as much as the common acerola.
	QUINCE *Cydonia oblonga*	2/221	**Astringent** and intestinal **anti-inflammatory.**
	LOQUAT *Eriobotrya japonica*	2/298	**Antidiabetic, astringent,** and **diuretic.**
	STRAWBERRY *Fragaria vesca*	2/103 EMP 575	**Potent antioxidant,** combats **arteriosclerosis.**

VOLUME 1 / 48

EMP = Encyclopedia of Medicinal Plants, EDUCATION AND HEALTH LIBRARY, Editorial Safeliz.

FRUITS OF THE WORLD – *continued*

Botanical Family	Food	Vol./Page	Description and Use
	MEDLAR *Mespilus germanica*	2/299	*Powerful **astringent** with antidiarrheal properties* due to its **tannin** content. *Reduces **cholesterol**.* Must be cooked before eating.
	PEAR *Pirus communis*	2/112	Combats **hypertension** and promotes **kidney** function.
	APPLE *Pirus malus*	2/229 EMP 513	*Protects the **intestine**, reduces **cholesterol**, and combats **arteriosclerosis.***
	APRICOT *Prunus armeniaca*	2/26	Rich in **provitamin A**, *promotes **vision*** and **healthy skin.** Antianemic.
	CHERRY *Prunus avium*	2/304 EMP 586	Satisfies the appetite and **cleanses the blood.**
	SOUR CHERRY *Prunus cerasus*	EMP 587	Somewhat more acid tasting than the cherry and a little sour. It is used as an **aperitif** and **a digestive tonic.**
	PLUM *Prunus domestica*	2/233	**Syn.** *Prune.* Known for its **laxative effect.** Also protects the **intestine** and lowers **cholesterol.**
	PEACH *Prunus persica*	2/75	Provides a balanced amount of vitamins and minerals (potassium, magnesium). Promotes **cardiac health, aids digestion,** and helps combat **obesity.**
	SLOEBERRY *Prunus spinosa*	EMP 372	**Syn.** *Sloe, Blackthorn plum.* Sloeberries are rich in **flavonoids** and **tannins.** They are used as **aperitifs, digestives** and **astringents.**
	BRIER HIP *Rosa Canina*	EMP 762	**Syn.** *Dog rose, Rose hip, Wild brier, Eglantine gall.* **Very rich in vitamin C,** enhances the **immune system.**
	BLACKBERRY *Rubus fructicosus*	EMP 541	**Syn.** *Bramble berry.* **Similar species:** *Rubus ulmifolius.* A good source of **folates, vitamin C, potassium, iron,** and **fiber** (5.3%). Is also **very rich in anthocyanins,** a type of flavonoid that helps to regenerate the pigmentation of the **retina** and *improves **vision.*** Additionally, blackberries contain **potent antioxidants** and are recommended for **cardiac disorders** (angina, heart attack) and for the prevention of **cancer.**
	ANDES BERRY *Rubus glaucus*		These are grown in Colombia. They are similar to the blackberry, but larger. They are rich in **provitamin A, vitamin C,** and **minerals.**
	RASPBERRY *Rubus idaeus*	EMP 765	**Syn.** *Black-cap, Purple raspberry, Thimbleberry.* Raspberries are a good source of **fiber** (6.8%), **folates, vitamin C, potassium, iron,** and **flavonoids.** They are useful in cases of **infectious diseases, constipation, and kidney and liver failure.** They stimulate **detoxification** processes throughout the organism.
	LOGANBERRY *Rubus x loganobaccus*		This **hybrid** of the **blackberry** and the **raspberry** has the beneficial qualities of both. It is grown on the West Coast of the United States. These berries can be eaten fresh or used to make jams, jellies, preserves, gelatins or juice.
	SERVICEBERRY *Sorbus domestica*		**Syn.** *Juneberry, Sorbapple, Shadblow, Shadbush.* These red **berries** are rich in **vitamin C** and **tannins.** They are astringent and promote digestive function. Serviceberries can be eaten fresh or in compote.

Loquat

Cherry

Apple

Blackberry

EMP = Encyclopedia of Medicinal Plants, EDUCATION AND HEALTH LIBRARY, Editorial Safeliz.

Botanical Family	Food	Vol./Page	Description and Use
RUBIACEAE This family if composed of more than 4,000 species of herbaceous and woody plants found all over the world. They produce **alkaloids**. The coffee (EMP 178) and quinine (EMP 725) trees are examples.	**INDIAN MULBERRY** *Morinda citrifolia*		**Syn.** *Malay custard apple, Morinda.* These small **aggregate** fruits are grown in the South Pacific and tropical regions of America and Asia. They are a good source of **provitamin A**.[15]
RUTACEAE This family is composed of more than 1,600 species, mostly trees. They are **rich in essential oils.** **Citrus:** This is the most important genus of the family Rutaceae. It consists of some 20 species with edible fruit, all **rich in vitamin C**, **flavonoids** and **essential oils.** The common characteristic of these fruits is that their endocarp is made up of various juice-filled cells.	**WHITE SAPOTE** *Casimiroa edulis*		**Syn.** *Mexican apple, Zapote.* **Fruit** similar to the **quince**, grown in Mexico and California. Its pulp is creamy, sweet, slightly bitter, and not acid. It is used in beverages and confection.
	LIME *Citrus aurantiifolia*	2/364	Very acid and aromatic. Ideal for refreshing beverages.
	SEVILLE ORANGE *Citrus aurantium*	2/364 EMP 153	**Syn.** *Sour orange, Bitter orange.* Aids **digestion.** It is used in confection and marmalade.
	BERGAMOT ORANGE *Citrus bergamia*		Similar to the Seville orange. **Essential oils** used as **perfuming agents** are extracted from the rind.
	SWEET LIME *Citrus limetta*		More acid and sweeter than the lemon.
	LEMON *Citrus limon*	2/124 EMP 265	**Detoxifies**, combats **infection** and **acts as anticarcinogen.**
	CITRON *Citrus medica*	2/364 EMP 267	This citrus has the least vitamin C of any but has the **highest calcium** content.
	CALAMONDIN *Citrus mitis*	2/364	This small fruit is very juicy and somewhat sour.
	GRAPEFRUIT *Citrus paradisi*	2/93 EMP 267	Protects the **arteries** and serves as a **depurative** and **detoxifier.**
	TANGERINE *Citrus reticulata*	2/359	This is the **best tolerated** of all citrus.
	ORANGE *Citrus sinensis*	2/360 EMP 153	**Immune booster,** increases the **blood fluidity.**
	KUMQUAT *Fortunella margarita*	2/364	The **smallest** of citrus fruits. The entire fruit is eaten, including the peel.
SAPINDACEAE Composed of more than 1,000 species of trees and bushes found in warmer climates throughout the world.	**AKEE** *Blighia sapida*		**Syn.** *Achee, Ackee, Vegetable brains.* When it is ripe this fruit has a soft, creamy pulp that tastes like hazelnut. The **unripe fruit** is **poisonous** since it contains hypoglycine, a toxic amino acid. They are grown in East Africa and tropical America.
	LONGAN *Dimocarpus longan*	2/366	Similar to the **litchi** but smaller and more acid.
	LITCHI *Litchi chinensis*	2/366	Useful against **infectious diseases.**

Lime

Tangerine

Litchi

FRUITS OF THE WORLD – continued

Botanical Family	Food	Vol./Page	Description and Use
	GENIPA *Melicoccus bijugatus*		**Syn.** *Akee, Honeyberry, Limoncillo, Spanish lime, Mamoncillo.* Fruit found in **bunches** on a small tree cultivated on Caribbean islands. Its cream-colored or orange-colored pulp is sweet and a little acid. It is used in blended beverages or in jam.
	RAMBUTAN *Nephelium lappaceum*	1/37	Its whitish, aromatic pulp is *similar* to the **litchi**. Its rind is covered with characteristic hairs.
SAPOTACEAE This family contains 600 species of trees producing **berries**. The **bark** of some of these trees has a **febrifuge** (fever-reducing) effect.	**SAPOTE** *Calocarpum sapota*	2/220	Rich in **carbohydrates** and **tannins**. Serves as an **astringent**.
	CAIMITO *Chrysophyllum cainito*	EMP 302	This beautiful Central American tree produces a round **fruit** with a purple or light green peel. Its gelatinous pulp is sweet and aromatic, reminiscent of the pear. It is useful against **traveler's diarrhea** because of its astringent effect.
	CHICOSAPOTE *Manilkara zapota*	2/220	This fruit has a soft, sweet, gelatinous pulp that is orange in color.
	LUCMO *Pouteria lucuma*		These are grown in Chile, Peru and Ecuador. Its rind is dark green. Its **pulp** contains **starch**. It is prepared by blending with water or milk.
SAXIFRAGACEAE Herbaceous and woody plants that grow in temperate and cold climates	**BLACK CURRANT** *Ribes nigrum*	2/329 EMP 468	Rich in **vitamin C** and **flavonoids**. Reduces *inflammation* in the **joints**.
	RED CURRANT *Ribes rubrum*	EMP 468	**Aperitif, digestive, depurative.**
	GOOSEBERRY *Ribes uva-crispa*	EMP 588	This fruit is used as an **aperitif, depurative** and **tonic**.
SOLANACEAE This family comprises about 2,300 species of **alkaloid-producing** American plants. Only about 30 are cultivated. Among these are the potato, the tomato, and tobacco (see more Solanaceae on Vol. 1, p. 111).	**TAMARILLO** *Cyphomandra betacea*	1/36	**Syn.** *Tomato tree.* Very similar to the **tomato** in appearance but with a **different taste**. They grow on a bush cultivated in Brazil, Colombia, and South Africa.
	WINTER CHERRY *Physalis alkekengi*	1/37 EMP 585	**Syn.** *Alkekengy, Bladder cherry.* Orange-colored **berry** about the size of a cherry. It *helps dissolve* urinary **stones**.
	CAPE GOOSEBERRY *Physalis peruviana*		**Syn.** *Groundcherry, Goldenberry.* Similar to **tomato** but smaller and with lower concentrations of **nutrients**. Rich in **provitamin A, Vitamin C**, and **iron**.
	PEPINO *Solanum muricatum*		**Syn.** *Melon pear.* Its appearance and flavor are similar to the **melon**. It is rich in **provitamin A**. It is grown in South America, New Zealand, and California.
VITACEAE This family is formed by around 600 species of climbing vines and bushes bearing **berries**. They are found in warm or tropical countries. **Vitis:** This genus is composed by some 20 species, most of them cultivated for their **fruit** (grapes) although some are raised for their **leaves**, which are used as a green.	**GRAPE** *Vitis vinifera*	2/78 EMP 544	The fruit of the vine acts as a tonic for the **heart** and improves **blood flow**. This assumes, of course, that one follows the advice of the great French scientist, Louis Pasteur, to **"take wine in pills"** as he did. In other words, by **eating fresh grapes** rather than those denatured through fermentation into wine (see Vol. 1, p. 379).

Lucmo

Gooseberry

Winter cherry

EMP = *Encyclopedia of Medicinal Plants*, EDUCATION AND HEALTH LIBRARY, Editorial Safeliz.

3

NUTS

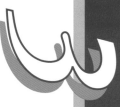

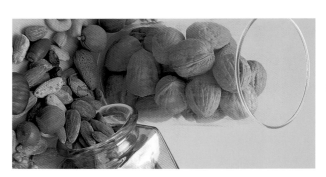

Recent scientific studies have demonstrated that oleaginous nuts are not harmful for cholesterol levels. To the contrary, they are beneficial.

N UTS provide *many calories, fats, and proteins;* as such, they should be considered important and nutritious foods, not mere snacks.

The high *energy* content of nuts makes them ideal during periods of exercise or during the winter months. They **combine** *very well* with **citrus,** which also are available during the colder months. These contain *vitamin C* and *provitamin A* that are lacking in nuts.

Nuts as Food

Until recently, many nutritionists felt that oleaginous (oily) nuts were harmful

to the heart and arteries because of their high fat content. We have come to realize, however that this is not the case. Diverse studies[1,2,3] have confirmed that they act to protect the arteries and reduce cholesterol levels, supporting the beliefs of many of the pioneers of natural diet as far back as the 19th century.

Nuts perform a very important role in two types of diets:

• **Mediterranean diet:** Together with fruit, vegetables, and legumes, nuts are foods typical of a healthy Mediterranean diet. The beneficial impact that this diet has on **cardiovascular health** is due, in large part, to the generous use of nuts.

Continued on page 54

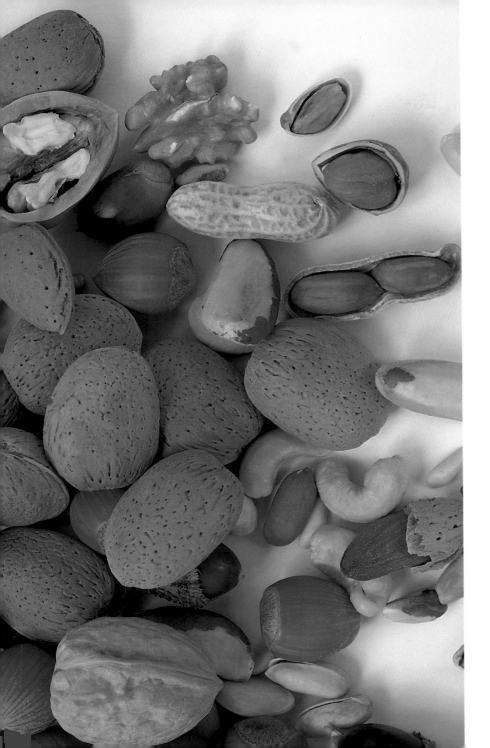

Nuts and Seeds

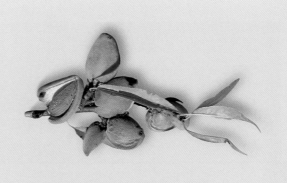

- **Nuts:** *This term describes an edible, dry seed enclosed in a hard shell containing very little water, but is rich in oils or starch. Nuts can be:*
  - **oleaginous,** *whose seed is rich in* **oil** *(Cashew, walnut, almond, hazelnuts, peanuts, etc.), or*
  - **starchy,** *whose seeds contain a large proportion of* **starch** *(acorn, chestnut, etc.). Nuts are the* **seed** *of a fruit, and not its fleshy part, which is typically inedible. For example, the part that we eat of the common* **walnut** *('Juglans regia' L.) is the seed. The portion that corresponds to the pulp of the fruit, or pericarp, is a tough, green, inedible exterior shell.*

  Most nuts come from trees not belonging to the leguminous family. The exception is the **peanut** *that grows underground from a leguminous plant. The peanut is classified as a nut rather than a legume because of its richness in oil.*

- **Seed:** *This refers to other seeds that are not considered nuts, such as sunflower seeds, pumpkinseeds or sesame seeds.*

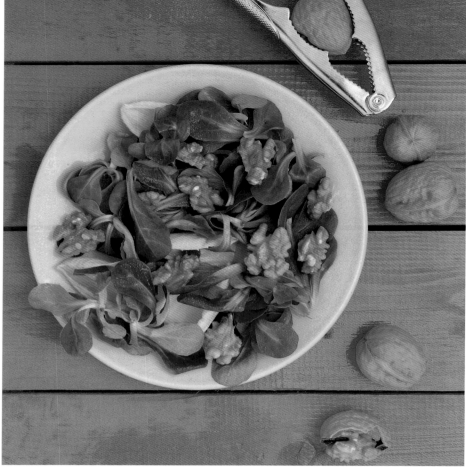

Continued from page 52

- **Vegetarian diet:** Because they have as *much or more protein* than **meat**, contain *no uric acid nor cholesterol*, nuts are a fundamental food for vegetarians.

The Processing of Nuts

It is best to naturally dry nuts after they have been shelled to facilitate storage. Once they have been well dried, they can be processed in a variety of ways to make them easier to eat.

1. Blanching in boiling water

Nuts become more tender and their indigestible peels are easier to remove when they are dipped briefly in boiling water. This is the *most healthful* way to eat nuts.

2. Roasting

Roasting brings the full flavors of nuts. However the heat of this process *destroys* up to 75% of the nut's *vitamin B₁*.

3. Salting

It is *unnecessary* to add salt to nuts since they are flavorful enough without it. Besides, salting does not aid in preserving them. The amount of salt consumed with salted nuts is unhealthful for children as well as adults.

World Nut Production

Coconuts and **peanuts** make up ninety-four percent of world nut production because their oils are commonly used in the production of margarine and sauces. The **coconut** (Vol. 2, p. 325 is the nut that contains the *most* **saturated fat** and, as a result, is the *least* **healthful**.

Almonds and **walnuts** are the next highest in production volume. Approximately one million metric tons are produced each year.

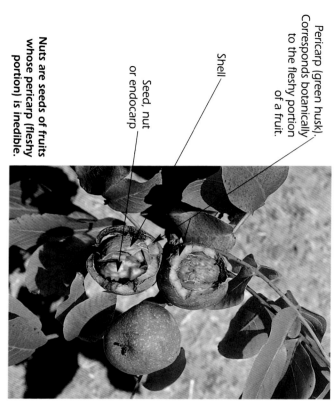

Pericarp (green husk). Corresponds botanically to the fleshy portion of a fruit.

Shell

Seed, nut or endocarp

Nuts are seeds of fruits whose pericarp (fleshy portion) is inedible.

Products Based on Nuts

Nuts remain fresh for only a limited time due to their high content of unsaturated fatty acids, which easily become rancid (oxidized). For this reason, particularly in Mediterranean regions, various methods have been developed to prepare them in ways that keep them useful longer and take full advantage of their flavor.

Turron

It is said that turron was invented in a besieged city to provide a dessert that would not spoil. From the Spanish city of Alicante on the shores of the Mediterranean, comes the best turron in the world, made from almonds (ground or whole) and honey.

Italian **"torrone"** is of Spanish origin and is made of almonds, walnuts, egg white, and acacia honey. French **"nougat"** is made from almonds or other nuts, honey, and egg whites.

Almond Milk

Almond milk has outstanding health properties, although provides less proteins and calcium than cow's milk (see Vol. 1, p. 216 and Vol. 2, p. 51).

Cremes

These are made by blending or grinding nuts, particularly almonds. These are particularly useful for children and the elderly since they require little chewing.

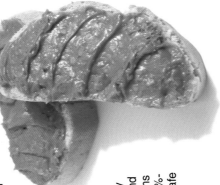

Peanut Butter

This is very popular in the United States and can be used as a substitute for dairy butter. It is made by grinding toasted peanuts and adding hydrogenated oils, sugar, salt, and antioxidants. It is rich in mostly unsaturated fat (50%) and protein (29%). It contains few carbohydrates (5%-7%), which makes it safe for diabetics.

Are Nuts Fattening?

*There are many who deprive themselves of the health benefits of nuts, simply because they are afraid that they will cause them to gain weight. **Calorie for calorie** nuts are **less fattening** than **meat, sausages,** milk fats (**cream, aged cheese,** etc.) or **refined sweets** (pastries, ice cream, etc.).*

*It is true that nuts have a high caloric content, but their oil is composed of **mono** or **polyunsaturated fatty acids, which are** **easily metabolized** and do not tend to be deposited in the body.*

The so-called RENO study[4] regarding heart-healthy diets that was carried out in the United States demonstrated that in general, those who regularly eat nuts are more health conscious and weigh less than those who do not eat them.

We can be assured that nuts are not fattening if they are eaten in place of other calorie-rich foods and not in addition to them.

Although it seems a paradox, given their high fat content, oil-bearing nuts reduce cholesterol levels.

Nutritional Value

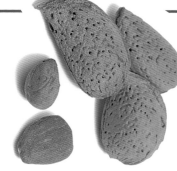

Almonds

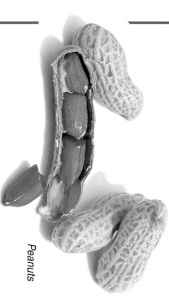

Peanuts

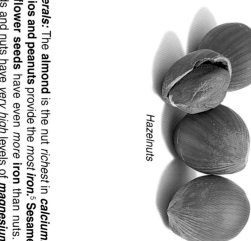

Hazelnuts

Nuts Provide:

- **Energy:** Of all natural foods, nuts provide the *most* **calories** in proportion to weight.

- **Fats:** Approximately *half* of their **weight** is liquid fat (oil) that is *very rich* in **mono and polyunsaturated fatty acids** (except the coconut whose fats are predominantly saturated).

Walnuts are particularly rich in linolenic acid, a precursor of the *omega-3* fatty acids. As a result, nuts *reduce* LDL cholesterol (harmful), *increase* **HDL cholesterol (beneficial)**, and protect against **arteriosclerosis.**

- **Protein:** Nuts follow only **legumes** (see Vol. 1, p. 84) in protein content. Their protein content is usually *greater than* **meat, fish, eggs,** and **grains.**

The proteins in nuts are *quite* **complete,** being deficient only in the amino acids lysine and methionine. They are well supplemented by **legumes** (rich in lysine) and **grains** (rich in methionine), as well as **milk.**

- **Minerals:** The **almond** is the nut *richest* in **calcium. Pistachios and peanuts** provide the *most iron.*[5] **Sesame and sunflower seeds** have even *more* **iron** than nuts. Both seeds and nuts have *very high* levels of **magnesium** and **phosphorus.**

- **Vitamins:** Nuts are a *good source* of vitamins B_1, B_2, B_6, E, pantothenic acid, and folates. About 75% of the vitamin B_1 is destroyed in the roasting process. Nuts are a *good source* of **choline,** a vitamin factor that forms part of lecithin, and improves liver function.

- **Trace elements:** Nuts are *very rich* in zinc, manganese, copper, and selenium.

- **Phytochemicals:** Nuts contain many substances that are very active throughout the organism:

  – **Ellagic acid, flavonoids,** and **phenolic compounds,** all of which are potent **antioxidants;**

  – **Phytosterols:** substances similar to cholesterol but of vegetable origin, that *block the absorption of* **cholesterol** in the intestine;

  – **Isoflavons:** similar to those contained in soy (see Vol. 1, p. 268), but in lower proportions. Isoflavons *protect against* **arteriosclerosis, osteoporosis, and cancer.**

Portion of Some Nutrients per 100 g of Nuts

Nut	Calories	Carbo-hydrates	Fats	Protein	Vitamin E	Calcium	Iron	Fiber
ALMONDS	586 kcal	11.8 g	52.5 g	20.4 g	20.3 mg α-TE	247 mg	3.63 mg	6.7 g
HAZELNUTS	632 kcal	9.2 g	62.6 g	13 g	23.9 mg α-TE	188 mg	3.27 mg	6.1 g
PEANUTS	567 kcal	7.64 g	49.2 g	25.8 g	9.13 mg α-TE	92 mg	4.58 mg	8.5 g
WALNUTS	642 kcal	13.5 g	61.9 g	14.3 g	2.62 mg α-TE	94 mg	2.44 mg	4.8 g

# of Nuts

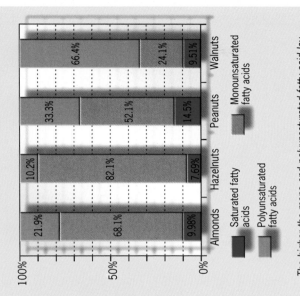

Walnuts

Nuts Do Not Contain:

- *provitamin A,* nor
- *vitamin C*

Fresh **fruits** and **vegetables** *compensate* for these vitamin deficiencies.

Fat Distribution in Nuts as a Percent

Legend:
- Saturated fatty acids
- Polyunsaturated fatty acids
- Monounsaturated fatty acids

Almonds: 21.9%, 68.1%, 9.98%
Hazelnuts: 10.2%, 82.1%, 7.69%
Peanuts: 33.3%, 52.1%, 14.5%
Walnuts: 66.4%, 24.1%, 9.51%

The higher the mono and polyunsaturated fatty acid levels, the greater the beneficial effect on cholesterol level.

Benefits of Nuts

- They provide **energy** and are *very* **nutritious.**
- They can be eaten **raw,** as nature intended, without need for further processing.
- They are a *healthful* **alternative** to **meat** given their richness in protein, minerals, and vitamins.
- In addition to containing *no* **cholesterol,** they are *effective* in **reducing** blood cholesterol levels. [1,2,3]
- They *protect* the **heart's health** by reducing the risk of coronary heart disease, such as **heart attack** and **angina pectoris.** This has shown to be the case in persons that eat nuts in place of other fatty foods.
- They *do not* **cause obesity.** To the contrary, they aid weight loss when nuts replace other high-calorie foods in the diet. **Calorie for calorie, they are** *less* **fattening** than high-fat foods such as sausages, aged cheeses, sweets, and pastries or ice cream.
- Due to their very low carbohydrate level, they are *well tolerated* by **diabetics.** [6]
- They *do not* **produce uric acid.**

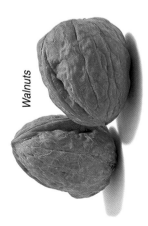

Drawbacks to Nuts

- They must be well chewed. Whole nuts may present difficulty for children and the elderly, who may eat them either in paste or creme.
- They may produce **indigestion** in persons with digestive system disorders. To improve tolerance they should be:
  - eaten raw or lightly roasted (not fried),
  - limited to eating no more than 50 g (about 2 ounces) at one time,
  - chewed well or ground, and the skin should be removed by blanching in scalding hot water (see Vol. 2, p. 50).
- They may cause **allergenic reactions** in small children and should not be given to infants under the age of 12 months. In any case they should be introduced gradually. The **pine nut** or **piñon nut** is the *best* **tolerated by small children.**

NUTS AND SEEDS OF THE WORLD

Botanical Family	Food	Vol./Page	Description and Use
ANACARDIACEAE Composed of 500 species found in warmer countries across Africa, India, and the Mediterranean. Their **fruits** are rich in **essential oils**. See other Anacardiaceae used as fruit in Vol. 1, p. 42.	**CASHEW** *Anacardium occidentale*	2/40	These **seeds** are roasted before eating and are **very rich** in **magnesium**.
	PISTACHIO *Pistacia vera*	2/135	This is the **richest** of all nuts in **iron** and the **lowest** in **fat**. Antianemic.
BETULACEAE Made up of some 70 species of deciduous trees found in the Northern Hemisphere. Their fruits contain **seeds that are rich in oil**.	**HAZELNUT** *Corylus avellana*	2/252 EMP 253	Prevents the formation of **kidney stones**.
COMPOSITAE These flowers are composed of many florets that may number in the thousands, as is the case of the sunflower. See other Compositae that are used as vegetables in Vol. 1, p. 103.	**SUNFLOWER SEEDS** *Helianthus annuus*	2/105 EMP 236	Combats **arteriosclerosis** and **fortifies the nervous system**.
CUCURBITACEAE Includes some 850 species of generally herbaceous plants, which are used as **fruit** (see Vol. 1, p. 44) or as **vegetables** (see Vol. 1, p. 107).	**SQUASH SEEDS** *Cucurbita pepo*	2/99 EMP 605	These may be eaten raw or lightly roasted in cases of **enlarged prostate**, **cystitis**, and **intestinal parasites**.
FAGACEAE This botanical family contains 400 species of trees and bushes whose fruit contains **seeds rich** in **starch**, **fats**, and **tannins**.	**CHESTNUT** *Castanea sativa*	2/322 EMP 495	Tones the muscles and combats **fatigue**; it is an **alkalizer**.
	BEECHNUT *Fagus silvatica*	EMP 502	This is the **seed** of the beechnut tree, which is found in Central and Northern Europe and North America. They are similar to the hazelnut in nutrition, although they are richer in **iron**. Edible **oil** is extracted from beechnuts, however it **must be heated** before it can be consumed. **Caution: raw seeds or oil** contain **a toxic** substance that causes headache and general indisposition. This toxic substance disappears with roasting or heating the oil.
	ACORN *Quercus ilex*	EMP 208	The oak produces this starchy nut. Because of their **high tannin** content, they have a bitter taste. Soaking or washing them removes most of the tannins. There are sweet varieties that are used as they are or to make a nutritious **flour**. They are rich in **carbohydrates**, and essential **fatty acids**. They are beneficial in cases of **gastroenteritis** or **diarrhea**.
JUGLANDACEAE Consisting of about 50 species of trees with large **leaves** that are rich in **tannin** and **oleaginous nuts**.	**PECAN** *Carya illinoiensis*		**Syn.** *Carya pecan.* This **nut** is produced by a tree native to North America. It is fifth in level of nut production in the United States. The husk of this nut is so soft that it can be removed with the fingers. The edible **seed** has an exquisite flavor and aroma. They have **very high nutritional content**, **particularly fat**. Their nutritional value is similar to the walnut, although somewhat **higher in calories**.
	ENGLISH WALNUT *Juglans regia*	2/64 EMP 505	Recommended for those with **heart disease**. It reduces **cholesterol** levels, balances the **nervous system**, and improves **sexual performance**.

Sweet acorn

EMP = Encyclopedia of Medicinal Plants, EDUCATION AND HEALTH LIBRARY, Editorial Safeliz.

NUTS AND SEEDS OF THE WORLD – continued

Botanical Family	Food	Vol./Page	Description and Use
LECYTHIDACEAE This family consists of some 130 species of large, majestic trees found in tropical regions. They are valued for their wood. The **nuts are oil-bearing.**	**BRAZIL NUT** *Bertholletia excelsa*	2/44	Recommended for disorders of the **nervous system** and tobacco detoxification due to their **high vitamin B₁** content.
LEGUMINOSAE This extensive family includes about 13,000 species characterized by **seedpods.** Even though the peanut is a **legume** from a botanical standpoint, it is considered a **nut.** Other plants of this family are used as **vegetables** (see Vol. 1, p. 91), **greens** (see Vol. 1, p. 109) and even as **fruit** (see Vol. 1, p. 46).	**PEANUT** *Arachis hypogea*	2/336	Rich in **niacin.** Promotes healthy **skin** and **mucous membranes.**
PALMAE In addition to shade and beauty, palm trees produce wonderful **seeds** such as the coconut that are used as much for their solid portions as for their liquid (see Vol. 1, p. 48 for other palms whose fruit pulp is used).	**COCONUT** *Cocos nucifera*	2/325	This seed is rich in **magnesium, calcium,** and **fat. Mineralizer.**
	KING COCONUT *Cocos nucifera*	2/328	Contains a great deal of **water** and is very aromatic.
	SEA COCONUT *Lodoicea maldivica*	2/328	Like the common coconut but much larger (up to 25kg).
PINACEAE This botanical family is comprised of about 215 **resin-producing** trees that produce **oil-bearing seeds.** The family *Pinaceae* is part of the *phylum* Conifers (inflorescences in form of a pine cone), a kind of Gymnosperms (plants whose seeds are not protected by a fruit husk). The **Chilean pine nut** is also classified in the family Araucariaceae.	**CHILE PINE NUT** *Pinus araucana*	2/47	Large, flavorful pine nut grown in Southern Chile.
	PINE NUT *Pinus pinea*	2/47	Rich in **fats, protein, vitamin B₁,** and **iron.** Recommended for **nervous disorders** and **anemia.**
PROTEACEAE Family consisting of some 1000 species, originally from Australia, with very bright flowers in bunches. Some are nut-producing trees such as the macadamia.	**MACADAMIA** *Macadamia integrifolia*	2/69	Reduces **cholesterol,** helps avoid arteriosclerosis.
ROSACEAE Includes more than 2,000 of herbaceous plants, bushes, and trees. The vast majority of Rosaceae is cultivated for their fruit (see Vol. 1, p. 48). The almond, however is raised for the **seeds** of their fruit.	**ALMOND** *Prunus amygdalus*	2/48	*Fortifies the* **nervous system,** *lowers* **cholesterol,** *and protects the* **heart.**

4

CEREALS AND GRAINS

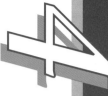

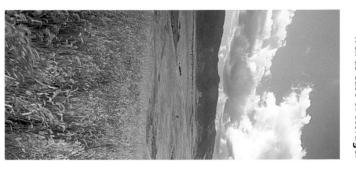

The development of human culture has always been linked to the cultivation, transformation and consumption of grains. This is due to the grains' enormous nutritional value; their capacity to adapt to varied environments, as well as ease of storage.

F ROM THE EARLIEST beginnings, the human race has depended on grains more than any other food product to satisfy their needs for protein and energy.

Because of their ease of cultivation and high caloric yield compared to surface area cultivated, grains have been ubiquitous in all human civilizations.

Grains: A Basic Food

From antiquity humans have used mechanical methods of grinding grain, even though their teeth are capable of performing this task, something that carnivorous animals cannot do. This grinding process produced a precious commodity, **flour**, which serves as a base in the preparation of such a basic food as **bread**.

Continued on page 62

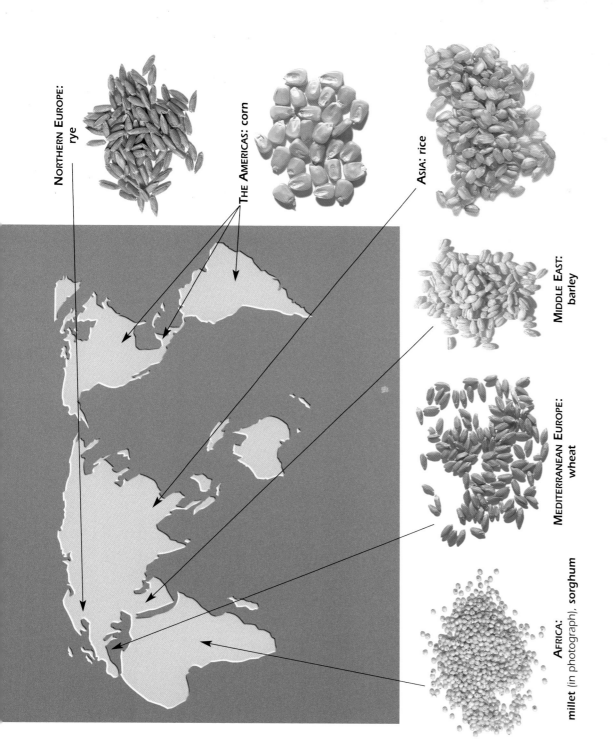

NORTHERN EUROPE: rye

THE AMERICAS: corn

ASIA: rice

MIDDLE EAST: barley

MEDITERRANEAN EUROPE: wheat

AFRICA: millet (in photograph), sorghum

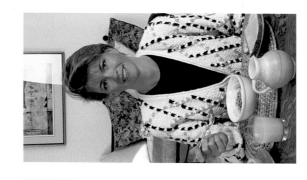

Cereals and Grains

Cereals are plants of the Gramineous family yielding an edible grain, such as wheat, corn rye, rice and oats.

Grains are the cereals plants belonging to the family 'Gramineae'.

*The grain is a special type of single seed fruit called caryopsis. It is formed by the homogenous union of the pericarp (**bran**) and the **seed** (endosperm) (see Vol. 1, p. 64).*

*In grains, fruit and seed appear to be a single unit. However, we prefer to say that the **grain is a fruit** and **not a seed**, since the word 'fruit' includes everything; bran (pericarp) and seed (endosperm).*

*There are plants that do not belong to the family 'Gramineae', but produce a grain that is similar, such as **buckwheat** (Saracen corn) and **amaranth** (see Vol. 1, p. 77).*

1

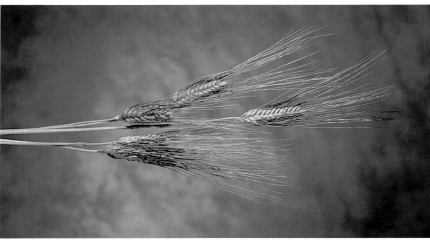

Grains represent the basic food for all of the world's peoples.

would be taking a life in pledge."[1] Without both millstones (both are necessary), there is no flour nor bread; without these human nutrition is at stake.

Whole Grains

Most of the flour produced up until the 19th century was made of all parts of the whole grain (see Vol. 1, p. 68). From antiquity, even such eminent physicians as Hippocrates or Galen considered this somewhat coarse flour and the dark bread that was made from it, inferior.

The Food of the Poor

In ancient Egypt, the higher the social status, the whiter and more refined the bread eaten. The upper classes of classical Greece and Rome used white flour as a symbol of prestige and social distinction, since only the wealthy had access to it.

Grindstones began to be replaced by **steel rollers** in 1870, and with this began the industrial production of refined white flour. Classic **grindstones**, as the name implies, *grind* the grain, while the modern **rollers** of metal or porcelain *crush* it. This new method makes *easier* to *remove* the **bran** and **germ**, and to obtain white flour. Millers were very satisfied because **white flour could be stored** *longer* before becoming rancid because of the germ, and was *more desirable* to consumers. Finally, everyone would have access to the extolled white flour and white bread.

Remedy for the Rich

Many decades passed before scientists and nutritionists noted that refined flour is not as healthful as that of whole grains. Doctor *Max Bircher-Benner,* of Swizerland, had noted in the second half of the 19th century what Doctor *Denis P. Burkit* demonstrated about a hundred years later: that the *natural fiber* missing in white flour is *necessary* for proper intestinal function.

Continued from page 60

From ancient times, **grindstones** were one of the most essential of household items. Grains and their flour were considered of such fundamental importance to sustain life, that the Law of Moses prohibited the use of grinding instruments as security for debt: *"No man shall take millstones, or even the upper one alone, in pledge; that*

World Cereal Production[2]

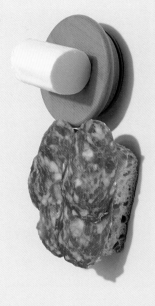

- Rice 26.6%
- Corn 24.3%
- Wheat 30.5%
- Barley 9.2%
- Sorghum 3.0%
- Oats 2.2%
- Rye 1.9%
- Millet 1.5%
- Other grains 0.8%

*This chart shows that **wheat, rice, corn** and **barley** make up **90%** of **world grain production**. The **total annual production of all grains** is about two billion metric tons. Grains alone represent 40% of world agricultural output.*

Today, we have sufficient scientific evidence showing that **whole grains** and the products made from them have *very real* **healing and preventive power** *over* what have come to be known as **diseases of civilization,** such as cancer, arteriosclerosis, diabetes, and dental caries.

Continued on page 67

Are Grain Products Fattening?

Grains are high-energy foods and provide abundant calories. However, even liberal use of these products does not produce obesity, providing one does not consume more calories than necessary.

*When compared with the energy content of other foods (caloric content), grains, particularly whole grains, and their products, lead to less fat accumulation than foods rich in fats (particularly animal products). In other words, **100 g** (about 4 slices) of **bread** which provide 250 calories is less fattening than **35 g** (about 1.25 ounces) of **butter** or **62 g** (about 2.2 ounces) of **ice cream,** each of which provides about 250 calories.*

*In reality, **what is fattening** about grain products is the **sugar** and **fat** that are added as they are prepared (sweet rolls, pies, etc.), as well as **what is often eaten** with bread: butter, prepared meats, or other products.*

Bread alone is not fattening, particularly if it is made from whole grain. However, if it is regularly eaten with butter or prepared meats they present many other drawbacks in addition to being fattening.
(see Vol. 1, pp. 204, 326).

Nutritional value

Some see grains and grain products as foods that only provide carbohydrates and calories. However, whole grains in particular are a good source of protein, minerals and vitamins.

Grains Provide:

- *Digestible carbohydrates* (50%–60% of grain weight): Most is in the form of *starch*, which is converted to *glucose* by digestive **enzymes**. The glucose is then absorbed into the blood through the small intestine and provides **energy** to the entire body.

- *Indigestible carbohydrates (cellulose fiber):* particularly in **whole grains** and their products.

- *Protein* (7.5%–17% of grain weight): Grain proteins are of a *sufficient quality* to meet the needs of **adults. Children,** on the other hand, need to *supplement* grain products with other *lysine-rich* foods such as **milk** or **legumes.**
  Oats and wheat are the *most protein-rich* grains in relation to their caloric content; **corn and rice** are the least.

- *Vitamins B₁, B₂, B₆, E, niacin and folates:* are found particularly in the **germ** and **bran**. This means that **refined** grains have *very little* of these nutrients.

- *Minerals and trace elements:* **whole-grain** products contain *much more* phosphorous, magnesium, iron, calcium, zinc, and selenium than those that are more refined.

- *Phytochemical elements:* lignans, phytoestrogens (similar to the isoflavons found in soy, see Vol. 2, p. 268), phytic acid and phytates (see Vol. 2, p. 311) and phenolic compounds that act as **antioxidants.**[3]

Grains *Do Not* Contain:

- *Provitamin A* (except corn),
- *vitamin C,*
- *vitamin B₁₂.*

On the other hand, **sprouts** from grain (see Vol. 1, p. 86) do contain *provitamin A* and *vitamin C.* As mentioned, these vitamins are missing in dried grains.

Grain: a Complete Unit

All grains are made up of three components: **bran, endosperm and germ** (see Vol. 2, p. 309).

According to the principles of Dr. *Bircher-Benner,* these three components form a complete unit whose nutritional value surpasses the nutritional value of the bran, endosperm or germ separately.

It is *wisest* to eat the **whole grain** just as it is provided by nature, since it contains the **ideal proportion of nutrients.**

1. **Bran:** rich in fiber, vitamins and minerals. The *most widely used* brans are that of **wheat** (Vol. 2, p. 311) for its laxative action, and those of **oats** (Vol. 2, p. 41) for its **cholesterol** *lowering properties.*[4] Bran from barley, rice, and corn are also used.

2. **Endosperm or nucleus:** Formed by granules of starch and proteins.

3. **Germ:** *very rich* in **B vitamins** and *vitamin E.* Wheat **germ** is the most used. (Vol. 2, p. 310).

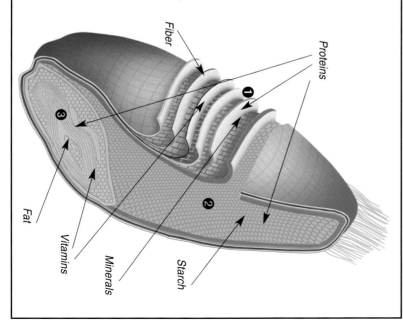

Fiber

Proteins

① ② ③

Fat

Vitamins

Minerals

Starch

# of Grains

Benefits of Grains
(particularly whole grains)

- They contain *more nutrients* than refined products, particularly more vitamins and minerals. *Eating whole-grain products* has *no adverse effect on the absorption of minerals.*[12] As a result; those suffering from iron deficiency anemia can safely use them. The use of *bran alone* does *reduce absorption of iron and zinc.* (see Vol. 2, p. 311).

- They are *rich in fiber:* This insoluble cellulose fiber that acts like a "broom" sweeping the digestive tract.

- They produce a greater sense of satiety because of their fiber content. The fiber swells in the stomach. This *helps* reduce additional food intake, thus *preventing obesity.*

- They help avoid constipation: eating whole grains improves intestinal function:[5]
  - Increases fecal volume
  - Accelerates fecal passage through the intestines
  - Facilitates the elimination of toxic substances, such as bile acids.

- They reduce cancer risk, especially that of the colon[6] and the breast, when whole-grains are eaten regularly.

- They help avoid coronary disease and arteriosclerosis: The protective effects of whole grains regarding cardiovascular disease[7] are due to high levels of:
  - *antioxidants*[8] (vitamin E, selenium, phenolic compounds, etc.),
  - *unsaturated fatty acids* (in the germ),
  - *trace elements,*
  - *phytochemicals* (lignans, phytoestrogens),
  - cellulose *fiber.*

- They prevent diabetes: A study conducted at Harvard University (USA) demonstrated that the more whole-grain products eaten, the lower the risk of non-insulin dependent diabetes.[9]
  Because the glucose in whole grains is released slowly, it does not produce abrupt increases in its blood level. As a result, diabetics **tolerate whole-grain products *better* than those of refined grains,** and can eat them without difficulty.

- They **do not contain cholesterol,** and contribute to the reduction of its level in the blood.

Drawbacks to Grains

- Their proteins are deficient in lysine. This deficit can be made up in two ways:
  - *Combining* them *with milk* or *legumes.*
  - Eating varieties of grains that have been genetically engineered to contain *high levels of lysine.* Since their protein is complete, they are *ideal* for infant diets. The problem with these hybrids is that they yield 10% to 15% less per planted area, and are therefore more expensive.

- They acidify the blood and the internal organs to some extent, but to a much lesser extent than cheese, meat or fish.

- Its abuse may cause malnutrition: Eating *excessive* quantities of grain products satisfies the appetite. While this may supply protein and calorie needs, *other foods containing necessary nutrients are neglected.* This can occur when infants are overfed with cereals. This creates a condition known as farinaceous dystrophy.

- Contraindicated in cases of celiac disease (gluten intolerance). *Only rice* and *corn* contain *no gluten* and can be safely eaten by those suffering from this disorder.

- Allergies: Some children with atopic eczemas and other symptoms of skin allergies improve when gluten is removed from their diet.[10]

- Anti-nutritive factors: Whole grain bran contain phytates that can interfere with the absorption of various minerals such as iron and zinc.
  However, *soaking, fermenting* (through the natural leavening process of bread-making), and *sprouting* of the grain virtually *eliminate* its phytate content[11] as well as other anti-nutritive factors that may be present in the bran (see Vol. 2, p. 311).

Grain Products

*A great variety of products are obtained from grains.
Usually, the more refined the lower the nutritional value and less healthful they are.*

Components Extracted From Grains

- **Flour** (Vol. 1, p. 68).
- **Bran** (Vol. 2, p. 311).
- **Germ** (Vol. 2, p. 310).
- **Germ oil** (Vol. 1, p. 127).
- **Gluten** (Vol. 1, p. 332, Vol. 2, p. 307).

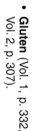

Natural rolled oats

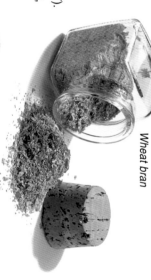

Wheat bran

Processed Grains

- **Popcorn** (Vol. 2, p. 239).
- **Flakes** (Vol. 1, p. 67).
- **Puffed cereals** (Vol. 1, p. 67).

• **Polished grains:**
Grains are polished to remove the bran. This is done with barley (Vol. 2, p. 162) and rice (Vol. 2, p. 225).

• **Parboiled grains:**
Also referred to as precooked, these grains are little refined so they are quite rich in vitamins, minerals and fiber. Rice (Vol. 2, p. 225) and Bulgur wheat (Vol. 2, p. 306) may be processed in this way.

• **Snacks:**
These are made with refined flour, fats, salt, sugar and flavorings. They are very tasty but *not* **healthful.**

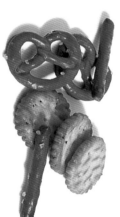

Manufactured Products

- **Bread** (Vol. 1, p. 70).
- **Pasta** (Vol. 1, p. 74).

Sprouted wheat

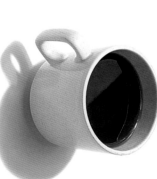

Sprouts
(Vol. 1, p. 86)

Alcoholic Beverages

Beer and whiskey are made by fermenting barley and other grains.

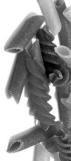

Malt
Made by roasting sprouted grains, generally barley (Vol. 2, p. 164).

Continued from page 63

Breakfast Cereals

The Western Health Reform Institute, later known as *Battle Creek Sanitarium,* was founded in 1866 in Michigan, USA, by a group of Seventh-day Adventists under the leadership of *Ellen G. White.* This institution caused a great impact on the medical world of its day because of its pioneering work in the practice of natural medicine and healthy lifestyle.

From the beginning, Seventh-day Adventists placed particular emphasis on healthful living, an emphasis that continues today. This served as a basis for the brilliant physician, *John Harvey Kellogg,* Director of Battle Creek Sanitarium, to develop the famous breakfast cereals that would revolutionize the eating habits of a large portion of the world's population.

Doctor Kellogg searched for a healthy substitute for the popular breakfast of bacon and eggs. He successfully produced a type of flake, called *granose,* based on whole grain that maintained its food value while being ready to use. Together with his brother *William,* he founded the Kellogg's Food Company, pioneer in breakfast cereal production.

Since then a multitude of companies have sprung up making breakfast cereals as good or better than those originally developed by the Kellogg brothers.

Whole-grain Cereal Flakes

Derived from Kellogg's primitive *granose,* this is the simplest and most healthful way to process whole grains. It is prepared in four steps:

1. **Cook** the whole grain in water.
2. **Dry** the grain until it reaches the optimum moisture content.
3. **Press** the grain with rollers, making them into flakes.
4. **Dry** or toast the flakes.

Flakes prepared in this way are ready to eat soaked in milk, yogurt, fruit juice or wa-

ter. They can also be boiled briefly in milk or vegetable broth.

Processed Breakfast Cereals (Corn Flakes)

These are not made from whole grain but from dough made from more or less refined flour. **Salt, sugar, malt** and various **extracts** are usually added to give flavor. Normally they are *enriched* with **vitamins and minerals** to *compensate* for those lost in the process of refining the flour.

These processed cereals are very, tasty, crunchy and appetizing, but they have these **drawbacks:**

- *high sugar* content,
- *lower nutritional value,* since the artificial enrichment process only replaces a portion of the lost nutrients.

Puffed Cereals

These are made by blowing compressed air into small bit of dough made from flours from various grains. They are light and crunchy but *less* **nutritious** than the whole grains.

Continued on page 70

The famous Swiss Doctor *Bircher-Benner* was the first to popularize the nutritional benefits of traditional robust Swiss country breakfasts toward the end of the 19th century.

'Muesli' is a healthful substitute for the poor breakfast based on coffee, sweet rolls and butter, or the typical English breakfast of bacon and eggs. Today, we know that a breakfast rich in grains and fruit improves physical and mental performance all morning.

'Muesli', eaten with fruit juice, milk or yogurt, contains the following ingredients:

- *crushed grain* grain *soaked* overnight (original version) or *grain flakes* (contemporary version),
- *nuts* (walnuts, almonds, hazelnuts, etc.),
- *dried fruit* (raisins, prunes, etc.) and *fresh fruit* (apple, pear, etc.).

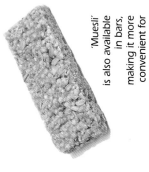

'Muesli' is also available in bars, making it more convenient for active people.

From Grain

Flour

This is the dry powder that results from the process of grinding or milling of grains.

Likewise, powders obtained from some nuts, tubers, or even fish, are also considered types of flour.

Extraction Ratio

During the refining process that accompanies milling, certain components of the grain are retained while greater or lesser amounts of the bran and germ are removed.

The extraction ratio is *the percentage of a grain that is converted to flour*. For example, if from 100 kg of wheat are extracted 70 kg of flour and 30 kg of bran and germ, the extraction ratio is 70%.

The finer and whiter the flour, the higher its extraction ratio and the lower its fiber, vitamin and mineral content.

Common Wheat Flours and Their Extraction Ratio

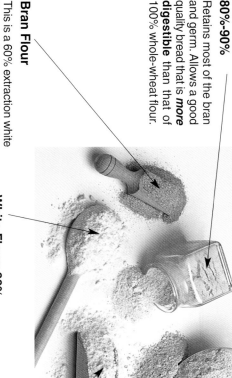

Semi-whole Grain: 80%-90%

Retains most of the bran and germ. Allows a good quality bread that is **more digestible** than that of 100% whole-wheat flour.

Bran Flour

This is a 60% extraction white flour with bran added. Because it contains no germ, it **cannot** be considered *true* **whole-wheat flour.**

White Flour: 60%

This can be stored for a longer period, but it is the *least* **nutritious.**

Enriched Flour

This is a 60% white flour that has had iron, B vitamins, and niacin artificially added up to the levels found in 80% whole-wheat flour. In spite of this, it will *never* reach the **nutritional** *levels* of whole grain.

Pure Whole-wheat: 100%

While this is the **most nutritious** of all flours, it is somewhat coarse and more **difficult to digest**, due to its high fiber content from the external layers of the grain.

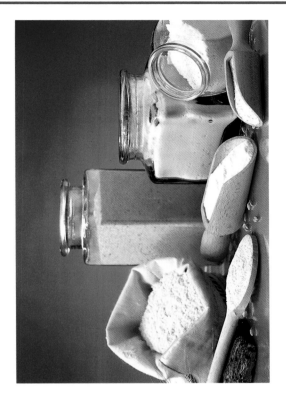

Flours of Various Grains

- **Wheat flour:** this is *the most valued* of all grains for its pleasant flavor and its *high gluten* content, which makes it *best for bread-making* since it rises perfectly during the fermentation process.

- **Toasted wheat flour:** This is a whole-wheat flour make from toasted grains of wheat or other grains.[14] It is used primarily as infant food with milk. It is typical of the Canary Islands (Spain) where it is known as "gofio" and used in other dishes as well.

- **Barley flour:** This flour is white with a delicate flavor. Dough made with it rises very little due to its *low gluten* content. It may be whole grain, removing only the husk or refined by polishing (See Vol. 2, p. 162).

- **Corn flour:** Also known as **cornmeal**, this flour is quite complete. It contains 8% fat (whole-wheat flower is less than 2% fat) and no gluten. It *must not be confused with* **cornstarch**, which is very refined.

- **Rye flour:** This is always dark, even if refined. It contains *little gluten* so its dough does not rise. Bread made from rye flour is very dense, but flavorful.

- **Rice flour:** This is made from polished rice (refined) and contains no *gluten.*

- **Oat flour:** This is *very rich* in **unsaturated fatty acids,** and poor in *gluten.* It is mixed with wheat flour in bakery products.

Semolina

This is made by coarsely grinding grain, not to the fineness of flour. It is made from refined grains that retain part of the bran. The *most common* grains for this purpose are **hard wheat** and **corn.**

- **Couscous:** This is coarse-grain semolina, generally wheat, although barley, millet or rice may be used, that is prepared using specialized techniques. It is a basic ingredient in a variety of dishes from countries of the Magreb (Morocco, Tunisia and Algeria).

Nutrients Found in Different Wheat Flours (per 100 grams)

*The higher level of refinement, the whiter the flour and the **higher** its carbohydrate content. However, it contains **less** protein, fiber, vitamins, and minerals.*

Level of refinement	Whole grain 100%	Semi-whole grain 80%	White 60%
Nutrients			
Carbohydrates (g)	60.4	64	73.6
Protein (g)	13.7	13.2	10.3
Fats (g)	1.9	1.4	1
Fiber (g)	12.2	8.6	2.7
Vitamin B₁ (mg)	0.45	0.25	0.12
Vitamin B₂ (mg)	0.22	0.08	0.04
Niacin (mg)	6.4	1.6	1.25
Vitamin B₆ (mg)	0.34	0.1	0.04
Vitamin E (mg α-TE)	1.23	1.02	0.06
Calcium (mg)	34	27	15
Magnesium (mg)	138	96	22
Iron (mg)	3.9	2.9	1.17
Zinc (mg)	2.93	2.1	0.7

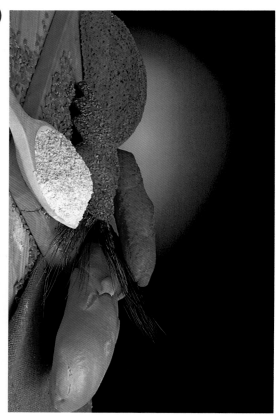

Continued from page 67

Bread, the Basic Food

Bread is a typically Mediterranean food. The Israelites and the Egyptians may have been the first to make leavened bread. From there its use spread to Greece and Rome and throughout the world. It can be truly said that bread from wheat flour has conquered the world.

Making Bread

Making everyday bread consists of three steps:

1. **Preparing the dough:** Flour is mixed with **water**, a **leavening** agent, and **salt.** Then it is kneaded until it becomes homogeneous. During the kneading process the water acts on the proteins of the gluten, giving it its typical elastic consistency. Wheat flour has the highest gluten content, followed by rye. Other flours have very little gluten (see previous page).

2. **Rising:** The leavening action of the natural yeast or other leavening agents forms **carbon dioxide** (CO_2), which swells the dough, causing it to "rise." The elasticity of the gluten is responsible for keeping this gas within the dough, forming small bubbles. In order for the dough to rise properly it must be:

   - *sufficiently* **elastic** to allow it to expand, and

   - *sufficiently* **strong** to keep the gases from escaping (if they do escape, the dough "falls" and becomes a solid, unbread-like mass).

3. **Baking:** The water is driven out of the dough by the heat and it acquires the firm consistency typical of bread.

Leavening With Natural Yeast

When dough is left in the open air for some days, it becomes colonized by wild bacteria and microscopic yeasts (specialized fungus) living in the air.

These microorganisms develop rapidly in the dough, transforming it into **sour-**

Bread: Universal, but With Limitations

Bread is a universal food, but even when it is whole grain, it has nutritional deficiencies (as it the case with grains in general).

- Its **protein** is deficient in **lysine.**
- It is relatively low in **calcium** (particularly white bread).
- Does not contain **provitamin A** nor **vitamin C.**

Lysine

Lysine is one of **22 amino acids** that form the proteins of our bodies. It is vitally important for **children** for healthy **bone, cartilage and muscle** development. Adults do not require as much lysine as children do.

Bread and **cereals** contain lysine (wheat germ more than the endosperm), **but not in sufficient quantities** to meet the needs of the body, particularly children. For this reason, children raised on bread, gluten (wheat protein), or cereals but with little milk or legumes display retarded growth and organic deficiencies.

- **Sources of lysine and calcium:** milk, whose protein contains twice as much lysine as that of grains, and legumes. **Milk** and **legumes** combined with **bread** or **any cereal** supplement the quality of their protein. This way, one receives **a protein that is equal or superior to that of meat.**

- **Sources of Provitamin A and vitamin C:** fruit and some fresh vegetables.

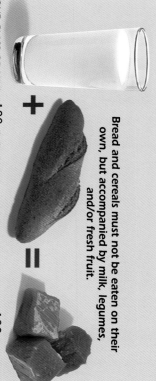

ONE GLASS OF MILK + 100 g OF BREAD = THE PROTEIN VALUE OF 100 g OF MEAT
The milk can be whole or skimmed. It is better if the bread is whole-grain.

Bread and cereals must not be eaten on their own, but accompanied by milk, legumes, and/or fresh fruit.

Recognizing Authentic Whole-wheat Bread

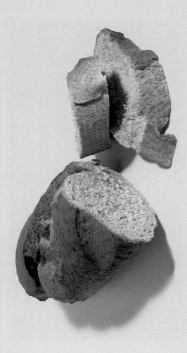

- Its **aroma** is strong, a little acid, but unmistakably pleasant.
- Its thick dark **crust** protects the interior of the bread and allows for longer storage.
- The **interior** of the bread is brown, more or less dark, and quite uniform. If the dough has been fermented with natural yeast, the bran is barely perceptible since the fermentation process has softened it. If the bran is noticeable, it may be because it has been artificially added to white flour to produce false whole-wheat bread or bran bread.
- The **bubbles** in the bread are irregular; industrially prepared breads are much more uniform in constitution.

True whole-wheat bread is made from whole grain flour (not from white flour and bran), and is leavened with natural yeast (starter).

It is slower and more expensive to produce, but it is more digestible, contains more B vitamins and allows the absorption of more minerals.

---

dough. A small portion of this is capable of leavening other loaves.

This process of using sourdough or natural yeast as leavening agent has only one *drawback*: **it is *slower*** than other methods because the dough must rest for several hours before being leavened. However, there are many benefits:

- The yeast cells ferment the dough by **partially decomposing** or *predigesting* **the starch** and *protein* in the dough, facilitating later digestion in the intestine.
- Simple carbohydrates are *converted* into *carbon dioxide* and *ethyl alcohol* by yeast. The carbon dioxide is a harmless gas that gives the bread its bubble texture; the small amount of alcohol that is produced evaporates during baking.
- Natural leavened bread contains *more B vitamins* (produced by the yeast) than other breads leavened with baking soda.
- Natural yeast also contains **bacteria** that *transform* carbohydrates into *lactic acid* (such as is found in sauerkraut and yogurt, see Vol. 2, p.197, Vol. 1, p. 201). The acidification of the dough improves the taste of the bread, and facilitates the action of the enzyme **phytase** that *destroys* **phytates** (see Vol. 2, p. 311). With virtually all phytates removed, naturally fermented bread permits greater mineral absorption in the intestine.

Artificial Yeasts and Leavening Agents

Artificial yeast consists of cell cultures of the yeast *Sacharomyces cerevisae*. Its **storage** and **use** are *easier* than that of natural yeast. It produces a rather rapid fermentation; but the quality of the **bread** is *inferior* due to lack of the acidifying bacteria found in natural yeast.

Baking Soda

It has been known from antiquity that adding wood ash to dough speeds the production of gas, causing it to rise. This is due to the ash's high content of sodium and potassium salts, which, when added to the dough, create carbon dioxide.

Modern baking powder contains *sodium bicarbonate* and various *acids*, which *rapidly* release *carbon dioxide* when moistened in the dough.

Baking soda causes dough to rise very rapidly due to the gas released (carbon dioxide), but there is *no* **fermentation.** The baking industry uses this leavening technique a great deal, particularly because it is fast. However, "rapid" baked goods are *less* **nutritious** than bread leavened by natural means.

Our Daily

Foods that are eaten daily, such as bread, have many more implications for our health than foods that are eaten less frequently. For this reason we must chose the bread for our tables with care.

True Whole-grain Bread

When we say that bread is *"the staff of life"*, we are *not* referring to modern industrial **white bread**, which is poor in nutrients, but rather to *true* **whole-grain** bread that is *almost* a **complete food** by itself (see Vol. 1, p. 70) and has been the **staple food** through millennia in the **Mediterranean diet.**

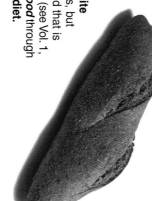

White Bread

White bread has been the desire of much of humanity for millennia. However, now that it is within reach of all, and is even cheaper than whole-grain bread, nutrition science has found that it is a *rather* **deficient food.**

The *regular predominant use* of white bread and baked goods made from refined flour *promotes* the so-called **diseases of civilization** (arteriosclerosis, diabetes, caries, cancer, etc.).

Unleavened or Unfermented Bread

This is the simplest bread to make. The dough does not rise since no leavening is used and no gas is produced. It is compact, not spongy, as is the case with leavened bread. It takes longer to digest than leavened bread.

Examples of unleavened bread are:

- **Chapati,** thin bread made from quite complete grain and cooked on a hot stone. These are typical of India and the Near East.

- **Tortilla** made from corn, typical of Central America and particularly Mexico (see Vol. 2, p. 241).

- **Matzo** or unleavened bread, eaten by Jews during Passover as a commemoration of their deliverance from Egyptian bondage some 3,500 years ago. The majority of Christians also use unleavened bread in the Communion service to commemorate the last supper of Christ and as a reminder of His death and second advent.[15]

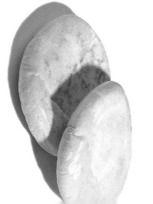

Bran Bread

This is a false whole-grain bread made from **white flour** to which **bran** has been *added*. It does not contain germ, which is the grain component richest in vitamins, minerals and essential fatty acids. It is *better* than white bread but of *lesser* **quality** than true **whole-grain** bread.

The large fragments of bran that it contains may irritate the bowel. It *should not be used* in cases of **colitis** or **irritable bowel.**

Rye Bread

This has less gluten than wheat. Therefore it makes denser bread since its dough traps less gas. It is very *nutritious and* **laxative** (see Vol. 2, p. 116).

Bread

Toasted Bread

Toast requires more chewing and less of it produces a feeling of satiety, it is *useful* in diets *against* **obesity.** Lightly toasted bread is better than darker since the more heat used, the greater the *loss* of two fundamental nutrients:

- *lysine* (see Vol. 1, p. 70) and
- *vitamin B₁.*

A beneficial effect takes place during toasting. Starch molecules are broken into smaller fragments called **dextrin,** which are *easier to digest* than starch.

Dextrinated bread is toasted bread made from dextrinated flour. Most of its starch has predigested and converted to dextrin.

Zwieback (German term for twice-baked bread) is small, thinly sliced very lightly toasted bread that can be stored for long periods of time. They are typical of Germany and Nordic countries. In some places they are known as **Swedish bread.**

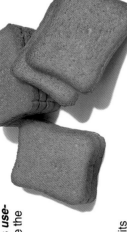

Bakery Products

These are generally prepared with an unhealthy combination of **white flour, saturated fat** (animal or vegetable), and **white sugar.** They should be *avoided* from a health standpoint. Their *regular use* provokes *increased* **cholesterol** level, *promotes* **diabetes** and creates conditions that *promote* dental **caries.**

Additionally, these products are made with **baking powder** (see Vol. 1, p. 71), which causes the dough to rise rapidly but makes them *less* **nutritious and digestible** than using natural yeast.

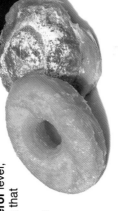

Special Breads

These are created by adding various ingredients to the dough:

- **Whole eggs** or egg whites: makes the dough more elastic and compensates for any lack of gluten;
- **Soy flour:** increases the nutritional quality of the proteins in the grains (see Vol. 2, p. 264);
- **Nuts, seeds other whole grains, dried fruit,** etc., with the goal of making the bread more appetizing and nutritious.

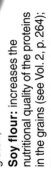

Drawbacks to Bread

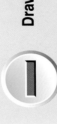

Bread can aggravate certain conditions, regardless whether it is whole-grain or white. Therefore, it should be eaten in *moderation or avoided* when one is suffering:

- **Digestive disorders,** in which toasted or dextrin bread is better tolerated;
  - **heartburn**
  - severe **gastroenteritis and colitis,** or
  - **flatulence** (excess intestinal gas).
- **Acidification** of the body. As with all grains and their derivatives, bread acidifies the blood and tissues (see Ch. 37).
- **Celiac** disease due to gluten intolerance.

Composition of Pasta

Necessary ingredients:

- **Semolina made from hard wheat:** hard wheat (see Vol. 2, p. 307) contains more gluten than soft or common wheat. This results in pasta with better consistency. Semolina from soft wheat can be used but it requires that an egg be added to the dough.

- **Water.**

Optional ingredients:

- **Egg:** gives more consistency to the pasta and makes it more nutritious. In some countries eggs are required for making noodles.

- **Vegetables:** These are blended to a paste or puree and added to the dough. They add vitamins, minerals and a touch of color. The most used vegetables are spinach, carrots, artichokes, and tomato.

- **Protein supplements,** such as soy flour, non-fat powdered milk or wheat gluten. Pastas that are prepared in this way are described as **fortified.**

- **Vitamin and mineral supplements:** Pastas that have these added are called **enriched** (see the next page). These supplements may be:
  - *artificial:* iron and B group vitamins, or
  - *natural:* brewer's yeast, torula yeast, wheat germ.

Benefits of Pasta

- **It stores easily** without need for refrigeration, except fresh pasta.

- **It is easy to cook.**

- Its **neutral flavor** allows it to be easily combined with a wide variety of sauces and other complements.

- It is **easily digested** and well tolerated by those with digestive difficulties.

- It is *rich* in **carbohydrates and protein,** but *low in fats,* which helps compensate for the fats present in the typical Western diet.

- It provides *sufficient* **calories,** which makes it an **excellent food** for **children,** those **active in sports and active people in general.**

Making Pasta

Although in many parts of Italy pasta making is done by hand, the usual industrial method consists of the following steps:

1. **Prepare semolina:** After soaking hard wheat to make bran removal easier, the grain is coarsely ground to a specific particle size. This, and not flour, is ideal for making pasta.

2. **Preparation of the dough:** Even though the main ingredient is semolina, some flour is usually added. The dough must not ferment. To avoid the formation of bubbles that would weaken the pasta, the dough is placed in a mechanical vacuum.

3. **Extrusion of the pasta,** which consists of forcing the dough under pressure through molds that give it the desired shape.

4. **Drying** and hardening. **Fresh pasta** pasta is sold without drying, but it cannot be stored as long as dry.

Drawbacks to Pasta

- Made from **refined grain:** Even though whole-grain pasta is available, it is generally made of refined wheat semolina that has had the bulk of the bran and germ removed. Therefore, as is the case with white bread, it is lacking in *fiber,* **B vitamins,** and *minerals.* This issue can be *compensated* for by:
  - **Enriching it** it with minerals and vitamins (generally iron, vitamins B_1 and B_2 and niacin). This only compensates for the loss of a few nutrients lost in the refining process.
  - Adding **brewer's or torula yeast** and/or **wheat germ,** as is done by some commercial manufacturers. This is a *better approach* than enrichment since all of these products are rich in vitamins, minerals and trace elements.
  - Eating it *with vegetables.*

- **Its protein is deficient in lysine,** as is the case with all grains and their derivatives (see Vol. 1, p. 70). This can be partially compensated for by *fortifying* it with egg or soy flour.

- It may *exacerbate* symptoms of **flatulence, acidification of the blood** and **celiac disease** and should be avoided by persons suffering from these conditions.

All Shapes

Types of Pasta

Italy, and Naples in particular, seems to be the birth-place of pasta. From there it has extended throughout the world. More than 300 kinds of pasta are made in its native land. These can be grouped in five types:

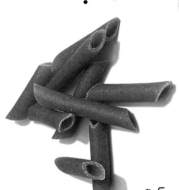

- **Dry:** 100g are more than enough for an adult. For example, 100 g of macaroni provide 72.3 g carbohydrates, 12.8 g protein, 1.6 g fat, 2.4 g fiber and 371 kcal.

- **Enriched and/or fortified:** adding egg, soy flour, brewer's yeast, wheat germ, or vegetables increases its nutritional value.

- **Filled:** This consists of laminated dough filled with various products such as cheese, meat, spinach, etc. **Ravioli** and **tortellini** are the best known.

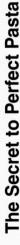

- **Fresh:** Since it has not been dried, it has a soft texture, which makes it easier to prepare, and takes less time to cook. But it can only be stored for a few days.

- **Whole-grain:** This is the richest in fiber, vitamins, and minerals.

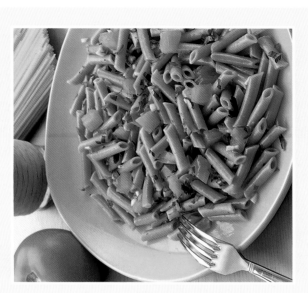

The Secret to Perfect Pasta

1. Place an appropriate, uncovered kettle on the stove with *one liter* (about 4 cups) *of water* for each *100 g* (about 4 ounces) *of pasta.*

2. Heat the water **to a boil. Add the pasta a *small amount at a time* so the water does not stop boiling. Add about *6 g* (about 1 teaspoon) of **salt** for each liter of water. Stir occasionally with a wooden spoon to prevent sticking.

3. Fresh pasta requires only 3 or 4 minutes of cooking.

4. Dry pasta should be removed from the heat when it is *al dente;* in other words, well cooked but firm in consistency.

5. **Drain** in a colander *without* rinsing with **cold water.**

6. After draining, add a little oil to keep the pasta from sticking.

GRAINS OF THE WORLD

Botanical Family	Food	Vol./Page	Description and Use
GRAMINEAE Taken together, this botanical family is **the most important** in the world for human nutrition. Their **fruit** represents the true **grains**, which represents 40% of the world's agricultural output by weight. Their botanical characteristics are: • Herbaceous plants, not woody with few exceptions. • They are monocotyledonous, which means that one cotyledon and not two forms their seeds, as is the case with most plants of dietary interest. • Their stalks are cylindrical and hollow. • Their leaves are narrow, long and with parallel veins. • Their **fruits** are dried grains, **rich** in **starch.**	**OATS** *Avena sativa*	2/41 EMP 150	This grain is the **richest** in **protein, fats, vitamin B₁, calcium,** and **iron.** It balances the **nervous system** and protects the **mucosa of the digestive tract. Diabetics** tolerate it is very well. Its **bran** is **very effective** in lowering **cholesterol** level.
	ADLAY *Coix lacryma-jovi*		**Syn.:** Job's tears, Adlay millet, Teargrass. This grain, originally from India, is cultivated throughout Asia and the Philippines. Its grains are in the shape of drops of liquid. It is eaten cooked or as flour. It is considered a food of poverty, even though its nutritional value is similar to that of **wheat.** It has antiasthmatic and diuretic properties.
	TEFF *Eragrostis tef*		**Syn.:** Lovegrass, Toff, *Warm-season/ annual bunch grass* This grain is very important in the diet of the peoples of Ethiopia and East Africa, as it adapts well to a dry climate. With the collaboration of the Swedish government, production has begun on a flour composed of teff, chickpeas and powdered milk, that has greatly improved the nutritional level of Ethiopian children.
	TEOSINTE *Euchlaena mexicana*		This **wild** grain of Mexico is similar to corn, with which it is often crossed. It is used the same as **corn.**
	BARLEY *Hordeum vulgare*	2/162	Improves digestion, reduces cholesterol, and is well tolerated by diabetics. Malt is made by toasting rye sprouts.
	RICE *Oryza sativa*	2/225	This is the grain with the **least protein content** and the **lowest in fats.** Boiled, it is effective in case of **diarrhea** and in the diet of those suffering from **cardiovascular** disease or **hypertension.**
	MILLET *Panicum miliaceum*		**Syn.** Bengal grass. Millet is the **principle source of calories** and **protein** for millions of inhabitants in Africa, India and China. It contains 11% protein, somewhat more than wheat, rice and corn. It has very little gluten, so it is of little use in making bread. Millet is used to make infant food and flat cakes, since the dough does not rise.
	RYE *Secale cereale*	2/116	Avoids **arterial degeneration** and **colon cancer.**
	SORGHUM *Sorghum bicolor*		**Syn.** Broomcorn, Grain sorghum, Great millet, Sudan grass. This **grain** is similar to **corn** in terms of its composition. It only differs in that it provides more protein and provitamin A, and a somewhat less fat. It is widely cultivated throughout Africa and Asia, and is the fifth grain in the world in terms of production volume. Its flour is used to make infant food, flat cakes (its dough does not rise due to its low gluten content) and bakery products mixed with wheat flour.
	WHEAT *Triticum aestivum*	2/306	**Nutritious** and easy **to digest.** The use of **whole-wheat** and flour made from it, protects against the so-called **diseases of civilization:** arteriosclerosis, diabetes, rheumatism and cancer.
	EMMER *Triticum dicoccum*		**Syn.** *Emmer wheat.* Cultivated in ancient times in the Mediterranean region. Its nutritional value is similar to that of **wheat.**
	KAMUT *Triticum polonicum*		This is the **wheat** of ancient **Egypt.** It is being cultivated once again. Its grains are larger and of a softer texture than common wheat.
	SPELT *Triticum spelta*		This is *rough* **wheat** with more fiber and a stronger flavor.

Wheat

Millet

Chap. 4: CEREALS AND GRAINS

VOLUME 1 / **76**

EMP = Encyclopedia of Medicinal Plants, EDUCATION AND HEALTH LIBRARY, Editorial Safeliz.

GRAINS OF THE WORLD – *continued*

Botanical Family	Food	Vol./Page	Description and Use
	CORN *Zea mays*	2/238 EMP 599	Protects the mucosa of the digestive tract, and *reduces* **cholesterol** level.
	WILD RICE *Zizania aquatica*		*Syn.* Indian rice, Water oats. Although it is called "rice", this grain is quite different from common rice. It is the only native grain in North America and had been cultivated by Native Americans of the Great Lakes region since well before the arrival of Europeans. It is **richer** in **protein, minerals, vitamins** and **fiber** than common rice and **lower** in **fat**. It takes longer to cook than common rice, and it is recommended that it soak in water for several hours prior.

Corn

EMP = Encyclopedia of Medicinal Plants, EDUCATION AND HEALTH LIBRARY, Editorial Safeliz.

PSEUDO GRAINS *

Botanical Family	Food	Vol./Page	Description and Use
AMARANTHACEAE This family consists of some 850 species of herbaceous and bushy plants that are characterized by very dense inflorescence made up of many small florets. Some species of the Genus *Amaranthus* produce edible **seeds** that are used in ways similar to those of true grains of the family Gramineae. Amaranthaceae are dicotyledonous, as opposed to Gramineae, which are monocotyledonous.	**AMARANTH** *Amaranthus caudatus*		*Syn.* African spinach, Pigweed, Redroot. The genus *amaranthus* **includes** various species of plants found in tropical regions of Central America, Asia, and Africa that produce **very nutritious seeds** that are reminiscent of **grain**.[16] Amaranth makes up part of the traditional diet of Mexico. It has a higher yield than corn per cultivated area. Amaranth **seed** contain high quality **protein**,[17] as well **as B complex vitamins**. It is *effective* in lowering **cholesterol** level.[19] The **leaves** are a good source of **vitamin C**.[18]
CHENOPODIACEAE This family is similar to Amaranthaceae. In addition to the pseudo grain quinoa, chard, spinach, beets (see Vol. 1, p. 104) and pazote (EMP p. 439) belong to this family.	**QUINOA** *Chenopodium quinoa*		*Syn.* Goosefoot, Quinua, Inca wheat. The **seeds** of this herbaceous plant, which grows in the Andes, constitute a good dietary source for those living in the region. Its nutritional value is *as good as or better* than that of true grains. It contains **more protein** than wheat or corn.[20,21] Its **starch** is easily assimilated.[22] Its flour is used to make bread.[23]
POLYGONACEAE This family contains about 800 species, among which is sorrel and rhubarb. Some, such as buckwheat, produce seeds that are similar to grain.	**BUCKWHEAT** *Fagopyrum esculentum*	2/102	*Syn.:* Saracen corn Its **protein is lysine-rich**, which is the opposite of true grains. It is of value in cases of **arteriosclerosis.**

* **PSEUDO GRAINS:** are certain plants that produce seeds with similar uses and nutritional value to true grains. However, they belong to other botanical families than *Gramineae*, which contains all true grains.

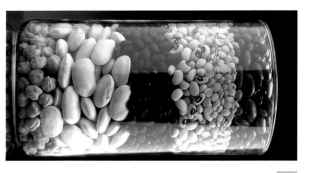

Legumes are one of the best vegetable sources of protein and iron.

5

LEGUMES

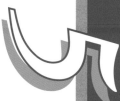

EGUMES are a fundamental element in the diets of Central America (the famous Mexican 'frijoles'), Asia (soy and its derivatives), and in Mediterranean countries where they constitute a true main dish of a meal.

Even though for quite some time, legumes were considered a rather lowly food, their use is increasing with recent discoveries concerning their many nutritional and therapeutic properties.

Processing Legumes

In their **natural state**, legumes are *inedible* because of their indigestibility and the toxic substances that they contain. As a result they must be processed in some way.[1,2] The most common methods are:

- **soaking and cooking** (see Vol. 1, p. 83);
- **sprouting** (see Vol. 1, p. 86);
- **fermentation**, which is used to derive some soy products;
- **industrial processing** (flours, oils, soy products, etc., see Vol. 1, p. 88).

A Well-matched Pair: Legumes and Grains

Pre-Columbian peoples of America traditionally grew beans and corn together. The bean vines clung to the thick stalks of the corn. Both foods, beans (a legume) and corn (a grain) formed the basis of the pre-Columbian diet.

Continued on page 80

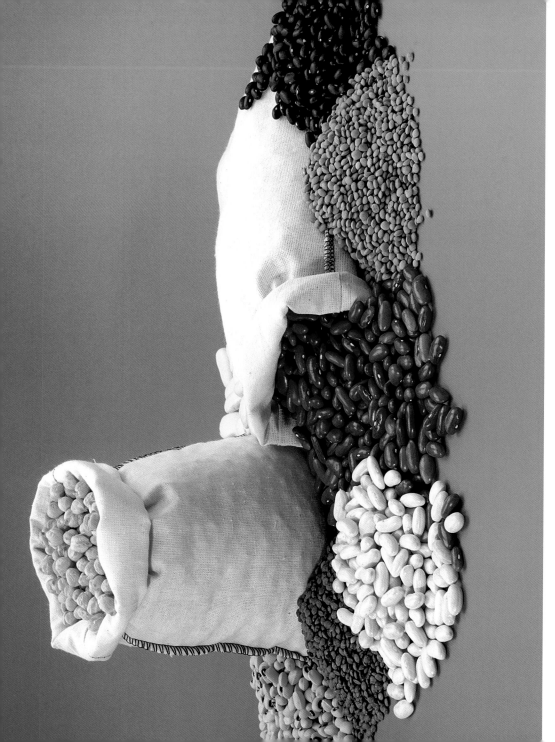

Today, the international scientific community has no doubt that the combination of legumes and grains provides biologically high-quality protein that contains all essential amino acids in proper proportion. This fact has lead to an increase in consumption of legumes.

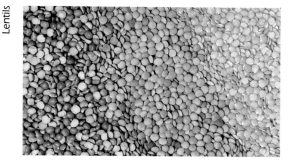

Legumes

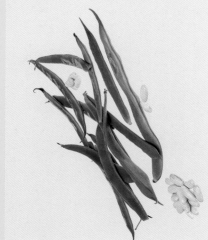

The word 'legume' is used with two meanings:

- **Botanical:** Refers to the fruit of plants of the family Leguminosae formed by a pod with seeds in its interior.
- **Dietary:** Legumes usually refer to the dry, hard seeds of plants of the family 'Leguminosae', which are eaten only after they have been prepared in the kitchen.

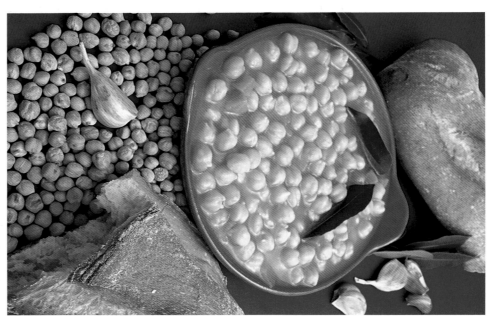

A simple piece of bread eaten with any legume increases the value of its protein. In this way the biological value of the combination of bread and legume protein is equal to or higher than protein from animal sources.

Continued from page 78

This native custom was noted by both Spanish and English 16th century explorers. Legumes and grains were grown together, and later eaten together.

Today we understand what Native Americans knew centuries ago: that legumes and grains go together very well in the field as well as on the plate.

In the Field

The plants of the botanical family *Leguminosae*, which produce legumes, have an extraordinary biological characteristic: bacteria of the genus *Rhizobium* develop in their roots. These have the capability to convert atmospheric nitrogen, an inert gas, into nitrogenous compounds such as ammonia or nitrates. The plant absorbs these compounds, which are then used to synthesize proteins.

For this reason the **cultivation** of legumes:

- *needs no nitrogenous fertilizer;*
- Can be done in soils whose nitrogen reserves have been depleted through the cultivation of other crops, such as grains;
- Leaves the soil prepared to plant other crops needing a great deal of nitrogen, such as grains.

Thanks to this property, legumes and grains combine well whether they are grown simultaneously or rotated.

On the Plate

The *proteins* found in **legumes** and **grains** combine very well from a nutritional standpoint, since their amino acids *supplement* each other:

- **Legumes** are deficient in methionine, but *rich* in *lysine.*
- **Grains** lack lysine but contain copious amounts of *methionine.*

Eating legumes and grains (either at the same meal or during the same day), our body gains the correct amounts of all amino

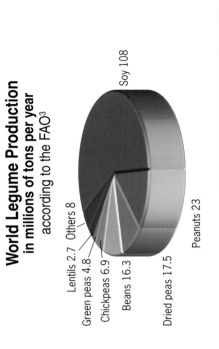

World Legume Production
in millions of tons per year
according to the FAO[3]

Lentils 2.7 Others 8
Green peas 4.8
Chickpeas 6.9
Beans 16.3

Dried peas 17.5

Soy 108

Peanuts 23

*As can be seen, the annual world production of **legumes**, excluding soy, is somewhat more than **79 million** tons a year; while more than **100 million** metric tons of soy is produced. Unfortunately, most soy is used as animal feed, resulting in an **enormous waste of dietary resources**, with practically no benefit in return.*

acids necessary to synthesize its own proteins. The result is the same as if one had eaten animal protein (meat, fish, eggs, etc.), with the advantage that grains and legumes contain little fat and no cholesterol.

Nitrogen, Indispensable for Protein Formation

The process of using atmospheric nitrogen in the roots of legumes, called **nitrogen fixation**, is essential to life on our planet.

Protein contains nitrogen as opposed to carbohydrates and fats that are formed of carbon, hydrogen and oxygen. Without nitrogen, plants cannot synthesize *amino acids* to make *proteins.*

The nitrogen content of the soil is limited, especially if it has not been fertilized. For this reason, the legumes' capacity to take advantage of the immense supply of atmospheric hydrogen makes them of special agricultural value.

There are only two types of life that are capable of fixing or utilizing atmospheric nitrogen for the synthesis of amino acids and proteins:

- **nitric bacteria**, such as those of the genus *Rhizobium* that develops in the roots of legumes, and

- **blue-green algae** or cyanobacteria that live in water, and are the most self-sufficient of all living things. They produce their own carbohydrates from carbon dioxide (CO_2) through photosynthesis, and their own proteins from atmospheric nitrogen.

As nitric bacteria in the roots of legumes fix or utilize atmospheric nitrogen, they transform it into ammonia, nitrites, and nitrates. These are necessary for the synthesis of numerous amino acids, including those that are essential. The proteins found in legumes are formed from these amino acids.

Legumes Without Gas

Legumes, *particularly* the thin **skin** that covers them, contain carbohydrates classified as oligosaccharides, whose molecule is composed of a few units of simple sugars such as galactose.

Humans do not possess enzymes capable of decomposing these oligosaccharides in the intestine. Nevertheless, he bacteria in the colon, particularly those of the genus *Clostridium*, are, indeed, capable of decomposing them, converting them into carbon dioxide, hydrogen, and methane.

There are various ways to *avoid* the formation of these gases and the flatulence that often results after eating legumes:

1. **Soaking:** After 12 hours of soaking, most of the gas-producing oligosaccharides are removed from the legumes. It is best to *change the water once or twice* during the process. Soaking is *more effective* if **boiling** water is poured over the legumes.

2. **Removing the skins** of the legumes:
   - Manually, before cooking (extremely labor-intensive).
   - By using a vegetable grinder, once they have been cooked.

3. **Taking a pharmaceutical preparation** known in some countries as *Beano.* These are rather innocuous tablets whose active ingredient is the enzyme *alpha-galactosidase*, which is able to disintegrate the oligosaccharides from the legumes before they arrive in the large intestine and are metabolized by gas-producing bacteria.[4]

Eating **bread** with legumes, whether whole-grain or white, *does not make them more flatulent*, as is popularly believed.

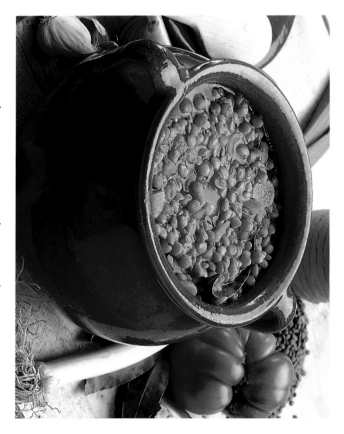

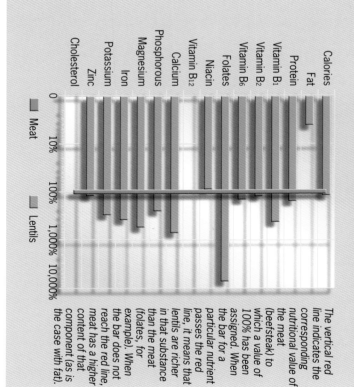

Relative Composition of Lentils Compared to Meat

Equal weight of edible raw material.

Calories
Fat
Protein
Vitamin B₁
Vitamin B₂
Vitamin B₆
Folates
Niacin
Vitamin B₁₂
Calcium
Phosphorous
Magnesium
Iron
Potassium
Zinc
Cholesterol

■ Meat   ■ Lentils

0   10%   100%   1,000%   10,000%

The vertical red line indicates the corresponding nutritional value of the meat (beefsteak) to which a value of 100% has been assigned. When the bar for a particular nutrient passes the red line, it means that lentils are richer in that substance than the meat (folates, for example). When the bar does not reach the red line, meat has a higher content of that component (as is the case with fat).

Legumes surpass meat in most nutrients, except fat (which is positive) and vitamin B₁₂.

The remaining higher plants depend exclusively on soil nitrogen to synthesize amino acids and proteins.

Lentils on Fridays

A diet of lentils on Friday is one of the characteristics that Miguel de Cervantes used to describe Don Quixote, the best-known character in Spanish literature. The Ingenious Knight probably ate lentils on Fridays because of the Catholic tradition of abstaining from meat on that day during Lent. But from a strictly nutritional point of view we might ask:

- *Are lentils really a good substitute for meat?*
- *Did Don Quixote win or lose by eating lentils on Fridays instead of meat?*
- *Which provides more nutrition, a portion of meat or a plate of lentils?*

The accompanying graph compares the composition of 100 g of raw meat (beef loin) with 100 g of dry lentils, a sufficient quantity for a serving. As can be seen, **lentils** provide:

- *carbohydrates and fiber,* neither of which is present in the meat;
- more *protein;*
- more *folates* and *vitamins B₁ and B₆;*
- more *minerals* (calcium, phosphorous, magnesium, iron, potassium and zinc).

For its part, the 100 g of **meat** provide:

- *vitamin B₁₂* and *cholesterol,* both missing in lentils;
- more *fat.*

Don Quixote certainly suffered no nutritional loss by eating lentils instead of meat on Fridays. Quite the opposite, he took in more carbohydrates, vitamins (except B₁₂), minerals and much less fat. Perhaps the Ingenious Knight was able to face his adventures vigorously because legumes replaced meat in part of his diet.

Cooking Legumes

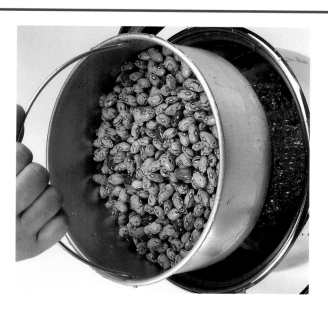

Legumes must be cooked for two fundamental reasons:

- To *eliminate toxic substances* that they contain when raw.[5]
- To *improve* their **digestibility**, thus taking better advantage of their nutritional properties.

The following steps should be followed to ensure proper cooking.

1. **Soaking:** The secret of properly cooked legumes is soaking them well. The purpose is to soften the skin so water reaches the interior of the seed. This may be done in two ways:

   – **Soaking for 6 to 12 hours.** The water poured over the legumes should be boiling to remove as much gas-producing oligosaccharides as possible.

   – *Rapid soaking:* It is possible to achieve the same result by **boiling** the legumes for *two minutes* and allowing them to soak for *one hour* before cooking resumes.

2. **Changing water:** Before starting cooking, it is necessary to discard the water in which the legumes have

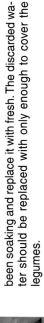

been soaking and replace it with fresh. The discarded water should be replaced with only enough to cover the legumes.

3. **Alkalizing the water:** if the water to be used for cooking is **hard**, in other words, if it has a great deal of dissolved mineral salts, the legumes will become tough. This is because the *calcium* and *magnesium* in the water *combine* with the *pectin* in the legumes, giving them a tough consistency.

   The addition of *one gram* of **sodium bicarbonate** *per serving* to the cooking water precipitates the salts and prevents them from hardening the pectin.

   Acidic substances, such as **vinegar** or **tomato sauce**, *must not be added* to the cooking water. Acids facilitate the combining of the salts and pectin, thus producing toughness.

4. **Cooking:** The *best results* are obtained using a pressure cooker (10 to 20 minutes are sufficient). However, one must be careful since the saponin in the legumes creates dense foam that can obstruct the escape valve of the pressure cooker.

   The formation this foam can be avoided by adding a tablespoon of oil to the cooking water before sealing the pressure cooker.

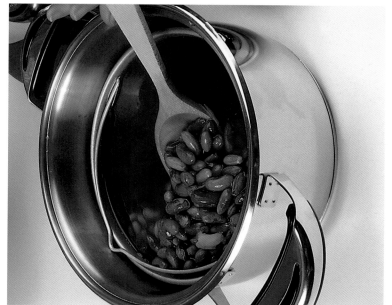

Nutritional Value

Legumes are genuine capsules of concentrated nutrition.
Their use has many benefits, not only for health, but also for the environment.

Legumes Provide:

- **Protein:** *No other* food is **as rich** in **protein** as legumes in their natural state. Soy contains 36.5% of its weight, although most other legumes contain between 20 and 30%. The **proteins** found in legumes contain *all* essential and non-essential **amino acids** in proportions very similar to those in animal protein. *Only* the sulfured **amino acid methionine** is found in *less* than ideal amounts. This minor methionine deficiency is less pronounced in **soy**, whose **protein** is the *most* **complete** of all legumes. Some experts feel that concern over the lack methionine in legumes has been exaggerated. This is because tests evaluating protein quality have been conducted on labo-

ratory rats. It has recently been shown that these animals require more methionine than humans.[6]

Grains are *rich* in **methionine**, and as such, are able to **supplement** the protein in legumes when they are eaten at the same meal, or even the same day (see Vol. 1, p. 70).

- **Vitamins B₁, B₂, B₆, niacin, and folates,** which are very important to the proper functioning of the nervous system and the skin.

- **Minerals,** particularly **iron:** All legumes contain *two to three times more* **iron** than **meat.** This is non-*hem* iron, which is not absorbed as well as the *hem* **iron** found in meat.

Drawbacks to Legumes

- **Uric acid:** Legumes contain **purines** that *convert* to **uric acid** in the body. They are foods that **acidify** the blood and the urine. If they are eaten *with* **fruits** and **vegetables,** which are **alkalizers,** and the kidneys function properly, the acidification produced by legumes presents *no problem* for health. This notwithstanding, legumes **should be avoided** in cases of **gout** or excess **uric acid.**

- **They cannot be eaten raw:** Because of the **anti-nutritional and toxic factors** (protease inhibitors, hemaglutinin, etc., see Vol. 2, p. 274), they cannot be eaten in their natural state. Fortunately, **soaking, cooking, sprouting** or other means of **processing** legumes *destroys* these undesirable substances.[7]

- **Their protein is deficient in methionine** (except soy): This deficiency is easily resolved by combining legumes with grains, thus gaining a complete protein. The *non-essential* **amino acid cystine** is

also present in lower than is ideal, however, the body can synthesize it, in addition to obtaining it from grain sources.

- **Vitamins:** Scarcity of **provitamin A and vitamin C,** absence of **vitamin B₁₂.**

- **Flatulence:** See information chart (Vol. 1, p. 81).

- **Diseases:** Consumption of certain legumes can cause these two diseases:

   – **Lathyrism:** Causes paralysis and nervous disorders. Eating large quantities of ill-cooked flour from the purple vetch produces it. The purple vetch (*Lathyrus sativus*) is a species of pea that is very drought-resistant which has been used during times of famine. If it is properly cooked, it loses its toxicity.

   – **Favism:** Destruction of the red blood cells in certain persons sensitive to Fava beans (see Vol. 2, p. 137).

# of Legumes

However, the *vitamin C* from other foods in the meal *increases* the **absorption** of non-*hem* iron of legumes to levels similar to *hem* iron of meat.

- *Fiber:* From 15% to 30% of legumes' dry weight is fiber, an amount *superior* to that of **whole-grains.** The fiber in legumes in contrast to bran fiber, is mostly *soluble, does not* **irritate** the bowel and has a greater **cholesterol-lowering** effect.

- *Phytochemicals:* All legumes, and especially soy, contain isoflavones, phytosterols, and other phytochemicals with healing properties (see Vol. 2, p. 267).

Benefits of Legumes

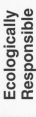

Nutritious

They provide abundant *protein and fiber,* while containing *very little fat* and *no cholesterol.* Legumes provide approximately the same caloric level as grains for the same weight, but two to four times more protein.

Economical

If the same amount of money used to buy a certain amount of meat were used to buy legumes, the amount purchased would be several times greater in terms of calories, proteins, vitamins, and minerals.

Ecologically Responsible

One hectare of land dedicated to legume production provides up to *seven times more calories and protein* than if it were used to raise livestock for meat or milk. In addition, legumes provide a natural fertilizer to the soil.

Medicinal

- **They reduce cholesterol:** Participants of medical studies who ate 120 g (about 4 ounces) of cooked beans

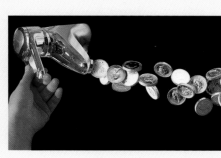

a day for three weeks had their cholesterol and triglyceride levels reduced by 10%.[8, 9, 10]

- **Antidiabetic:** Legumes have a low glycemic index, which means that they raise blood glucose levels very little. Additionally, they reduce the need for insulin in diabetics, and constitute a bona fide **diabetes** *preventive.*[11, 12]

- **They help avoid constipation:** They promote proper bowel function due to their *high* **fiber** content.

- **They help avoid arterial hypertension,** given their *high levels of potassium* and *low sodium levels.*

- **They combat iron-deficiency anemia,** given their *richness* in this mineral, in addition to copper, zinc, and other trace elements.

- **They lower the risk** of **gallstones** (cholelithiasis),[13] since they promote elimination of bile salts through the feces. These salts are the raw material in the formation of gallstones.

- **They reduce the risk of colon cancer,** due to their *fiber* content.

Sprouts:

Persons who cannot tolerate cooked legumes can, however, eat their sprouts, which are germinated seeds.

Changes that Take Place During Sprouting

When a seed has the water, oxygen, and heat necessary, it begins to sprout to form a new living thing, a new plant, which will in time produce more seeds. Sprouting begins with numerous chemical processes facilitated by enzymes. Thanks to this the following changes in the seed take place:

• **Transformation** of reserve substances;

– Large **starch** molecules are broken into smaller ones, such as **dextrin** and **maltose**, which will be converted into **glucose** in the digestive system.

– The **proteins** are transformed into fragments with smaller numbers of **amino acids** (peptides) and **free amino acids.**

– The **fats** release the **fatty acids** of which they are composed.

• **Synthesis** of new substances, such as:

– **vitamin C,** which was not present in the seed;

– **chlorophyll,** which is very healthful.

• **Elimination of antinutritional factors** that are found in the seed, particularly in legumes, such as **hemaglutinin, phytic acid, and protease inhibitors** (see Vol. 1, p. 84). It is necessary to cook legumes to deactivate these substances, but they **disappear** with **sprouting.**

Sprouting Technique

Although sprouts are available commercially, it is an interesting experience growing them at home following the following steps:

1. Use only seeds intended for domestic sprouting. **Seeds** destined for **agricultural use** may be treated with **pesticides** or other **chemical products.**

2. Put the seeds to soak in a glass (*never in metal*) container covered with a fine cloth such as cheesecloth. The amount of water should be three or four times the volume of the seeds.

3. Place the container in a **warm, dark place for about 12 hours.**

4. After 12 hours, discard the water and **rinse the seeds with tepid water.** After that, **rinse the seeds and change the water two or three times a day** until they sprout (this usually takes 2 to 5 days).

Benefits of Sprouts

• **They are living foods:** Even though fruit, grain, and vegetables are living foods in their natural condition, in sprouts **life** is present **with all of its vigor.** This means that sprouts are *rich* in substances that are of **great biological value** necessary for our bodies, such as **vitamins** and **enzymes.**

• **They are predigested:** the enzymes that are synthesized during the sprouting process **begin** the **digestion** of **starch, protein,** and **fats** that are in the seeds. This chemical process is similar to what takes place in the body during digestion. For this reason, sprouts are *easy* to **digest** and are **assimilated** *very well.*
They contain *many* **nutrients** and proportionately *few* **calories,** which makes them useful in diets against obesity.

• **They have medicinal properties:**
– They stimulate the digestive process.
– They regenerate intestinal flora.
– They are antioxidants, depurative and mineralizing.

• **They are simple to prepare** and may be eaten just as they are raw in salads or in a variety of cooked dishes.

• **They make us aware** of the value of natural life processes. Watching the sprouting of a simple seed makes us appreciate more how extraordinary the phenomena of life are.

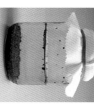
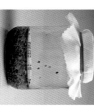
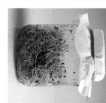

Living Foods

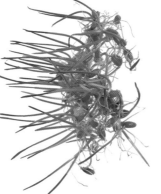

The Most Valued Sprouts:

Any legume or grain seed can be sprouted, however, the most valued for their tenderness and flavor are those obtained from:

- Legumes:
  - **mung bean** (also known as green gram, see Vol. 2, p. 266),
  - **alfalfa** (see Vol. 2, p. 131).

- Grains:
  - **wheat**
  - **barley**

It is also possible to sprout seeds of watercress, radish, pumpkin, sunflower, flax, sesame, etcetera.

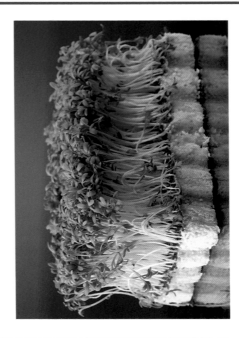

MUNG BEAN, SPROUTED
Composition
per 100 g of raw edible portion

Energy	30.0 kcal = 126 kj
Protein	3.04 g
Carbohydrates	4.13 g
Fiber	1.80 g
Vitamin A	2.00 µg RE
Vitamin B₁	0.084 mg
Vitamin B₂	0.124 mg
Niacin	1.37 mg NE
Vitamin B₆	0.088 mg
Folate	60.8 µg
Vitamin B₁₂	—
Vitamin C	13.2 mg
Vitamin E	0.010 mg α-TE
Calcium	13.0 mg
Phosphorus	54.0 mg
Magnesium	21.0 mg
Iron	0.910 mg
Potassium	149 mg
Zinc	0.410 mg
Total Fat	*0.180 g*
Saturated Fat	*0.046 g*
Cholesterol	—
Sodium	*6.00 mg*

1% 2% 4% 10% 20% 40% 100%

% Daily Value (based on a 2,000 calorie diet) provided by 100 g of this food

P E R C E N T A G E   C O M P O S I T I O N

Fiber **1.80 %**
Minerals **0.440 %**
Carbohydr. **4.13 %**
Fat **0.180 %**
Protein **3.04 %**
Water **90.4 %**

Possible Drawbacks to Sprouts

- **Toxic:** *Raw* legumes contain toxic *antinutritional factors,* such as hemaglutinin. For this reason they **must always be cooked.** Sprouting with appropriate soaking, as has been described, removes these toxic substances entirely.[14, 15, 16] **Alfalfa** sprouts contain a small amount of a non-protein amino acid (l-canavanine, see Vol. 2, p. 130), which can produce toxic effects to those suffering of erythematous lupus.

- **Phytates:** Raw legumes and grains contain phytates (see Vol. 2, p. 311), which have, in spite of being anticarcinogens, the undesirable effect of *interfering* with the **absorption** of *iron, calcium,* and *zinc.* However, during **sprouting,** these *disappear* for the most part.[17]

- **Saponins:** These substances found in seeds, *increase* during the sprouting process. Saponins were found to destroy red blood cells in *in vitro* laboratory experiments. For this reason they were considered toxic. However, today it has been proved that *in vivo,* that is, in the human body, they do not produce hemolysis (the destruction of blood cells). To the contrary, *saponins* are *beneficial,* since:
  - They *reduce* the level of blood **cholesterol,**[18,19]
  - they are **anticarcinogens.**[20]

- **Bacterial contamination:** There have been cases of alfalfa seeds and sprouts contaminated with the bacteria *Salmonella stanley.*[21] Treatment with chlorinated antiseptics can reduce the number of bacteria, but do not eliminate them completely.[22, 23] It is advisable to use sprouts from a reliable and hygienic source.

Soy

Soybean is the legume richest in nutrients, and the one from which the most dietary products are made. All of them have interesting nutritional and therapeutic properties.

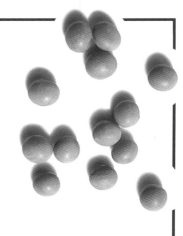

Traditional Products

Traditional soy products are made from the entire soybean, as contrasted with industrially produced items that use only part or an extract of soy. Traditional soy products have their origin in China, Japan, and other Far Eastern countries, although they are now quite easily found in the West.

Unfermented

- **Soy milk**, whose legal name within the European Union is **soy beverage**, is obtained, either at home or industrially prepared, as follows:

  Soy beverage, *compared to* **cow's milk**, contains:

  1. Soak soybeans.
  2. Blend the beans to a puree and cook.
  3. Press the puree to obtain an aqueous solution that is the "milk" or soy beverage.

  — *less* **fat** and **calories**,
  — *more* **iron** and *less* **calcium**,
  — **lecithin** and *more* **polyunsaturated fatty acids**, and
  — **isoflavons** (phytoestrogens, see Vol. 2, p. 268).

  On the other hand, it **does not** contain:

  — *Neither* **lactose** (sugar) *nor* **casein** (milk protein), which can produce allergies and intolerance;
  — *nor* **cholesterol;**
  — *nor* **vitamin B₁₂**, although various soy beverages fortified with this vitamin and/or calcium are commercially available.

  Soymilk or soy beverage can be used in the same way as cow's milk, which it can replace. Additionally, it is **especially useful** in cases of:

  — **lactose intolerance,**
  — **allergies, eczema,** and **atopic dermatitis** caused by cow's milk or milk products (see Vol. 1, p. 194),
  — high levels of **cholesterol, hyperlipemia** (excess fat in the blood), **arteriosclerosis, cardiovascular disease,**
  — **gallstones.**

- **Tofu':** is a term from Japanese, which means '**meat without bone.**' It is to soymilk what cheese is to cow's milk. It is made by coagulating soymilk, usually with calcic salts.

Its texture is *similar to* **cottage cheese.** Due to its *easy* **digestibility** and **neutral** flavor, it lends itself well to a variety of dishes, both salted or sweet.

- **'Tofu'** is quite *rich* in **protein** (8%), **calcium** (105 mg/100 g), **iron** (5.37 mg/100 g), and **zinc** (0.8 g/100 g). It is one of the soy **derivatives** *richest* in **isoflavons.** For this reason 'tofu', along with the soybean itself, are *highly recommended* **to prevent** the following disorders and diseases:

  — symptoms of **menopause;**
  — **arteriosclerosis** and **cardiovascular disease;**
  — **osteoporosis;**
  — **cancer,** particularly of the breast[24], prostate, and colon.

Fermented Soybeans

Fermented soybeans have been used in the Far East for millennia. This method achieves:

— improvement in the **taste** of the soybean,
— *elimination* of **toxic substances** and **antinutritional factors** contained in the raw soybean
— the *emergence* of **vitamin B₁₂**, synthesized by the microorganisms responsible for fermentation.

- **'Tempeh':** is obtained by soaking and cooking soybeans and later adding the fungus *Rhizopus oligosporus,* which causes them to ferment. After about 18-24 hours, it has turned to a paste. *'tempeh',* which is served fried, roasted, or as a hamburger. **'Tempeh'** is a *good source* of:

  — **protein:** contains 19%, an amount equal or greater than that of **meat,**
  — **vitamin B₁₂:** 1 μg/100 g, approximately *half* that of meat and three times that of **cow's milk,**
  — **iron:** 2.26 mg/100 g, approximately the same as **meat.**

- **'Miso':** This is produced in much the same way as 'tempeh' but the fungus *Aspergillus oryzae* is used for fermentation. The soybeans are typically mixed with rice or barley before fermentation. 'Miso' is a paste of a consistency similar to peanut butter.

- **'Tamari':** is a very flavorful sauce made from fermented soy. It is *rich* in **enzymes** and **vitamin B₁₂.**

Products

Products Extracted From Soy

- **Protein:** In 1937, scientists at the Ford Motor Company first extracted soy protein with the objective of using it as a textile fiber. However, they soon realized that it was of greater value as a food than as a cloth. Some years later the North American chemical engineer **Robert Boyer** patented the process for extracting an almost pure soy protein extract.

Finally, humanity had a source of high quality dietary protein in very large quantities and at a very low price.

There are various protein-rich soy products that are used to enrich the protein value of bread, rolls, cookies, and various other food products:

- **Soy flour:** Contains from 40% to 50% proteins.

- **Soy protein concentrate:** contains 70% protein.

- **Isolated soy protein:** it reaches a protein level of 95%.

- **Texturized soy protein:** Using a variety of industrial processes, soy protein is given the appearance and texture of meat. In granular form, its protein content is between 70% and 90%. When flavorings are added, it lends itself to the manufacturing of various meat analogs.

- **Soy oil:** This is generally obtained by mixing a solvent (hexane) with hot, blended soybeans. The industry guarantees that following processing, no hexane, which is toxic, remains in the resultant oil. This oil is rich in *linoleic acid* (polyunsaturated) and is insipid. It is used primarily in the manufacturing of margarine and sauces.

- **Lecithin:** This is a phospholipid whose molecule is formed by combining various *fatty acids* (stearic, palmitic, and oleic) with *choline* and *phosphoric acid.*

- **Source:** Lecithin that is used as a dietary supplement, or that is used in the food industry, is derived from soy oil, which contains it in an approximate proportion between 1% and 3%.

- **Other sources:** Although the soybean is possibly the *richest natural source of lecithin,* it is also found in the **seeds** of *many* other **plants** as well as in egg **yolks.** Our bodies can produce lecithin in cases where its dietary intake is deficient. Liver cells and those of the nervous system are those that contain the most lecithin.

- **Use as an additive:** Lecithin is an *effective* **emulsifier** that disperses oils into fine droplets and causes these to mix in aqueous solutions or water. For this reason it is used in mayonnaise, sauces, chocolate, and many other products.

- **Use in diet therapy:** Although there is limited scientific evidence to confirm the therapeutic effects of lecithin, it is used in the following situations:

  ✓ **Increase in blood cholesterol level:** It is assumed that regular use of lecithin lowers cholesterol level, but *there is no proof of this.*

  ✓ **Liver disease:** Lecithin contains *choline* (see Vol. 1, p. 408), a vitamin factor necessary in inhibiting fatty deposits in the liver. Even though the body can produce choline, most is taken in through foods or as nutritional supplements. Lecithin *avoids* **fatty degeneration in the liver.** It is useful in case of viral **hepatitis, alcoholism, toxic hepatitis** because of certain medications, or **abnormal liver function** from any cause.

  ✓ **Disorders of the nervous system:** *Lecithin* and *choline* are present in the neurons, where they contribute to the transmission process of nerve impulses. *Acetylcholine,* a derivative of choline, is one of the *principal* **neurotransmitters** (substances that allow neurons to chemically communicate with each other). Use of lecithin can be useful in cases of various nervous system disorders, including **depression,** even though there is *no conclusive evidence.*

Even though the therapeutic effects of lecithin are not proven, its use as a nutritional supplement presents no risk, since it *completely* **lacks** undesirable or toxic **side effects.**

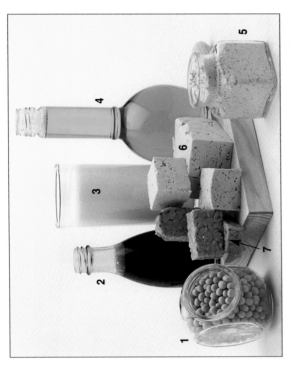

1. grains, 2. 'tamari', 3. milk, 4. oil, 5. flour, 6. 'tofu', 7. 'tempeh'

LEGUMES OF THE WORLD

Botanical Family

LEGUMINOSAE

This botanical family consists of more than 800 genera and some 13,000 species spread across the world. They have adapted to the most varied of habitats. They are grown in humid tropical regions, deserts and savanna, as well as mountainous areas.

Legumes constitute the third most important family of phanerogams or flowering plants, after composite plans and orchids. They represent everything from modest herbs and climbing vines to bushes and large trees. Their fruit is characterized by pods containing several seeds.

Only 50 species of legumes are of dietary interest, including those described here. These plants, together with **grains**, are the **richest** in **nutrients** of any that grow on the earth, and are those that **contribute the most** to the **proper nutrition** of humanity.

There are other leguminous plants that are used as:

- **fruit**: purging cassia (EMP p. 494), carob (EMP p. 497), guama, and tamarind (Vol. 1, p. 46);
- **vegetables**: peas and fava beans (Vol. 2, p. 73, 137);
- **nuts**: peanuts (Vol. 2, p. 336).

Pigeon peas

Chick peas

Food

	Vol./Page	Description and Use
PIGEON PEA *Cajanus cajan*		*Syn. Cajan, Gungo pea.* These are **seeds** of a bush cultivated in India, tropical Africa, and the Caribbean islands. It is very drought-resistant. It is used like any other legume. Its nutritional value is comparable to **lentils.**
CHICK PEA *Cicer arietinum*	2/91	*Syn. Garbanzo bean.* These beans reduce **cholesterol,** avoid **constipation,** and strengthen the **nervous system.**
JACK BEAN *Canavalia ensiformis*		*Syn. Horsebean, Cut-eye bean, Sword bean.* These beans, originally from Mexico, are cultivated throughout Central America for their **seeds** as well as for their **pods,** which is the part used for human consumption. They contain less provitamin A and vitamin C than green beans. The **seeds** are **nutritious,** but somewhat **indigestible.** *Caution:* These beans contain **more antinutritional factors** than any other legume. They must be **soaked** for 6 to 12 hours, with various changes of **water,** and **cooked well** to **eliminate** them.
GUAR *Cyamopsis tetragonoloba*		*Syn. Clusterbean.* The green **pods** of this legume are similar to those of peas and are used as a vegetable in India and Southeast Asia. **Guar gum** is extracted from the **seeds.** This is a natural additive used as a thickener and as a complement in the treatment of **diabetes** (slows the absorption of glucose, thus avoiding excessively high levels in the blood).
LABLAB *Dolichos lablab*		*Syn. Hyacinth bean, Bonavist bean.* This is cultivated in Africa, Central America, and India for their **pods** and their **seeds,** which have a nutritional value similar to other **beans.**
YARD-LONG BEAN *Dolichos sesquipedalis*		*Syn. Asparagus bean, Asparagus cowpea.* These are cultivated in Southeast Asia and Central America for their long **pods,** which are sweeter than European green beans. Their **seeds** are also edible.
SOYBEAN *Glycine max*	2/264	Soybeans are the **richest** of all legumes in **protein, fats, vitamins,** and **minerals.** Additionally, they contain **phytoestrogens** that **balance** the **endocrine** system and protect against **cancer.**
LATHYRUS PEA *Lathyrus sativus*		*Syn. Grass-pea, Chickling vetch.* These are grown in India and South America, although they are originally from the Mediterranean region. **Flour** is made from this, one of the **most nutritious** legumes. It was eaten during periods of famine in Europe. *Caution:* The **seeds** contain a **toxin** that produces a disease called **lathyrism** (Vol. 1, p. 84). **Soaking** and **cooking** removes **most** of this toxin.
LENTIL *Lens culinaris*	2/127	Very rich in **iron** and **fiber,** they are useful in cases of **anemia, constipation, diabetes,** and elevated **cholesterol** levels.
LUPINE *Lupinus albus*	2/303	Antidiabetic, diuretic, and vermifuge (destroys intestinal parasites).

EMP = *Encyclopedia of Medicinal Plants,* EDUCATION AND HEALTH LIBRARY, Editorial Safeliz.

LEGUMES OF THE WORLD – *continued*

Botanical Family	Food	Vol./Page	Description and Use
	ALFALFA *Medicago sativa*	2/130 EMP 269	Alfalfa seeds contain **antinutritional factors** (see Vol. 2, p. 273) that make them unfit for human consumption. However these toxins **disappear** during the **sprouting** process. Alfalfa **sprouts** are **antihemmoragic, mineralizing,** and **improve resistance** to infection.
	TEPARY BEAN *Phaseolus acutifolius*		These are cultivated in Mexico for their **seeds**. These beans require longer cooking time than others do. They are the **least flatulent** of all beans.
	COMMON BEAN *Phaseolus vulgaris*	2/343	These protect the **skin** and the **mucosae,** and lower **cholesterol.** See their varieties in Vol. 2, p. 343.
	ADZUKI *Vigna angularis*	2/266	This is similar to **soy**, but softer and sweeter when eaten cooked.
	MUNG BEAN *Vigna radiata*	2/266	Commercially available **soy sprouts** come from this bean.
	BAMBARA GROUNDNUT *Voandzeia subterranea*		**Scientific syn.** *Glycine subterranea.* **Syn.** *Congo goober, Ground pea.* These are grown in West Africa (Mali) and Central Africa (Zambia), where they are replacing the peanut. It grows below the ground. The dried **seeds** are toasted and the **pods** are cooked. They are a good source of **calories** and **protein** in African countries.

Azuki

Botanical Characteristics of Leguminosae

- **Fruit:** Botanically, they are called **legumes.** They are formed by a pod containing seeds.

- **Pod (1):** These can be of different consistencies (fleshly in the case of common beans or green beans, starchy in the case of carob or even woody), and of varying sizes (from one millimeter up to almost a meter, as the case of the yard-long bean). Legume **pods** contain **provitamin A** and **vitamins B, C,** and **E,** as well as minerals, particularly **iron.** Some species, such as carob and tamarind, have thick **pods** that are rich in **starch.**

- **Seeds (2):** They are referred to culinarily as **legumes,** as well. They are found inside the pods, and are formed by a **skin,** two **cotyledons,** and an **embryo.** They are very rich in **protein, vitamins,** and **minerals.** Some, such as soy or the peanut, are also rich in fats. The seeds of legumes also contain toxic **antinutritional factors** that disappear with soaking or cooking (see Vol. 1, p. 84).

- **Roots:** Almost all herbaceous legumes of agricultural interest have special **nitrogen-fixating bacteria** in their roots that are capable of converting atmospheric nitrogen into nitrates. These nitrates, in turn, are used by the plant to form **amino acids and proteins.** For this reason, legumes **do not need fertilizer,** and, indeed, leave the soil prepared for other crops (see Vol. 1, p. 80).

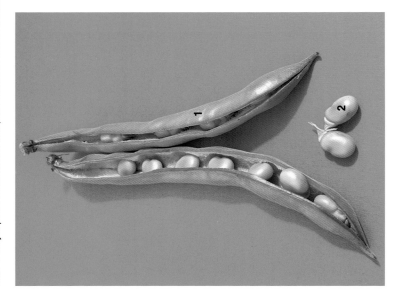

VEGETABLES

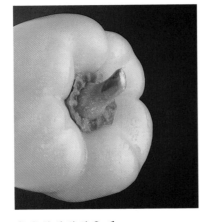

Vegetables should not be considered a mere side dish to the "main course", quite to the contrary. Vegetables, together with grains and fruit, should be principal elements of a truly healthful and nutritious diet.

EVEN THOUGH vegetables such as garlic, leeks, and onions were widely used in ancient Egypt[1] fifteen hundred years before the birth of Christ, their use in the West was considerably more limited. Vegetables have been little valued in Europe except in the countries around the Mediterranean.

The Consumption of Vegetables

This was not the case in Asia, where from antiquity peoples throughout the region have made abundant use of a wide variety of vegetables. Nor was it true on the American continent where pre-Colombians used potatoes, tomatoes, and peppers as staples in their diet.

During the same period, in Anglo-Saxon cultures of Europe, meat consumption was considered evidence of wellbeing and progress. Those persons who ate vegetables were considered too poor to afford meat or too ill to eat it. Vegetables that are so common today such as the potato and the tomato, imports from the Americas, were viewed with suspicion in countries such as France, Germany, and England.

Vegetables and the Mediterranean Diet

Arabs from North Africa introduced and promoted the cultivation and use of many vegetables into Western Europe during the Middle Ages. Some, such as the eggplant, were imported from as far away as India.

Today vegetables remain *fundamental ingredients* in the **Mediterranean diet**, possibly because of almost a thousand years of Arabic cultural influence in Southern European regions.

Continued on page 94

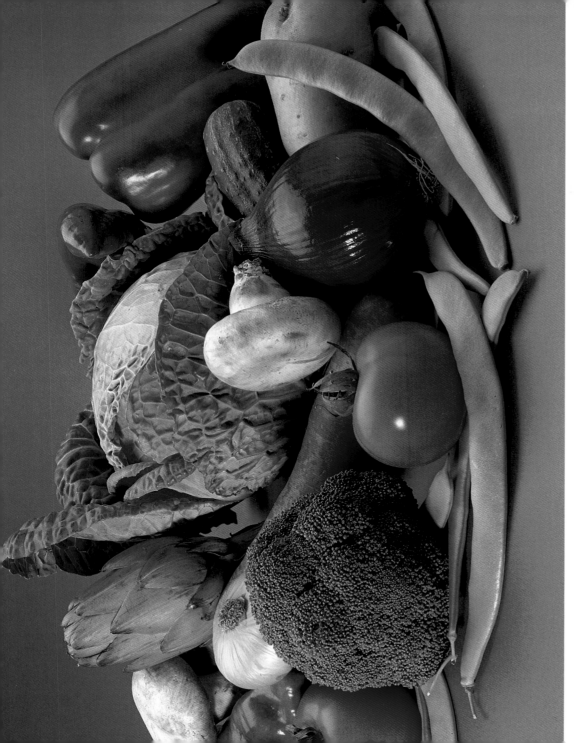

Human nutrition as well as that of all higher animals, especially cattle, depends in the first place on vegetables. Even carnivores could not survive if their prey could not find vegetables to eat. This means that vegetables are at the base of the food chain of Planet Earth.

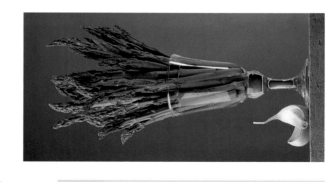

Vegetables

ⓘ

- **Vegetables:** are generally herbaceous (non-woody) plants that are cultivated in the market gardens or truck farms as well as kitchen gardens for home use. Usually, all the botanical parts of these plants such as leaves, buds or flowers, fruit, stalks, roots, etc., can be eaten.

  Plants whose dried seeds are called **legumes** or pulses belonging to the leguminous family are not considered as vegetables in this work (see Vol. 1, p. 78).

  The word vegetable refers to the whole plant as well as to its edible parts.

- **Leafy greens** or just greens are a special variety of vegetables characterized by their green color, resulting from their chlorophyll content. **Leaves, stalks,** and some **flowers** or **buds** of these plants fall into this category.

> Getting children to eat vegetables often requires a complete strategy involving the preparation and presentation of these foods as well as appropriate information about their nutritional value in the diet.

Continued from page 92

An Example of Changing Diet: Greater use of Vegetables in the Former East Germany

Today the situation is somewhat different. The use of vegetables and vegetable products in countries of Anglo-Saxon extraction is increasing while, unfortunately, Mediterraneans are increasing their consumption of meats and meat products. For example, in the former East Germany the diet was characterized by:

- extensive use of sausages, animal fats, and butter, and

- proportionally less use of vegetables, fruits, and vegetable oils than in West Germany.[2]

However, since German reunification in 1989, the use of fresh vegetables and fruits

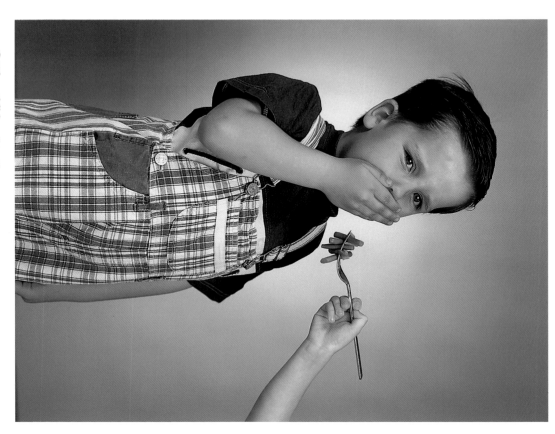

has increased dramatically in the former East Germany. As a result, there has been a decrease in death rate from cardiovascular disease, which had previously been very high.

"Five a Day"

"Five a Day" is the slogan used in a broad educational campaign begun in the United States in 1991 under the auspices of the National Institute of Health. Through the use of the various media, Americans of all ages were urged to eat *at least* five servings of fresh fruits and vegetables a day. This ambitious effort to change the nation's dietary habits was based on:[3]

- The **pleasing flavor** and **attractiveness** of fruits and vegetables.

- The **health benefits** derived from their increased use in the diet.

The results of this campaign were not long in coming. Cholesterol levels and the incidence of cardiovascular disease are decreasing markedly in the United States. While one must bear in mind other factors such as the positive effects of lowered tobacco use, increased interest in a Mediterranean-style diet in the United States and other developed Western countries is having a significant positive impact on the health of their citizens.

Children and Vegetables

Most mothers complain at one time or another that their children do not want to eat vegetables. In fact, a study by the National Cancer Institute of the United States revealed that the vegetable of choice for children and adolescents is French-fried potatoes.[4] Only one in five children eats five or more servings of fruit or vegetables a day.

It is true that adults need the nutrition provided by vegetables more than children do with their high energy and growth demands. However, vegetables contain calcium and iron, as well as **pro-vitamin A**, all of them necessary for healthy growth and development.

Psychosocial factors greatly influence the consumption of vegetables.[5] Nutrition experts recommend these and other *strategies* to encourage children to **eat more of these important foods:**[6]

- They should be presented on the table as attractively as possible. Many children prefer a **fresh salad** rather than cooked vegetables, vegetable roasts, or vegetable soups.

- **Information appropriate to the age of the child** should be presented at home, school, and the media about the benefits of vegetables and fruits.

Continued on page 102

Weight Loss With Vegetables

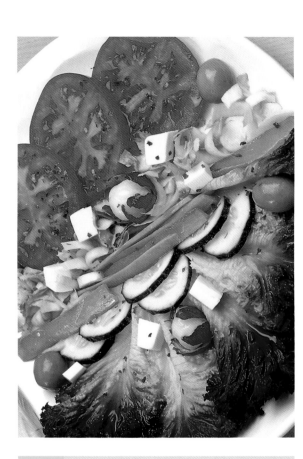

No vegetable is fattening even when eaten in large quantities *(an exception is fried vegetables). Because of this, vegetables should be at the top of the list for diets for losing and maintaining weight.*

Vegetables produce a much greater feeling of satiety than other foods when one compares the amount eaten with calories taken in.

*For example, to consume **300 calories:***

- *one can eat a small **ice cream** (70 grams or 2.5 ounces), or a slice of **bread with cheese;***

- *however, one would have to eat **1.9 kilos** (8 pounds) of **lettuce**, or **1.2 kilos** (2.65 pounds) of **cauliflower**, or **1 kilo** (2.2 pounds) of baked **eggplant** (without oil or dressing).*

Eating vegetables leaves one feeling comfortably full without a heavy feeling. However, only a few calories have been taken in. Learning to feel satisfied eating foods with low caloric content is all a matter of taste.

A Pharmacy on Your Plate

*In addition to vitamins, minerals, and fiber, vegetables contain hundreds of substances that are active all over the organism. These are called **phytochemicals** (see Vol. 1, p. 410).*

*Although much research remains to be done regarding these elements, science has confirmed their **preventive powers against cancer and arterosclerosis.**[7]*

Types of

Depending on which part of the plant is used, each type of vegetable has particular properties that should be understood

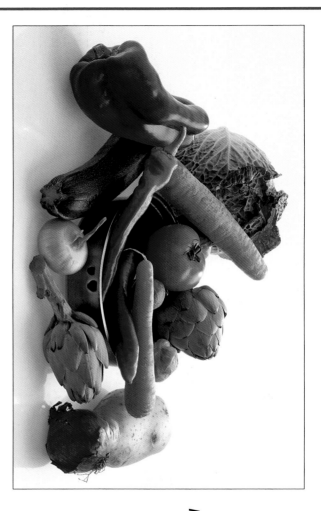

Stalks

These, such as **asparagus** and **leeks**, are *rich in* ***fiber*** and are generally **diuretic. Sugar** cane is a stalk that stores great quantities of a type of sugar called sucrose. In some cases only parts of some stalks, called shoots, are eaten. Examples are **bamboo shoots** and palm **hearts.**

Leaves

These are more nutritious than one might believe. The leaves of **turnips, parsnips,** and **cabbage** are good sources of ***calcium.*** **Spinach** is a good source of ***iron.*** They also contain between 1% and 3% ***protein.***

Some leaves, such as **spinach** and **sorrel** contain ***oxalic acid*** that can interfere with the absorption of calcium (see Vol. 1, p. 103).

Cabbage leaves contain **anti-carcinogenic phytochemicals** (see Vol. 1, p. 410).

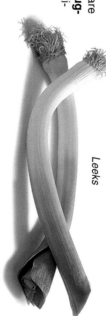

Leeks

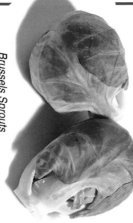

Brussels Sprouts

Flowers and Buds

Artichokes, cauliflower, and **broccoli** are inflorescent vegetables, meaning that they are made up of tightly bunched florets. They contain ***provitamin A*** as well as ***vitamins B and C.***

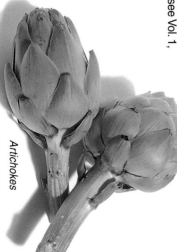

Artichokes

Vegetables

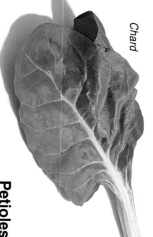

Chard

Petioles

These are the stems connecting the leaves to the stalk. In some plants, such as **cardoon** and **chard**, they are so developed that they become very tender and flavorful. Like stalks, petioles are rich in *cellulose.*

Fruits

From the bright red of the **toma-to**, the brilliant purple of the **eggplant**, the orange and yellow of **pumpkins** and **squash** to the varied greens of **cucumbers, zucchini**, and **avo-cado**, these vegetables are notable for their colors.

The **avocado** is a special fruit since it contains be-tween 15% and 17% **fat**. We consider it a vegetable because of the way it is used, even though it comes from a tree rather than a herbaceous plant (see Vol. 2, p. 108).

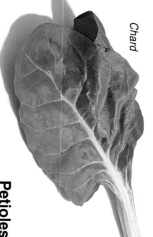

Cucumbers

Seeds

Peas and **beans** are the seeds of plants of the *Legu-minosae* family that are used as vegetables. As with all seeds, they are a *good source of protein.*

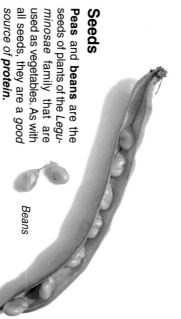

Beans

Tubers

These are not roots but rather specialized underground en-largements of the plant's stalk. They are the storage site for **starch**, which is the *primary reserve substance in vegetables.* They contain some level of *protein* as well as *vitamin C* (for example, the **potato**) and *provita-min A* (**sweet potato**).

Tubers should *not* be eaten *raw* since they contain **tox-ic substances**, which are removed by cook-ing (see Vol. 1, p. 103).

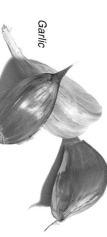

Potatoes

Roots

These contain carbohydrates (**starch**), **fiber, and minerals.** Some, such as **carrots** and **red beets**, contain beta-carotene (**provitamin A**).

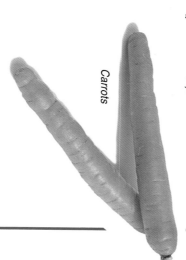

Carrots

Bulbs

Bulbs are an underground thicken-ing of the stalk that is formed by nu-merous layers. They contain sul-furous (**onions, garlic**) or aromatic (**fennel**) substances.

Garlic

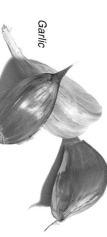

Salads: the Perfect Appetizer

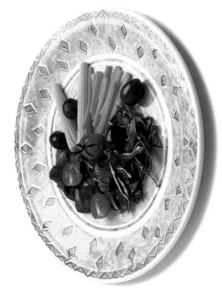

A SALAD A DAY PROTECTS AGAINST HEART ATTACK

Researchers from Oxford University (UK) have shown through a broad epidemiological study that eating one salad a day reduces the death rate from heart attack by 26%.[8]

Ingredients

Almost any *raw* vegetable works well in a salad, as long as it is **ripe and tender. Tubers** are the *exception* (potatoes, sweet potatoes, tapioca, yucca, etc.). These should not be eaten raw (see Vol. 1, p. 97). For example:

- **leaves:** lettuce, escarole, endive, etc.;
- **fruit:** tomatoes, cucumbers peppers, avocado, etc.;
- **flowers:** cauliflower, broccoli, artichoke;
- **stalks:** asparagus, celery, etc.;
- **roots:** carrots, red beets, etc.;
- **bulbs:** onion, garlic, fennel, etc.

Sunflower seeds, **nuts** such as walnuts, cooked **legumes** or **cereals** such as corn or rice prepared in different ways *add a great deal* to salads. They also increase the nutritional value of salads, making them truly substantial dishes.

Dressing

There are many ways to dress a salad, but the ideal from a nutritional standpoint is this:

- **Oil:** preferably cold-pressed virgin olive oil.
- **Salt:** Even though it is not necessary to add salt, given the *abundant mineral* salts contained in vegetables, it does add to the flavor. Refined table salt (NaCl, sodium chloride) is not recommended. If salt is to be added, it is *preferable* to use **sea salt,** which contains *potassium* and *magnesium,* or salts made with **garlic, celery,** or

other vegetables; these contain *potassium* and other *minerals.*

- **Lemon** juice, whose *vitamin C* and *organic acids:*
  – *prevent* **oxidation** and *help* **protect vitamins and minerals** of vegetables, and
  – *enhance* the **absorption** of iron.
- *Aromatic herbs*

Vinegar is a poor substitute for lemon juice in salads. While its acidity does protect the vegetables, it lacks vitamins and antioxidant properties (see Vol. 1, p. 337).

Dressings based on hydrogenated vegetable oils typically contain *trans*-fatty acids that can promote arteriosclerosis. These preparations may also contain other additives that can be unhealthful.

When To Eat Salads

Doctor *Bircher-Benner* of Switzerland developed a whole school of dietetic thought regarding the value of **raw and live foods.** This was based on a very broad experiential base during the first half of the twentieth century. It had, and continues to have great influence in Europe. He arrived at the conclusion that:

- To maintain good health it is necessary to eat at *least* one **salad a day** consisting of raw vegetables.
- The best time to eat **salad** is at the *very beginning* of the main meal of the day.

Advantages of a Salad at the Beginning of a Main Meal

- They provide *digestive enzymes,* which are *only* present in **live foods** and aid digestion of other foods that have higher protein content, carbohydrates, and fats.
- **Prevents digestive leucocytosis:**[9] this is an inflammation process which occurs in the intestines after beginning a meal with cooked foods.
- They produce a greater **feeling of satiety** than cooked foods with higher caloric content. Therefore salads make *special* sense in diets where one desires to **lose or maintain weight.**

Raw Salads and Pollution

Polluted water is used in many developing countries to irrigate vegetable gardens. The result is contamination by organisms transmitted through feces such as *Vibrio cholera.*

The use of **chlorine** (bleach) is very effective in disinfecting raw vegetables, as is **limewater.** Lettuce or cabbage that has been soaked for five minutes in limewater is completely free of cholera bacilli and can be eaten with complete safety.[10]

The Art of Cooking Vegetables

Eating raw vegetables in salads is the best way to take advantage of their nutritional properties. However, if one wishes to cook them, here is information to help maintain their food value.

The primary nutrients of vegetables are *vitamins and minerals.* The cooking process affects these as follows:

- **Light** and **heat** degrade *vitamins.*
- *Minerals* and their salts are **dissolved** in water and are removed in the cooking liquid.

Cooking in Water

One can minimize the loss of vitamins and minerals in the cooking process by following these simple suggestions in preparing vegetables:

- Use as **little water as possible** when cooking.
- **Place vegetables into boiling water** rather than into water while it is being heated.
- **Cook vegetables as little as possible,** leaving them *al dente,* like pasta.
- **Do not leave** vegetables **in water** after they are cooked. This prevents the further dissolving of mineral salts.
- **Save the water used for cooking vegetables.** It is rich in minerals and can be used to make soups and other dishes.

Roasts

Although roasting enhances the flavors of vegetables, the process causes them to lose approximately 25% of their vitamins, more than cooking.

Frying

This method causes the **greatest** *loss* of nutrients. Fried vegetables also absorb fats that make them *less digestible* and very high in **calories.**

The **cooking methods** that **minimize** loss of nutrients are:

- **by steaming,** as shown in the illustration below (the vegetables are separated from the water by a colander); or,
- **in a microwave oven.**

Processing Vegetables

- Light and heat degrade vitamins. For this reason, the **refrigerator** is the *best place* to store vegetables.
- When vegetables are **chopped or pureed,** the cellular walls are broken down. This results in a great *loss* of **nutrients.** Therefore, **purees** should be **eaten** *immediately* after preparation.

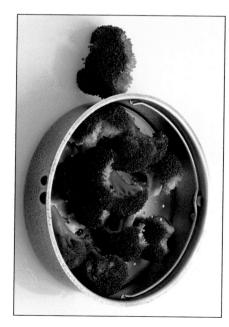

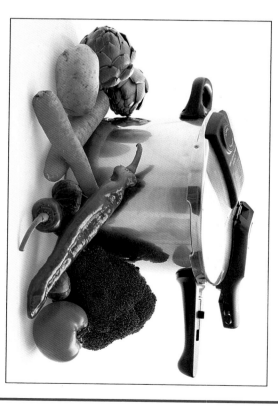

Nutritional Value

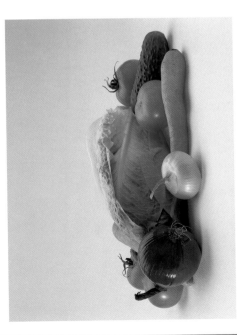

Even though the bulk of their weight is water, vegetables represent a veritable natural pharmacy of minerals, vitamins, and phytochemicals.

Vegetables Provide:

- *Water:* Most vegetables contain 90% to 95% water. This is even more than milk, which contains less than 88%. But this does not mean they are low in nutritional value. The remaining 5% to 10% of solids contain substances of great biological and therapeutic value.

- *Minerals:* Vegetables are a **good source** of *all* minerals. This explains their **alkalizing** effect and resulting benefit on the blood and tissues. The minerals most abundant in vegetables are:

  – *Potassium:* important for **diuretic and hypotensive** effect (lowers arterial blood pressure).

  – *Calcium:* Cabbage, for example, contains between 35 and 77 milligrams (mg) of calcium per 100 grams (g) of weight. This is a relatively important amount when compared with milk, which contains 119 mg per 100 g. Additionally, the body easily **absorbs** the *calcium* found in **cabbage.**[11]

  – *Iron:* **Spinach** contains 2.71 mg/100 g, which is more than the iron contained in **meat. Lamb's lettuce, fava beans, peas,** and **beets** are also good sources of iron. The *vitamin C* in these vegetables enhances the **absorption** of iron.

- *Vitamins:* in particular *provitamin A* (beta-carotene that is found in orange and red-colored vegetables), and *vitamins C, B* (except B₁₂), and *K* (found in alfalfa, cabbage, and spinach).

- *Folic acid and Folates:* These are *abundant* in *leafy green vegetables*, particularly in **spinach.** *Folic acid is an essential* nutrient for **pregnant women.**

- *Fiber:* Contributes to the feeling of satiation and satisfaction associated with eating. It also works to *prevent* **constipation.**

- *Proteins:* Vegetables contain significant amounts of protein that should not be overlooked. These proteins are generally superior to those found in fruits, although inferior to those in grains and legumes. Keeping in mind that a serving of vegetables may be as much as one cup, it becomes evident that such serving may provide a fair amount of proteins. For example, consider the milligrams of protein per 100 grams of some common vegetables: lettuce, 1.62; potatoes, 2.07; asparagus, 2.28; spinach, 2.86; Brussels sprouts, 3.38; peas, 5.42.

The proteins found in vegetables contain all of the essential and non-essential *amino acids* with two important considerations:

– Vegetables do not provide an adequate level of *methionine* to meet the body's need. However, **grains** are very *rich* in this essential amino acid.

– Vegetables contain *abundant lysine,* an essential amino acid that is found in very *low levels* in **grains.**

Vegetables and grains *together* provide *complete protein* thanks to the phenomenon of **supplementation.** The *protein* in **potatoes** is the *most complete* found in any vegetable.

- *Carbohydrates:* Only tubers such as the **potato** contain significant amounts.

- *Chlorophyll:* This is the green pigment found in all plants. While its effect in the body is not well known, it is thought to facilitate blood production.

- *Phytochemicals:* These constitute a very recent discovery in nutrition science. (see Vol. 1, p. 410). **Vegetables,** together with **fruit** and **legumes,** are the foods richest in these elements. Even though they are found only in very small amounts, they act as powerful **antioxidants** that help in the prevention of **cancer** and **coronary disease.** The vegetables *richest* in these elements are those that belong to these two botanical families:

  – **Cruciferae:** cabbage, radish, turnip, and watercress.
  – **Liliaceae:** onions, garlic, and leeks.

The phytochemicals found in these two groups are rich in sulfur, which gives them their piquant taste.

# of Vegetables

Benefits of Vegetables

They are a Complement to Grains and Legumes

Vegetables provide nutrients that are lacking in the other two types of foods: *Pro-vitamin A, vitamin C,* and *folates.*

Beans

Natural Laxatives

The *fiber* content of vegetables increases the volume of fecal matter and facilitates its passage through the digestive tract. When vegetables are not tender, their fiber may be indigestible. In this case, they are best eaten grated or cooked.

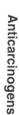

Ideal in Cases of Obesity

Maintain your weight by eating vegetables. They contain almost no *fat* and their *caloric content* is *very low.* However, they produce a sensation of satiation that substantially relieves feelings of hunger.

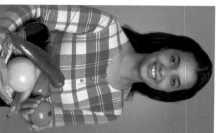

Appropriate For the Elderly

Because of their low caloric content, their **calcifying action,** and their **anti-carcinogenic** effect they are an excellent food for older persons.

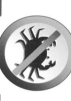

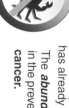

Source of Minerals

Turnip greens contain more *calcium* than **milk,** in addition to *magnesium, phosphorous,* and other minerals. **Cabbage** is also a good source of *calcium.* In general, stalks and leaves vegetables are rich in the *minerals* that build bone tissue. As such, they are recommended in cases of **osteoporosis** and other **calcium deficiency** disorders.

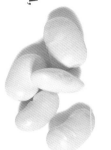

Diuretics and Antihypertensives

Because of their *potassium* content they *increase* urine production and *reduce* arterial **blood pressure.**

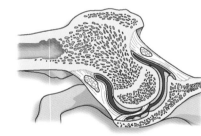

Antianemic

All vegetables, but particularly **beets, fava beans, spinach, watercress,** and **lamb's lettuce** facilitate the production of **red blood cells** due to their high **iron** content (whose absorption is facilitated by the simultaneous effect of *vitamin C* in the digestive system), as well as *trace elements* and *chlorophyll.*

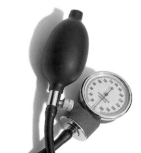

Lamb's lettuce

Anticarcinogens

All vegetables, especially those of the family *Cruciferae* (**cabbage, radish, and turnip**) and *Liliaceae* (**onions, garlic, and leeks**) families, contain substances which have been shown to be **effective** *in vitro,* as well as *in vivo* to:

- *neutralize* the action of **carcinogenic substances** that promote cellular degeneration and,
  - *slow* the **growth** when the cancer process has already begun.

  The *abundant use* of vegetables is useful in the prevention as well as the treatment of **cancer.**

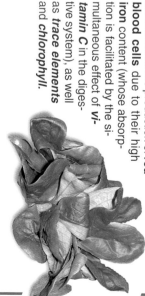

the **nutritional and curative properties** of vegetables is to eat them **raw in salads.**

These are some of the most common processing methods used with vegetables in addition to cooking, which is described in this chapter (Vol. 1, p. 99).

- **Artificial ripening:** Due to commercial needs, many tomatoes are ripened artificially in special chambers. Consumers know from experience that their flavor is inferior to those that are vine-ripened. Additionally, it has been demonstrated that artificially ripened tomatoes contain *33% less vitamin C* than those ripened naturally.[12]

- **Freezing:** *Conserves most* of the *vitamins* and other properties of vegetables.

- **Canning** is the *least* effective processing method from a nutrition standpoint. However, it is the **safest** and has the longest shelf life of all.

- **Chopped or grated:** Cutting the vegetable's tissues accelerates the loss of nutrients. For this reason vegetables prepared in this way should **be eaten *immediately*** rather than stored.

Drawbacks to Vegetables

None of the drawbacks associated with vegetables is significant enough to justify eating less of them. However, no matter how slight they may be, it is worthwhile being aware of them.

Flatulence

The *fiber* in certain vegetables such as **leeks** and **cabbage** can produce flatulence (gas), since they are partially metabolized by intestinal bacteria.

Indigestion

Some persons do not tolerate vegetables with piquant *sulfurated components* such as **cabbage, radishes, or onions.**

Continued from page 95

The Processing of Vegetables

Vegetables in general, with the exception of tubers and some fruits such as the eggplant, can be eaten raw in their *natural* **state**. The **best way** for persons without digestive problems to take **full advantage** of

---

Gazpacho: a Mediterranean Way To Eat Vegetables

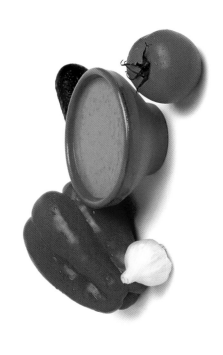

For some it is a blended salad; for others it is a cold vegetable soup; and for others still it is a refreshing drink. Gazpacho is all of these. The popular conception is that the people from Southern Spain "invented" it as a food that quenches the thirst while providing minerals and vitamins during the hot summer months.

*Gazpacho is prepared, with minor regional differences in Andalusia, from a base of **tomato, pepper, cucumber, garlic, and olive oil**. These are all liquefied in a blender to a homogenized thick liquid. It should be served well chilled.*

Gazpacho has many advantages from a nutritional standpoint:

- *It is an **unique way** to eat vegetables that may be more attractive to those who do not normally eat them, for example, some children.*

- *The maximum vitamin content of the vegetables is maintained since they are all in a **raw state**.*

- *It is **easily digested** since all the vegetables are liquefied. They require almost no chewing.*

Of course, to take full advantage of these nutritive and curative properties, gazpacho must be eaten as soon as possible after it is prepared.

Toxic Substances

Some vegetables contain certain toxic substances. Although they are not generally dangerous, it is good to be informed about them:

- **Alkaloids: Solanine** is found in *unripe* vegetables of the family *Solanaceae* (**potatoes, eggplants, tomatoes, and peppers**). There is *no risk* of solanine poisoning from eating these vegetables ripe. If they are not **ripe**, potatoes and eggplants contain very high levels of solanine. **Cooking** partially *destroys* solanine.

- **Hydrocyanic acid:** This is released while cutting certain tropical tubers such as the **yam, tapioca, and** some **sweet potatoes.** It is also present in **bamboo stalks. It *disappears* with washing and cooking.**

- **Oxalic acid:** is found in **rhubarb, chard, spinach, and sorrel.** It produces a disagreeable numbing effect on the tongue, but above all, if it is taken in large quantities it:

  – interferes with the absorption of calcium and iron, and
  – can lead to the development of kidney stones.

  Most of the oxalic acid **disappears** when the **water used to cook** these vegetables is *discarded.* At any rate, the body tolerates and easily eliminates certain levels of the oxalic acid found in many vegetables and fruits.

- **Goiter-producing agents:** These are found in the family *Cruciferae,* primarily **cabbage** (see Vol. 2, pp. 191-197) and **turnips** (see Vol. 2, p. 320). It has been demonstrated that the *excessive* consumption of these foods during *long periods* can slow or stop the proper functioning of the thyroid, thus causing **goiter.**

  Persons who do not suffer from hypothyroidism (diminished thyroid activity) are not at risk from eating cabbage and turnips in reasonable amounts since these vegetables are very beneficial.

- **Nitrates and nitrites:** *All* vegetables **naturally** contain these salts, especially **beets, radishes, spinach,** and **lettuce.** Some think that the use of chemical fertilizers can raise the concentration of these substances. However, even if this were so, it has not been shown dangerous.

  Vitamin C helps **eliminate** nitrates and nitrites through the urine,[14] at no risk to the health.

  On the other hand, nitrites and nitrates used as preservative **additives** in **sausages** and **hams** are indeed dangerous. They can react with certain proteins and form **nitrosamine,** which is a powerful **carcinogen** (see Vol. 1, p. 326).

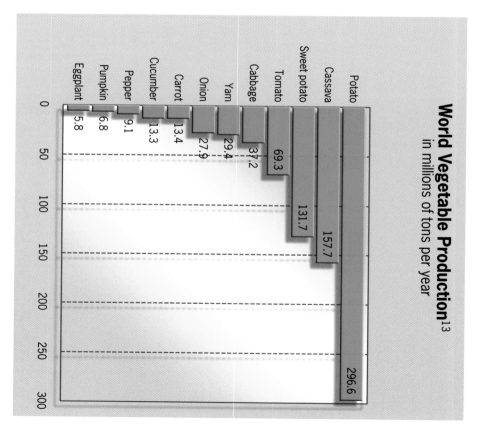

World Vegetable Production[13]
in millions of tons per year

Vegetable	Millions of tons
Potato	296.6
Cassava	157.7
Sweet potato	131.7
Tomato	69.3
Cabbage	37.2
Yam	29.4
Onion	27.9
Carrot	13.4
Cucumber	13.3
Pepper	9.1
Pumpkin	6.8
Eggplant	5.8

Because of their high-energy content from carbohydrates (starch), tubers (potato, cassava, and sweet potato) are the most cultivated vegetables in the world.

VEGETABLES OF THE WORLD

Botanical Family	Food	Vol./Page	Description and Use
AMARANTHACEAE This family comprises approximately 800 species of herbaceous and shrub-like plants found in temperate and tropical regions. **Amaranthus:** Genus that includes 60 species. Twelve of these are cultivated for their **leaves** that are eaten as greens, or for their **seeds** (see Vol. 1, p. 77).	**AMARANTH** *Amaranthus tricolor*		**Syn.** *Chinese spinach, Callaloo, Amaranthus spinach.* The **leaves** of these and other species of amaranthus form a group of the **most nutritious** vegetables in the tropical regions of America, Africa, and Asia. They are a good source of **protein, folates, vitamin C, calcium, iron, and potassium.** Their composition and preparation are similar to **spinach.**
ARACEAE This family comprises approximately 1,500 herbaceous tropical or subtropical plants. Many of these have thick, edible **tubers** or **leaves.**	**TARO** *Colocasia esculenta*		**Syn.** *Tarro, Tara, Tarrow, Dasheen.* This is a **staple** of the lower classes in the humid tropical regions of Central America, Southeast Asia, and Oceania The **tubers** of this plant are similar in appearance and food value to the **potato.** They are prepared (cooked, roasted or fried) in the same way. Taro **leaves** are very high in nutrients, more, in fact, than the tubers. They are possibly the **most nutritious** leafy **vegetables** known They contain an abundance of **protein** (5%), **provitamin A** (483 μg RE/100 g), **vitamins B, C, and E,** and **minerals.** A troublesome aspect of taro is that it contains a great deal of **calcium oxalate** that is irritating to the digestive system. By cooking the leaves or the tubers and changing the water several times, most of the oxalate is removed.
	MALANGA *Xanthosoma sagitifolium*		**Syn.** *Tannia, Cocoyam, Yautia.* These are grown in the same areas as taro. However they require less moisture. Only the **cooked tubers** of these plants are eaten.
BORAGINACEAE This botanical family contains approximately 1,500 species of plants that usually consist of stalks and leaves covered with rough hair-like structures. They produce **mucilage.**	**BORAGE** *Borago officinalis*	2/358 *EMP 746*	**Sudorific, diuretic,** and **blood depurant.**
CHENOPODIACEAE Consists of some 1,400 species of herbaceous plants from coastal or temperate saline soils. They have a drawback: they produce **oxalates.**	**CHARD** *Beta vulgaris*	2/297	**Digestive aid, diuretic,** and **depurant.** *Recommended for treatment of* **obesity.**
	RED BEET *Beta vulgaris*	2/122	**Antianemic, anticholesterol,** and **anticarcinogenic.**
	MARSH SAMPHIRE *Salicornia europaea*		**Syn.** *Glasswort, Samphire, Sea salicornia.* These herbaceous leafless plants grow wild on the coasts of Northern Europe. Their tender **stalks** are eaten either raw or cooked slowly. Their flavor is similar to seaweed.
	SPINACH *Spinacia oleracea*	2/28	*Protects the* **retina** *and reduces* **cholesterol.**

Taro

EMP = *Encyclopedia of Medicinal Plants,* EDUCATION AND HEALTH LIBRARY, Editorial Safeliz.

VOLUME 1 / **104**

COMPOSITAE

This is the **most important family** of all **dicotyledonous** plants. It contains more than 1,000 genera and more than 20,000 species. It is characterized by flowers that are composed of the fusion of up to thousands of florets, as is the case of the sunflower.

The plants in this family represent a wide variety of vegetables: **leafy** (chicory, lettuce), **stalk** (cardoon), **flower** (artichoke), **tuber** (Jerusalem artichoke).

Cardoon

Artichokes

CONVOLVULACEAE

This family includes some 1,600 species of tropical and subtropical plants. The Latin name of this family refers to the form in which their stalks grow, which is twisted, rather than straight. (Convolvere = convoluted in Latin).

Botanical Family / Food	Vol./Page	Description and Use
SEA ASTER *Aster tripolium*		This **wild** plant grows along the coasts of Northern Europe and Asia. Its **leaves** are narrow and fleshy and are used as a vegetable.
ENDIVE *Cichorium endivia*	2/176	Aids **digestion** and **gall bladder** function.
BELGIAN ENDIVE *Cichorium intybus*	2/175	Used as an appetizer, aids **gall bladder** function.
RADICCHIO *Cichorium intybus*	2/176	*Syn. Red-leaf chicory.* This is an **endive** with similar properties as the others but with red leaves.
CHICORY *Cichorium intybus*	2/176 EMP 440	There are a number of varieties of wild and cultivated chicory such as leaf chicory or catalonga These benefit **liver function.**
CARDOON *Cynara cardunculus*	2/177	Useful for those suffering from **liver dysfunction** or **diabetes.**
ARTICHOKE *Cynara scolymus*	2/178 EMP 387	Detoxifies the **liver, antidiabetic, and** lowers **cholesterol.**
JERUSALEM ARTICHOKE *Helianthus tuberosus*	2/300	Aids with **diabetes** and **gout.**
LETTUCE *Lactuca sativa*	2/45	Aid to **sleep** and **digestion.**
SCORZONERA *Scorzonera hispanica*		*Syn. Black salsify, Black oyster-plant, Viper-grass.* This plant is cultivated for its **roots** in Belgium, France, and Holland. Historically it has been used for medicinal purposes only. It is cylindrical and about 30 to 40 cm long. It is cooked in a variety of ways and has a flavor reminiscent of walnut. It is rich in **protein** and **carbohydrates.**
SALSIFY *Tragopogon pratensis*	EMP 243	*Syn. Oyster plant, Vegetable oyster.* Similar to black salsify but with a shorter, more branched root. It is diuretic, sudorific, and depurant. It is recommended for **arteriosclerosis, hypertension,** and **gout.** Diabetics will also find it useful.
JICAMA *Exogonium bracteatum*		*Syn. Mexican potato, Yam bean.* This tuber is similar to the sweet potato, but less sweet. It is grown in Mexico and California. It is eaten raw in salads, or cooked like a potato. Its composition is similar to that of the **potato** but with a lower nutrient content. It is **very rich** in **fiber** (4.9%).
SWEET POTATO *Ipomoea batatas*	2/301	Produces a sensation of satiety and helps with **weight loss.**

EMP = Encyclopedia of Medicinal Plants, Education and Health Library, Editorial Safeliz.

VEGETABLES OF THE WORLD – *continued*

Botanical Family	Food	Vol./Page	Description and Use
CRUCIFERAE This important family of herbaceous plants contains some 380 genera and some 3,000 species grown in temperate or cold regions of the Northern Hemisphere. The morphological characteristic that identifies them is that their flowers have four petals arranged in the form of a cross. The importance of this family is in the fact that sulfurated (containing sulfur) anticarcinogenic **phytochemicals** have been discovered in their **roots** and **leaves.** Plants of the family *Cruciferae* are considered some of the **most effective anticarcinogens** whether eaten raw or cooked.	**CABBAGE** *Brassica oleracea*	2/191 *EMP 433*	Serves as a healing agent for the **skin** and gastroduodenal **ulcers.** Prevents osteoporosis due to its rich **calcium** content. **Anticarcinogen.** Varieties of cabbage such as Savoy cabbage, red cabbage, and white cabbage are described in Vol. 2, pp. 192, 193.
	BRUSSELS SPROUTS *Brassica oleracea*	2/192	This cabbage has **the highest levels of *carbohydrates* and *protein.*** It is also rich in *vitamins* and *minerals.*
	CAULIFLOWER *Brassica oleracea*	2/154	This is the **most digestible** of the cabbages. **Anticarcinogen.**
	KOHLRABI *Brassica oleracea*	2/193	The **bulbs** as well as the **leaves** of this plant are eaten. They are rich in *minerals* (particularly *magnesium*) and *vitamins.*
	BROCCOLI *Brassica oleracea*	2/63	Ideal for those with **heart disease. Anticarcinogen.**
	ROMANESCA CAULIFLOWER *Brassica oleracea*	2/155	This is a variant cauliflower, yellow-green in color.
	CHINESE CABBAGE *Brassica pekinensis*	2/193	This cabbage is the **lowest** in **calories** of any. It can be eaten raw in salads or cooked.
	TURNIP *Brassica rapa*	2/320	**Turnip greens** (leaves) are the **richest** of all greens in **calcium.**
	SCURVY GRASS *Cochlearia officinalis*	EMP 356	*Syn.* Spoonwort. This plant grows **wild** along the coasts of Northern Europe. Its fresh **leaves** and **stalks** are eaten in salads. It is an **aperitif, depurative,** and, due to its high **vitamin C** content, it combats scurvy.
	ARUGULA *Eruca sativa*		*Syn.* Rocket, Rugula, Rucola. The **leaves,** which are similar to those of the radish, are eaten in salads because of their delicate flavor. They are **digestive** and **diuretic.** They are grown around the Mediterranean, the Near East, India, and Brazil.
	WATERCRESS *Nasturtium officinalis*	2/132 *EMP 270*	Blood **purifier, invigorating, and expectorant.**
	RADISH *Raphanus sativus*	2/181 *EMP 393*	Regenerates the **liver,** combats **sinusitis** and **bronchitis.**

Broccoli

Turnip

EMP = Encyclopedia of Medicinal Plants, EDUCATION AND HEALTH LIBRARY, Editorial Safeliz.

VEGETABLES OF THE WORLD – continued

Botanical Family	Food	Vol./Page	Description and Use
CUCURBITACEAE Comprised of some 850 species of climbing or ground-crawling plants, virtually all of which are herbaceous. They usually produce large fruit that is protected by a hard rind. Some are used as **fruit** (melon, watermelon, etc. see Vol. 1, p. 44). Others described here are used as **vegetables**.	**CUCUMBER** *Cucumis sativus*	2/339	**Moisturizes** the skin, **depurative**, and **aids in weight loss**.
	SQUASH *Cucurbita pepo*	2/97 EMP 605	*Protects* the **arteries** by combating **hypertension** and **arteriosclerosis**. Helps avoid **acid** stomach and **constipation**.
	ZUCCHINI *Cucurbita pepo*	2/159	Recommended in cases of **indigestion** and **cardiovascular disease**.
	SQUASH BLOSSOMS *Cucurbita pepo*	2/100	**Syn.** *Pumpkin flowers.* Rich in **provitamin A** and **antioxidant flavonoids**. Helps prevent **arteriosclerosis** and **cancer**.
	BOTTLE GOURD *Lagenaria siceraria*		**Syn.** *Calabash gourd.* This is grown in tropical and sub-tropical regions of America and Asia. It is similar to the zucchini and is always eaten cooked.
	LUFFA *Luffa acutangula*		**Syn.** *Angled loofah, Ridged loofah, Silk gourd.* This is grown in India and the Caribbean islands. It is similar to the cucumber, although longer, with ten longitudinal veins. It is eaten either raw or cooked.
	SPONGE GOURD *Luffa cylindrica*		**Syn.** *Angle luffa, Chinese okra, Loofah, Vegetable sponge.* This is like the luffa but without veins and bitter taste.
	BITTER MELON *Momordica charantia*		**Syn.** *Bitter gourd, Balsam pear.* These are grown in India, Southeast Asia, and the Caribbean. The fruit is like a long cucumber with a type of 'warts' and grooves on the rind. It is very bitter when raw; thus it is eaten boiled, generally with rice. The **leaves** are also eaten as a vegetable. Studies indicate that the bitter substance in this melon is **toxic to the liver**.[15] It should be eaten **cooked** and in **very moderate** amounts.
	CHAYOTE *Sechium edule*		**Syn.** *Vegetable pear, Mirliton, Buddha's hand, Christophene.* This is grown in Southern Mexico and Central America. Although it is pear-shaped, it is similar to the zucchini. It contains **very few calories** (24 kcal/100 g) and some vitamins and minerals particularly **iron** (0.4 mg/100 g). It is a **diuretic**, facilitating proper **kidney** function. It is also of value in **weight-loss** diets. It is eaten cooked.
CYPERACEAE Herbaceous plants that grow in wet, swampy areas all over the world. They are monocotyledons like the *Gramineae*, with which they are related.	**TIGER NUT** *Cyperus esculentus*	2/160	**Syn.** *Chufa, Earth Almond.* This small **tuber** is rich in **nutrients** and digestive **enzymes**. It is used to prepare a refreshing and nutritious beverage: **Tiger nut horchata**.
	CHINESE WATER-CHESTNUT *Eleocharis dulcis*	2/323	This small **tuber** is grown in China. It is quite nutritious and somewhat astringent.
DIOSCOREACEAE This family consists of some 600 tropical species and receives its name from Dioscorides, the famous Greek physician and botanist from the 1st century of the Christian era.	**YAM** *Dioscorea alata*	2/101	Lowers **triglyceride** levels and helps prevent **arteriosclerosis**.
	SWEET YAM *Dioscorea trifida*		**Syn.** *Cush-cush yam, Indian yam.* Similar to the yam but with better flavor. They are grown in the Caribbean.

Cucumber

Chayote

EMP = *Encyclopedia of Medicinal Plants*, EDUCATION AND HEALTH LIBRARY, Editorial Safeliz.

Botanical Family	Food	Vol./Page	Description and Use
EUPHORBIACEAE This family is comprises more than 7,000 species spread throughout the warmer regions of the entire world. Some are used as **fruit** (see Vol. 1, p 45). They produce **alkaloids** and other **toxins.**	**CASSAVA** *Manihot esculenta*	EMP 460	**Scientific syn.** *Manihot utilissima.* **Syn.** *Yuca, Manioc.* This is the **tuber** of a bush that is grown in tropical regions of America, Africa, and Asia. It is eaten cooked like potatoes, and constitutes a **staple** in the diets of many in the Third World. It is **very rich** in **carbohydrates** (25.3%), **B vitamins, vitamin C** (48.2 mg/100 g), **magnesium, potassium, iron,** and **calcium.** It does not contain provitamin A or vitamin B₁₂, and contains very little fat. It has **anti-thyroid** effects (slows thyroid function).[16] *Caution:* The tubers and **raw leaves** of the cassava are **toxic** due to the prussic acid that they contain. **They must be washed** in water and **boiled** or **dried** before they are edible.[17]
	SWEET CASSAVA *Manihot dulcis*		This species of cassava does not produce prussic acid and may be eaten raw without further processing. **Tapioca** is the **flour** obtained from the tubers of both species of cassava. It can be cooked with milk or vegetable broth. It contains 88% **carbohydrates (starch)** and **very little protein** or **fat.** It is very easily **digested** and **rich** in **calories.** It is particularly beneficial is cases of: • **Digestive disorders:** Tapioca flour retains a great deal of water due to its **mucilage** (soluble fiber) content and it is an **excellent emollient** (softener) and protector of the digestive lining. It is recommended in cases of excess stomach acid, gastritis, gastro-duodenal ulcer, and all types of colitis. • **Celiac disease:** Contains no gluten. • **Liver disease:** Tapioca provides easily assimilated carbohydrates and virtually no fat or protein. This facilitates liver function. • **Convalescence** from serious disease or surgery and reinitiating solid foods after a period of fasting. *Tapioca*
GRAMINEAE This botanical family contains more than 10,000 species, among which are the grains (see Vol. 1, p. 76).	**BAMBOO SHOOTS** *Phyllostachys pubescens*		The tender shoots of the bamboo plant are harvested much in the same way as asparagus. They are approximately 30 cm in length. They contain protein (2.6%), vitamins B, C, and E (but not provitamin A) and minerals, above all **potassium.** *Caution:* **Raw** bamboo shoots are **toxic** due to their prussic acid content. **Soaking** and, above all, **cooking** eliminate the toxin.
	SUGARCANE *Saccharum officinarum*	EMP 332	**Syn.** Noblecane, White sugar. **Molasses** (see Vol. 1, p. 174) and **cane sugar** (Vol. 1, p. 174) are obtained from sugarcane. Chewing the fresh cane releases a sweet, pleasant juice that is rich in mineral salts. *Sugarcane*
LABIATAE This family comprises some 3,000 species, mostly herbaceous, among which are many **aromatic** and **medicinal** herbs such as rosemary, lavender, and thyme.	**CHINESE ARTICHOKE** *Stachys sieboldii*	2/180	These are caterpillar-shaped **tubers** with a flavor similar to black salsify. They are grown in China and Japan.
LAURACEAE This contains a group of woody plants used for their **essence** that grow in warm regions. Laurel, camphor, and cinnamon belong to this family. The only specie that provides edible fruit is the avocado.	**AVOCADO** *Persea americana*	2/108 EMP 719	Avocados are rich in **protein, fats, vitamins B₆** and **E,** and **iron.** Their use reduces **cholesterol.** Although avocados are considered fruits botanically, from a culinary point of view they are used as vegetables in salads, cremes, soups, etcetera.

EMP= Encyclopedia of Medicinal Plants, EDUCATION AND HEALTH LIBRARY, Editorial Safeliz.

VEGETABLES OF THE WORLD – *continued*

Botanical Family	Food	Vol./Page	Description and Use
LEGUMINOSAE This family includes herbaceous and woody plants and trees spread throughout the world. Most are cultivated for their seeds, called **legumes** (see Vol. 1, p. 78). The **pods** and **seeds** of these four legumes are used for human consumption. *Garden pea*	**GREEN BEAN** *Phaseolus vulgaris*	*EMP 584*	*Syn. String bean, Fresh bean, Snap bean.* These are the tender **pods** that cover the fruit of this plant. They are harvested before they develop their interior seeds (beans). They are **diuretic**, invigorate the **heart**, and reduce the blood glucose level. *Caution:* These should **not** be eaten **raw.** They contain a **toxin,** known as phaseolin, which disintegrates with **cooking.**
	PEA *Pisum sativum*	2/73	Useful in cases of **coronary disease** and **nervous system** disorders.
	SNOW PEA *Pisum sativum*	2/74	This is a pea whose fleshy pod is eaten as well.
	FAVA BEAN *Vicia faba*	2/137	Fava beans are *rich* in **iron** and, as a result, are **antianemic.**
LILIACEAE This family contains about 3,500 herbaceous plants and trees. **Allium:** is the most important genus of this family from a dietary standpoint. Many of its species form **bulbs** (underground enlargements of the stalk) and all of them are rich in sulfurated **essential oils,** which are very volatile and piquant. Thanks to these substances, plants from the genus *Allium* lower **cholesterol** and act as **anticarcinogens.** *Welsh onion*	**SHALLOT** *Allium ascalonicum*		*Syn. White shallot.* This is the **mildest and most delicate** of all the onions. Its composition and properties are very similar to those of the common onion.
	ONION *Allium cepa*	2/142 *EMP 294*	Loosens **bronchial mucus** and facilitates its **expectoration.** Prevents **arteriosclerosis** and **cancer.**
	WELSH ONION *Allium fistulosum*	2/144	This falls between the **onion** and the **leek,** tenderer than the common onion, but with all of its properties.
	LEEK *Allium porrum*	2/319	Leeks are **diuretic, alkalizing,** and **laxative.**
	GARLIC *Allium sativum*	*EMP 230*	**Antibiotic,** lowers **cholesterol,** increases **blood** fluidity, **anticarcinogenic.**
	CHIVE *Allium schoenoprasum*		The stalks and cylindrical leaves of chives share the properties of the **onion,** but with a delicate flavor. They are used **fresh** as a healthful **condiment.** Dried they lose almost their entire aroma. Chives are rich in **provitamin A, folates, vitamin C,** and **iron.**
	BEAR'S GARLIC *Allium ursinum*	*EMP 233*	These grow **wild** in the north of Europe and Asia. It is similar to the **garlic** in terms of composition and properties. Its **fresh stalks and leaves** (they lose their aroma when dried) are used as a condiment.
	ASPARAGUS *Asparagus officinalis*	2/250 *EMP 649*	Asparagus stimulates **kidney** function; it is a **depurative** and **detoxifier.**
MALVACEAE This family consists of 900 herbaceous plants and bushes. They produce abundant **mucilage,** which acts as an emollient (softener), making them very viscous when cooked. They contain no toxic substances.	**OKRA** *Hibiscus esculentus*	2/200	The **mucilage** released by cooking okra softens the mucosa of the digestive tract and the throat.
MARANTACEAE This family contains some 360 species of herbaceous tropical plants. Their **rhizomes and roots** are rich in **starch.**	**ARROWROOT** *Maranta arundinacea*		*Syn. Maranta.* A very **starch rich flour** (84.8%) is made from the **rhizomes** of this plant from the Antilles. However it is low in **protein** (0.3%) and **vitamins.** Its starch grains are very fine and easily digested. They are used in the Antilles islands in case of **diarrhea,** and to feed the feeble and children. However, its lack of protein makes it inappropriate as an **infant food.**

EMP = Encyclopedia of Medicinal Plants, EDUCATION AND HEALTH LIBRARY, Editorial Safeliz.

VEGETABLES OF THE WORLD – continued

Botanical Family	Food	Vol./Page	Description and Use
MORINGACEAE This family contains only one genus and four species of trees found in Eastern Africa and Southeast Asia.			
	BENOIL TREE *Moringa oleifera*		**Syn.** Drumstick, Moringa nut. All parts of this Afro-Asiatic tree are used due to their high nutritional value. Its elongated **fruit** is **very rich** in **vitamin C** (141 mg/100 g) and is used as a vegetable. The **leaves** are **very rich in proteins** (9.4%), **provitamin A, B vitamins**, and **minerals**, especially magnesium (147 mg/100 g) and iron (4 mg/100 g). They are used extensively in the Philippines as a green due to their excellent nutritional value.[18] The **seeds** are eaten roasted. **Oil** is extracted from them, as well. The **root** is used as a condiment.
OXALIDACEAE This family is composed of around 900 species of herbaceous plants and small trees that produce **oxalic acid** (see Vol. 1, p. 103) in their green parts (leaves).			
	LUCKY CLOVER *Oxalis tetraphylla*		**Syn.** Goodluckplant. This plant, originally from Mexico, is cultivated in Europe for its turnip-shaped **roots** and tart tasting **leaves.**
	OCA *Oxalis tuberosa*		**Syn.** Occa, Ulluco. This herbaceous plant is grown in South America for its **tubers,** which are similar in flavor and nutritional value to the **potato.**
PALMAE Most of the food species of this family are raised for their **fruit.** However, at least two species are grown for their terminal **shoots,** which are used as a vegetable.			
	DWARF PALM *Chamaerops humilis*		These white, **tender shoots** are from a small palm that grows in the Mediterranean area. They are invigorating and somewhat astringent.
	HEART OF PALM *Euterpe edulis*		**Syn.** Swamp cabbage. Hearts of palm are the terminal shoots of a palm found in the American tropics. This white, soft delicacy is **not ecologically sound,** since their harvest causes the death of the palm (hence the name **'heart of palm').** One to two trees of about ten years of age are required to harvest one kilogram of heart of palm. They contain relatively high levels of **protein** (2.5%), **iron** (3.13 mg/100 g), **calcium, magnesium,** and **fiber** (2.4%).
POLYGONACEAE Some 800 species of generally herbaceous plants from around the world are included in this family. Buckwheat (see Vol. 2, p. 102) belongs to this family. Some of the *Polygonaceae* produce **oxalic acid** (see Vol. 1, p. 103) as do Oxalidaceae.			
	RHUBARB *Rheum officinale*	EMP 529	**Syn.** Pieplant, Chinese rhubarb. The **peduncles** (bases of the leaves) of these plants are a valued green in the cooler regions of North America and Europe, particularly Switzerland, where they are eaten as if they were asparagus. They are aperitif, digestive, laxative, and promote drainage of the gallbladder. The **root** is used as a **laxative** medicinal plant. Caution: Rhubarb **leaves** and **roots** contain a great deal of **oxalic acid** (see Vol. 2, p. 103). Discard **cooking water** to eliminate excess amounts of this acid.
	SORREL *Rumex acetosa*	EMP 275	**Syn.** [Sour] dock, Sour grass. This plant grows **wild** in the cooler regions of North America and Europe, although it is **cultivated** on a small scale. Its very pleasant, slightly tart leaves are used in salads and soups. Sorrel is **very rich** in **provitamin A** (400 mg RE/100 g), **vitamin C** (48 mg/100 g), **potassium, magnesium,** and **iron.** Caution: Sorrel should be eaten in **moderation,** because of its high **oxalic** acid content.

Rhubarb

EMP = *Encyclopedia of Medicinal Plants,* EDUCATION AND HEALTH LIBRARY, Editorial Safeliz.

VEGETABLES OF THE WORLD – *continued*

Botanical Family	Food	Vol./Page	Description and Use
PORTULACACEAE Consists of some 300 species of herbaceous or bushy plants found on the American continent. Many have fleshly **leaves** that are rich in **mucilage**.	**WINTER PURSLANE** *Montia perfoliata*		Its **leaves** are eaten in salads or cooked much in the same way as spinach. It is **very rich in vitamin C.**
	PURSLANE *Portulaca oleracea*	*EMP 518*	**Syn.** *Cuban spinach, Miner's lettuce.* The fleshly and slightly tart **leaves** of this wild plant are used in salads or cooked much in the same way as **spinach.** Purslane is raised as a crop in France and Belgium. It is a good source of **Provitamin A** (132 mg RE/100 g), **vitamins, B, C** and **minerals**, especially **iron** (2 mg/100 g). It is **laxative, emollient, depurative,** and **antioxidant.** It has been recently discovered that purslane is a good source of essential polyunsaturated fatty acids **omega-3** (some 300 mg/100 g), which protect against **cardiovascular** disease and **cancer.**[19]
SOLANACEAE **The great majority** of the 2,000 species found in this family of American plants are **poisonous,** such as tobacco, belladonna, Jimson weed, or henbane. Only very few Solanaceae have any part sufficiently free of toxic alkaloids to be eaten. In spite of this, Solanaceae have achieved great relevance in the human diet: the tomato, the pepper, and the potato seem **indispensable vegetables** to us today, even though they were unknown outside the Americas before the 16th century. See more Solanaceae in Vol. 1, p. 51.	**PEPPER** *Capsicum annuum*	2/198 *EMP 354*	**Aperitif** and **digestive. Very rich** in **antioxidant vitamins,** particularly **C.**
	TOMATO *Solanum lycopersicum*	2/275	Protects the **prostate,** *enhances* the **immune system, anticarcinogen.**
	EGGPLANT *Solanum melongena*	2/256	*Stimulates the filtering action of the* **kidneys,** *aids* **digestion.**
	POTATO *Solanum tuberosum*	2/201	**Almost complete** and **balanced** food. *Neutralizes excess stomach* **acid.**
UMBELLIFERAE Only about 70 of the 3,000 species of this family are of agricultural interest. They are easy to recognize by these characteristics: • Their **inflorescence** (groups of flowers) is arranged in **umbel,** which means that all of their peduncles (stalks) rise from the same site. • Some produce aromatic **essences** (for example anise or angelica), and others **alkaloids** (for example, hemlock). • Many of them have thick **bulbs** or **tubers** that are used as food. *Caution:* **Hemlock** *is a toxic* Umbelliferae *that* **can be confused** *with* **parsley, celery,** *or* **carrots** (*see EMP p. 155*).	**CELERY** *Apium graveolens*	2/248 *EMP 562*	**Blood** *depurant and reduces* **cholesterol.**
	PERUVIAN PARSNIP *Arracacia xanthorrhiza*		This is the **root** of a plant from Peru that is *similar* to **celery.** It is cultivated in Central America. It has a pleasant aroma and is rich in **starch.** It is cooked in various manners. Because it is **easy to digest** and *rich* in **calories,** it is appropriate for **children** and **convalescents.**
	TURNIP-ROOTED CHERVIL *Chaerophyllum bulbosum*		This **tuber,** grown in Northern Europe, has a very pleasant flavor and is **rich** in **minerals.** It can be baked or cooked as if it were a **potato.** There are other species of chervil, whose leaves are used as condiments.
	CARROT *Daucus carota*	2/25 *EMP 133*	Protects the **retina,** *enhances the* **skin, anticarcinogen.**
	FENNEL *Foeniculum vulgare*	2/161 *EMP 360*	**Syn.** *Florence, Finocchio, Sweet anise.* *Aids* **digestion** *and helps fight* **constipation.**
	PARSNIP *Pastinaca sativa*		This is a **root** similar to the **turnip** with a slightly piquant flavor. It is *rich* in **fiber** (4.9%), and **minerals,** particularly **potassium.** It is grown in Europe and North America; however, it is being replaced by potatoes and carrots in many of the dishes in which they were previously used.
VALERIANACEAE This family consists of about 350 species found in Europe and America. Among them is **valerian,** which is noted for its sedative properties (see *EMP* p. 172).	**LAMB'S LETTUCE** *Valerianella locusta*	2/136	This is a green with a delicate flavor that is rich in **provitamin A, vitamins B, C,** and **iron. antianemic.**

Celery

EMP = Encyclopedia of Medicinal Plants, EDUCATION AND HEALTH LIBRARY, Editorial Safeliz.

7

OILS AND MARGARINE

OILS and margarine are two types of *fats* of **vegetable** origin that are used to make foods tastier.

In reality, the custom of adding fats to foods is rather superfluous, since **all foods, *except* vegetables**, already contain a certain amount of *fat*.

Although they are ***not* indispensable** from a strictly nutritional point of view, oils and margarine are a desirable addition that makes foods more appetizing and flavorful. They also possess in themselves some nutritional value.

Oils

Source of Oils

Oils are *fats found within the cells of seeds and of some fruits*. These fats are in tiny globules in the cells called vacuoles.

When the cell walls of the fruits or seeds are broken through the grinding process, the oil globules are released, forming oil. Thanks to various methods of physical and/or chemical processing, the oil is isolated from the remaining material that forms the fruit or seed.

Seeds

All seeds contain a certain amount of oil, but the most used are the following:

- **Legumes:** soy, peanut.
- **Grains:** the **germ** of corn and wheat.
- **Nuts:** walnuts, almonds, hazelnuts, coconut.
- **Other seeds:** sunflower, grape, sesame.

Continued on page 114

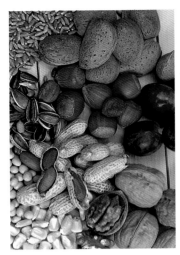

Oils are in reality extracts of certain seeds or fruits. Their nutritional value, particularly in the case of refined oils, is only a portion of the value found in the complete seed or fruit.

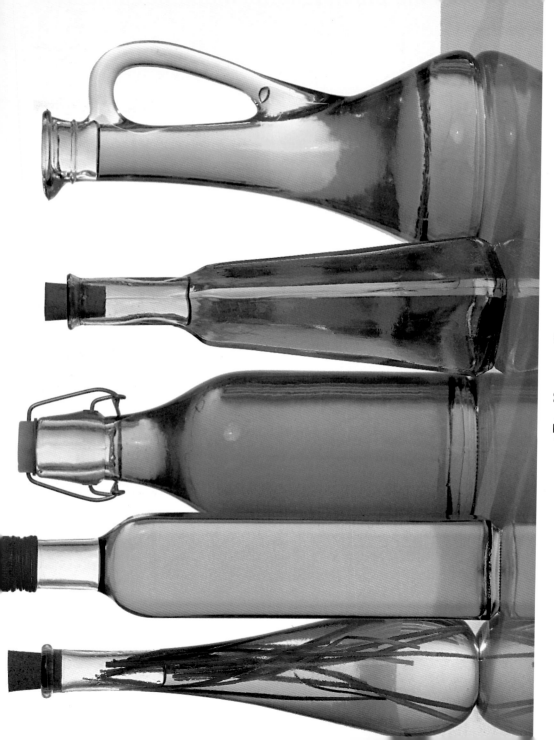

The King of Oils

Olive oil is considered the king of oils for its flavor as well as its medicinal properties (see Vol. 1, p. 119).

Thanks to its high levels in monounsaturated fatty acids, such as oleic, olive oil protects against the most harmful effects of excess cholesterol in the blood: arteriosclerosis[2]. When this affects the coronary arteries that supply the heart muscle, the feared myocardial infarction or heart attack occurs.

For this reason olive oil is considered the most heart-healthy of all vegetable oils.

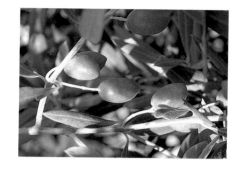

Oils and Margarine

- **Oils:** Fats from **vegetable** sources that are **liquid** at room temperature. They are produced from seeds such as soy, or from fruits such as the olive.

- **Margarine:** Fat that is solid at room temperature and similar in appearance to dairy butter. It is produced primarily from vegetable oils (corn and soy).

1. Extraction

Extracting oil requires the **breaking** of vegetable cells through **milling**, and later **isolating** the fatty portion (oil) from the other components of the seed or fruit.

- **Milling:** This is done using rollers or grinders to create a homogeneous paste.

- **Pressing:** The oil contained in the paste is squeezed out using mechanical pressure. This can be done **cold** or **hot** (see the Informational chart on the next page).

- **Extraction with solvent:** The paste residue left after pressing still contains 10% to 20% oil, which the industry is loath to discard. The following processes are are used to recover this oil:

  – The paste is treated with *solvents* (ethylene chloride, hexane) that wash out the residual oil.

  – *Removal of the solvents:* The solvents evaporate when the residual oil is heated, leaving pure oil. Both **ethylene chloride** and **hexane** are *extremely toxic.* They must be totally eliminated from the oil. Theoretically, the heating process accomplishes this, but in practice some vestiges of solvent may remain. Additionally, **the heating process destroys** the *vitamins* and other active substances that might remain in the oil.

2. Refining

Impurities and substances that produce **undesirable flavors** to the oil develop as a consequence of the physical and chemical processes of pressing, heating, and treating with solvents. The most important of these are free fatty acids, which, when present in a proportion higher than 2% (2° acidity), they give the oil a very strong unpleasant flavor.

The stronger the extraction using pressing and heat, the more free fatty acids the resultant oil contains, and the greater need for refinement to eliminate them.

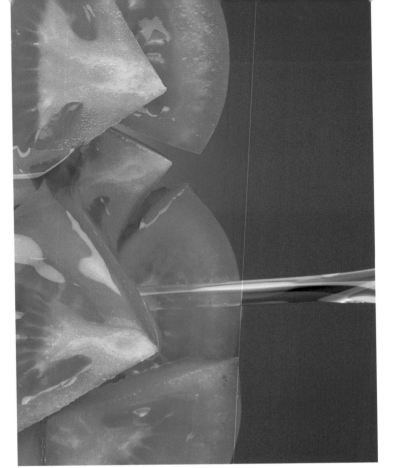

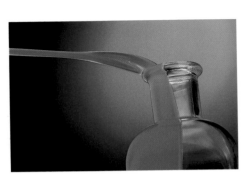

An oil's acidity is measured as a percentage of free fatty acids that it contains. The best quality virgin olive oil, shown above, has a maximum acidity of 0.2%, or 0.2°.

There is nothing healthier and more delicious than preparing salads and vegetables with a generous amount of virgin olive oil.

Continued from page 112

Fruits

Only a *few* fruits contain enough oil in their fleshy portion (mesocarp) to allow extraction: **olive, oil palm,** and **avocado.** The latter is used very little due to its high cost and strong flavor.

Production of Oils From Seeds

The following steps are followed during the industrial production of oils from seeds:

Hot and Cold Pressing

*The paste that is produced by milling the seeds or fruit is pressed to squeeze out the oil. This may be done either hot or cold and the difference is **very important** from a nutritional standpoint.*

- *Hot pressing: The paste is heated before pressing. **More oil is obtained** by this method, but a significant **portion of the vitamins and phytos-terols** contained in the oil is **destroyed**.*

- *Cold pressing: The paste is pressed at room temperature, yielding a **lesser amount** of oil, but **richer** in unsaponifiable substances (see Vol. 1, p.116). These substances are the non-fatty components of the oil, such **vitamins and phytosterols**, which give it its flavor and many of its med-icinal properties.*

*Cold-pressed oils do not require the same level of refining as hot-pressed oils. Cold-pressed oils lose fewer vitamins and phytosterols and are rich-er in active ingredients. For this reason cold-pressed oils are **recom-mended** for therapeutic diets.*

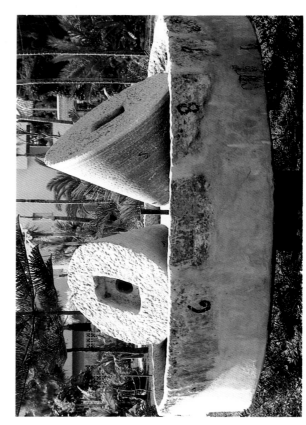

Complex processes of extraction and refining convert olive oil in-to a purified fatty substance. It stores very well, but it is insipid and does not have healing power. On the other hand, cold-pressed, unrefined (virgin olive oil), such as the one extracted with this old mill, is true seed or fruit juice, which contains vitamins, phytosterols, lecithin, and other medically active ingredients.

Refining the oil produces the following changes:

- The **acid level is reduced** through the elimination of free fatty acids.

- **Flavor is lost**, making them more mild and neutral.

- **Reduction in the amount** of unsaponifi-able (nonfat soluble) substances (*vita-mins, phytosterols* and others, see Vol. 1, p. 116). These substances give the oil part of its aroma and medicinal properties.

Refining is a rather complex process whose objective is the elimination of every-thing other than fat, leaving, basically, triglycerides (pure fat). The refining process consists of the following steps:

- **Clarification** using citric or phosphoric acid. This eliminates carbohydrates, pro-teins, resins, and phospholipids (lecithin), which are industrially consid-ered "impurities". It is precisely these "impurities" that contain a large portion of the oil's medicinal properties. The sediment that is formed by these sub-stances is precipitated from the oil and processed commercially as *lecithin.*

- **Neutralization** to eliminate the free fatty acids responsible for the acidity of the oil. This is done by adding caustic soda, which forms soaps from the free fatty acids, which are then eliminated by cen-trifugation.

- **Purification** using clay or charcoal to fil-ter out carotenoids, minerals such as iron and copper, and any other natural substances that the oil may contain.

3. Solidifying

Hydrogen and a metallic catalyst are ap-plied to oils rich in polyunsaturated fats to make them less fluid and to increase their stability and resistance to becoming rancid. The *great disadvantage* of this process is the formation of **trans fatty acids.**

Vitamin E and Phytosterol Content of Various Oils

Oil	Vitamin E mg α-TE/100 g	Phytosterols mg/100 g
Wheat germ	192.4	553
Sunflower	50.6	100
Safflower	43.1	444
Cottonseed	38.3	324
Corn (germ)	21.1	968
Soy	18.2	250
Peanut	12.9	207
Olive	12.4	221
Sesame	4.1	865

Refined oils retain some quantity of non-fat soluble substances, such as **vitamin E** and **phytosterols**. Olive oil is the one that loses the most of these substances in the refining process.

The Composition of Oils

Triglycerides

These are the most common type of fat found in nature. They form the virtual total weight of oils and margarines, both made from triglycerides.

Each triglyceride **molecule** is formed by:

- *one* molecule of *glycerin* or *glycerol*, and
- *three fatty acid* molecules.

The triglycerides of all oils may be differentiated by the types of fatty acids that they contain. There are *three types of fatty acids*: **saturated, monounsaturated and polyunsaturated**, depending on whether their molecule contains no double or triple bonds, just one of them, or more than one. The monounsaturated and polyunsaturated fatty acids are called together **unsaturated**.

The *more unsaturated fatty acids* found in the composition of an oil, it will be:

- *more **fluid*** at room temperature;
- more reactive, in other words, *less* **stable** and more susceptible to become rancid;
- *more* **effective in lowering cholesterol levels** and a better protector against **arteriosclerosis.**

Unsaponifiable substances

These are substances other than fats, which although found in very small quantities in oils, are **very important**, since they provide:

- flavor and aroma
- vitamin and mineral content
- medicinal properties.

Taken together they represent between 1% and 2% of the weight of unrefined oils. Substances in oil that are not triglycerides are defined as unsaponifiable.

The refining process has as its specific objective, the elimination of most of these substances that are considered *industrially* as **impurities**, even though some of them are of *great value in therapeutic diets*. The most important unsaponifiable substances are:

- *Free fatty acids:* These do not rise above 1% in cold-pressed extra virgin olive oil. Processed oils may have as much as 5%, which necessitates refining to eliminate these fatty acids since they give the oil a very strong flavor.

- *Volatile substances* such as hydrocarbons and long-chain alcohols: More than 70 distinct compounds have been identified. These are responsible for the aroma and flavor of the oil, together with the free fatty acids.

- *Vitamin E:* This is present in almost all vegetable oils, but it is most abundant in **wheat germ** and **sunflower seed oils.** It is a *powerful antioxidant.*

- *Provitamin A:* Unrefined oils contain small amounts of **beta-carotene** and other *carotenoids* that are transformed into vitamin A in the body (see Vol. 1, p. 389)

- *Phytosterols:* These are substances similar to cholesterol, but of vegetable origin. The *most important* of these is called *sitosterol.* They *inhibit* the *absorption of cholesterol* in the intestine. Each milligram of sitosterol, found in foods, avoids the absorption of one milligram of cholesterol.[1]

- *Lecithin:* This is only present in unrefined oils, particularly soybean oil (see Vol. 1, p. 89). It *protects* the **liver** and the **nervous system.**

CHOLESTEROL IN OILS

Minute quantities of cholesterol are found in vegetable oils. In the case of olive oil this is about 0.3 mg/100 g.

These cholesterol levels are **nutritionally insignificant,** and in no way affect the beneficial effect of vegetable oils on blood cholesterol level.

Nutritional Value of Oils

Oils, broadly speaking, only provide significant amounts of two types of nutrients:

- **Simple fats**, which are formed by different fatty acids linked with glycerin (triglycerides). Some, such as linoleic acid, are considered essential, since the body cannot synthesize them. Oils in general, and seed oils in particular, are good sources of these essential fatty acids that we **must eat every day.**

- **Vitamin E.**

Since one gram of oil contains about 9 calories (=9 kcal), the caloric value of oils is very high (884 kcal/100 g).

Oils **lack:**
- protein,
- carbohydrates,
- minerals (except virgin olive oil, which contains iron), and
- fiber.

Oils, like all fats, **contribute to the transport** of liposoluble vitamins (A, D, E, and K) and **promote** their **absorption.**

- *Minerals:* Virgin olive oil (unrefined) is the only oil with an appreciable amount of iron (0.38 mg/100 g).

Drawbacks to Oils

Unbalanced food

As with flour, oils are **extracts** containing only part of the original seed or fruit. This extraction breaks down the natural equilibrium of the nutrients, as they exist in the natural food source. Therefore, they **are not a balanced food,** something that must be kept in mind when using them. Their *only* **nutrients** are *fats* and *vitamin E.*

The nutritional imbalance of oils *worsens* when they are **refined,** since these process remove most of the non-fatty substances found in the oil.

Carriers of toxic substances

Organic phosphate insecticides, such as DDT (now prohibited in many countries), and the many other pesticides used in intensive agriculture are **liposoluble;** in other words, they are soluble in fats such as oil.

If the chemical treatments applied to oil-bearing seed or fruit crops have not been properly done, the oil produced will contain significant amounts of toxic pesticides.

Organic farming *avoids* this problem. Unfortunately, there are very few oils made from seeds or fruit that have not been treated with pesticides.

They are easily adulterated

Oils, particularly olive oil, lend them themselves quite easily to adulteration. The *most common* type of fraud is **mixing** with some other type of cheaper oil, with the accompanying loss of dietary and nutritional value.

In other cases, the fraud consists in selling oil designated for industrial use as if it were for human consumption. This fraudulent oil is processed with various chemicals to hide its origin. This may lead to massive poisonings, such as what happened in Spain in the 1980s.

Antinutritive factors

Undesirable antinutritional factors can form in oils from seeds rich in polyunsaturated fatty acids, under certain circumstances:

- *Peroxides:* These are formed as a reaction between the polyunsaturated fatty acids and the oxygen in the air. The oil becomes rancid and loses its nutritional value. Contact with air, light, heat, or metals such as iron or copper promote peroxidation, which is *more prone to happen in* **seed oils.** Peroxides act as *free radicals, destroying vitamin E and promoting* **arteriosclerosis.** It is possible to avoid the formation of peroxides by:

  – adding **antioxidants,**

  – storing the oil in **tightly closed** containers protected from light and heat,

  – **using caution when frying with oils** (see Vol. 1, p. 122).

- *Trans-fatty acids:* These are formed when oils are hydrogenated to make them more solid. Their greatest drawback is that they *promote* **arteriosclerosis.**

Continued on page 120

POISONING FROM ADULTERATED OILS

Rapeseed oil that is for industrial use is marked as such with a dye. In Spain in the 1980s a group of swindlers processed some of this oil with chemicals to remove the dye. The resulting oil was sold as olive oil.

A chemical reaction unforeseen to the swindlers caused the formation of toxic substances when they processed the industrial rapeseed oil. The result was a massive poisoning of the Spanish population resulting in 2,000 deaths and 20,000 persons left with disabilities.

Olive Oil:

Advantages of Olive oil Over Seed Oils

- **Ideal composition:** Main nutrients found in olive oil are:
  - triglycerides formed from glycerin and various fatty acids,
  - vitamin E: 12.4 mg α-TE/100 g and
  - iron: 0.38 mg/100 g

  Its distribution of fatty acids, with monounsaturated **oleic acid** prevailing, *comes the closest to the optimum according to the American Heart Association,* as can be seen in the graphs following graphs.

- **Better flavor:** The aroma and flavor of olive oil are more pronounced than those of seed oils, which are quite insipid. Although some persons are not used to the flavor of olive oil and prefer other oils with a neutral flavor, very few do not come to appreciate the *bouquet* of an excellent virgin olive oil.

- **More natural:** Its production process is simpler and more natural than that of seed oils. Virgin olive oil is **not refined** nor is it processed with **solvents**, as most seed oils are. Additionally, olive oil does not contain **trans-fatty acids.**

- **More stable:** Since it contains fewer **polyunsaturated fatty acids,** it is more stable than seed oils. It lasts longer before becoming rancid and producing dangerous **peroxides** (see Vol. 1, p. 117).

- **Better for frying:** Resists **higher temperatures without decomposing.** For this reason, it is appropriate for frying.

- **Greater medical value:** A black legend has been about for quite some time in certain Anglo-Saxon regions suggesting that olive oil raises blood cholesterol.
  Fortunately, **studies** regarding the Mediterranean diet *have demonstrated* that olive oil **protects the heart** *more* than any other, thus leading, on the whole, to the cardiac benefits of the Mediterranean diet.

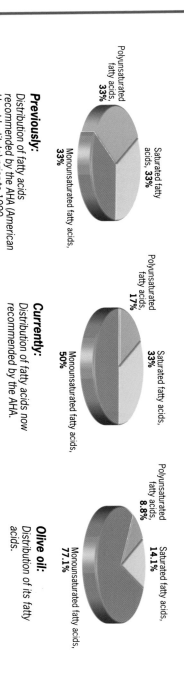

Previously:
Distribution of fatty acids recommended by the AHA (American Heart Institute) prior to 1990.

Polyunsaturated fatty acids, **33%**
Monounsaturated fatty acids, **33%**
Saturated fatty acids, **33%**

Currently:
Distribution of fatty acids now recommended by the AHA.

Polyunsaturated fatty acids, **17%**
Monounsaturated fatty acids, **50%**
Saturated fatty acids, **33%**

Olive oil:
Distribution of its fatty acids.

Polyunsaturated fatty acids, **8.8%**
Monounsaturated fatty acids, **77.1%**
Saturated fatty acids, **14.1%**

As can be seen, olive oil's composition comes the closest of any to meeting the recommendations for the prevention of heart disease.

Proportional Distribution of Different Types of Fatty Acids

*With the objective of preventing cardiac disease (angina and myocardial infarction), the American Heart Association (AHA)[2] recommends that **fats represent no more than 30%** of dietary calories. This percentage is less than that of the average Western diet, which averages 40% of its calories from fats.*

For a 2,000 calorie diet, the 30% is 600 calories; these are obtained from 67 g of fats (65 g to facilitate calculations). Until the 1990s, the AHA recommended that these 67 grams of fats should be distributed in equal portions among saturated, monounsaturated and polyunsaturated.

However, in light of the latest studies, which highlight the importance of monounsaturated fatty acids, the AHA has modified the percentage distribution of the different fatty acids.

*Now the AHA says that rather than one third, fully **one half** of the daily intake of **fatty acids** should be **monounsaturated.** Olive oil and avocado are the healthier source of oleic acid, the main **monounsaturated** fatty acid of diet. These AHA recommendations coincide with those of the WHO (World Health Organization).[3]*

the Ideal Formula

Olive oil is superior to seed oils as much for its dietary therapeutic properties, as for its flavor and aroma.

Medicinal Effects of Olive Oil

- **It promotes heart health.** Regular consumption of olive oil *protects* against coronary disease **(angina and myocardial infarction)**.

  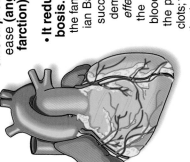

  - **It reduces the threat of thrombosis.** In a study in South Africa by the famous cardiac surgeon Christian Barnard, the first to perform a successful heart transplant, demonstrated that olive oil is *as effective* as fish oils in *reducing* the level of **fibrinogen** in the blood.[4] This protein substance is the primary component of blood clots; the higher its level, the greater the threat of **thrombosis** (formation of clots).

- **It controls cholesterol level.** It is true that olive oil does not reduce total cholesterol levels as much as seed oils. In reality, it does very little to reduce harmful LDL cholesterol and total cholesterol. It does, however, raise HDL (beneficial cholesterol) levels.[5]

  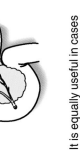

  Olive oil

  This does not mean, however, that olive oil is less beneficial than seed oils, as was once thought. The use of olive oil provides *greater protection* against **arteriosclerosis** and **coronary disease** (angina and infarction) than *any other* oil, because it inhibits the oxidation of lipoproteins.

- **It inhibits the oxidation of lipoproteins.** It is known that the oxidation of low-density lipoproteins (a type of fat that circulates through the blood and contains a great deal of cholesterol), known by the initials LDL, is the *main* mechanism in the production of **arteriosclerosis.**

Numerous studies have demonstrated that *monounsaturated* fatty acids, such as oleic acid from olive oil, are more effective than *polyunsaturated* fatty acids in inhibiting oxidation of lipoproteins.[6,7]

In other words, **olive oil** is *more effective* than those of **seeds** in the prevention of arteriosclerosis, even though seed oils reduce cholesterol levels to a greater degree.[8,9,10]

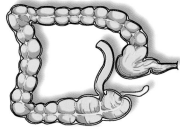

- **It reduces the risk of breast cancer.** Investigators from the Spanish National School of Health (Escuela Nacional de Sanidad, Madrid, Spain) were the first to propose that olive oil reduces the risk of breast cancer.[11] Another joint study by the University of Athens (Greece) and Harvard University (USA),[12] confirmed that an increase in olive oil consumption (more than once a day) lowered risk of breast cancer by 25% to 35%. On the other hand, the use of **margarine** is associated with a *higher* **risk** of this disease.

  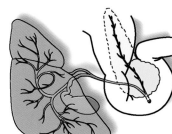

- **It protects the liver.** Olive oil promotes liver function and is *particularly* useful in case of some types of **hepatic insufficiency** due to hepatitis, cirrhosis or toxins from medications or from other sources. This has been confirmed experimentally with laboratory animals.[13]

It is equally useful in cases of **gallbladder** disorder due to its cholagogue effect (it aids drainage of the bile).

- **It helps avoid constipation.** It serves as *a mild, effective* laxative, particularly when it is taken on an empty stomach (one to two tablespoons are sufficient).

  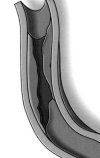

Olestra: Oil "Without Fat"

After 25 years of scientific investigations and discussions the FDA (Food and Drug Administration) of the United States approved the use of **Olestra** in 1996 as a substitute for oil and other dietary fats. At present its use is limited to potato chips and other snack foods.

Olestra is a special type of oil that passes unabsorbed through the digestive tract. It is the realization of a dream of an opulent society: the ability to eat fatty and flavorful foods without the risk of weight gain. However, Olestra has drawbacks, as well, that must be taken into account.

Chemically, Olestra is a polymer of esters of sucrose and fatty acids. It is produced through a complex industrial chemical process, using common **sugar** or sucrose and edible **seed oils**.

Advantages

• *Its appearance is identical to oil:* Its flavor and texture are indistinguishable from any refined oil.

• *It is appropriate for frying and cooking:* It is stable at high temperatures, allowing excellent quality cuisine.

• *The body does not absorb it:* Our digestive tract lacks the enzymes to hydrolyze and digest Olestra molecules. As a result, this type of oil is eliminated through the feces without passing through the blood. Because of this,
– It provides no calories.
– When it is used to replace other oils, it produces a minor reduction in blood cholesterol level.

Drawbacks to Olestra

• It may produce minor **digestive disorders**, such as flatulence, intestinal pain and involuntary fecal emission.

• Causes the **elimination of provitamin A** (beta-carotene and other carotenoids), and **vitamins A and E**, which Olestra dissolves and removes through the feces. In the United States legislation demands that products containing Olestra be fortified with these vitamins because of this.

Time will tell if the benefits of Olestra truly outweigh its drawbacks.

Continued from page 117

Types of Olive Oil

Virgin Olive Oil

This is produced by grinding olives to a paste, then cold-pressing them to squeeze out the oil. Virgin olive oil is **not refined**. *Only* **physical processes** are used to remove suspended solid particles and leave the oil transparent: sedimentation, centrifugation, and/or filtration.

The *fewer* free **fatty acids** the oil contains, depending on the characteristics of the fruit, the *higher* the **quality and delicacy** of its flavor:

• **Extra:** Acidity lower than one degree (1% of free fatty acids). Its flavor and aroma are fruity, very delicate and exquisite.

• **Fine:** The same as *extra* but may have 1.5° acidity.

• **Ordinary:** May contain up to 3° acidity.

• **Industrial:** Contains more than 3° acidity. It is not edible due to its strong taste, and it must be refined.

Refined Olive Oil

Oil that contains high levels of free fatty acids, due to the use of hot pressing in its production, or that has come from low quality fruit, must be refined to make it edible. After refining,

• its acidity does not reach 0.2% (0.2°), resulting in almost no flavor;

• it is very pale in color;

• contains almost no vitamins, phytosterols or substances responsible for aroma (see Vol. 1, p. 116).

Pure Olive Oil

Pure olive oil, or simply **olive oil**, is produced by mixing virgin olive oil with refined olive oil, whose acidity cannot exceed 1° (1%). It is an intermediate between the first two types of oil, and is *the most common* in the market.

Oil From Olive Residue

This is produced by applying a solvent, generally hexane, to the residue left after pressing. It is of *low quality*, and must be refined to reduce its acidity to a maximum of 0.3°.

The more refined an oil is, the lighter its color. Virgin olive oil typically has a yellow-green hue.

Margarine

Margarine is an **emulsion of fat and water, solid at room temperature**, with the following characteristics:

- Its fat is derived *primarily* from **vegetable oils** that have been treated industrially to make them denser. On occasion, **animal fats**, such as slaughterhouse waste or fish oil, may *also* be used.
- Its **fat** content must be *above* 80% although **light margarine** may contain less than **70%** fat.

Production Process

Margarine is a very artificial food, in the sense that its production requires a number of industrial processes:

1. **Selection of oils:** Those most used are from soy and corn, followed by palm, peanut, cottonseed and others. These seed oils are produced by hot pressing, solvents, and later refining.

2. **Hydrogenation:** To convert the oil into a thick semisolid, it is heated to about 200°C (392°F) and is injected with hydrogen in the presence of nickel catalysts. In this way part of the unsaturated fatty acids are converted into:

   – saturated fatty acids and
   – *trans* fatty acids.

   Both types of fatty acids are dense at room temperature. They also generate more cholesterol in the body.

3. **Additives:** Antioxidants, synthetic vitamins, yellow dyes, flavorings and emulsifiers are then added with a certain amount of water to the hydrogenated paste.

A Broad Debate

Even though margarine is commercially represented as a healthful food and "without cholesterol" (this is the primary argument in its favor), it is *inferior* to oil in **nutritional value and in dietary therapeutic properties.**

There is an ongoing, broad debate among scientists concerning whether or not margarine is *preferable* to dairy **butter.** In reality, each has its advantages and disadvantages. *Neither of these two* foods is truly **appropriate** for a healthful diet.

Even though margarine is a vegetable-based food, that does not necessarily mean it is healthful.

The industrial processing of seeds to obtain refined oil inevitably results in the loss of nutritional and therapeutic properties. However, converting this oil into margarine lowers levels even more.

Margarine and Butter Compared

	Margarine	Butter
NATURAL FOOD	No	Yes
TOTAL FAT CONTENT	70%-80%	81%
PERCENTAGE OF SATURATED FAT	15%	50.5%
ESSENTIAL POLYUNSATURATED FATTY ACIDS	25%	3%
TRANS FATTY ACIDS	20%-30%	4%-5%
CHOLESTEROL	0	219 mg/100 g
VITAMIN OR PROVITAMIN A	799 µg RE/100 g	754 µg RE/100 g
VITAMIN E	12.8 mg α-TE/100 g	1.58 mg α-TE/100 g
RELATION TO HEART DISEASE	For some, consumption of **trans-fatty acids**, which is present in large quantities in margarine, does **not** increase coronary risk.[14] According to the American Heart Association, **margarine**, especially **light** margarine is **preferable** to butter.[15,16]	For other investigators, such as Doctor Willett, of Harvard University, the animal fat in butter is not as harmful as once thought. On the other hand, consumption of foods rich in **trans-fatty** acids (margarine, bakery goods) are, indeed, associated with greater risk of coronary disease[17, 22] and breast cancer.[12]

Fried Foods:

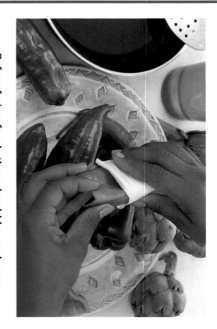

Before frying foods they should be as dry as possible, since water hastens the decomposition of the oil.

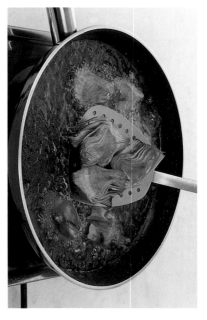

All oils decompose during the frying process, but olive oil is the slowest to be affected. As a result it is the best oil for this process.

Changes Created by the Frying Process

Frying is a complex process from a physicochemical[18] standpoint, in which changes take place in the oil as well as in the food:

• **Changes in the oil:** *all are negative* and lead to the formation of undesirable substances:

– **Saturation of fatty acids:** unsaturated fatty acids are converted to saturated fats (like animal fat), thus *losing their* **beneficial properties,** *particularly that of* **lowering** cholesterol.

– **Formation of peroxides and hydroperoxides:** These are derived from fatty acids and act as free radicals, which promote **arteriosclerosis.**

– **Formation of** *trans***-fatty acid,** which *raises* **cholesterol** levels.

– **Formation of free fatty acids** through hydrolysis of triglycerides, that give the oil a disagreeable flavor.

– **Formation of volatile** *irritants,* such as acrolein, various hydrocarbons, ketones, and alcohols.

• **Changes in the food:**

– **Evaporation of** the food's **water** content.

– The food becomes **saturated** with the oil from 5% to 40% of its total weight. Fried potatoes contain roughly 40% oil.

– **A crust is formed** consisting of coagulated proteins and caramelized carbohydrates. This crust provides a pleasing flavor and texture but lacks nutritional value.

Recommendations for Frying Foods

• Use **olive oil:** It is the *most appropriate* for frying because:

– It **remains** *stable* at the higher **temperatures** (160° to 200°C = 320° to 392°F) used in frying.

– It is *more stable than seed oils,* and **it decomposes** *slower.*

– It **saturates foods** *less* than seed oils.

• **Avoid overheating:** Frying must be done at the lowest possible temperature. Under no conditions should the temperature be above 170°C (338°F). If one is using an electric fryer the thermostat should be set at a low to medium temperature. Oil is overheated when:

– it smokes and/or

– turns dark in color.

• **Avoid introducing water:** Foods to be fried should be *as dry as possible,* since water promotes hydrolysis and decomposition of the oil.

• **Filtering:** This should be done *each time the oil is used* to remove food particles that remain floating in it. These particles promote oxidation and decomposition of the oil.

• **Change oil frequently:** Oil should *not* be used *more than two or three times,* especially if it has been heated to the smoking point.

• **Do not fry meat or meat products:** This produces carcinogenic substances.

Tasty But Dangerous

Carcinogenic Substances in Fried Foods

The incidence of lung cancer is quite high among Chinese women, even among those that do not smoke. This fact aroused the interest of the National Cancer Institutes of the United States, whose specialists collaborated in epidemiological studies trying to discover the causative factors of these tumors.

The results were unmistakable: The **smoke** of fried foods that the Chinese women inhaled in the kitchen contains **carcinogens.**[19]

The oils most used in China are soy and grapeseed, which are very polyunsaturated, and, as a result, decompose easily. Add to this the custom of heating the oil to a very high degree, 240° to 280°C (464° to 536°F). All of this contributes to the formation of many toxic substances, some of which are carcinogenic.

Fried Meat and Its Smoke

The smoke of fried foods is not the only carcinogen involved. Certain fried foods, such as meats, contain **mutagens** that *promote* the development of **malignant tumors.** This has been demonstrated experimentally in laboratory animals,[20] and epidemiologically in various studies:

- The Social Security Institute of Finland conducted a follow-up review of all cancer cases presented over a 24-year period.[21] One of the most noteworthy conclusions of this study is that the consumption of **fried meat** is related to increased *risk* of suffering from the following types of tumors in females:

  – breast cancer,
  – endometrial cancer,
  – ovarian cancer.

- The Department of Environmental Toxicology at the University of California (USA) has analyzed the **smoke** produced by frying certain foods.[23]

  – **Meats and meat products:** The **smoke** from these foods is *highly mutagenic* (promotes cancerous mutations in the cells), and contains *elevated levels of heterocyclic amines* (intensely carcinogenic substances).

  – **Vegetables:** Their smoke produces **no mutagens.**

  Curiously, not all smoke from meats has the same mutagenic properties. **Pork** (*bacon*) is eight times more mutagenic that that of **beef.**

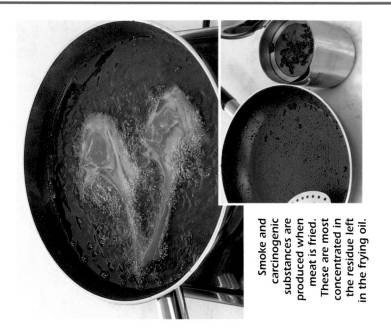

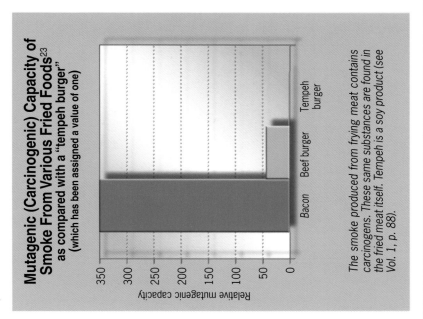

Smoke and carcinogenic substances are produced when meat is fried. These are most concentrated in the residue left in the frying oil.

Mutagenic (Carcinogenic) Capacity of Smoke From Various Fried Foods[23] as compared with a "tempeh burger" (which has been assigned a value of one)

Relative mutagenic capacity

350 300 250 200 150 100 50 0

Bacon   Beef burger   Tempeh burger

The smoke produced from frying meat contains carcinogens. These same substances are found in the fried meat itself. Tempeh is a soy product (see Vol. 1, p. 88).

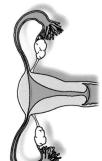

Women that regularly eat fried meat are at greater risk for breast, uterine, and ovarian cancers.[21]

OILS OF THE WORLD

Oil	Plant Part	Uses	Benefits	Drawbacks
PEANUT *Arachis hypogea* 32 g · 16.9 g · 46.2 g	Seeds	Raw. Frying, due to its stability Processing sauces and **margarine.**	*Following only olive and rapeseed oils,* this is the *richest in monounsaturated* **oleic acid,** thus it is quite **stable** for frying and is **heart healthy.** Provides **vitamin E** (12.9 mg α-TE/100 g) and phytosterols (270 mg/100 g). Its flavor is somewhat sweet and pleasant.	Virtually all peanut oil available commercially has been **refined.** It becomes cloudy at low temperatures.
CANOLA OR RAPESEED *Brassica campestris* and other species of this genus, which also contains the turnip and the cabbage 7.1 g · 29.6 g · 58.9 g	Seeds	Raw. In sauces and **margarine.**	This oil contains the *fewest* **saturated fatty acids** of any, and one of the *richest* in monounsaturated **oleic acid,** which protects against **arteriosclerosis.** Together with walnut oil (see Vol. 1, p. 126), it is the richest in **linoleic acid omega-3** (9.3%). A genetically selected variation of rapeseed called **CANOLA** has been developed in Canada that does **not** contain toxic **erucic acid.**	This oil comes from the common rapeseed plant contains a long-chain fatty acid known as **erucic acid** that is toxic to the coronary system. The **refining** process **eliminates** virtually all of it. Canola oil contains no erucic acid. It must be **refined** before it can be consumed. It has almost no taste. Canola oil has a very bad reputation in Spain, due to the massive poisoning from the consumption of canola oil destined for industrial uses (see Vol. 1, p. 117).
SAFFLOWER *Carthamus tinctorius* 9.1 g · 12.1 g · 74.5 g	Seeds	Raw, in Salad dressings. Processed, in sauces and **margarine.**	Its composition is similar to that of **olive oil,** but with somewhat more linoleic acid and less saturated fatty acids. This oil contains one of the lowest levels of **saturated fats,** second only to canola oil. It is the richest in the **essential fatty linoleic acid.** Only wheat germ and sunflower oil contain more **vitamin E** (43.1 mg α-TE/100 g). It provides a significant amount of **phytosterols** (444 mg/100 g), which combat cholesterol. It is of value in cases of: **prostate hypertrophy** (due to its high linoleic acid content), in **cholesterol** reduction diets, as a **laxative,** and **rheumatic disease.**	It must always be **refined.** It becomes rancid very easily, and must be **protected from contact with the air.** It contains little monounsaturated oleic acid with its cardiac safeguarding action.
COCONUT *Cocos nucifera* 1.8 g · 5.8 g · 86.5 g	The white pulp from the inside of the seed, known as **Copra.**	Sauces, **margarine** and frying.	It is very **stable** at high temperatures. Its high content of medium-chain saturated fatty acids, such as lauric, myristic, and palmitic, makes it easily **digestible,** and *highly recommended for* **pancreatic and intestinal disease.**	Coconut oil contains the most **saturated fats** of all vegetable oils, resulting in a semisolid oil at room temperature. In spite of its elevated saturated fatty acid content, it **does not increase cholesterol** levels as much as one might expect if these were of animal origin (see Vol. 2, p. 325).

OILS OF THE WORLD – *continued*

Oil	Plant Part	Uses	Benefits	Drawbacks
PALM *Elaeis guineensis* 9.3 g 49.3 g 37 g	Pulp: produces an orange-colored oil. Seed: produces a pale yellow oil.	In the food industry in **margarine,** sauces, and industrial baked goods.	Unrefined palm oil contains beta-carotene (provitamin A), but this almost completely disappears during the refining process.	This vegetable oil or fat (it solidifies easily) is second only to coconut oil in **saturated fatty acids.** Those with elevated **cholesterol** levels should **avoid** its regular use.
SOYBEAN *Glycine max* 14.4 g 23.3 g 57.9 g	Seeds	Raw. Processed in margarine and sauces. Bakery products and cookies.	It contains, above all, **polyunsaturated fatty acids,** that reduce cholesterol level. It is one of the oils, together with canola and wheat germ (see Vol. 1, pp. 124, 127), richest in **linolenic acid** (6.8 g /100 g), a polyunsaturated fatty acid of the **omega-3** type, similar to that found in fish oil. It is recommended in cases of elevated **cholesterol** and those at risk for **thrombosis, arteriosclerosis, and coronary disease.**	As is the case with all seed oils, soy oil is **extracted with solvents** (see Vol. 1, p. 114). Since it is always used **refined**, it has lost its lecithin and other non-fat soluble components. Its flavor is quite insipid, which for some, is an advantage.
COTTONSEED *Gossypian hirsutum (American cotton); G. barbadense (Egyptian cotton); G. arboreum (Asian cotton) and other similar species*	Seeds, after they are separated from their textile fibers.	Cottonseed oil is the one least similar to **olive oil** in terms of its composition and appearance. Until recently, it was only used in chemical processes and as a fuel. Present-day refining techniques have made it edible. Raw as salad dressing. Processed, in **margarine** and ice cream.	This is a good source of essential **polyunsaturated fatty acids,** such as linoleic acid. It is a very good source of **vitamin E** (38.3 mg α-TE/100 g): two tablespoons of cottonseed oil (30 g) contain about 10 mg α-TE, an amount that meets the RDA (Recommended Dietary Allowance).	Raw cottonseed oil contains a toxic yellow pigment called **gosipol,** which gives it a strong sharp taste. This pigment is removed thanks only to modern chemical refining techniques, thus making this oil fit for consumption. Due to the intensity of the refining process, cottonseed oil is virtually colorless, odorless, and tasteless. It is one of the oils with the lowest levels of **monounsaturated fatty acids,** such as oleic (which safeguards the cardiovascular system).
SUNFLOWER *Helianthus annuus* 25.9 g 17.8 g 51.9 g 10.3 g 19.5 g 65.7 g	Seeds	Raw. For cooking and frying. Processed for sauces and **margarine.**	This oil contains very few **saturated fatty acids.** It is second only to safflower oil in **linoleic acid,** an essential polyunsaturated fatty acid that lowers **cholesterol** level. It follows only wheat germ oil in **vitamin E** content (50.6 mg α-TE/100 g): one tablespoon of sunflower seed oil provides the RDA. This oil is of great value in diets of **coronary disease victims,** due to its high vitamin E content and its beneficial effect on **cholesterol** levels.	Most commercial sunflower oil has been extracted using **solvents** and **refined.** It contains *little* monounsaturated **oleic acid,** which safeguards the cardiovascular system.

OILS OF THE WORLD – continued

Oil	Plant Part	Uses	Benefits	Drawbacks
WALNUT *Juglans regia*	Seeds	Raw, as a salad dressing.	This oil is produced through cold pressing and needs no refinement. Walnut oil is the *richest of any in linoleic acid* (10.4%), an **omega-3** type polyunsaturated fatty acid similar that found in fish oil. It safeguards the **cardiovascular system** by reducing **LDL** (harmful **cholesterol**) and increasing **HDL** (beneficial **cholesterol**). It also lowers the **triglyceride level** (a form of fat) in the blood, reducing the tendency of **platelets to aggregate** and form clots. It is a good source of **unsaturated fatty acids,** such a linoleic acid (polyunsaturated) and oleic acid (monounsaturated).	Walnut oil oxidizes and becomes rancid very easily.
OLIVE *Olea europaea*	Fruit (Olives)	Raw, as a salad dressing and for all vegetables. For cooking all types of dishes. For frying, because it is the most **stable** of all at high temperature.	This is *the most **aromatic** and **flavorful** of all oils.* It can be used without **refining** and a *minimum* of industrial **processing.** It is *the best oil for **frying.*** Although its use does not reduce cholesterol levels as much as seed oils, olive oil provides the most **protection** against **arteriosclerosis** and **coronary disease.** Olive oil, together with sesame oil, possesses the most **medicinal properties** of any (see Vol. 1, p. 119).	Its strong flavor may discourage some that are not accustomed to it.
POPPY *Papaver somniferum*	Seeds	Raw.	Poppy seed oil can be used unrefined. Even though the capsules or fruit of the poppy contains a latex from which opium is extracted, the seeds contain no alkaloids. This oil is *quite rich **in linoleic acid,*** which lowers cholesterol levels.	Its use is quite limited. It must always be use **unheated.**
SESAME *Sesamum indicum*	Seeds	Ideal raw as a salad dressing.	Together with olive oil, sesame oil is one of the few that can be used **unrefined.** Its **composition** is very **well balanced,** since it contains approximately the same proportion of oleic acid (safeguards the cardiovascular system) and linoleic acid (lowers cholesterol levels). Its aroma and flavor are quite pleasant. It is second only to corn oil (968 mg/ 100 g) in **phytosterols** (865 mg/100 g). It contains a natural **antioxidant,** known as **sesamol,** which makes it very **stable** and resistant to **oxidation.** It can be stored for several years **without turning rancid.** It is possibly the most effective of any oil in reducing **cholesterol** levels.	

OILS OF THE WORLD – *continued*

Oil	Plant Part	Uses	Benefits	Drawbacks
WHEAT GERM *Triticum aestivum*	The germ of the grain	Raw. In capsules and other pharmaceutical preparations.	Wheat germ oil contains the highest concentration of **vitamin E** (192.4 mg α-TE/100 g). One tablespoon (15 ml) contains three times the RDA for this potent **antioxidant.** The essential fatty acid, **linoleic acid,** is the *predominant* fatty acid in this oil, with its lowering effect on **cholesterol** levels. It is a *good source* of **linolenic acid** (6.9%), similar to soy (6.8%) but less than rapeseed (9.3%) and walnut (10.4%). This is an **omega-3** type fatty acid similar to that found in fish oils, and it is a *very effective* **safeguard** for the cardiovascular system. Wheat germ oil possesses preventive and *healing* properties involving **arteriosclerosis, thrombosis, and cardiovascular disease.**	Technically, it is difficult to extract wheat germ oil using a cold process; therefore most of what is available on the market is **refined.** This results in the expected loss of healing properties.
GRAPESEED *Vitis vinifera*	Seeds of the fruit	Raw. For frying.	Grapeseed oil has a very delicate and pleasant flavor. When used for **frying** it does *not produce* the irritant **acrolein,** although it is best not to heat it beyond 170°C (338°F). It is very rich in **linoleic acid,** an essential polyunsaturated fatty acid which reduces **cholesterol** levels.	This cannot be extracted cold and requires a certain level of refining.
CORN *Zea mays*	The grain, especially the germ	Raw, as a salad dressing and cooked in different dishes. It should not be used for **frying,** since it **decomposes** very easily. Processed, in **margarine.**	Its composition is *predominantly* **polyunsaturated** (linoleic acid) and monounsaturated (oleic acid) **fatty acids,** which reduce **cholesterol** levels. It is a *good source* of **vitamin E** (21.1 mg α-TE/100 g): One hundred grams provides more than double the RDA. It is one of the vegetable oils *richest* in **phytosterols,** particularly beta-sitosterol (see Vol. 1, p. 116), which prevent the absorption of **cholesterol** in the intestine.	Corn oil is quite unstable and decomposes easily at high temperatures. Only **refined** oil is available on the market.
PUMPKIN OR SQUASH (SEEDS)	Pumpkin or squash seeds (see Vol. 2, p. 99)	Raw to dress salads. As a nutritional supplement (2-3 teaspoons daily)	Rich in vitamin E, linoleic acid, zinc and iron. It soothes prostate and urinary bladder. It expels intestinal worms (take an spoon with empty stomach).	Not suitable for cooking, because it breaks down with heat. It must be used only raw.

Wheat germ: 61.7 g, 18.8 g, 15.1 g. Grapeseed: 69.9 g, 9.6 g, 16.1 g. Corn: 58.7 g, 12.7 g, 24.2 g. Pumpkin: 50 g, 14.6 g, 30.8 g.

TYPES OF FATTY ACIDS

saturated fatty acids *monounsaturated fatty acids* *polyunsaturated fatty acids*

NOTE: The pie charts represent the percentage distribution of different types of fatty acids in each oil. The values indicate the grams of fatty acid in 100 grams of oil.

8

SEAWEED

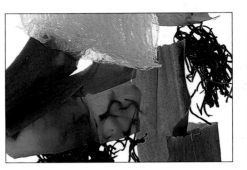

Seaweed is fairly uncommon as a food in the Western world. However, since more than three-fourths of our planet is covered with water, many scientists believe that seaweed might be a solution to the dietary needs of a large portion of humanity. In addition, some types of seaweed lend themselves very well to controlled cultivation.

LGAE form a wide variety of life forms that grow in salt and fresh water. Their size varies from a few thousandths of a millimeter (Spirulina), up to several meters (such as some Laminaria) or more. Most edible algae grow in the sea and are referred to as seaweed.

Algae derive nourishment from the simple elements found in the air and water. By means of sunlight they produce, first, glucose, then other carbohydrates, proteins, fats, and hundreds, perhaps thousands of other substances.

Algae are the most self-sufficient of all plants. They require no irrigation, fertilizers, or pesticides to thrive. They constitute, at least theoretically, an *almost unlim-*

ited **reserve** of **food** for fish and other aquatic creatures, as well as for humans willing to eat them.

Products Derived From Algae

In addition to being used directly as food, various algae become raw materials for use in the **food, pharmaceutical, and chemical industries.**

The cell walls of land vegetables are formed of cellulose and other substances indigestible for humans. However, marine vegetables or algae contain other types of indigestible material in their cellular walls. These are **gums** or **mucilage,** which are considered a special type of fiber in spite of their gelatinous appearance, so different

Continued on page 130

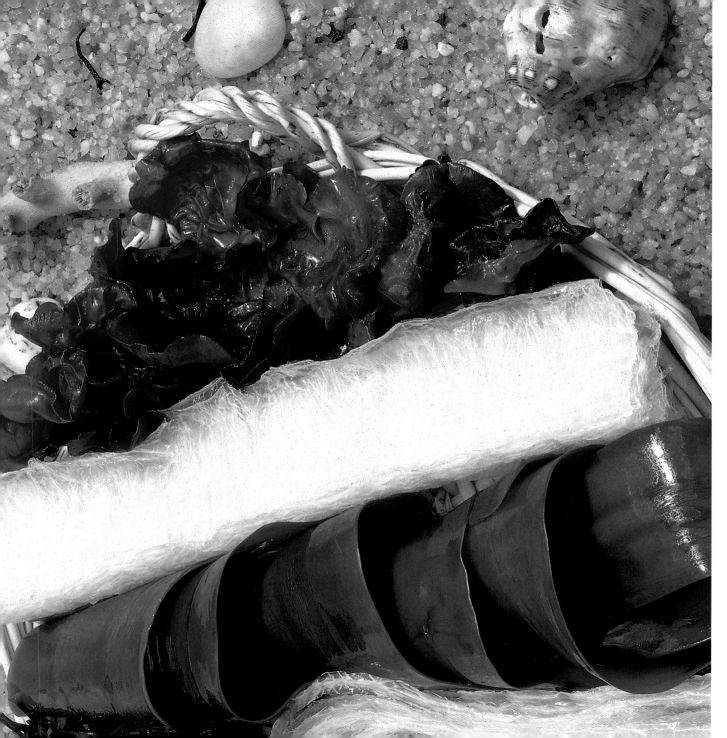

Seaweed
represents
a good source
of minerals,
particularly
iodine, calcium,
iron, and
magnesium.
It is also a source
of folates.

Seaweed and Algae

These are **aquatic plants** used as food. Most are **multicellular** (formed of many cells) and grow in the sea.

Others are **unicellular,** for example Spirulina, and grow in ponds and lakes.

The multicellular seaweeds do not possess roots, flowers or fruit, but only a vegetative body or **thallus** that is generally eaten cooked.

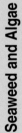

All algae contain chlorophyll, but this does not necessarily mean that they are all green. Some 'Rhodophyceae' that are commonly used in the diet, contain red or brown pigmentation.

Continued from page 128

from that of bran, for example. This is because the composition and properties of the *gums* found in algae are *similar* to those of *cellulose*.

The gums extracted from algae are widely used as additives in the food industry, as well as medications in the pharmaceutical industry.

- **As additives:** They give foods a smooth texture and are very effective **thickeners, emulsifiers,** and **coagulators.**

- **As medications:** Although they are composed of polysaccharides, which are indigestible, they perform an important physiological function. Because of their water retention and gel-forming characteristics, they increase the dietary bolus throughout the entire digestive tract. This produces:
  – a feeling of satiety in the stomach,
  – softer feces, making them easier to eliminate.

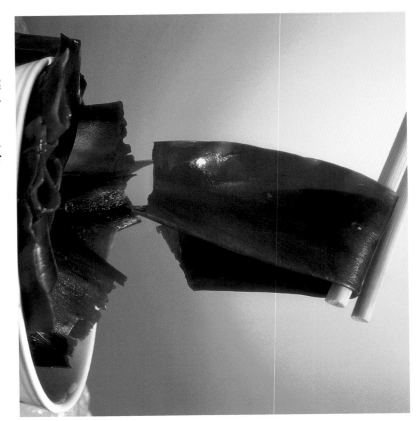

The **three** most important **types of *gums* or *mucilage*** derived from seaweed are agar-agar, alginates, and carrageenan.

Agar-agar

This is also called simply **agar**. It is a *vegetable gelatin* extracted from various seaweed species of red algae, particularly *Gelidium corneum*. This seaweed is collected during low tide along the coasts of Japan and Korea, although the best quality is "harvested" under water. Efforts have begun to "cultivate" agar seaweed along the Atlantic coast of Europe, particularly along the shores of Galicia in Spain.

- **Production:** First, the seaweed is boiled. The liquid that results is filtered, bleached, and dehydrated, converting it into a dry substance. When boiling water is added to dehydrated agar, it forms a compact, gelatinous mass when it has cooled, which is agar.

- **Composition:** Compared to animal gelatin, which is composed of incomplete proteins, agar or vegetable gelatin is a complex mixture of various substances of great dietary interest:

  – *Polysaccharides:* Carbohydrates derived from glucoronic acid, which make up 75% of the dry weight of agar.

  – *Minerals:* Agar is a *good source of magnesium* (67 mg/100 g) and *iron* (1.86 g/100 g). It also contains potassium, calcium, and iodine.

  – *Vitamins:* It is *rich in folates* (84.8 µg/100 g). It contains vitamin E (0.87 mg α-TE/100 g), but not provitamin A or vitamin C.

Alginate

These are generally sodium-based salts of alginic acid. This substance is an nonabsorbable polysaccharide, whose chemical formula is $[C_6H_8O_6]_n$. It is obtained from various brown algae from the genus *Laminaria*.

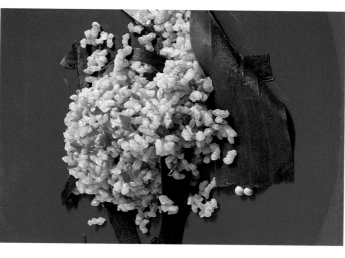

Seaweed cooked with rice is a typical Far Eastern dish, and one that may be enjoyed throughout the world. Both foods, seaweed and rice, complement each other in terms of nutritional value.

Both alginic acid and its salts alginates are used as natural **additives** in ice cream and various other desserts, because of their thickening, emulsifying, and coagulating properties.

Carrageenan

This is derived from a red alga called Irish moss (*Chondrus crispus*, see *EMP* p. 301), that grows along the northern coasts of Europe and America.

It gives a firm, yet smooth and creamy, consistency to foods. For this reason it is used as an **additive** in bakery products, pasta, dairy products, puddings, and jellies among others.

It is also used in syrups for lung congestion and coughs due to its **soothing** and **expectorant** properties.

Agar-agar: Advantages of Vegetable Gelatin

*Agar-agar, or simply agar, is a **healthful alternative to** animal gelatin (see Vol. 1, p. 317).*

- *It retains up to 8 to 10 times its weight in water.*

- *Its **gelling capacity** is 6 to 8 times that of animal gelatin. It forms a clear firm, tasteless, gelatinous mass that gives foods a soft texture without altering their flavor.*

- *It is an **effective thickener, emulsifier, and stabilizer,** which does not lose its characteristics with heat or other foods. It is very useful in thickening soups, stews and desserts (it must be added hot).*

- *It **contains no calories** (animal gelatin, however, does), and is slightly filling and laxative.*

- *In contrast to animal gelatin, it a **good source of folic acid**, minerals (**magnesium and iron**) and trace elements such as **iodine**.*

Seaweed:

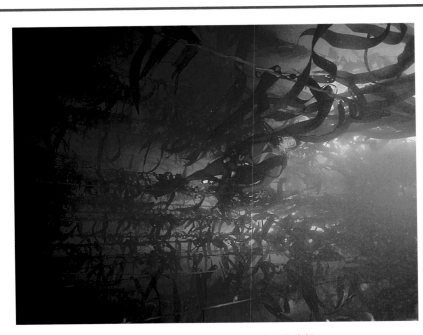

Seaweed highly concentrates the minerals found in the water that surrounds it.

For example, iodine concentrated in *Laminaria* ('kelp') represents 0.3%, 50,000 times more concentrated than in seawater, which contains only 0.000005% iodine.[2]

Seaweed Provides:

- **Carbohydrates:** Part of these are indigestible (gums and mucilage), and give seaweed satiating and laxative qualities.

- **Protein:** Fresh seaweed contains 1.68 mg/100 g, somewhat less than the potato. Most of this protein is of **low quality**. An exception is **Spirulina**, which, when dried, contains up to 70% **high quality** protein.

- **Sodium:** There is between 100 and 300 mg of sodium in 100 g of seaweed, which is quite high and comes close to the daily recommended maximum of 500 mg.

- **Calcium:** One-hundred grams of fresh *Laminaria* seaweed (kelp) contain 168 mg of calcium, considerably more than the 114 mg contained in 100 ml (approximately 100 g) of milk.

- **Iron:** Most fresh seaweed provides between 2.5 and 3 mg of iron per 100 grams. This is *equal to* or *greater than* that of **meat**.

- **Magnesium:** One hundred grams of fresh *Laminaria* seaweed *(kelp)* provides 121 mg of magnesium, which is more than *one-third* of the **daily requirement** of this mineral.

- **Iodine:** Seaweed is the *best source* of **iodine**. One hundred grams of dried *Laminaria* seaweed (kelp) provides 62,400 µg of iodine, about *one thousand times more than*

the adult daily requirement.[1] Fish, although a good source of iodine, only contains 150 to 350 µg/100 g.

- **Vitamins:** Seaweed contains **vitamins B₁, B₂, E, niacin,** and **folates;** the latter two are very abundant. Provitamin A and vitamin C are virtually absent.

- **Vitamin B₁₂:** Seaweed in and of themselves do not contain vitamin B₁₂. However, the bacteria accompanying certain algae species such as Spirulina, produce this vitamin in significant quantities. We now know that **bacteria** are in reality the ones that **synthesize** vitamin B₁₂ while **herbivores** merely **accumulate it** in the liver and other tissues. Unfortunately, only a small portion of the vitamin B₁₂ that accompanies Spirulina seaweed is used by the body.[3] In spite of this, seaweed must not be disregarded as a source of vitamin B₁₂.

Uses of Seaweed

- **Cooked:** It is usually boiled for 20 to 30 minutes, or added to rice or legumes just as any other vegetable. They may also be used in vegetable pastries, pizzas, and omelets.

  – **Take care with the amount:** Normally seaweed is sold dehydrated and its weight and volume are quite small. They must be used in small quantities, since when placed in contact with water, they swell to an unexpectedly large volume.

  – **Add little or no salt:** Seaweed heightens the flavor of foods in which they are cooked, and in many cases it is unnecessary to add salt.

- **As dietary supplements:** They are prepared as tablets or powder. The latter is added to salads, soups or stews to increase their mineral content.

- **As a substitute for common salt:** Pulverized seaweed can be used to season foods in place of salt, with the added advantage that it contains less sodium and more minerals, particularly magnesium, calcium, and iodine.

Vegetables From the Sea

KELP
Composition
per 100 g of raw edible portion

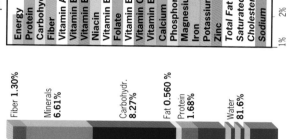

Energy	43.0 kcal = 180 kj
Protein	1.68 g
Carbohydrates	8.27 g
Fiber	1.30 g
Vitamin A	12.0 µg RE
Vitamin B₁	0.050 mg
Vitamin B₂	0.150 mg
Niacin	1.27 mg NE
Vitamin B₆	0.002 mg
Folate	180 µg
Vitamin B₁₂	—
Vitamin C	3.00 mg
Vitamin E	0.870 mg α-TE
Calcium	168 mg
Phosphorus	42.0 mg
Magnesium	121 mg
Iron	2.85 mg
Potassium	89.0 mg
Zinc	1.23 mg
Total Fat	*0.560 g*
Saturated Fat	*0.247 g*
Cholesterol	—
Sodium	*233 mg*

% Daily Value (based on a 2,000 calorie diet)
provided by 100 g of this food

1% 2% 4% 10% 20% 40% 100%

*Composition of fresh (not dehydrated)
Laminaria seaweed (also called 'kelp').*

PERCENTAGE COMPOSITION
- Fiber **1.30%**
- Minerals **6.61%**
- Carbohydr. **8.27%**
- Fat **0.560 %**
- Protein **1.68%**
- Water **81.6%**

Benefits of Seaweed

- **Prevents goiter:** When too little *iodine* is taken in with foods, as occurs in some interior mountainous areas, the thyroid gland becomes greatly enlarged and forms a swollen area on the throat known as a goiter. A handful of dried seaweed added to any dish more than satisfies the iodine needs of an entire family and prevents the possibility of suffering goiter.

- **It provides minerals:** Seaweed is a *good source of calcium, magnesium and iron.*

- **It satiates the appetite:** the *gums* or *mucilage* of seaweed retains up to ten times their weight in water, thus filling the stomach and producing a full feeling. This makes them *very useful* in reducing the appetite in **weight loss** diets.

- **It aids with excess stomach acid:** the *gums* or *mucilage* absorb gastric juices and act as **a natural antacid.**

- **It has laxative properties:** the *gums* or *mucilage* of seaweed increase the volume of and soften the feces, thus facilitating **smoother more natural evacuation.**

- **It increases metabolic rate and prevents obesity:** Due to seaweed's *iodine* content, it promotes hormone production in the thyroid gland. These hormones accelerate combustion of carbohydrates and fats. For this reason it should be part of every weight-loss diet.

- **Reduces cholesterol:** One of the effects of the *gums* or *mucilage* of seaweed is that of *impeding* the absorption of **cholesterol** in the intestine. Therefore, the *regular* consumption of seaweed *reduces* the cholesterol level in the blood.

Drawbacks to Seaweed

- **Flavor:** It is reminiscent of fish, and not appreciated by some persons.

- ***Elevated*** **sodium content:** Those suffering from **hypertension** should eat seaweed sparingly.

- **Should not be used by those suffering from hyperthyroidism:** The *high iodine* content of seaweed is beneficial to everyone except those suffering from hyperthyroidism (excessive thyroid function). In these cases, seaweed should be *avoided.*

Seaweed and Algae From Lakes and Seas

Cyanoficeae or Blue-green Algae

These are microscopic algae found in fresh water and now called **cyanobacteria**, since they are considered bacteria and not algae. These are their characteristics:

– They are **unicellular organisms**, in other words, formed of a single cell.

– They are **prokaryotes**, which do not have a true nucleus, like bacteria.

– They are **autotrophic**, capable of synthesizing their own organic matter, thanks to the chlorophyll that they contain. This is used in photosynthesis and releases great quantities of oxygen into the atmosphere.

Some 2000 species of blue-green algae exist, but the only one that is of dietary importance is Spirulina (*EMP* p. 276).

- **Spirulina** (*Spirulina maxima*): In spite of its biological simplicity, this alga is capable of synthesizing very valuable nutritional substances, which are stored in its cytoplasm. In particular, it contains:

– *Very high quality **protein*** (5.9% in fresh algae and 57.5% if dehydrated).

– *Minerals*, primarily *iron* (2.78 mg/100 g in fresh algae and 28.5 in the dehydrated).

– *Trace elements* such as copper, zinc, and others. Spirulina is **of value** in the following situations:

– As a **weight-loss treatment**, since it contains protein, minerals and vitamins, but very few calories (26 kcal/ 100 g fresh algae, 190 kcal/100 g dehydrated).

– In **nutritionally challenging events:** pregnancy and growth spurts.

– In cases of **anemia and malnutrition.**

– In cases of **arteriosclerosis,** due to it **antioxidant** action and its content of *omega-3 fatty acids.*

– *Vitamins*, particularly *B_1, B_2, E, niacin, folates* and *B_{12}* (see Vol. 1, pp. 390-397).

– Polyunsaturated *omega-3 fatty acids* (gamma-linolenic acid).

Phaeophytae or Brown Algae

These are seaweeds found in cold or mild regions of the Atlantic and Pacific oceans. They have the following characteristics:

– **Multicellular:** They are formed of many cells.

– **Eukaryotic:** Their cells contain a well-defined nucleus, as do all superior plants and animals.

– **Autotrophic:** They contain chlorophyll and perform photosynthesis.

– **Pigmented:** Their cells contain a brown pigment, called fucoxanthin, whose color obscures the green of the chlorophyll.

– Composed of **differentiated tissues** that form organs that are reminiscent of leaves, stalks, and roots, even though they are not.

– **Contain alginic acid** that accumulates in its cell walls. Of the 2,000 known species of brown algae, these are the *most used* in the human diet:

- **Laminaria** (see *EMP* p. 652): These are known generically as **kelp.** There are various species of the genus *Laminaria* (*L. saccharina, L. digitata, L. hiperborea, L. ochroleuca, etc.,* see *EMP* p. 652), so called for its ribbon-like shape.

– Pressed and dried, they form *Kombu*, a mixture of seaweed that is highly valued in Oriental cuisine.

– They are used as greens because of their fleshy consistency. Adding them to grain or legume dishes makes them easier to cook and gives them a pleasant flavor.

It can measure up to 2.5 m in length.

- **Bladderwrack or Fucus** (*Fucus vesiculosus,* see *EMP* p. 650): This seaweed, which is between 30 and 60 cm in length, is found along the Atlantic coast of Europe. It has air-filled bladders that resemble floats. It is very rich in *alginic acid* and other mucilaginous polysaccharides. They are used in capsules and other pharmaceutical preparations for the following situations:

– in **weight-loss diets**
– **excess** stomach acid and **gastritis**
– **constipation**
– **hypothyroidism** due to lack of iodine.

- **Alaria or wing** (*Alaria esculenta*): This seaweed grows in

Kombu

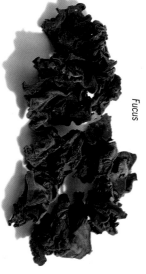

Fucus

EMP = Encyclopedia of Medicinal Plants, EDUCATION AND HEALTH LIBRARY, Editorial Safeliz.

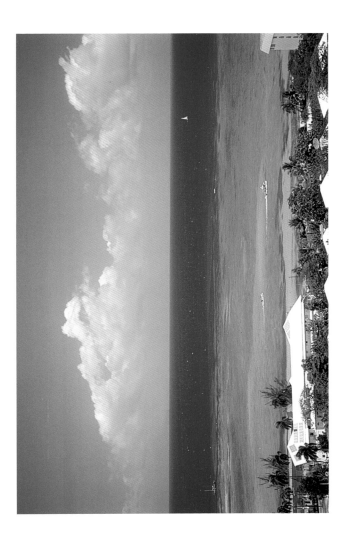

the North Atlantic, and is rich in iodine and other trace elements.

- **Himanthalia** or **Sea's spaghetti** (*Himanthalia elongata*): This seaweed reaches up to 2 meters in length. It has a delicious fish-like flavor. It is fermented and used much like sauerkraut. It is noted for its high iron content.

  - **Iziki:** (*Hizikia fusiformis*): This seaweed is from the Pacific Ocean. It forms long filaments up to a meter in length. It is tough in consistency and has an intense flavor. It is *particularly rich in calcium and trace elements*.

Iziki

Rhodophyceae or Red Algae

This is a genus of seaweed whose color varies from bright red to violet (although some are green or blackish) due to phycoerythrin pigmentation. They are found in temperate and tropical seas.

They are multicellular (except a few that are monocellular), eukaryotic and autotrophic. Of the 4,000 known species of red algae, these are the ones of the greatest dietary importance:

- *Gelidium cordeum*, is used as a source of **agar-agar** much the same as other species of red algae (see Vol. 1, p. 130).

- **Irish moss:** (*Chondrus crispus*, see *EMP* p. 301): **Carrageenan** is extracted from this seaweed, which is used as a medicine.

- **Nori** (*Porphyra umbilicalis*): This seaweed attaches itself to rocks by means of a central disk in the shape of an umbilicus. Its harvest takes place at low tide along the Korean coast. It is very tasty, and can be used in a variety of ways:
  - toasted and crumbled over salads or soups;
  - wrapped around balls of rice much as a croquette;
  - served raw cut in small pieces and seasoned with soy sauce.

Nori

- **Dulse** (*Palmaria palmata*): This seaweed measures some 20 cm in length. Its flavor and texture are quite agreeable. It is *rich in protein and iron*, as well as *iodine*. It is one of the **most versatile** of seaweeds for **cooking**, since it may be used:
  - raw in salads, combined with other vegetables
  - it goes well in potato salad
  - toasted
  - cooked just as any other vegetable.

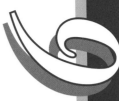

MUSHROOMS

A PASSION FOR MUSHROOMS

There are mycophiles and mycophobes around the world. In some places there are many mycological societies (mycology: the study of fungus) that spend many hours collecting, studying, and eating them, while in other areas they are unappreciated or completely ignored.

Mushrooms often taste delicious. However, they can be toxic or even deadly poison... and sometimes these can be confused with each other (see Vol. 1, pp. 148-150). It is easy to understand why many innate fears endure regarding mushrooms.

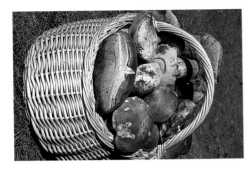

CHAPTER SUMMARY

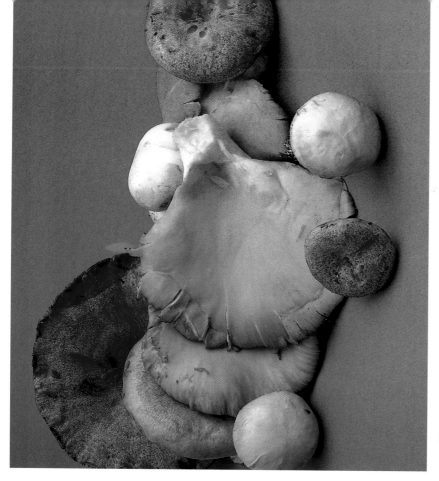

The mushroom is the visible, edible portion of certain fungi, which are formed by the mushroom and the mycelium. Their nutrients include protein, B group vitamins, and minerals.

M USHROOMS are a very special type of food. They are renowned for their variety of shapes, colors and aromas, which excite mycophiles that collect them, as well as gourmands that eat them.

However, mushrooms also produce revulsion among those who fear being poisoned by eating them. This is not irrational, since each autumn there are a number of poisonings among devotees who collect them in the wild. Some of these prove fatal.

Most mushrooms do not have special nutritional or healing powers. Their *appeal* is, above all, their **flavor.**

Since mushrooms are not an essential food, it is even more important that we avoid anything that may be harmful or that may result in disease. For this reason it is **vitally important** that all mushroom lovers and collectors know how to **identify** poisonous species, and to **avoid eating** any about which there is *the least doubt.*

Mushrooms are not independent living things. They are, in reality, only the **visible portions** of organisms known as **fungi.** Thus, it is important to understand the characteristics of fungi.

The Fungi Kingdom

Fungi are stationary organisms that were classified as vegetables for many years. During the second half of the 20th century they were grouped into a separate **kingdom**; that of **fungi**, since they are neither true vegetables nor animals. Although they are closer to vegetables, they possess certain characteristics found in animals:

• The **membrane** of fungi cells contains *cholesterol,* as do animal cells, although not in nutritionally significant amounts. In the **cellular wall** of fungi cells there is *chitin,* the same substance that forms the exoskeleton of insects and crustaceans.

Fungi and Mushrooms

Higher fungi are multicellular organisms that consist of two well-differentiated parts:

• *Mycelium: This is formed of a dense network of underground filaments that are normally invisible. They grow in concentric circles and may cover several square meters.*

• *Mushroom: The mycelium produces fruiting bodies, called mushrooms, during its reproductive phase. Reproductive spores spread from these. When the spores germinate they create new mycelia. It can be said that mushrooms are the sex organs or fruit of these higher fungi.*

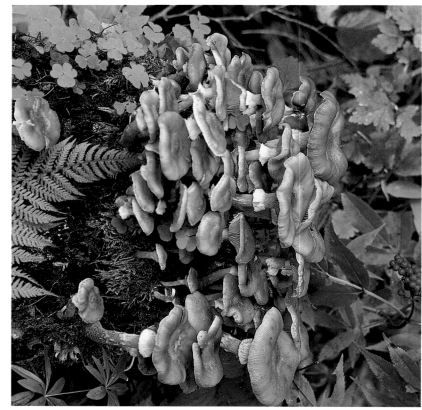

Raw mushrooms are dangerous, even if they are edible species. **They must always be cooked before eating to make them more digestible and eliminate any toxins that they may contain.**

For example, Armillaria mellea (honey mushroom) illustrated in the photograph, is only edible after it has been thoroughly cooked. Only the pileus (cap) should be eaten. The stipe (stem) should be discarded.

- They do *not* contain *chlorophyll*.
- They are **heterotrophic**, that is, incapable of synthesizing their own organic material. Vegetable plants form their own carbohydrates, proteins and fats using mineral elements. However, fungi must absorb these organic elements from the environment as do animals.

Fungi are classified according to the way they are nourished. They are:

- **Saprophytes:** These fungi nourish themselves on dead organic material (manure, dead leaves, etc.), and act as veritable plant "scavengers".

- **Parasites:** These live at the expense of other living things, including humans, to whom they cause a variety of diseases.

- **Symbiotic:** Even though they are nourished from other living things, the association is mutually beneficial. For example mycorrhiza is an association between the fungus mycelium and the roots of a tree. The tree provides sugars, and the fungus provides water and mineral salts.

Most **edible mushrooms are saprophytes,** which grow on manure or humus, or of fungi that form **mycorrhizas** with forest trees.

Fungi, True Chemical factories

There are some 100,000 known species of fungi. They can develop anywhere in the world, whether in the depths of the ocean, the arctic tundra, or the desert; as long as decomposing organic material or some living thing to parasite are available. Their size is variable from thousandths of a millimeter (monocellular yeasts), to many square meters (mycelia of higher fungi).

Fungi, particularly saprophytes, are true chemical factories. They are capable of decomposing organic substances for nourishment (fermentation process), and generating new ones. Their cells are provided with *powerful* tools, **enzymes,** to carry out these reactions. Due to these enzymes, fungi perform two simultaneous processes:

- **Decomposition or fermentation:** Fungi transform organic material (carbohydrates, proteins, and fats) into simpler

Continued on page 140

Anatomy of a Mushroom

Mushrooms are the **edible portions** of certain higher **fungi**, which emerge from the underground **mycelium** during certain times of the year. Botanically they constitute the **fruit** of the fungus.

The biological function of mushrooms is the release of **spores** formed in their **hymenium**.

Pileus (cap): The pileus is the fleshly portion of the mushroom. Its lower part constitutes the **hymenium**.

Scales: These are remains of the volva left on the pileus, as is the case with the toxic mushroom *Amanita muscaria*.

Hymenium: This is the reproductive site for **millions** of **spores** that spread from each mushroom. It may be formed of lamellae (gills), tubes, folds or spines. The hymenia of the **most poisonous** mushrooms are formed of **lamellae** (gills).

Annulus (ring): This structure is not present in all mushrooms. However, the **most poisonous** species *always* have an **annulus**.

Volva: This is a sac-like structure that covers the base of the stipe of some mushrooms. **All of the most poisonous mushrooms have a volva.** The volva can easily go unnoticed if the mushroom is not harvested carefully.

Stipe: (stem)

Mycelium: This is the vegetative portion of the fungus (the mushroom is the reproductive portion). It is formed by a network of fine filaments, called **hyphae**, which grow underground in concentric circles. It is estimated that ten cubic centimeters of forest soil can contain up to one thousand meters of mycelium filaments from various fungi.

How To Recognize the Most Poisonous Mushrooms

Death can result from eating even small amounts of the most poisonous mushrooms, which belong to the genus Amanita. They are relatively easy to recognize since all of them possess the following characteristics:

- *Hymenium: This is formed of white or light-colored lamellae.*
- *Annulus: The annulus is always present.*
- *Volva: The volva is always present.*

*The **most dangerous** poisonous mushrooms **always** have these three characteristics. One can avoid deadly poisoning by avoiding them.*

However, there are some species that are edible, and even highly valued, that have lamellae, annulus and volva. This is the case with the Caesar's mushroom (Amanita caesarea), which only specialists in mycology should attempt to identify.

Substances Produced by Fungi

Beneficial Substances

- **Antibiotics** such as **penicillin**, produced by various microscopic fungi from the genera Penicillium and Aspergillus.

- **Medications** such as **cyclosporin**, produced from soil molds (microscopic fungi formed of filaments or hyphae). Cyclosporin is used to avoid tissue rejection in organ transplant patients.

- **B complex vitamins** produced by various **yeasts** (unicellular microscopic fungi). One of the yeasts that produces the most vitamins is Saccharomyces cerevisae (see Vol. 1, p. 380), used to ferment malt to make beer.

- **Yeasts that ferment bread dough** (see Vol. 1, p. 71) **produce simple carbohydrates.** These are more easily digested than the starch from which they are derived. These unicellular, microscopic yeasts also produce carbon dioxide gas and B group vitamins.

- **Protein, vitamins, and nutritional mineral salts:** These are produced by higher fungi, and accumulate in mushrooms or fruiting bodies, which constitute the edible portions of these fungi.

various **molds**, such as Penicillium roqueforti, during the cheese making and aging process.

- **Ergotamine** is a toxic alkaloid produced by Claviceps purpurea, which is a parasite on rye and other grains.

- **Psylocibin:** This hallucinogenic produced by the Psilocybe mexicana fungus is similar to the drug LSD.

- **Toxic or deadly alkaloids:** These are produced by a variety of higher fungi, particularly those from the botanical class Basidiomycetes. They accumulate in the mushrooms or fruiting bodies.

- **Mycotoxins are toxins** produced by mold-type fungi, which are found on poorly stored foods. They produce a variety of toxic effects in humans and animals that are not always properly diagnosed. The most frequently encountered mycotoxins are **aflatoxins and okratoxins**, which are produced by molds of the genus Aspergillus. Aflatoxins cause a variety of liver diseases, including liver cancer.

— Mycotoxins in **plant foods:** The molds that produce mycotoxins grow on peanuts, legumes and grains that have been poorly stored. Modern storage methods for these foods avoid the formation of these toxins. Most serious mycotoxin poisonings occur in third-world countries.

— Mycotoxins **in animal products:** Meat, milk, and eggs from animals that have been fed moldy feed contain mycotoxins. This type of contamination happens rather frequently, even in developed countries. The harmful health effects of this small quantity of mycotoxins in meat, milk, and eggs are still being studied.

Harmful substances

- **Ethyl alcohol** is a toxic substance produced by various yeast-type fungi as they decompose or ferment natural sugars in fruit, or the carbohydrates in grain.

- **Hypertensive amines, ammonia,** and other **toxic by-products** resulting from the degradation of proteins, as well as fats, that form due to the action of

Continued from page 138

substances. In this manner they perform an *important* **ecological recycling** role. Fungi can, for example, decompose or ferment fruit scraps or juice, dead tree trunks, or animal excrement.

- **Synthesis:** This is the generation of new substances that are totally different from those found in the medium in which the fungi develop.

As they act upon the vegetable or animal organic matter through the processes of decomposition and synthesis, fungi produce numerous chemicals. Some of these are beneficial, while others are toxic, as can be seen in the chart on this page.

There are a great variety of fungi, each with its own enzymes and great capacity to produce chemical substances. This means

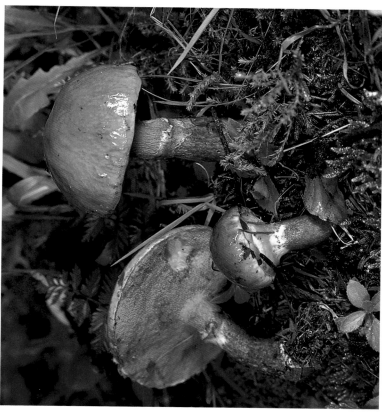

The *Suillus grevillei* or *Boletus elegans* only grows near the larch tree, with which it forms a symbiotic mycorrhiza. It is edible, although not very highly valued.

Some microscopic fungi, yeasts, are involved in the making of alcoholic beverages, cured cheeses, and bread.

Due to their considerable biochemical activity, many microscopic fungi or yeasts can produce a variety of harmful substances in addition to alcohol.

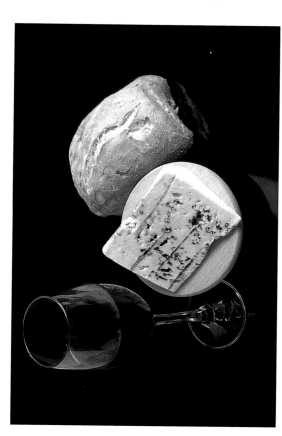

that, as a result of their activity, they can, produce harmful substances quite unpredictably. Some examples are:

- **Alcohol fermentation:** Yeasts (microscopic fungi) decompose fruit sugars and grain carbohydrates converting them into ethyl alcohol. They can also produce other, even more toxic substances, such as methanol.

- **Molds that develop in foods and animal feed:** These tend to produce very dangerous mycotoxins such as **aflatoxins** (see chart on preceding page).

  Meat, milk and eggs contain mycotoxins with greater frequency than do vegetables.

- **Curing and aging cheese:** The fungi that bring this about produce a large number of chemicals whose action is quite unpredictable; some of these are harmful to the health (see Vol. 1, p. 207).

- **Mushroom-producing fungi:** Substances that these fungi produce through metabolism are concentrated in the mushroom. Thus, normally edible species may produce toxins in some cases (generally in the mature phase), to the consternation of the diner.

This highlights the fact that there is always some *risk* in consuming foods or beverages in which fungi are involved. For example:

- aged cheese,

- alcoholic beverages or

- parts of fungi, such as mushrooms.

While **bread** is prepared with yeast (microscopic fungi), it seems an exception to the risk described above. It may be that the oven heat volatilizes any toxic substances from the fungi involved. This is what happens with the small amount of ethyl alcohol produced during the fermentation of the dough (see Vol. 1, p. 71).

Continued on page 146

Wild Mushrooms:

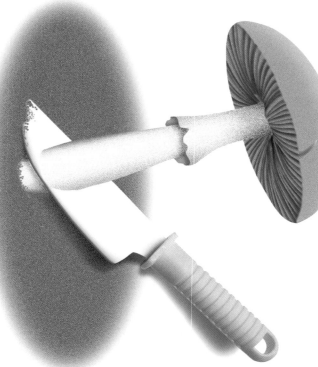

Mushrooms should be harvested using a knife to cut the stipe, rather than pulling them from the ground. This avoids damaging the invisible portion of the fungus. The network of underground filaments. If this network, called mycelium, is left intact, it will continue to produce mushrooms for years.

Additionally, one must bear in mind that mushrooms concentrate chemical contaminants from their environment. For this reason they should not be collected near roads, contaminating industries, or garbage dumps.

How To Harvest Mushrooms

- **Do not harvest** mushrooms that grow **near chemically contaminated sites**, since mushrooms concentrate toxic substances from the environment within their tissues. It is **particularly important to avoid** areas such as:

  - **Highways and expressways:** Investigations have shown that there are elevated **lead** levels in the soil within 300 meters of areas used by motor vehicles. Mushrooms concentrate this heavy metal to a greater degree than do plants.

  - Large **cultivated areas:** These are usually treated with various **pesticides** that also reach collateral fields.

  - **Chemical industries.**

  - **Garbage dumps** and **incinerators.**

- **They should be cut with a knife at the base of the stipe,** including the volva whenever possible. This structure is important in the identification of mushrooms. If the mushroom is pulled out of the ground rather than cut, the underground mycelium may be damaged, thus retarding the development of new mushrooms.

- When hunting mushrooms, **do not disturb the top layers of the humus** that covers the forest floor. This will damage any mycelium that may be there.

- **Discard any overripe specimens,** those that have been eaten by insects or show any signs of decay. These tend to have higher concentrations of natural toxins.

- **Use a wicker basket to carry harvested mushrooms.** They break and rot more easily when carried in plastic, cloth or paper bags.

- **Do not carry them upside down.** Dirt gets into the lamellae.

- **Do not step on or destroy unidentified mushrooms** or those supposed to be poisonous. They are also necessary to the balance of the ecosystem.

How to prepare and eat mushrooms

- **Identification:** *never eat* mushrooms until they have been positively identified as edible. Check with a specialist in mycology, if necessary. If there is the slightest doubt, it is preferable to discard the specimens.

  - They may contain **carcinogens** such as the agaratine of champignon.

- **Cooking:** Many edible mushrooms in their natural state contain toxic substances:

  - Substances that are **irritants** to the digestive tract, which can cause nausea and vomiting.

  These harmful substances disappear with the heat. This is why cooking for at least five minutes is important for wild, as well as domestic mushrooms. **They should *never* be eaten raw.**

- **Additional precaution:** When eating wild mushrooms it is a good practice **to keep** at least one intact specimen of each type in the refrigerator for 48 hours. This way it is possible to identify any mushroom responsible in case anyone becomes ill.

Safety First

How To Recognize Inedible or Poisonous Mushrooms

*In some cases it is relatively easy to recognize inedible or toxic mushrooms based on their characteristics. For example, the **stinkhorn mushroom** (Clathrus ruber), shown in the photograph smells of rotten meat, which clearly indicates that it is not fit for consumption.*

However, in many other cases, inedible or poisonous mushrooms appear, smell, and even taste completely normal. For this reason it is necessary to positively identify the species of each wild mushroom collected before eating.

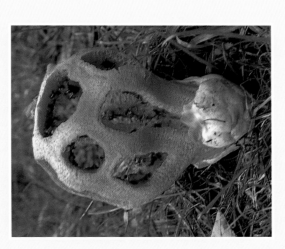

'Clathrus ruber'
(stinkhorn mushroom),
is an inedible mushroom.

Myths About Mushrooms

- **If one cooks mushrooms in water or oil with a piece of silver, and it turns black, the mushrooms are poisonous.**
  In reality only a few overripe mushrooms turn silver black due to the sulfur that they release, which reacts with the silver, turning it black. Deadly Amanitas do not blacken silver.

- **All mushrooms with an annulus on the stipe are edible.**
  There are edible mushrooms with annulus. But the most poisonous amanitas also have this structure.

- **Mushrooms with pleasant aroma and flavor are edible.**
  The deadly Amanita phalloides has a very pleasant sweet flavor, especial when young.

- **Mushrooms that have been eaten by snails or rodents are edible.**
  The digestive juices of mollusks and some small mammals such as rats and squirrels contain enzymes that destroy the poisons found in amanitas and other poisonous mushrooms. Therefore, they may eat them with no ill effects.

- **Mushrooms marinated in water, salt and vinegar lose their toxic properties.**
  Such marinating may reduce the bitter or piquant taste of some edible mushrooms, but does not eliminate the poisonous substances that they may contain.

- **Prolonged cooking or dehydrating eliminates poisons.**
  This is the case with very few slightly toxic species. The toxins found in the deadly amanitas are very resistant to both cooking and drying.

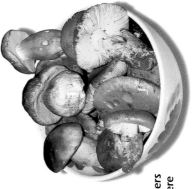

There is a popular saying that *"there are old mushroom eaters and there are bold eaters of mushrooms; but there are no old, bold mushroom eaters."*

Nutritional Value

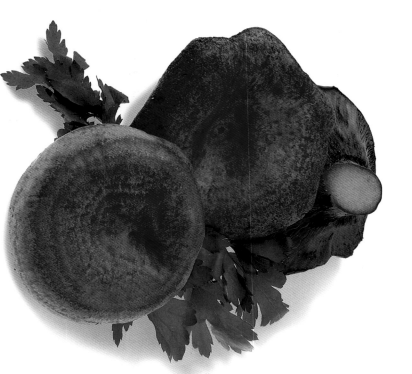

The milk mushroom (Lactarius deliciosus, Vol. 1, p. 154) is a mushroom highly prized for its exquisite flavor and digestibility. They are harvested in the wild, and have the advantage over other mushrooms of being easily distinguished from poisonous species.

Mushrooms Provide:

- **Water:** Between 80% and 92% of a mushroom's weight is water.

- **Protein:** Between 2% and 3% of weight is protein. It is greater than that of potatoes and most vegetables, but less than foods of animal origin, legumes, nuts, or grains. Mushroom proteins are of **biologically high quality.**

- **Carbohydrates:** Between 3% and 5% of their weight. These carbohydrates are made up primarily by **glycogen** (a type of starch found in animals) and short-chain **polysaccharides.**

- **Fats:** Very little: 0.2% to 0.5%.

- **Vitamins:** Particularly **B₁, B₂, B₆, niacin,** and **folates,** so 100 grams of mushrooms provide approximately one-fourth of the MDR of vitamin B2 and niacin. Mushrooms also provide from 1 to 3 µg of vitamin D, an amount similar to butter, but less than fish.

- **Minerals:** Above all phosphorus, potassium, and iron. Copper and zinc are among the **trace elements** that they provide.

- **Fiber:** They contain 2% to 3% **cellulose,** which is more than many vegetables and fruits.

- **Calories:** They have between 25 and 30 kcal/100 g, an amount well below most other foods except for green leafy vegetables and stalks, which provide approximately 15 to 25 kcal.

Mushrooms Contain Little or No:

- provitamin A, and vitamins B₁₂ and C;
- calcium;
- cholesterol.

Caution

- **Children, the elderly and the sickly** must exercise great care in eating wild mushrooms, since they are more sensitive to any toxins that may be present.

- **One should not eat more than 500 g** (about 1 pound) of wild mushrooms per week (200 g [less than half a pound] for children and pregnant women). Even though they may come from relatively uncontaminated areas, they always contain some level of heavy metals (lead, cadmium, mercury) and other chemical contaminants.

# of Mushrooms

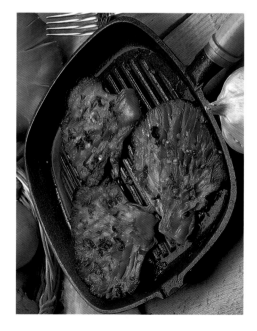

Positive Aspects of Mushrooms

- **Flavor:** Mushrooms contain aromatic substances that give them a very pleasant flavor that reminds some of meat.
- **Weight-loss diets:** Baked, broiled or cooked (but *not fried*, since they retain a great deal of oil) mushrooms are very appropriate for weight-loss diets because they
  - contain very little fat;
  - contain a significant amount of nutritional protein, vitamins, and minerals, but with the advantage that they are low in calories;
  - contain a significant amount of fiber, which provides a feeling of satiety.
- **Medicinal effects:** Some mushrooms contribute therapeutically, for example
  - **Champignon** (*Agaricus bisporus,* Vol. 1, p. 152): antidiabetic.
  - *Shiitake* (*Lentinus edodes,* Vol. 1, p. 151): immune booster, anticarcinogen, antiviral, reduces cholesterol, general tonic.

Drawbacks to Mushrooms

- **Poisoning:** When one eats wild mushrooms, there is always the risk of confusing edible mushrooms with poisonous ones. Unfortunately, every year there are poisonings, some fatal. This risk does not exist with domestic, cultivated mushrooms.
  Poisoning may be avoided by positively identifying each species of wild mushroom harvested and discarding any that may be in doubt. In many cases it may be necessary to consult an expert in mycology (the study of fungi).
  There are about 160 species of poisonous mushrooms. Some, such as the apparently harmless *Amanita phalloides* (see Vol. 1, p. 148), can cause death after eating only a small portion.
- **Chemical contamination:** Mushrooms are true **repositories** of chemical pollutants. They have the ability to *concentrate* toxic chemical substances found in the environment, *particularly* **heavy metals** (lead, cadmium, mercury) and **pesticides.** For this reason, the *only* mushrooms that should be **eaten** are those found in **uncontaminated areas.**
- **Radioactive contamination:** Mushrooms also *concentrate* radioactive elements that may be in the environment. For this reason eating mushrooms from anywhere there has been any type of radiation release, whether from accidents, faulty storage, or other cause, is unadvisable.
- **Allergies:** Certain species of mushrooms produce allergic reactions in sensitized individuals, while others tolerate them well. Because of this, it always best to eat only a small amount of any new species and eat no other species during the following 48 hours. This allows time for allergies, if any, to manifest.
- **Indigestible:** Mushrooms are not easily digested, and should be eaten with moderation to avoid digestive disorders. Fried mushrooms are particularly indigestible; they are much better tolerated roasted or boiled.
- **Uric acid:** Mushrooms contain nucleoproteins that form uric acid, although less than meat, fish, seafood, and legumes. Thus, those suffering from gout and excess uric acid should avoid them.

Some mushrooms that originally grow in the wild are cultivated in dark chambers on a mixture of straw and manure. There is no risk of poisoning from these cultivated, or domestic, mushrooms since they represent known, safe species.

This photograph illustrates the Elm oyster mushroom (see Vol. 1, p. 156).

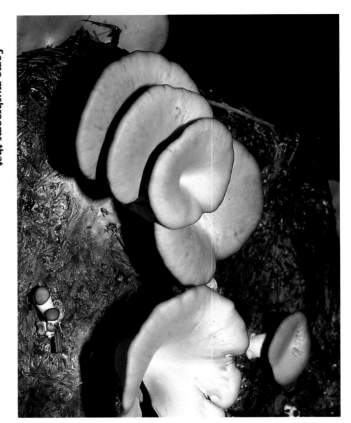

Continued from page 141

Mushroom Poisoning

In areas where collecting wild mushrooms is customary, poisoning is not infrequent. These may be more or less serious, some resulting in death.

There are about 160 known species of toxic mushrooms, a few of which contain truly life-threatening poisonings (see Vol. 1, pp. 148-150).

The most dangerous mushrooms are those of the genus *Amanita*, particularly *Amanita phalloides*. These are responsible for 90% of mushroom poisoning deaths in Europe.

There are at least four causes of wild mushroom poisoning:

1. Eating poisonous species of mushrooms

This is **the most common cause** and most serious of poisonings. Most of these cases are involuntary, accidental poisonings.

There are two types of poisonings, depending on the time that symptoms appear:

- **Precocious poisoning:** symptoms appear between one-half hour and six hours af-

ter eating poisonous mushrooms. This is *not usually fatal*; however, it can be serious, particularly when it affects the nervous system. The **symptoms** are of two types:

- *Digestive* symptoms are the most common. They include vomiting; abdominal pain, and diarrhea. They usually disappear spontaneously within two or three days.

- *Neurological:* These are accompanied by more or less intense digestive problems. In poisonings by the species *Amanita muscaria* and *Amanita pantherina*, the symptoms are nervous excitement, delirium, rapid pulse, pupil dilation, and dry mouth (atropine reaction). In poisoning by other mushrooms, such as the genus *Inocybes*, the opposite symptoms are produced: slowing pulse rate, pupil contraction, hypersecretion of saliva, and sweating.

There are **antidotes** for both of these that must be administered by healthcare professionals in the proper setting.

- **Slow-developing phalloidin poisoning** is most serious and is often fatal. The mushroom implicated most often is *Amanita phalloides*, whose powerful toxins produce massive liver damage. *Amanita verna, Amanita virosa* and certain species of the genus *Lepiota*, which are quite small, can also produce phalloidin poisoning. Eating one specimen or only a small portion of one may be sufficient to cause death.

Symptoms of phalloidin poisoning appear in three phases:

- *Gastrointestinal phase:* Between eight and twelve hours after eating, the victim experiences vomiting, abdominal pain, and bloody diarrhea.

- *Apparent improvement phase:* During the second day the digestive symptoms abate, and the victim may mis-

What To Do in Case of Mushroom Poisoning

1. ***Take*** the victim to a **hospital as quickly as possible,** or seek the aid of a physician, even though the symptoms appear minor at first.

2. If medical **assistance is slow** in coming or unavailable:
   – Have the victim **rest.**
   – Induce ***vomiting*** (the **ideal** procedure is **gastric lavage,** also referred to as stomach irrigation).
   – Give the victim **charcoal** and **sugar water.**

3. ***Determine when the mushrooms were eaten.*** If it is suspected that this occurred more than eight hours before the appearance of the symptoms, it is possibly a slow-developing phalloidin poisoning. If so, the prognosis is much more serious.

4. ***Keep*** a **specimen** of the suspected mushroom so it may be identified later by specialists.

takenly believe that recovery is taking place.

– *Visceral aggression phase:* By the third day and beyond jaundice sets in followed by hepatic coma and death.

There are *no* specific **antidotes or treatments** for phalloidin poisoning. However, some specialized hospitals have saved the lives of some victims. Hence, the importance of:

– avoiding poisoning by discarding all suspicious specimens (see Vol. 1, pp. 148, 149),

– or, if poisoning has already occurred, recognizing early symptoms and taking the victim to a **hospital** *as rapidly as possible.*

2. Consumption of certain mushrooms together with alcoholic beverages

Some mushrooms are well tolerated if they are not eaten with alcoholic beverages. However, when they are eaten with beer, wine, or liquor, they produce certain symptoms known as the **antabuse effect:**

- tachycardia,
- redness of the face,
- ringing in the ears,
- dizziness.

The mushroom most associated in this effect is the *Coprinus atramentarius.*

3. Eating raw mushrooms

Most species of mushrooms are irritating to the stomach when eaten *raw,* even those that are edible. Normally they produce minor digestive disturbances that pass with no long-term consequences. Some, such as the champignon or meadow mushroom, may have carcinogenic effects (see Vol. 1, p. 152).

However there are some mushrooms that are toxic and produce digestive and/or nervous symptoms when eaten raw, but when cooked they become well tolerated. For example:

- blusher mushroom (*Amanita rubescens,* see Vol. 1, p. 153),
- false milk mushroom (*Lactarius torminosus* see Vol. 1, p. 154),
- fluted white elfin saddle (*Helvella crispa*) and fluted black elfin saddle (*Helvella lacunosa*).

4. Eating overripe or decomposing mushrooms

Many species of edible species of mushrooms can produce toxic reactions if they are overripe or have begun to decompose. This is due to the fact that mushroom-producing fungi at this stage of development synthesize toxic substances that are not normally present.

The poisoning that results from these *tends* to be **minor** with digestive manifestations (vomiting, diarrhea and abdominal pain) and general malaise. These symptoms usually disappear spontaneously in one or two days.

The following pages contain a selection of the most common edible and poisonous mushrooms found in Europe and America.

Amanita phalloides

Death cap, death angel

Habitat: Beech, birch or oak forests. Rarely found among pines or fir.

Characteristics: Greenish pileus. White or light-colored lamellae with annulus, and volva as with all deadly mushrooms.

Poisoning: This is the **most poisonous** of all mushrooms. Eating a portion of one is enough to produce death. The first symptoms appear between 8 to 12 hours after eating (see Vol. 1, p. 146).

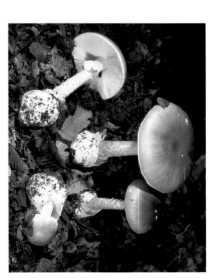

Mushrooms that May Be Confused With Amanita phalloides

	Mushroom	Vol./Page	Pileus	Lamellae	Annulus	Volva
☠	**AMANITA PHALLOIDES**	1/148	Greenish	White or light-colored	Yes	Yes
➡	RUSSULA VESCA	1/157	Reddish or violet	White	No	No
➡	AGARICUS CAMPESTRIS	1/152	White, pink or brown	Pink or purple	Small, incomplete	No

Amanita verna

Habitat: Broadleaf forests and less frequently, coniferous forests. They grow in spring.

Characteristics: The pileus is first hemispherical, later flattened. It is whitish to yellowish in color. The lamellae are white, annulus, and volva.

Poisoning: Slow phalloidin type (the first symptoms appear 8 to 12 hours after eating; (see Vol. 1, p. 146). It is as **deadly** as Amanita phalloides.

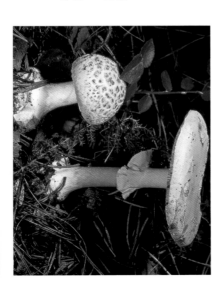

Mushrooms that May Be Confused With Amanita verna

	Mushroom	Vol./Page	Pileus	Lamellae	Annulus	Volva
☠	**AMANITA VERNA**	1/148	Whitish or yellowish	Whitish	Yes	Yes
➡	LEPIOTA PROCERA	1/155	Brown, with fixed scales	Whitish	Yes	No
➡	CAMPESTRIS	1/152	White, pink or brown	Pink or purple	Small, incomplete	No

Mushrooms

Amanita muscaria
Fly agaric

Habitat: Coniferous forests (fir, pine, etc), as well as broadleaf forests (beech, chestnut, birch, etc.).

Characteristics: Bright red or orange pileus with white scales. If the scales are missing these can be confused with Caesar's mushroom (*Amanita caesarea*, Vol. 1, p. 152). It has white lamellae, annulus, and volva.

Poisoning: Precocious onset poisoning. Mild neurological and digestive symptoms appear 2-3 hours after eating (see Vol. 1, p. 146). *It is **not** usually **fatal.***

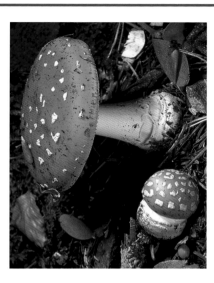

Mushrooms that May Be Confused With *Amanita muscaria*

Mushroom	Vol./Page	Pileus	Lamellae	Annulus	Volva
AMANITA MUSCARIA	1/149	Red, white scales	Whitish	Yes	Yes
AMANITA CAESAREA	1/152	Red, orange, without scales	Golden yellow	Yes	Yes

Amanita pantherina
Panther mushroom

Habitat: All types of forests.

Characteristics: Brown pileus with whitish scales that may be removed by rain. It has annulus and volva, and its flesh is white. Its odor is pleasant, reminiscent of radish.

Poisoning: Precocious onset poisoning (the first symptoms appear a few hours after eating), similar to *Amanita muscaria*, but more serious. ***Not** usually **fatal.***

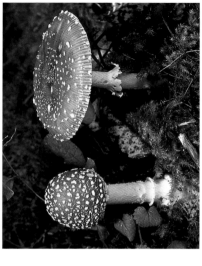

Mushrooms that May Be Confused With *Amanita pantherina*

Mushroom	Vol./Page	Pileus	Lamellae	Annulus	Volva
AMANITA PANTHERINA	1/149	Brown, whitish scales	White	Yes	Yes
AMANITA RUBESCENS	1/153	Reddish brown, spherical white scales	Pink	Yes	Small
LEPIOTA PROCERA	1/155	Brown, with fixed scales	Whitish	Yes	No

Poisonous Mushrooms (cont.)

▲ Boletus satanas

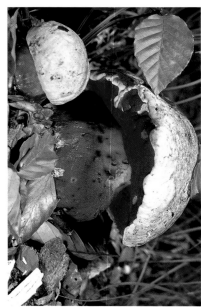

Habitat: Clearings in beech and other broadleaf forests.

Characteristics: Very large, light-colored pileus, it can reach 30 cm in diameter. Its hymenium is formed of tubules (as is all of the genus *Boletus*) which are reddish in color.

Poisoning: Precocious onset poisoning, with *minor* **diges-tive symptoms.**

Paxillus involutus ▶

Habitat: All types of forests, near trees.

Characteristics: Brown or yellow pileus and lamellae, with the edge turned under. This mushroom does not have an an-nulus or volva.

Poisoning: Some books list this mushroom as edible. It has been shown that it can produce a serious type of hemolytic anemia in predisposed persons.

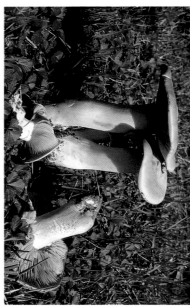

▲ Entoloma lividum

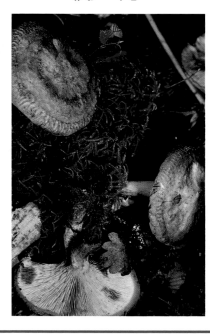

Scientific synonyms: *Rodophyllus sinatus* = *R. lividus.*

Habitat: Oak, beech, and chestnut forests.

Characteristics: Light gray or cream-colored pileus 10 to 15 cm in diameter. It has a thick cream or salmon-colored lamellae. It does not have an annulus or volva. It has a flour-like odor.

Poisoning: Precocious onset poisoning, with digestive symptoms.

Gyromitra esculenta ▶

Scientific synonym: *Physomitra esculenta.*

Habitat: Conifer forests; these mushrooms grow in spring like a brain

Characteristics: This mushroom's ochre-colored pileus looks like a brain

Poisoning: Some years ago this mushroom was considered edible. However, its **toxicity** has been shown to have a **cu-mulative effect.** Each time it is eaten, the more dangerous it becomes. It can produce **serious** poisoning or even death.

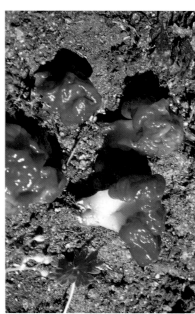

Medicinal Oriental Mushrooms

Mushrooms have been present in the Oriental kitchen as well as in Chinese, Japanese, and Korean **traditional medicine** for millennia. In recent decades there has been considerable growth in interest in Oriental mushrooms as their curative properties have become known in various studies.[1]

These Oriental mushrooms are available in Western countries in various forms: **fresh, dehydrated,** in various types of **preserves,** or **as extracts.**

Shiitake
Lentinus edodes

This is one of the most valued of Oriental mushrooms be-

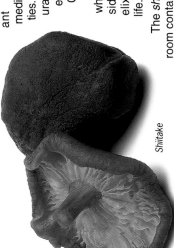

Shiitake

cause of its pleasant taste and medicinal properties. It grows naturally in forested areas in China, Korea and Japan, where it is considered as an elixir for long life.

The *shiitake* mushroom contains proteins, B vitamins and minerals, as do all mushrooms. However, additional substances have been found that provide therapeutic action. Among these, the following are notable:

- **Lentinan:** This polysaccharide acts in the body to *stimulate* the production of a type of defensive cells known as **T lymphocytes.** These lymphocytes are also referred to as killer cells, since they are able to destroy cancer cells. In addition to retarding the development of cancer, T lymphocytes defend against microbes.

- **Eritadenin:** This substance *reduces* **cholesterol** levels.

- **Interferon inductor:** *Shiitake* mushrooms contain a substance that induces the synthesis of interferon in the body.[2] Interferon acts as an **antiviral** and **anticarcinogenic** agent.

- **Superoxide dismutase:** This is an enzyme with *powerful antioxidant* properties. It is found in grains and sprouts, as well. It prevents the peroxidation of the lipids that cause **arteriosclerosis.**

Shiitake mushrooms and their extracts are used in traditional Chinese medicine as in other parts of the Far East in the following situations:

- **Infectious** diseases, particularly viral such as flu, hepatitis, and AIDS;
- **Cancer;**[3]
- Elevated **cholesterol** levels, **arteriosclerosis,** and **coronary disease.**[4]

Enoki
Pholiota nameko

This white, noodle-like mushroom is enjoying increased use in the West. It is eaten in soups. Enoki also stimulates the **immune system** and it is attributed with anticarcinogenic properties.

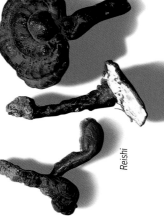

Enoki

Maitake
Grifolia frondosa

Scientific synonyms:
Polyporus frondosus = Calyporus frondosus.

This mushroom contains a polysaccharide derived from glucan attributed with **anticarcinogenic, antihypertensive,** and **antidiabetic** properties.[5]

Cordyceps
Cordyceps sinensis

This tiny fungus lives on the larvae of various insects in the Himalayan region. Traditional Chinese medicine uses it as:

- **Antiasthmatic** and **bronchodilator** (some Chinese athletes use it to improve performance in sporting events);

- **Aphrodisiac** and as an erectile **stimulant.**

Reishi or ganoderma
Ganoderma lucidum

This mushroom has a tough consistency and grows on tree trunks. It is found in the Far East as well as warmer regions of Europe and America. It is used in the preparation of macrobiotic foods or as a tea. It contains the **immunostimulant** and **anticarcinogen, lentinan.** It is important not to take more than 20 grams of dried ganoderma a day, since it can cause diarrhea.

Reishi

Edible Mushrooms

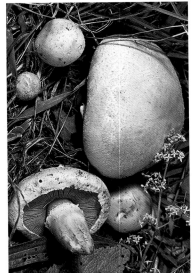

▲ Agaricus campestris

Scientific synonyms: *Psalliota campestris.*
Champignon, meadow mushroom

Habitat: Open fields and meadows, particularly areas that are rich with horse manure.

Characteristics: White pileus and flesh. Pink or brown lamellae. Small, incomplete annulus. No volva.

Use: This wild mushroom has a stronger flavor than the cultivated champignon. It is important to **avoid mature specimens**, due to their high **agaratine** content, a possibly carcinogenic substance.[6,7] It must **always be cooked** before eating, since the agaratine disappears with the heat. This is useful in the diets of **diabetics** and those **losing weight.**

Agaricus arvensis ▲

Scientific synonym: *'Psalliota arvensis'.*
Horse mushroom

Characteristics: This mushroom is very similar in all aspects to the *Agaricus campestris*, but it is whiter in color.

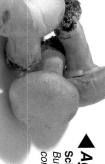

▲ Agaricus bisporus

Scientific synonym: *'Psalliota bispora'.*
Button mushroom, common champignon, common mushroom (see Vol. 2, p. 294).

Agaricus xanthodermus ▲

Scientific synonym: *Psalliota xanthoderma.*

Characteristics: These mushrooms are similar to other types of champignon of the genus *Agaricus*, but with two distinct characteristics:

– it is larger (it can reach 15 cm in diameter);
– its flesh turns a bright yellow when it is cut.

Use: This mushroom is **very indigestible** and *some* consider it **toxic**. However, there are those that tolerate it well.

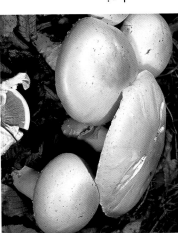

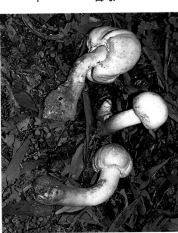

Amanita caesarea ▲

Caesar's mushroom

Habitat: Sunny Mediterranean forests.

Characteristics: Brilliant red or orange-colored hemispherical pileus with fine skin. The shape flattens as it matures. Its lamellae are yellow as contrasted with the poisonous *Amanita muscaria*, whose lamellae are white. It has an annulus and a volva.

Use: According to many experts, this is **the most exquisite** of all mushrooms.
Confusion: With *Amanita muscaria* (see Vol. 1, p. 149).

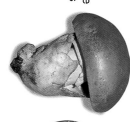

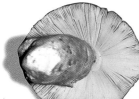

▼ Amanita rubescens

Blusher mushroom

Habitat: All forest types. They reproduce in spring and autumn.

Characteristics: Reddish brown pileus with pearly white spherical scales. It has an annulus and a small volva.

Use: This mushroom has an excellent flavor when it is well cooked, but it is **toxic** if eaten **raw.**

Confusion: *Amanita pantherina* (Panther mushroom, Vol. 1, p. 149), which is poisonous.

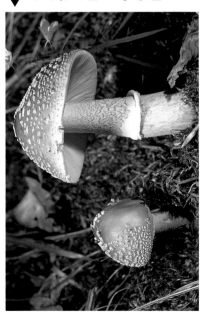

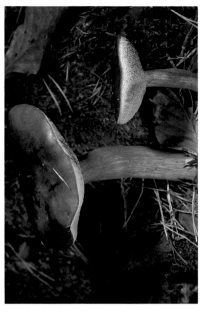

Boletus badius ▶

Bay bolete

Characteristics: The same as *Boletus edulis* but with firmer flesh. When the tubules of the hymenium are pressed, they turn blue-green in color.

▼ Boletus edulis

King bolete, cep, cepe

Habitat: Pine and broadleaf forests.

Characteristics: Hemispherical pileus that is light to dark brown in color and has a velvety surface. The hymenium is formed of small tubules, as is the entire genus *Boletus*. In this species they are whitish at first, then they turn yellow-green. The stipe is strong and thick. It has neither an annulus nor a volva.

Use: Excellent food. Its flavor is reminiscent of hazelnuts. They can be dehydrated for storage.

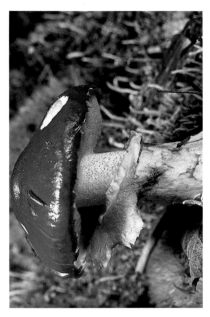

Boletus luteus ▶

Characteristics: Similar to those of *Boletus edulis*, but with bright yellow tubules. It is best to remove the cuticle that covers the pileus, since it has a bitter taste.

Edible

▲ Cantharellus cibarius

Chanterelle

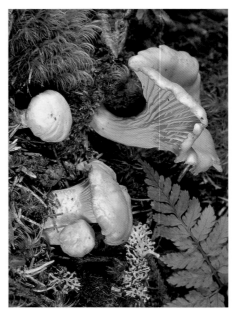

Habitat: A variety of forest settings, particularly among ferns.

Characteristics: This mushroom has a yellow pileus, with curled, irregular edges. Its hymenium is formed of irregular yellow pleats. It has neither annulus nor volva.

Use: This mushroom has an excellent flavor, although its flesh tends to be tough. It stores well **dehydrated.**

Lactarius deliciosus ▼

Milky cap mushroom

Habitat: Pine forests.

Characteristics: The orange pileus of this mushroom is concave on top. Its lamellae and the liquid it releases when cut are also orange. It has neither annulus nor volva.

Use: Excellent food. Its natural pigments turn the urine red a few hours after eating. However, this presents no health risk.

Confusion: This mushroom cannot be confused with any poisonous species.

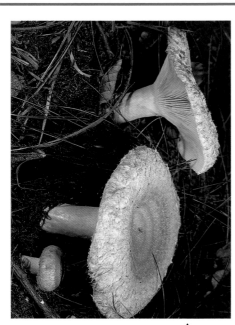

▲ Lactarius torminosus

False milk mushroom

Habitat: Sandy soil and birch forests.

Characteristics: The pileus of this mushroom is similar to that of Lactarius deliciosus but of a lighter color. It releases a whitish sour liquid when cut.

Use: If eaten **raw** this mushroom **irritates** the digestive tract. When cooked, however, it has a **pleasant flavor,** and is valued in Northern and Eastern Europe.

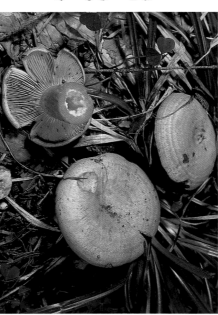

Mushrooms (cont.)

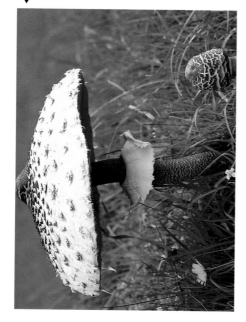

▶ Lepiota procera

Scientific synonym: *Macrolepiota procera.*

Habitat: Sunny forests and meadows.

Characteristics: This mushroom has a brown pileus with permanent scales. Its early shape is ovoid, then conical and finally hat-shaped, with a diameter of up to 25 cm. It has whitish lamellae and a fleshly annulus that is easily removed. It does not have a volva.

Use: Excellent food when eaten **young.**

Confusion: This mushroom may be confused with *Amanita pantherina* (see Vol. 1, p. 149) and other smaller, very poisonous, species of the genus *Lepiota.*

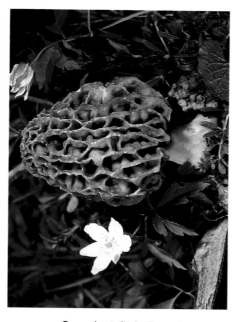

Morchella esculenta ▶

Scientific synonym: *Morchella vulgaris.*
Morel

Habitat: This mushroom is found in meadows, close to rivers and near ash trees.

Characteristics: Ovoid pileus that is covered by a honeycomb shaped hymenium. The stipe is thick and hollow. The morel, together with the truffle, are the only edible mushrooms from the Ascomycete botanical class presented here. None of the species of the genus *Morella* is poisonous.

Use: Morels must **not** be eaten **raw**. Cooked, they have a **delicate flavor.**

▶ Pholiota mutabilis

Scientific synonym: *Kuehneromyces mutabilis.*

Habitat: This mushroom grows on dead tree trunks.

Characteristics: Pholiota mutabilis has a cinnamon-colored or brown pileus, the same as its lamellae. Its stipe has an annulus but no volva.

Use: Edible, valued for its **pleasant**, somewhat sweet, **flavor.**

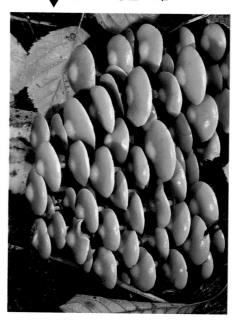

Edible

Pleurotus eryngii ▲

Elm oyster mushroom

Habitat: This mushroom grows wild in pasturelands in Southern Europe, close to *Erynigium campestris*. These are widely **cultivated** in Europe (see photograph).

Characteristics: Dark brown pileus with a typical indentation near the off-center stipe. The white lamellae are decurrent, curving partly down toward the base of the stipe and attached to it.

Use: These edible mushrooms are **much appreciated** for their **delicate,** somewhat sweet flavor.

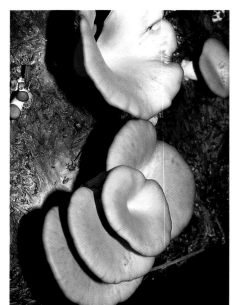

Pleurotus ostreatus ▼

Oyster mushroom

Habitat: This mushroom grows on the living or dead trunk of broadleaf trees (chestnut, beech, oak, etc.). It is widely **grown commercially** in Europe, America and Asia.

Characteristics: *Pleurotus ostreatus* has a dark brown or gray pileus in the shape of an oyster shell. Its lamellae are decurrent on the stipe, which is short and off center. There is no annulus or volva.

Use: Edible, **highly valued** for its **delicate flavor.**

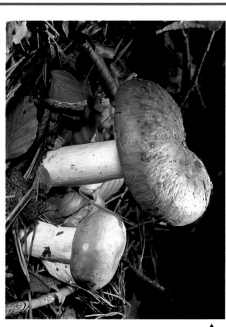

▲ Russula aeruginea

Grass-green russula

Characteristics: Similar to those of *Russula vesca* but greenish in color. Its flesh is somewhat tough and of lower quality than *Russula vesca.*

Confusion: *Amanita phalloides* (see Vol. 1, p. 148).

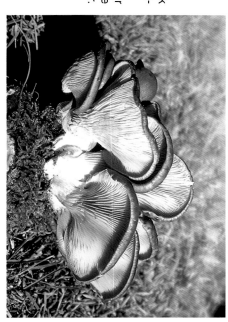

Russula cyanoxantha

Characteristics: Similar to *Russula vesca* but blue-violet in color.

Mushrooms (end)

▶ *Russula vesca*

Bare-toothed mushroom

Habitat: Beach and conifer forests.

Characteristics: Reddish or violet pileus with white lamellae. Has neither annulus nor volva.

Use: Edible, valued for its **delicate flavor** reminiscent of hazelnuts.

Confusion: *Russula vesca,* as with all the species of the genus *Russula,* may be confused with the dangerous *Amanita phalloides* (see Vol. 1, p. 148).

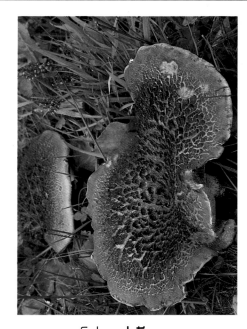

Sarcodon imbricatum ▶

Habitat: Conifer forests

Characteristics: Dark brownish pileus that may reach 25 cm in diameter, with tile-like scales. The light gray hymenium is covered with spiny structures.

Use: Only young specimens are used. This is a **very flavorful** mushroom and is used as a **spice or condiment** in a variety of sauces, stews, and other dishes.

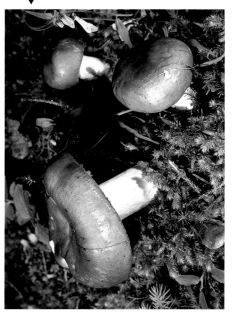

▶ *Tuber nigrum*

Scientific synonym: *Tuber melanosporum.*
Black truffle

Habitat: The truffle grows underground in oak forests in central and southern Europe.

Characteristics: The truffle is dark in color and has a shape similar to a small potato. Since they grow **underground,** trained dogs and pigs are used to find them. These animals are sensitive to their exquisite aroma.

Use: As a **condiment,** due to their **exquisite aroma.**

Related species: *Tuber aestivum* (summer truffle) and *Tuber magnatum* (white truffle).

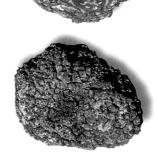

10

HONEY, SUGAR, AND CHEMICAL SWEETENERS

A LL HUMANS have an innate craving for sweets. But it has not always been as easy to satisfy as it has been for the last two hundred years since the invention of refined sugar. Before then anyone wishing something sweet had only two options:

- eat **honey**, or
- fresh **fruit**, or, even better, dried fruit.

In either case, satisfying this desire was healthy.

Appetite For Sweets Today

Unfortunately, the situation today is very different. Although it is still completely possible to satisfy this desire with honey or fruit, few choose this option. The majority, particularly children, prefers pastries, chocolates, and other sweetened foods.

Sweeteners vary widely in origin and chemical composition. The only thing they have in common is that they are sweet to the taste. Some have healing properties when eaten in moderation. Others, such as refined sugars and chemical sweeteners, are potentially harmful.

Some sweeteners can end up making life bitter for those who look for sweet pleasure in them. It isgood to understand and to use them with care. Keep in mind that *there is* **nothing sweeter** than **good health.**

Continued on page 160

Types of Sweeteners

In the broadest sense, 'sweeteners' are all natural or synthetic substances that stimulate the sense of taste by producing a sweet sensation. This includes honey, sugars, syrups, and certain chemical products.

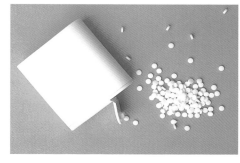

Sugars (Vol. 1, p. 168)

These substances are part of the natural composition of higher plants and milk. They are extracted from these sources for dietary or additive use.

Chemically they are either ***mono*** or ***disaccharide carbohydrates.***

The term **common sugar**, or simply sugar, refers to a white refined product extracted from **sugarcane** or **sugar beets**, which is composed *almost completely* of ***saccharose.***

Honey

(Vol. 1, pp. 160,164)

Honey is the **oldest known sweetener** and is attributed with the ***most healing* properties.** Bees make it naturally from the nectar of flowers and other plant secretions.

Chemically it is a mixture of ***glucose, fructose,*** and small quantities of ***saccharose,*** in addition to many other ***active ingredients.***

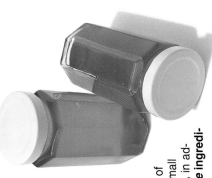

Natural Syrups

(Vol. 1, p. 174)

These are viscous liquids formed from various sugars dissolved in water. Those of *natural origin* are *rich in **vitamins*** and ***minerals.***

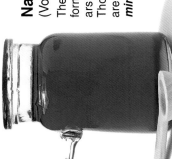

Chemical Sweeteners

(Vol. 1, p. 176)

These sweeteners are produced from other substances or by chemically modifying natural substances. They are used as **additives to foods**, giving them a sweet flavor. They have very little or no nutritional value.

The three most commonly used groups of chemical sweeteners are **polyols, intense sweeteners** and certain **amino acids.**

Although they are not sweeteners in the strict sense of the word, sweet fruits represent the most healthful means of consuming sugar (see Vol. 1, p. 38).

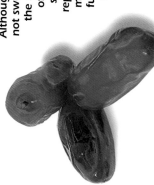

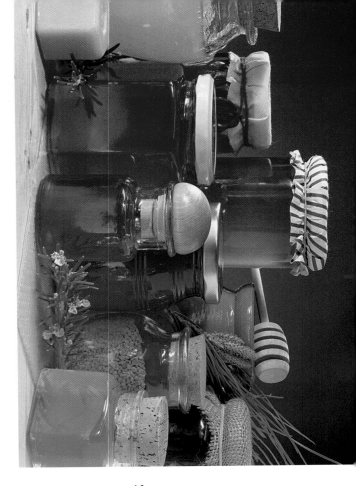

Continued from page 158

Honey

For many, honey is more than a natural sweetener. The numerous medicinal properties attributed to it, both in internal and external use, make it a *sweet medicine*. As is the case with the various types of sugars, honey is composed primarily of simple carbohydrates, in other words, sugars. However these are of a different chemical composition than that of common sugar.

Honey is unique in that it is a food between animal and vegetable in origin. Although the raw material used to make honey is of vegetable origin (flower nectar), it is predigested by animals: bees.

The Production of Honey

Honey production by bees involves three phases:

1. **Gathering:** Bees suck **nectar**, a sugary substance produced by flowers and other open parts of plants. To a lesser degree, bees also suck the **sweet secretions** of certain insects that feed on plant sap. Plant nectar is made up of 10% to 50% *saccharose* and *small amounts of* **vitamins** and **mineral** salts.

Unscrupulous beekeepers provide sugary liquids for the bees that weaken the vitamin and mineral content of the honey.

2. **Predigestion:** Bees store the nectar in a widening of the esophagus called honey stomach. There it mixes with enzymes secreted from the hypopharyngeal glands, primarily invertase, which transforms the saccharose into glucose and fructose, based on this chemical reaction:

$$C_{12}H_{22}O_{11} + H_2O = C_6H_{12}O_6 + C_6H_{12}O_6$$
saccharose + water = glucose + fructose

Upon arrival at the beehive, the bees regurgitate the contents of their honey stomach and pass it on to other bees, which continue the predigestion process in their own honey stomachs. After three or four such transfers, the predigested nectar is placed in cells in the honeycomb.

3. **Reduction:** Newly deposited predigested nectar is about 50% water. The heat and ventilation of the beehive evaporate the water until it becomes **honey**, which has a *water* content of 17% to 20%. The cells are then sealed with wax to preserve the honey.

The Processing of Honey

Once the bees have finished the honey, it is submitted to these human processes:

- **Extraction** of the honey from the honeycomb. This may be done by any of the following processes:

– *Centrifugation* of the honeycomb: This is the *ideal* method, since it does *not alter* the properties of the honey.

– **Pressure:** The honeycomb is pressed, generally at higher temperatures. This method produces *greater* **quantities** of honey than centrifugation, but the heat **destroys** the antiseptic and antibiotic substances in the honey.

- **Filtration,** to remove wax fragments.

- **Thermal shock:** In some cases industrially processed honey is heated to 80°C (176°F) to make it more fluid and to keep it from crystallizing. However, this process causes the honey to **lose** some of its **properties.**

PRODUCTS OF THE BEEHIVE

In addition to honey, bees produce other things that have medicinal properties described in Chapter 16, "Nutritional supplements": **pollen** (Vol. 1, p. 359), **royal jelly** (Vol. 1, p. 360) and **propolis or bee glue** (Vol. 1, p. 361).

Comparison of Honey, Molasses, and Various Types of Sugar (per 100 g)

Honey, brown or raw sugar, and maple sugar contain small, but nutritionally significant amounts of vitamins and minerals. Common or white sugar is practically pure saccharose. Blackstrap molasses is much richer than any in minerals (see Vol. 1, p. 175).

	Honey	Molasses	Raw sugar	Maple sugar	White sugar
Calories (kcal)	304	260	376	354	387
Carbohydrates (g)	82.2	68.8	97.3	90.9	99.9
Protein (g)	0.3	0	0	0.1	0
Vitamin B_1 (mg)	0	0.041	0	0	0
Niacin (mg)	0.121	0.930	0.008	0.009	0
Vitamin B_6 (mg)	0.024	0.670	0.082	0.04	0
Folates (µg)	2	0.026	0.026	0.003	0
Vitamin C (mg)	0.5	0	1	0	0
Calcium (mg)	6	205	85	90	1
Phosphorus (mg)	4	31	22	3	2
Magnesium (mg)	2	2	29	19	0
Potassium (mg)	52	1.464	346	274	2
Iron (mg)	0.42	4.72	1.91	1.61	0.06
Zinc (mg)	0.22	0.290	0.18	6.06	0.03
Sugars	Glucose and fructose	Saccharose	Saccharose, fructose, and glucose	Saccharose, fructose, and glucose	Saccharose
Damage tooth enamel	No	Yes	Yes	Yes	Yes
Antiseptic effect	Yes	No	No	No	No
Allergies	Yes	No	No	No	No
Bacterial spore contamination	Yes	No	No	No	No

Composition of Honey

Honey is more than sugar. It is formed of more than **70 bioactive substances**, most from the nectar and some from the hypopharyngeal glands of the bees, such as enzymes and inhibin:

• *Water:* Normally, honey contains less than 20% water. The *ideal* consistency of honey is reached when water contents ranges between *17%* and *18%*.

• *Carbohydrates:* From 80% to 82%, formed by a mixture of 31% glucose (dextrose), 38% fructose (levulose), 1-2% saccharose, and others. Both glucose and fructose are simple sugars (monosaccharides) that do not require digestion.

— *Glucose:* This simple sugar passes *directly* from the small intestine to the **bloodstream**. From there it is distributed to all the cells of the body, where it is oxidized or metabolized, producing large amounts of energy that is stored as ATP (adenosinetriphosphate). Glucose metabolization *requires* the hormone **insulin** to enter the cells and be burnt.

— *Fructose:* The absorption of fructose is **slower** than that of glucose. When eaten in *large amounts*, the fructose in honey *can cause* abdominal discomfort and **diarrhea** in some persons due to malabsorption.[26]

• *Protein:* These are present in very small amounts, from 0.3% to 1%.

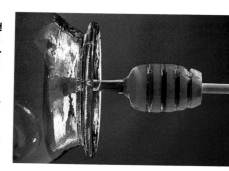

The clearer and more fluid honey is, the more likely that it has been industrially processed or adulterated.

HONEY
Composition
per 100 g of raw edible portion

		% Daily Value (based on a 2,000 calorie diet) provided by 100 g of this food
Energy	304 kcal = 1273 kj	
Protein	0.300 g	
Carbohydrates	82.2 g	
Fiber	0.200 g	
Vitamin A	—	
Vitamin B_1	0.038 mg	
Vitamin B_2	0.188 mg NE	
Niacin	0.024 mg	
Vitamin B_6	2.00 µg	
Folate	—	
Vitamin B_{12}	0.500 mg	
Vitamin C	—	
Vitamin E	—	
Calcium	6.00 mg	
Phosphorus	4.00 mg	
Magnesium	2.00 mg	
Iron	0.420 mg	
Potassium	52.0 mg	
Zinc	0.220 mg	
Total Fat	—	
Saturated Fat	—	
Cholesterol	—	
Sodium	4.00 mg	

Crystallization of Honey

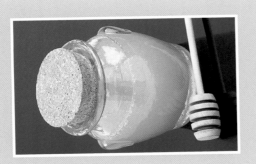

Crystallization in honey is a guarantee of its quality and purity. Since it is a saturated sugar solution, the natural tendency of honey is to spontaneously crystallize, becoming solid.

*It is **normal** for honey to crystallize. If a honey never does so, it may be due to heating during extraction or during bottling. In this case, the honey is usually heated in excess of 40°C (104°F), which destroys the inhibins and makes it lose its antiseptic properties.*

If one wishes to return the honey to a liquid state, although this is unnecessary, it is enough to warm it in a water bath no hotter than 40°C (104°F) so as not to destroy the inhibins and their antibacterial properties.

Honey must be stored away from light in as cool a place as possible to conserve all of its medicinal, particularly antibiotic, properties.

- *Minerals:* In small quantities, such as iron, phosphorus, magnesium, calcium, and potassium. It also contains trace elements, such as zinc, copper, and manganese.

- *Vitamins:* Small amounts of all the B vitamins (except B_{12}) and vitamin C.

- *Organic acids:* primarily formic acid, maleic acid, acetic acid, and succinic acid. These all come from the nectar that serves as raw material. Taken together they form about 0.3% (0.3 g/100 g).

- *Enzymes:* The most important of these is **invertase**, which converts saccharose into glucose and fructose.

- *Inhibins:* Thermolabile and photolabile (destroyed by heat and light) substances that give honey its **bactericidal** properties.

- *Other components:* Aromatic substances, a substance *similar* to *acetylcholine*, various proteins and amino acids, pollen grains, and many others not well understood.

Healing Properties of Honey

Honey is the subject of conflicting opinions among various groups:

- Some idealize it, attributing all types of healing properties to it.

- Others view it with disdain, considering it nothing more than "expensive sugar."

Taking the composition of honey into account, it can be concluded that:

- The numerous nutritive and bioactive substances, in addition to sugars, must affect the body in some way.

- The fact that these substances are present only in small amounts is no reason to ignore them. There are continuous discoveries of new and unexpected beneficial effects of substances that are found in tiny amounts in foods, such as the phytochemicals found in plants (see Vol. 1, p. 410).

Even though more study is needed, it seems reasonable to accept that honey possesses healing properties. This view is held by distinguished physicians such as Dr. *Ernst Schneider*[27] in Germany and Dr. *Yves Donadieu* in France,[28] among others, that have realized the medicinal effects of honey (Vol. 1, p. 164) in their daily medical practice.

Continued on page 168

The Bee: a Flying Laboratory

Bees produce a variety of nutritional and healing substances.

The honey bee (Apis mellifica) in the most surprising of all of the 200,000 known insect species due to its ability to produce food and medicinal products.

Posterior intestine

Anus

Medial intestine

Hind legs: these have hair-like structures used to transport **pollen** grains (see Vol. 1, p. 359), which bees use to feed their young.

Honey stomach, where nectars from flowers are stored and predigested during the **honey**-making process.

Digestive tube

Proboscis

Hypopharyngeal glands: are located in the insect's head. They produce:

- The enzymes that predigest nectar to form honey;
- Various proteins, among which are antibacterial inhibins found in honey;
- **Royal jelly** (see Vol. 1, p. 360), which worker bees feed to the larvae of future queens.

Products From Bees

- **Royal jelly** (Vol. 1, p. 360) and **wax** are secreted from its own glands.
- **Honey, pollen** (Vol. 1, p. 359), and **propolis** (Vol. 1, p. 361) are the result of mixing its secretions with various vegetable products.

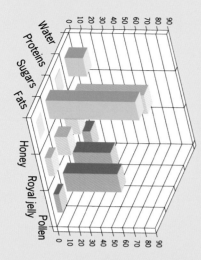

Composition of the Products of the Beehive in %

Water
Proteins
Sugars
Fats
Honey
Royal jelly
Pollen

0 10 20 30 40 50 60 70 80 90

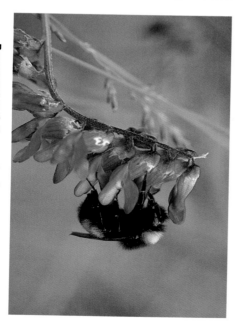

Bees must suck the nectar from two to six million flowers to produce one kilo of honey.

Honey:

Honey can benefit children, those that are active in sport or other activities requiring high energy, and those suffering from fatigue or exhaustion.

If honey is taken at the beginning of a meal, it can take away appetite.

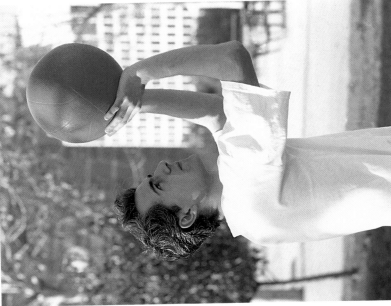

Therapeutic Uses For Honey

- **Asthenia,** either physical or nervous fatigue or exhaustion. Additionally, it provides **energy** to **muscle cells,** particularly if it is accompanied by vitamins and minerals, as occurs with honey.

- **Insomnia:** Two tablespoons of honey *augment* the effect of any **sedative infusion.** Honey helps avoid muscle spasms and facilitates relaxed sleep.

- **Underweight.**

- **Constipation,** due to its gentle laxative action, possibly due to insufficient fructose absorption.[26]

- **Infectious diarrhea:** 3 or 4 tablespoons of honey dissolved in water helps control infectious diarrhea associated with gastroenteritis caused by salmonella. Honey is also effective in cases of infectious colitis normally caused by *Escherichia coli* bacteria, due to its antibacterial action.

- **Respiratory disease:** Honey acts as a gentle **expectorant and antitussive.** If taken *regularly* (20-30 g daily) *it can help avoid* **asthma** attacks in some cases. The pollen grains found in honey have been attributed with desensitizing capabilities. They act as a type of **vaccine.**

- **Inadequate liver function** due to hepatitis, alcoholism, or other causes. The *fructose* found in honey *promotes* the production of **glucogen** in liver cells. This starch-like substance stores energy.

- **Applied directly to the skin,** honey promotes healing of infected wounds, ulcers, and burns. When used as a **gargle,** it relieves throat irritations, tonsillitis, and pharyngitis.

> *Glucose* is the **neurons'** *primary* nutrition source.

Honey: Not For Babies

Honey should not be given to children ***younger than*** **one year of age,** *since it may:*

- *provoke* ***allergies,***

- *cause* **botulism** *(see "drawbacks..." on the following page). Although infrequent, this is a real risk (in Italy a nine-week-old infant contracted botulism after its pacifier was dipped in honey).*[32] *The bacterial toxin causing botulism is very potent, even more so than tetanus, and is almost always fatal.*

A study carried out at the Centers for Disease Control and Prevention (Atlanta, USA) revealed that of the 68 identified cases of infantile botulism during two years in the United States, 16% (11 cases) were caused by honey.

Sweet Medicine

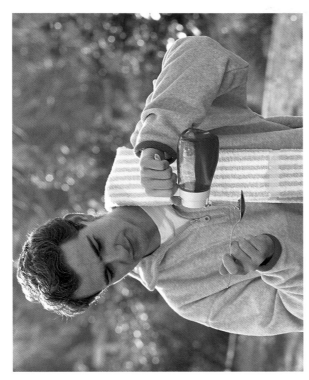

Since honey is such a concentrated food, one should not take in more than 50 grams per day. It should also be eaten little by little to avoid digestive disturbances.

 Benefits of Honey

- **Provides energy** (304 kcal/100 g = 1,270kj/100 g) **very rapidly.** Its **sugars** (glucose and fructose) *do not need to be processed* in the digestive tract; thus, they are quickly absorbed into the bloodstream distributing energy to all the cells of the body.

- It **contains** small quantities of *B* group *vitamins* and *minerals* (calcium and phosphorous) that aid in the metabolism of sugars in the cells.

- **Antiseptic:** When applied to the skin or mucosa (interior of the nose, mouth, pharynx) it destroys pathogens due to its:
  – *elevated sugar concentration*, which inhibits bacterial development;
  – content of specific substances (**inhibins**) that destroy many pathogens such as the staphylococcus and the diphtheria bacillus.

- **Does not deteriorate dental enamel:** Even though honey has an acidic pH and is very rich in sugars, it does not attack dental enamel[31] nor does it promote dental caries.

- **It has healing properties.**

 Drawbacks to Honey

- **Botulism:** Although honey does not contain bacterial pathogens, it may contain spores of certain microorganisms such as *Clostridium botulinum*.[29] In the favorable conditions found in the human intestine, these spores transform into the pathogens causing botulism. This *generally* occurs in **infants**, due to their lower resistance level. It is for this reason giving honey to **infants** *less* than *one year* of age is **not** advised (see caution on the preceding page).

- **Allergies:** These may manifest themselves in a variety of ways: itching in the mouth, digestive disorders, or even severe anaphylactic shock. This is due to the proteins secreted by the bee's glands, as well as the pollen grains in the honey.[30]

- **Diabetes:** Even though honey is better tolerated than white sugar, it must be used with *great* **caution.**

- **Toxic honeys:** Bees naturally avoid nectars from toxic plants. However there have been cases of honeys containing stramonium alkaloids (*Datura stramonium*) or glucosides from digitalis (*Digitalis purpurea*). The expertise and care of good beekeepers insure that these cases are extremely rare.

Types of Honey

Honey produces a pleasant sensation of pleasure and wellbeing, which is enhanced when the aroma of the flowers from which the nectar has been taken, is preserved.

Orange Blossom Honey

Orange blossom honey has a very delicate flavor and a *particularly* **sedative** effect.

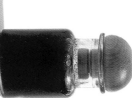

Heather Honey

This honey is disinfectant and anti-inflammatory in the urinary tract. It is useful in case of **cystitis, urinary stones,** and **prostate disease.**

Lavender Honey

Antiseptic, expectorant, and sedative: advised in case of **bronchitis, colds** of the upper respiratory system, and nervous spasmodic **cough.**

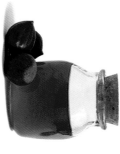

Pine and Fir Honey

Tends to be dark. Advised for **respiratory disease.**

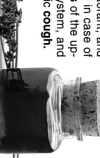

Rosemary Honey

General tonic in case of **stress** and **exhaustion.** *Promotes* proper liver function.

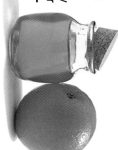

Oak Honey

Somewhat dark, but *very rich* in **mineral** salts.

Eucalyptus Honey

Effective against cough and **respiratory disease.**

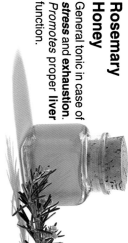

Thyme Honey

Antiseptic and digestive aid, and it is appropriate in case of **gastroenteritis.**

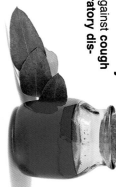

Chestnut Honey

Very rich in **iron,** however this honey has a rather strong flavor.

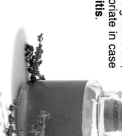

The Best Sweets: Fruit

Fruit is the most healthful way to eat sugars and satisfy the natural craving for sweets.

In Addition to Sugars, Fruits Contain:

- *Vitamins and minerals* that *facilitate* the **metabolism of sugar**, transforming it into energy.

- *Fiber*, which slows the absorption of sugars. For this reason, *less* **insulin** is required when eating fruit than when eating sugar alone or in refined products lacking fiber.

The less insulin is secreted, the *less* **fat** is produced, since one of insulin's effects is promotion of lipogenisis, in other words, the synthesis of lipids or fats in the body.

Due to all of this, the **natural** or intrinsic **sugar** found in fruit has two great advantages over extrinsic sugar added to foods, particularly if they are refined:

- it is better tolerated by diabetics,
- it is less fattening.

Calorie for calorie, natural fruit sugar is **better utilized by the body and is less fattening than common sugar.**

One large apple (200 g) = 25 g of sugar

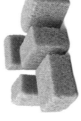 =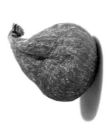

20 g of raisins = 15 g of sugar

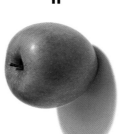 =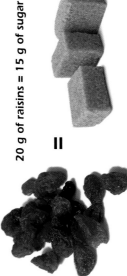

One dried fig (20 g) = 10 g of sugar

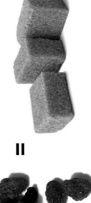 =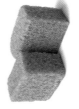

Nutritional Value of Different Natural Sweets

Very High

- **Dried fruits**, which are very rich in fiber, minerals, and vitamins.

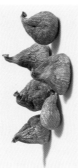

High

- **Molasses,** which is very rich in minerals, particularly iron and calcium.

Acceptable

- **Maple syrup, maple sugar, and brown sugar:** Contain small quantities of vitamins and minerals.

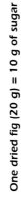

- **Honey,** in addition to being sweet, contains enzymes and proteins endowed with medicinal properties.

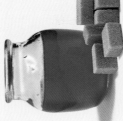

Low

- **Common sugar and other sugars** are almost completely void of nutritional elements. Thus its value is reduced to the *'empty'* **calories** that they contain.

Sugar; Is It Really Harmful?

Where does the truth reside? Is sugar harmful or beneficial? These questions can only be answered correctly by objective and balanced judgement.

Sugar Is Not Harmful For What It Contains...

Sugar in and of itself is a natural substance that makes up part of many healthful foods such as fruits and vegetables from which it is derived. It provides energy that allows the body's cells to function. It should not be said that sugar itself is harmful to health.

... But Rather For What It Does Not Contain and the Way It Is Used

The health problems associated with sugar are not caused by its own composition, but rather:

- **What it does not provide:** The problem with sugar is not what it contains (saccharose), but what it does not contain. It has no vitamins, minerals, fiber, antioxidants nor any of the other nutritious substances found in plant foods that provide protective effects. This is why it is said that sugar's **calories** are **"empty."**

 Because sugar is a more or less refined or purified extract, the nutritional balance found in the original, natural product from which it is made is profoundly altered. From a nutritional point of view, its value is *very partial* and *unbalanced.*

- **For the amount that is consumed:** Average sugar consumption in developed countries is between 80 and 100 grams a day per person.[8] This is much higher than the 50 grams accepted as maximum intake for a healthy 2,000 calorie diet).

- **For the products with which it is associated:** Sugar is usually added to rather

---

Hidden Sugar

Visible sugar added to foods to make them sweeter is only a **small part of** the total that is hidden in various types of processed foods such as soft drinks, ice cream, pastries, fruit yogurt, chocolates, etcetera.

Sugar is the **most commonly** used food **additive.** Many processed foods contain considerable quantities of added sugar. It is important to bear this in mind in order to assure that one does not exceed the 50 daily grams considered acceptable (for a 2,000 calorie diet).

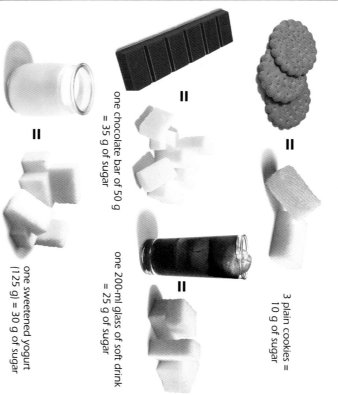

3 plain cookies =
10 g of sugar

one chocolate bar of 50 g
= 35 g of sugar

one 200-ml glass of soft drink
= 25 g of sugar

one sweetened yogurt
(125 g) = 30 g of sugar

Continued from page 162

Sugar

Few food products have been the object of as much lively controversy as sugar. Some see the growing consumption of sugar as responsible for most of the evils of modern society, from dental caries to cardiac disease and diabetes. Others see sugar simply as a chemical compound that can sweeten our lives and provide energy to our cells.

Common sugar is an artificial extract that contains only a tiny portion of the food value of the foods from which it is derived.

As with white flour and refined oil, the nutritional value of white sugar is partial and unbalanced.

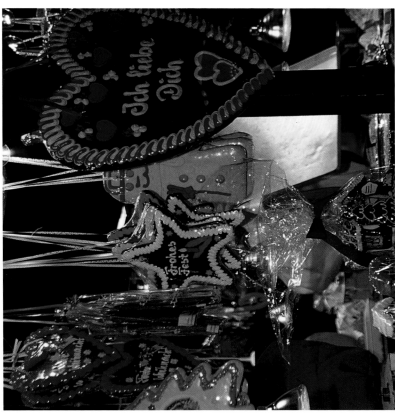

In Germany, an average of the population takes in 49% of carbohydrates from sugars, according to a study conducted at the University of Giessen. This proportion should be no more than 20% for a healthy diet.

Glucose CH₂OH

Fructose HOH₂C

Saccharose: Its molecule represents the combination of a molecule of glucose and another of fructose.

unhealthful products, such as pastries, ice cream, refined and processed foods, and artificial beverages. For this reason, eating a great deal of sugar possibly entails consuming many products that are also undesirable from a health standpoint.

Is Sugar Fattening?

Each gram of any type of sugar provides some 4 calories when it is metabolized or burned in the cells of the body. When one eats excessive amounts of sugar above the body's energy requirements, *part* of that sugar is transformed into **fat** in the liver. Each gram of excess sugar becomes about 0.4 grams of fat. This fat is then deposited throughout the body, leading to weight gain.

An even greater fat increase occurs when sugar is eaten together with fats, as with pastries or chocolate, and the excess calories are not metabolized.

Any type of sugar, particularly common table sugar or any refined sugars, is fattening if the energy they provide is not utilized

How Much Sugar?

- **Minimum:** No healthy person needs to eat sugar to maintain good health. In fact, the less sugar we eat, the better. In a balanced diet, the sugar provided by fruits and vegetables is more than sufficient to meet the possible demands of intense physical activity.

- **Maximum:** According to the World Health Organization (WHO)[9] total sugar in the diet (from fruits, vegetables, and added sugar) should not make up more than 10% of total caloric intake. For a 2,000 calorie diet, this represents 200 calories from sugar, or 50 grams of sugar (each gram of sugar provides some 4 calories).

Continued on page 174

Common Sugar

Also referred to as **white sugar, refined sugar, granulated sugar,** or simply **sugar.**

- **Origin:** Sugarcane or sugar beets.
- **Composition:** 99.8% **saccharose,** a disaccharide formed by the union of two monosaccharides: glucose and fructose.
- **Digestion and absorption:** Saccharose cannot pass directly to the bloodstream without first being digested by intestinal **disaccharase,** enzymes that *break it* into its two components, **glucose** and **fructose,** which are then rapidly absorbed.
- **Use:** This is the most widely and commonly used additive found in human foods. Its **drawbacks** are described in Vol. 1, p. 172.

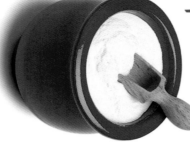

Powdered Sugar

This is manufactured by grinding common sugar crystals and mixing the resulting powder with starch to prevent it from clumping.

Invert Sugar

- **Production:** When common sugar (saccharose) is heated in the presence of enzymes or a weak acid, it decomposes into its two monosaccharides, glucose and fructose.
- **Composition:** Invert sugar is used as a **syrup.** It is formed of *equal parts glucose and fructose.* Honey is composed basically of invert sugars.

Maple Sugar

- **Production:** Maple syrup is the first product when maple sap is boiled down (see Vol. 1, p. 174). As the boiling process
- **Use:** It is **sweeter** than common sugar. It is used as an additive in baking and desserts due to its ability to keep buns and cookies fresh.

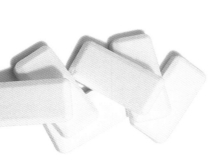

Brown Sugar

- **Production:** Most of what is sold today as brown sugar is simply white sugar mixed with a molasses extract. This gives it its color and particular flavor in addition to a very small proportion of vitamins and minerals, primarily iron and calcium.

  Authentic brown sugar, also known as **raw sugar,** is obtained through the crystallization of sugarcane juice without further processing or refining. Only it can be properly called **whole sugar.** When it is minimally processed to remove impurities and dirt, it is then referred to as **turbinado sugar.** Both are *rich in* **calcium** and **iron,** but less than molasses.

- **Nutritional value:** Commercial brown sugar is much inferior to molasses in terms of mineral content, and its nutritional value is only slightly greater than common sugar.

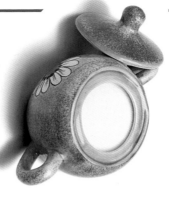

Glucose

Also called **dextrose.**

- **Origin:** This sugar is found in many fruits, particularly grapes. It is prepared industrially by fermenting starch.
- **Digestion and absorption:** Glucose does *not require di-gestion* to be absorbed; in other words, it passes directly into the bloodstream without requiring any type of transformation. Nevertheless it does require the hormone **insulin** in order to be metabolized by the cells of the

continues, followed later by condensation and crystallization, the result is maple sugar.

- **Composition:** *Saccharose, fructose, glucose,* and a small proportion of minerals and vitamins. It is *very rich* in **zinc** and other *trace elements,* as is maple syrup.
- **Use:** It can be used much as common sugar. It has a unique flavor, somewhat reminiscent of honey.

Sugar

body to produce energy. *Excess glucose is transformed into **glucogen** and **fats** in the liver.*

Glucose is the ***most important*** for the body. However, this does not mean that it is the most appropriate sweetener.

- **Use:** Even though it is less sweet than common sugar or saccharose, it is used as an **additive** in the food industry.

Fructose

This sugar is also called **levulose.** Its molecule is formed by the same atoms as glucose but in different spatial positions. Because of this glucose (dextrose) and fructose (levulose) are called isomers.

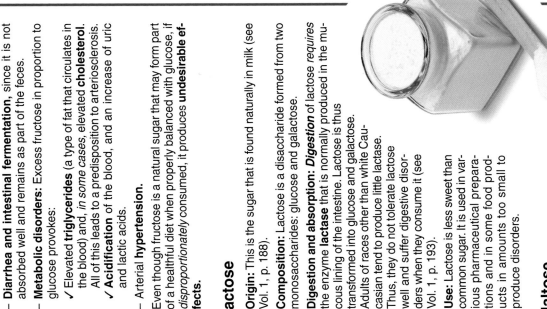

- **Origin:** This is one of the sugar types found naturally in fruits, but not the only one.

- **Composition:** Some might think erroneously that fructose contains part of the normal components of fruit, since that is its source. However, fructose is a *refined and purified* product formed only by the monosaccharide fructose.

Fructose, together with glucose, forms saccharose or common sugar.

- *Benefits:*
  - Fructose is **sweeter** than common sugar (saccharose).
  - It **dissolves *better*** in water.
  - It is ***better* tolerated by diabetics**, since it does *not* raise blood glucose level as much and requires less **insulin** to be metabolized.[4] However, this does not mean that diabetics can use fructose in large amounts: a portion of the fructose is transformed into glucose in the liver, which does require insulin; besides, excess use presents serious drawbacks.

- *Drawbacks:* When fructose and glucose are eaten in similar quantities, as occurs with common sugar, honey or fruit, it is absorbed well and causes no disorder.

However, when fructose is eaten in *much greater proportion* than other sugars, the following disorders occur:[1,6]

- **Diarrhea and intestinal fermentation,** since it is not absorbed well and remains as part of the feces.
- **Metabolic disorders:** Excess fructose in proportion to glucose provokes:
  - ✓ Elevated **triglycerides** (a type of fat that circulates in the blood) and, *in some cases*, elevated **cholesterol.** All of this leads to a predisposition to arteriosclerosis.
  - ✓ **Acidification** of the blood, and an increase of uric and lactic acids.
  - Arterial **hypertension.**

Even though fructose is a natural sugar that may form part of a healthful diet when properly balanced with glucose, if *disproportionately* consumed, it produces **undesirable effects.**

Lactose

- **Origin:** This is the sugar that is found naturally in milk (see Vol. 1, p. 188).

- **Composition:** Lactose is a disaccharide formed from two monosaccharides: glucose and galactose.

- **Digestion and absorption:** *Digestion* of lactose *requires* the enzyme **lactase** that is normally produced in the mucous lining of the intestine. Lactose is thus transformed into glucose and galactose. Adults of races other than white Caucasian tend to produce little lactase. Thus, they do not tolerate lactose well and suffer digestive disorders when they consume it (see Vol. 1, p. 193).

- **Use:** Lactose is less sweet than common sugar. It is used in various pharmaceutical preparations and in some food products in amounts too small to produce disorders.

Maltose

- **Production:** Maltose is produced by the decomposition of starch by yeast enzymes.

- **Composition:** This is a disaccharide whose molecules are formed by the union of two glucose molecules.

- **Use:** Maltose is *much less sweet* than common sugar. It is used in the baking industry.

Pros and Cons of Sugar

Sugar provides precisely what we generally have too much of (calories, 4 per gram), while it lacks what we need most (vitamins and minerals).

Benefits of Sugar

- **It produces a sense of wellbeing:** When the blood glucose level is low (**hypoglycemia**) due to intense physical exercise, fasting, metabolic problems, or more frequently, an inadequate breakfast, sugar consumption quickly alleviates the sense of anxiety and unease. However, it is *much better to avoid* hypoglycemic situations with a correct diet based on grains, preferably whole, since their **starch** releases sugar (glucose) over a period of various hours in the intestine.

- **It provides quick energy:** The saccharose in common sugar digests easily, and rapidly converts to glucose and fructose that pass to the bloodstream.

- **It is hypoallergenic:** Since it is a highly purified product, common sugar produces no allergic reaction. On the other hand, natural products such as honey and syrups can.

Drawbacks to Sugar

These drawbacks apply primarily to common sugar, since it the most prevalent. However they also apply to the other refined or purified sugars.

- **Nutritionally unbalanced:** *all* types of sugar are made of *only* **carbohydrates**, which are *practically* pure. They provide about 4 calories per gram. They contain no protein, fats, vitamins, minerals, nor fiber.

- **Metabolic imbalance:** Sugar **metabolism**, which results in energy, requires **B complex vitamins** (particularly **B₁**) and **minerals** (calcium in particular). When sugar (which contains no vitamins or minerals), or refined foods (that are poor in these) are consumed, the body is forced to use its own reserves, thus overtaxing them. This is why sugar is referred to as a **calcium "thief."**

  Liberal use of any refined sugar without the correspondent amount of vitamins, minerals, and fiber found naturally in foods, alters the metabolism of carbohydrate, fats, and proteins producing negative effects in the body.[10]

- **Displaces other foods:** Sugar satiates and reduces appetite. This leads to a reduction in the consumption of necessary healthy foods.

- **Dental caries:** *All* sugars, including natural sugars in fruits, promote tooth decay (dental caries). This is because the bacteria normally found in the mouth convert sugars into acids that attack dental enamel.

  The removal of bacterial plaque by tooth brushing and the fluoride in toothpaste may avoid the harmful effects of sugar on the teeth.[11]

  However, *it is not clear* that greater sugar consumption leads to more caries, according to an important study conducted at Reading University (UK), which analyzed data from 90 countries. In addition to sugar there must be *other* **dietary** or **genetic factors** that promote dental caries.[12]

- **Triglycerides:** Sugar consumption *increases* the level of these fatty substances in the blood, which, in turn, promotes arteriosclerosis and heart disease.[13]

- **Obesity:** Sugar and sugared foods are *important causes* of obesity in children and adults.

- **Hyperactivity:** In spite of the seeming relationship between sugar consumption and certain behavioral disorders such as hyperactivity or attention deficit, it *has* not been proven in any study to date.[14,15] It *has* been shown that **additives**, particularly food colors, can alter the behavior of certain children.[16] Current knowledge indicates that overall diet plays a vital role in children's behavior, but not specifically sugar.[17]

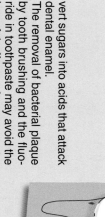
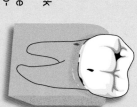

The Bitter Side of Sugar

Can it produce disease?

More Sugar and Less Fiber = Disease

Although sugar alone has no toxic or carcinogenic effects, there are studies that relate consumption of large amounts (more than 50 g a day) of sugar with various chronic diseases. It is possible that in many cases, the harmful effect of sugar is primarily due to a lack of fiber and certain vitamins and minerals displaced in the diet when a great deal of sugar and sugared products are eaten.[18]

This chart illustrates some of the diseases related to a diet that is high in sugar and low in fiber and other nutrients.

Gallstones

A long-term follow-up study conducted by the National Institute of Public Health in Bilthoven (Netherlands) showed a relationship between sugar consumption and increased risk of cholelithiasis.[19]

Crohn's Disease

The combination of a great deal of sugar and little fiber is one of the causative factors of this disease.[18]

Gastroduodenal Ulcer

The use of sugar, together with a diet of refined foods poor in fiber, increases this risk.[20]

Diabetes

There are no studies that prove that the liberal use of sugar is a cause of diabetes, but evidently it does make it worse and more serious.

Bone Brittleness

A high fat, high sugar diet depletes the calcium reserves in the body. This causes the bones to become brittle and fracture according to a study conducted at University of Southern California in Los Angeles (USA).[24]

Stomach Cancer

A study carried out in Marseilles (France) demonstrated that sugar, saturated fat, and, and calcium increased the risk of stomach cancer. On the other hand, a diet that is rich in raw vegetables, fresh fruit, and vegetable oil reduces this risk.[21]

Colon Cancer

According to the Mario Negri Institute of Pharmacological Investigation in Milan (Italy), the consumption of sugar between meals stimulates the proliferation of the epithelial cells of the intestine. This promotes the formation of cancers.[22] Additionally, a study in Iowa (USA) involving 35,215 women found that the more sugar one eats the higher the risk of colon cancer.[23]

Retarded Fetal Growth

A study at the University of New Jersey (USA) shows that pregnant adolescents who consume excess sugar, have a probability of giving birth to low weight babies.[25]

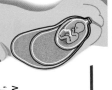
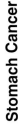
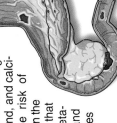
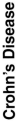
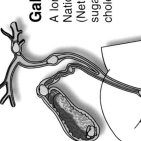
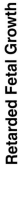

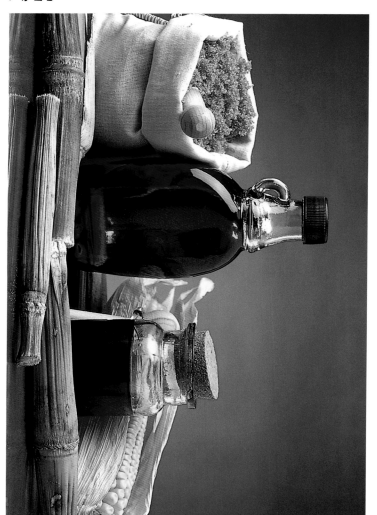

From left to right: Brown sugar, maple syrup, and molasses. In the foreground, sugarcane.

Continued from page 169

Syrups

Syrups are viscous liquids formed from various sugars dissolved in water. Syrups prepared from sugar have no nutritional advantages over sugar. However, syrups obtained from **natural** sources have the following **advantages** over sugar:

- They have a *more pleasant*, sweet flavor;
- They contain less sugar, thus, *fewer calories;*
- They provide *more vitamins* and *especially minerals.*

Types of Natural Syrups

Maple Syrup

- **Production:** Maple syrup is made by heating the sap from the sugar maple (*Acre saccharum*), a tree found in parts of North America. In early spring small

orifices are tapped in the trunk, from which comes this valued sap. A healthy tree can produce some 150 liters of sap per season, which is then cooked down to about four liters of syrup.

The **sap** is filtered and boiled until it acquires the proper consistency for **syrup.** If boiling continues, it crystallizes and becomes maple **sugar** (see Vol. 1, p. 170).

- **Nutritional value:** Maple syrup contains 67.2% sugars, principally *saccharose,* and a certain amount of *minerals* (calcium, magnesium, iron, potassium and particularly zinc). It provides virtually *no vitamins* as opposed to molasses, which is rich in vitamin B_6. It is a *healthy* natural sweetener, but of *less nutritional value* than **molasses.**

- **Uses:** Maple syrup can be used in a great number of desserts and recipes. It also makes a refreshing drink when mixed with water.

Natural syrups are healthful sweeteners. They sweeten due to their sugar content, but they also provide a variety of minerals and some vitamins.

Molasses, made from sugarcane or sugar beets, is particularly rich in iron, calcium, and other minerals.

Corn Syrup

- **Production:** Corn syrup is derived from cornstarch, which is processed with enzymes (amylase) or by heating and the addition of a weak acid. Both methods partially decompose or digest the large *starch* molecules, converting them into various sugars, primarily *maltose* and *glucose*. Some corn syrups contain a high proportion of *fructose*.

- **Nutritional value:** Its food value is in its *sugar* composition. It contains small amounts of minerals, although much less than maple syrup or molasses.

- **Uses:** Although it is less sweet than sugar, corn syrup is used as an **additive** in a wide variety of food products. It is noted for its ability to retain moisture and keep foods fresh.

Molasses

- **Production:** When sugar cane or sugar beet are crushed to make sugar a **juice** is obtained. **Molasses** is a dark, viscous syrup that remains after part of the sugar dissolved in the juice is extracted by means of heating and centrifugation. After all of the crystallized sugar is removed from molasses it becomes darker and more concentrated. This is referred to as **blackstrap molasses.**

- **Nutritional value:** Molasses contains the same nutritional compounds of the sugarcane or the sugar beets, except that a portion of the sugar has been removed through crystallization. In addition to sugars (*saccharose, glucose,* and *fructose*), molasses is a *very good source* of vitamin B_6, calcium, magnesium, iron, potassium, and trace elements. One hundred grams of molasses provides:

  - *one third* of the RDA (Recommended Dietary Allowance) for *vitamin B_6,*
  - *one fourth* of the RDA for **calcium,**
  - more than *two thirds* of the RDA for *magnesium,*
  - almost *half* of the RDA for *iron.*

Blackstrap molasses contains more than *triple* the amount of *calcium* and *iron* of regular molasses.

- **Uses in diet therapy:** Molasses is recommended for many diseases, even though there is insufficient research as to its efficacy. Its use is indeed justified in instances where there is a need to increase mineral and trace element levels:

  - **anemia** due to lack of iron,
  - **osteoporosis,**
  - **skin** disorders: dermatitis, eczema, and psoriasis,
  - brittle **nails** and **hair.**

- **Uses:**

  - As an **additive** in the baking industry. It gives sweet rolls and pastries a very pleasant flavor and helps maintain their moisture and freshness.
  - In a variety of **culinary** preparations, accompanying beans or potatoes.
  - As a kitchen and table **sweetener** in the same way as honey.

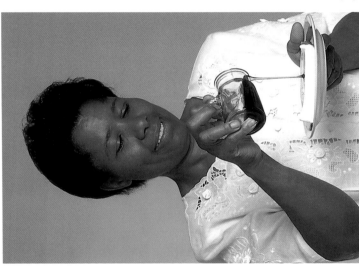

Foods sweetened with molasses are suitable in cases of anemia and osteoporosis.

Molasses, like bran from grains, was considered a basically worthless byproduct. Both of them were used as animal feed.

But now we know that molasses contains the vitamins and minerals that are missing from sugar in the same way that bran contains the fiber that is missing from flour.

Sweetening Power of Various Substances

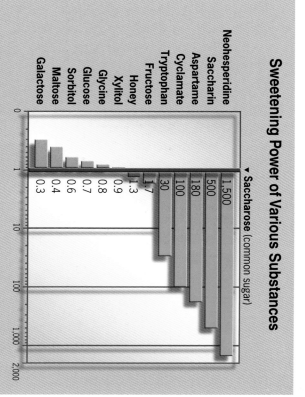

▼ Saccharose (common sugar)

Neohesperidine	1,500
Saccharin	500
Aspartame	180
Cyclamate	100
Tryptophan	30
Fructose	1.7
Honey	1.3
Xylitol	0.9
Glycine	0.8
Glucose	0.7
Sorbitol	0.6
Maltose	0.4
Galactose	0.3

The sweetening power, or capacity to stimulate a sensation of sweetness of a particular substance, is established by comparing it to common sugar or saccharose.
When equal weights are compared, substances that sweeten more than sugar or have a higher sweetening index, those that sweeten less, a lower index. Therefore comparing equal weights:

- Intense sweeteners sweeten much more than common sugar.
- Honey and fructose are slightly sweeter than common sugar.
- Polyols and the remaining sugars sweeten less than common sugar.

themselves: soft drinks, preserves, ice cream, chocolate-based beverages, etcetera.

Most chemical sweeteners used as additives belong to these three groups: polyols, amino acids, or concentrated sweeteners.

Polyols

These are also called polyhydric alcohols, sugar-alcohols or **polyalcohols**, since they are carbohydrates with two or more alcohol-type (–OH) chemical processes in their molecules.

In spite of their chemical similarity to ethyl alcohol (a monoalcohol), they do not act on the central nervous system as does ethyl alcohol and do not produce any drunken or euphoric effects.

Many polyols are found naturally in some fruits, though in small quantities. They are usually produced *industrially* using **cornstarch**. Their **safety** as additives has been the object of many studies.[5]

Benefits of Polyols

- They are sweeteners, although less than saccharose or common sugar.
- They are **very little absorbed** by the body, thus providing *fewer calories* than sugars.
- They do *not raise* blood *glucose* levels, and are *well tolerated* by **diabetics**.
- They do **not foster** dental **caries**.
- They retain water and keep food products moist and fresh. For this reason they are used as **additives** in ice cream, sauces, preserves, chewing gum, various sweets, and foods for diabetics.

Drawbacks to Polyols

- When used in *large quantities* (more than 40 g daily), they can produce **flatulence** and/or **diarrhea**.
- They should *not* be given **to children** less than **three years of age**, since they cause intestinal disturbances.

Chemical Sweeteners

Chemical sweeteners are produced from a variety of chemical processes or from vegetable sources.

Today, the food industry has more than 200 chemical substances at its disposal that are capable of producing a sweet flavor when they are added to foods or beverages, while adding virtually no calories.

The use of these substances is growing, due to the increasing interest in the developed world in lowering caloric intake. Nevertheless they pose a health risk for two reasons:

- All have undesirable secondary effects.
- Some of the foods that are often sweetened in this way are not healthful in

Types of Polyols

The most common are:

- **Sorbitol:** This is found in the service-berry.

- **Mannitol:** This is derived from a liquid that seeps from certain types of ash trees. It is called **manna** (see *EMP* p.669).

- **Xylitol:** This is found in plums, strawberries, and other fruits. It is used to sweeten sugarless chewing gum. A study conducted in Finland has shown that children that chew gum sweeten with xylitol tend to have *less* dental caries and *fewer* cases of **otitis media**.[3]

Amino Acids

Glycine and **tryptophan** are two amino acids (constituents of protein) that provide a sweet flavor and used as sweetening additives.

There is no concrete data on their possible toxicity.

Intense Sweeteners

This is the name given to the most powerful of chemical sweeteners. Their flavor is so sweet that very few milligrams are enough to sweeten a product.

The possible toxicity of these sweeteners has been the object of intense scientific debate, in an environment of commercial and political pressure. The famous Delaney Clause and successive regulations in the United States prohibit the use of food additives potentially carcinogenic to humans or laboratory animals. These regulations have been used to ban **cyclamates** and **saccharine** on the basis of causing cancer in laboratory animals and *removed* them from the list of **GRAS additives** (Generally Recognized as Safe). Saccharin is now back on the GRAS list.

However, the discussion continues. While the health risk of intense sweeten-

---

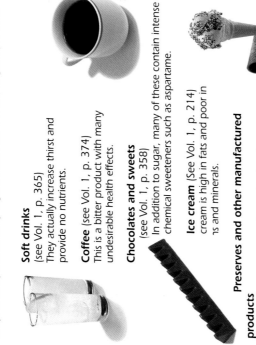

Sweetened Products

*Products with added sweeteners are generally **less suitable** from the point of view of a healthy diet. Eating them is more a search for pleasure than for health. The undesirable effects of sweeteners (sugar or chemical products) are actually higher than those of the original product.*

Soft drinks
(see Vol. 1, p. 365)
They actually increase thirst and provide no nutrients.

Coffee (see Vol. 1, p. 374)
This is a bitter product with many undesirable health effects.

Chocolates and sweets
(see Vol. 1, p. 358)
In addition to sugar, many of these contain intense chemical sweeteners such as aspartame.

Ice cream (See Vol. 1, p. 214)
cream is high in fats and poor in 's and minerals.

Preserves and other manufactured products
These are rich in salt and poor in vitamins, minerals, and fiber.

Healthy foods do not need chemical sweeteners.

There is no sweeter pleasure than enjoying good health.

---

ers is virtually nonexistent for some, for others it is vitally important and adds the many other risks we already suffer as a consequence of chemical pollution.

Types of Intense Sweeteners

- **Artificial or synthetic:** Saccharine, cyclamates, aspartame, and acesulfame K are the most commonly used sweeteners by the food industry as well as by individuals. They are also the most criticized.

- **Natural origin:** These sweeteners are extracts of various plants and are used either directly or after some chemical modification. They are little used at present due to their high cost and the fact that many of them are still in the research phase.

"Light" Products: Solution or Trap

*Even though they have fewer calories, there is no conclusive evidence that artificial chemical sweeteners such as the **aspartame** used in "light" products help avoid obesity. In some cases, in fact, they can have the opposite effect by **increasing the appetite**, with its accompanying weight gain.*

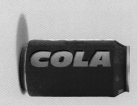

Can of regular soft drink (33 cl)
Contains 35 g of sugar = 140 calories.

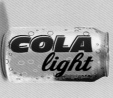

Can of "light" soft drink (33 cl)
Contains 300 mg of aspartame = 1 calorie.

Benefits of Intense Sweeteners

- They do **not** provide *calories*
- They are **easy to use**, since a very small amount is sufficient to produce an intense sweetening effect.

Drawbacks to Intense Sweeteners

- **They are non-nutritive:** They provide no nutrients whatsoever, nor do they provide any health benefits. They *merely* provide a sweet **flavor.**
- **They pose health risks:** All synthetic intense sweeteners present some risk of undesirable effects, from nervous disturbances to carcinogenic effects. There is an ADI (Acceptable Daily Intake) for each of these that should not be exceeded.
- **Paradoxical effect:** Contrary to what would be expected of these sweeteners, they could produce an *increase* in **appetite**, with its accompanying weight gain.

How Safe Are Intense Artificial Sweeteners?

A study conducted in Germany shows that 99.8% of persons tested did not exceed the ADI (Acceptable Daily Intake) of saccharin, aspartame, or cyclamates.[7]

These results may convince some, but the question remains about the reliability of the ADI values. What are the long-term health consequences after years of consuming the ADI?

Until firm answers to these questions are in hand, the most prudent course is to forego the non-caloric sweet taste of intense artificial sweeteners.

"Light" Products

Products labeled *light* are those containing the **highest level of intense sweet-**

ener. Sweeteners providing sweetness but not calories replace all or part of the sugar that would normally be in these products. In some cases fat levels are also reduced.

Benefits of "Light" Products

- Since they contain fewer calories, sugars, and saturated fats, "light" products may be useful for those persons suffering from obesity, diabetes, arteriosclerosis, or other metabolic diseases, but do not wish to give up their favorite foods.

Drawbacks to "Light" Products

- **Processed foods:** Most *light* products are manufactured using foods containing preservatives and have lost portions of their natural vitamins. Additionally, they contain many additives. Because of all of this, they are rather **unhealthful.**
- **Greater consumption:** Many persons unconsciously consume larger quantities of *light* products to reach a level of satiety or satisfaction to which they are accustomed. The result is that the total caloric intake through *light* products is equal to or greater than normal, with the disadvantage of a greater number of additives.
- **Paradoxical effect:** A sweet taste is a promise of energy: It notifies the nerve centers in the brain responsible for regulating physiological activity and metabolism of the imminent arrival of important fuels (sugars in the bloodstream). If these sugars do not arrive in the expected amounts, the neurohormonal system acts as if it has received them, enhancing weight gain.
  Although some deny this effect, it is particularly *notorious* with **aspartame**, the sweetener most used in *light* foods. It has been shown that its use can increase appetite, causing one to eat more, leading to the tendency toward obesity; instead of helping to avoid it.[2]

Intense Sweeteners

Sweetener	Characteristics	Drawbacks	RDA
SACCHARIN E 954	Saccharin was the first zero calorie sweetener discovered. It excited great expectations among diabetics and the obese. Quite accidentally the young German chemist Constantin Fahlberg, who was studying at Johns Hopkins University (USA) discovered an extremely sweet tasting derivative of coal tar in 1879, which he called saccharin. Saccharin was on the first GRAS (generally recommended as safe) list in the United States in 1959.	Saccharin leaves a somewhat bitter aftertaste. In 1972 it was removed from the GRAS list in the United States since it had been shown that *large doses* (equivalent to that contained in 250 cans of soft drink per day) caused **cancer** of the urinary bladder in laboratory animals. Currently, products containing saccharin sold in the United States must bear a warning label. This product is still accepted in the European Union.	2.5 mg per kilo of body weight per day (175 mg for a person who weighs 70 kg). This is the amount of saccharin in a two-liter bottle of carbonated soft drink.
CYCLAMATES (Sodium or calcic salts of cyclamic acid) E 952	Cyclamates were discovered in 1937. It was noted that it increased the potency of **saccharin**. As a result it is usually mixed with it to enhance its sweetening power and reduce saccharin's aftertaste.	Cyclamates were banned in the United States in 1969, when they were shown to cause **cancer** in laboratory animals. They are allowed in many European Union countries.	11 mg per kilo (kg) of weight per day.
ACESULFAME K (Organic salt) E 950	Acesulfame K is a recent discovery; it is not metabolized in the body, and is eliminated in the urine just as it is. It has a very pleasant sweetness.	There are some *doubts* regarding its **harmlessness,** and many feel that it has not been adequately tested.	9 mg per kilo (kg) of weight per day.
ASPARTAME (Two amino acids, aspartic acid and phenylalanine, and methylic alcohol) E 951	Aspartame was discovered in 1965. Its flavor is very similar to that of sugar. It degrades with cooking. It was accepted in the United States as a GRAS additive in 1981.	May cause an **increase in appetite** with its accompanying weight gain. The amino acid *phenylalanine* that it contains is **very toxic** to the nervous system, if it is not rapidly eliminated from the bloodstream. Because of this, aspartame is **harmful** to: • Those suffering from **phenylketonuria**, who cannot metabolize phenylalanine. • **Sensitive individuals** who suffer of headaches and nervous agitation when taking aspartame.	40 mg per kilo (kg) of weight per day.
THAUMATIN E 957	Thaumatin is derived from an African plant called *Thaumacoccus danielli*. It is 2,000 times sweeter than sugar and used in candy making.	The sweet taste of this product is not perceived immediately, but after a few seconds.	Not established.
NEOHESPERIDINE E 959	Neohesperidine is derived from the peels of citrus fruits. It is used in chewing gum and toothpaste.	Like thaumatin, its sweetness is perceived only after a few seconds.	Not established.

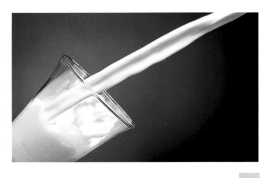

11

MILK AND DAIRY PRODUCTS

Milk and its derivatives enjoy great popularity as essential foods. While it is very important to recognize their great nutritional and culinary value, it is also important to recognize their drawbacks. Fortunately, today those who wish to substitute other products for milk and dairy products may do so without any concern that their health or their cooking will suffer in any way (see Vol. 1, p. 216).

CHAPTER SUMMARY

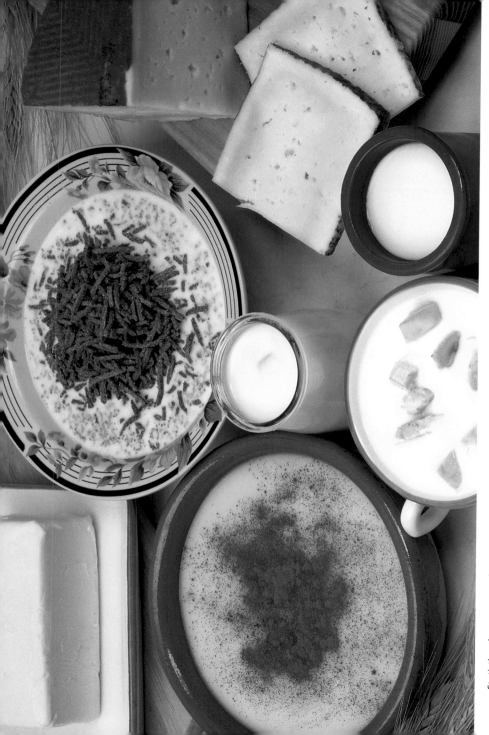

Statistics demonstrate that **dairy products** are the most **valued and used** of any **animal-based food products** in all developed and developing societies.

Milk and its derivatives (yogurt, cream, cheese, butter, etc.) have become so highly valued in the human diet because of their **nutritional value** and their **culinary possibilities.**

Dairy products contain nutrients of great nutritional value, such as **protein** and **calcium,** which are necessary during periods of rapid growth.

However, milk is one of the most fragile of foods. It can only be stored for a brief period without spoiling, especially in warmer climates.

As a consequence, a whole series of **hygienic measures** are applied to overcome these drawbacks, but at the expense of a certain **loss of nutritional value** (see Vol. 1, p. 184).

Therefore there is legislation in all advanced countries prohibiting the sale or use in manufacturing of dairy products of any milk that has not been properly sanitized in a duly authorized dairy plant.

Dairy products are innumerable. It is said that in France alone there are 300 kinds of cheese. But there is not only one kind of milk (see Vol. 1, pp. 186-187), **although cow's milk is the best known and most widely used.**

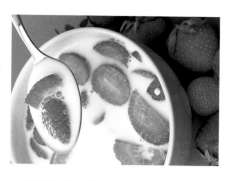

Milk and Dairy Products

- **Milk:** This is a liquid secreted by the mammary glands of female mammals, for use in feeding their young.
  When no other designation is used, the use of 'milk' refers to **cow's milk.**
- **Dairy products:** These are the various products derived from cow's milk or that of other female mammals.

From Feed to Milk

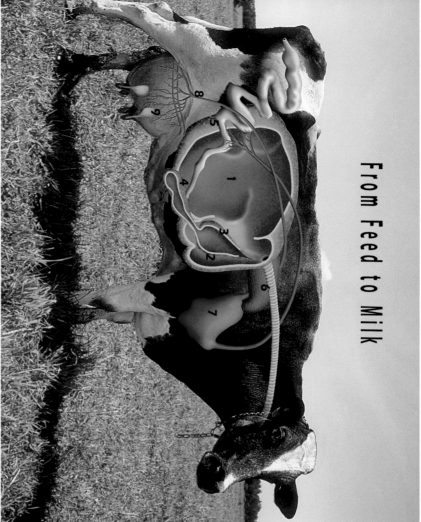

1. **Rumen:** This is the first of four stomach compartments of ruminants, where freshly eaten feed first arrives.

2. **Reticulum:** This is the second compartment. From here it is regurgitated for rumination.

3. **Omasum:** This is the organ that receives the ruminated food.

4. **Abomasum:** This is the fourth and final gastric chamber. Here the conversion of cellulose (vegetable fiber) into glucose and amino acids is completed. Rennet used in cheesemaking is taken from the lining of the abomasum.

5. **Small intestine:** This is where glucose and amino acids are absorbed into the bloodstream.

6. Glucose is transformed into fatty acids in the **liver,** and then returned to the bloodstream.

7. **The heart** circulates the blood.

8. **Five hundred to 1,000 liters of blood** must circulate through each mammary gland for its secreting cells to produce **one liter of milk.**

9. **The udder** is where the milk accumulates before it leaves through the teats.

The cow has been called humanity's adoptive mother, even though the milk that it secretes is quite different from that of the human female.

It may correctly be said that milk-secreting cells are, after those responsible for **photosynthesis,** those that contribute the most to sustaining life on our planet.

Milk

After giving birth, female mammals feed their young with milk secreted from mammary glands. This process continues for a certain length of time as long as the nipples are stimulated. The true protagonists of this process are the secreting cells of these **mammary glands.** Each of these tiny globes measures a few hundredths of a millimeter and produces complete milk. Each cell is capable of synthesizing hundreds of chemical substances from blood plasma. Millions of these perfectly organized cells are grouped to form the mammary gland.

A True Milk Factory

Through genetic selection and physiological manipulation, the female of the species *Bos taurus,* the cow, has been converted into a true milk "factory."

In the 19th century a good milk cow could produce up to 4,000 liters of milk a year. Today, it is not unusual for an animal to produce 6,000 liters up to as much as 10,000 liters annually (some 27 liters daily).

One might well ask if the milk produced so intensively by specialized animals in completely unnatural circumstances, maintains its nutritional value, or if it contains chemical contaminants that make it unfit for human use.

Continued on page 184

Types of Cow's Milk

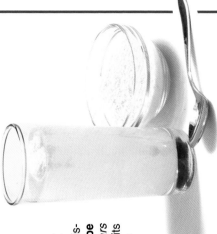

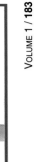

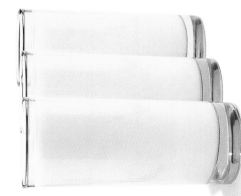

Whole Milk

This milk contains its entire original **fat content,** which must not fall below **3%.** All of its other **solid components** (carbohydrates, protein, minerals, vitamins, etc.) must not fall below **8.2%** by weight.

Because of its *high fat* content, whole milk is *not recommended* for **adults.**

Lowfat Milk

This milk contains only **0.5%** to **2% fat.** Because of this, it retains most of the flavor of whole milk but with *less fat* and *calories.*

Skim Milk

Whole milk with milkfat content reduced to **0.5%.**

Nonfat Milk

Most of the *fat* has been removed from this milk leaving a proportion of **0.18%** (its containers usually indicate *"fat content less than 0.2%").* It is less flavorful but *easier* to **digest** and has *fewer* **calories.**

In USA nonfat milk refers to skim milk.

Evaporated Milk

Evaporated milk is produced by heating whole milk to 55°C (131°F) in a vacuum until it has lost 60% of its water content. After this, it is heated to 115°C (239°F) for 15 minutes to sterilize it.

Its primary advantage is its *long* **storage capacity,** although it has lost from **25% to 50%** of its hydrosoluble *vitamins.*

Powdered Milk

This milk has 5% moisture content. **It can be stored** for *three years or more. A portion* of its hydrosoluble **vitamins** *is lost* in the dehydration process.

Condensed Milk

After removing 60% of the water from whole milk through evaporation, 40% to 45% *sugar* (saccharose) by weight is added. The need for **sterilization** is thus avoided, since the high sugar concentration inhibits bacterial proliferation.

This milk has the advantage of a **long storage life** with less vitamin loss than evaporated milk. However, its *high sugar content* makes it *difficult* to **digest.**

A Glass of Milk (200 ml) Provides:

- **Whole: 6.7g of fat and 123 calories** of which 49% are from fat.
- **Lowfat (2%): 3.84g** of **fat** and **99 calories,** of which 35% are from fat.
- **Nonfat: 0.36g** of **fat** and **70 calories,** of which 4.6% are from fat.

Nutrient Loss in Milk Due to Various Sanitizing Techniques

	Type of sanitizing		
	Pasteurization 74°C*, 15 sec.	**UHT Sterilization** 130°-150°C, 3-5 sec.	**Classic Sterilization** 120°C, 20 min.
Lysine	1%	1%	10%
Vitamin B$_1$	5%	10%	50%
Vitamin B$_6$	—	10%	20%
Folic Acid	5%	20%	30%
Vitamin B$_{12}$	10%	20%	80%
Vitamin C	25%	30%	50%
Length of storage	One week, refrigerated	Several months at room temperature, 3 days refrigerated once container has been opened	

*74°C = 165.2°F; 130°-150°C = 266°-302°F; 120°C = 248°F

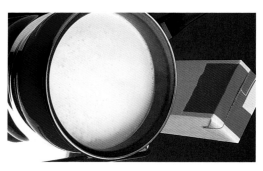

Continued from page 182

Milk Processing

Today, most of the milk used in industrialized countries has been homogenized and sanitized before it is sold for use.

Homogenization

Homogenization consists of *passing hot milk through very fine sieves under very high pressure (100-150 atmospheres)*. This way, the *large* milk **fat globules** are finely split into much *smaller* **globules** that are evenly dispersed throughout the liquid and tend not to float. This results in:

- *No* **fat** (cream) **layer** *forms* on the milk.
- The milk is *easier* to **digest,**
- The milk **curdles** *more easily* through the action of heat or acids. For this reason, *more caution* must be exercised in **storage.**

Today, pasteurization or sterilization of milk for market is mandatory in all developed countries. This represents a great advance in public health, since many diseases are transmitted through raw milk.

Boiling milk for two minutes eliminates all bacteria except those that form spores. However, it also destroys bacteria responsible for acidic fermentation, and alters proteins as well, which degrades its flavor.

Sanitizing

In its natural state, milk poses two significant concerns due to its high microorganism content:

- it is quite unstable and spoils easily;
- it transmits disease.

In the past, milk was boiled at home, which was effective. However, today, other industrial methods are used:

- **Pasteurization:** The French scientist Louis Pasteur discovered in 1860 that it was not necessary to boil milk —which changes its flavor and properties— to preserve it without spoiling. Pasteur found that heating the milk to 57°C (134.6°F) for a specified time is sufficient to accomplish this.

  Today, milk pasteurization is described as a process of heating milk to a particular temperature for a period that:
  – **destroys** all **pathogens** (but not their spores) and
  – **reduces** the number of **microbes** that cause **spoiling** or **fermentation.**

  There are various time and temperature combinations that accomplish the pasteurization of milk, but the most widely used is heating it to 74°C (165.2°F) during 15 seconds.

- **Sterilization: destroys all microorganisms and their spores** including those responsible for lactic fermentation, as well as pathogens. Sterilized milk is packaged in sterile containers.
  – **Classic sterilization:** *Greatly prolongs* **shelf life** of milk, but *considerably erodes* its **flavor** and **nutritional content,** particularly certain essential amino acids, such as lysine and vitamins B$_1$ and B$_{12}$.
  – **UHT (Ultra High Temperature) sterilization:** This method achieves the same result as classic sterilization, but with *less* **flavor and nutritional loss.** It consists of submitting milk to very high temperatures for very brief periods (2.5-5 seconds).

Continued on page 190

Microorganisms in Milk

Freshly produced **raw milk** is an **optimal medium** for the *development* of **microorganisms.** It normally contains several hundred thousand bacteria per milliliter (ml), an amount that can reach several million in summer, especially in warmer climates. The ideal bacterial count is not above 10,000 per milliliter (ml); however, this is very rarely achieved.

These are some of the bacteria that milk may contain.

Modifying Bacteria

These are not pathogenic bacteria. In other words, they do not cause disease, but they do produce certain changes in milk. Pasteurization reduces their number, particularly coliforms, but does not eliminate them completely:

- **Acid-producing bacteria:** These bacteria produce the acidification of milk by *fermenting* the *lactose* and converting it to *lactic acid.* These bacteria serve as the basis for acidified milks and cheese. They are **streptococci** (*Streptococcus lactis* and *Streptococcus cremoris*) and **lactobacilli** (*Lactobacillus bulgaricus* and *Lactobacillus casei*).

- **Coliforms:** These bacilli are of fecal origin, and give bad odors and flavors. These belong to the genera *Escherichia* and *Enterobacter.*

- **Butyric acid-forming bacteria:** These anaerobic (not needing oxygen) spore-producing bacteria belong to the genus *Clostridium.* They also produce lactic acid, in addition to carbon dioxide (CO₂) and hydrogen.

- **Enzyme-producing bacteria** decompose fats and proteins, and produce bitter, rancid taste. Their characteristics are:
  - They belong to the genera *Bacillus* and *Pseudomona*
  - Their spores survive pasteurization.
  - Some of these so-called psychrophilic bacteria thrive at temperatures in the 7° to 12°C (44.6° to 53.6°F) range. Therefore, it is essential to store raw or pasteurized milk at less than 7°C = 44.6°F (ideal is between 3° and 4°C = 37.4° to 39.2°F).

Pathogenic Bacteria

Pathogenic bacteria, as the name indicates, cause disease, some of which are very serious. Fortunately, their presence in milk has become quite rare due to mandatory pasteurization and other means of sanitizing.

Pathogenic bacteria in milk can come from:
- The **mammary gland** of an infected animal;
- **external contamination** from filth on the udder or on milking instruments.

Viruses

It has been known for some time that milk can transmit the **poliomyelitis** virus and infectious **hepatitis A.** Besides it can transmit the virus of two bovine diseases:[1,2]

- **bovine leukemia** virus, and

- **bovine immunodeficiency** virus, which causes a disease similar to AIDS in cattle.

The *possibility* that these viruses may be **pathogenic** to humans has not been demonstrated; however there are ongoing investigations on the subject.

Sterilization eliminates all the viruses found in milk if it has been properly performed. It has been proven that **pasteurization,** while not as effective as sterilization, destroys certain viruses, such as that of bovine immunodeficiency.[3] In the same way that certain bacteria such as Listeria resist pasteurization,[4] there may be other viruses that also survive this process.

Bacteria	Disease
Mycobacterium bovis	human and bovine tuberculosis
Brucella abortus	brucellosis (Maltese fever)
Salmonella typhi	typhoid fever
Shigella dysenteriae	bacterial dysentery
Escherichia coli	colitis
Corynebacterium diphtheriae	diphtheria
Streptococcus pyogenes	scarlet fever
Vibrio cholerae	cholera
Campilobacter jejuni	gastroenteritis, gastroduodenal ulcer
Listeria monocytogenes	listeriosis

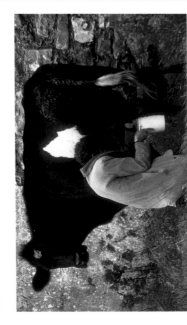

Raw milk is a true breeding ground for numerous pathogenic microbes. Drinking it before it has been sanitized presents a great health risk.

Most of the bacteria found in milk come from the udders of milk-producing animals, which tend to have fecal contaminants on their outer surface, even if they have been washed.

The Milks Most Utilized

The milk of each species is designed to meet the needs of its own young. Humans, child or adult, have the capacity to consume milk from other species of mammals that is quite different in composition from that of humans. This provides abundant nutrients; however, it also has some drawbacks (see Vol. 1, p. 193).

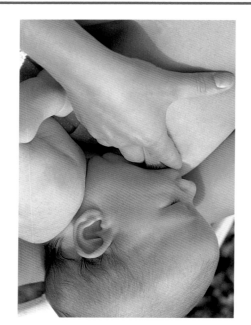

Goat Milk

Although goat milk represents only 3% of the milk consumed by humans, in some Asian countries (Turkey, Iran, India, China, etc.), it is used as much or more than cow's milk.

- **Composition:** Goat milk is *very similar* to **cow's** milk. The most important *difference* is that the fat **globules** of goat milk are smaller than those found in cow's milk. Thus, they tend to stay in suspension rather than float to the surface and form cream. Therefore, goat milk does not need to be homogenized.

- **Properties:**

  - It is *more flavorful* and somewhat sweeter than cow's milk.

  - It is *whiter* than cow's milk, since the goat converts all carotenoids (yellow and orange vegetable pigments) into **vitamin A.** Cow's milk contains carotenoids, which gives it a yellowish color.

  - It is *more digestible* than cow's milk, since its fat globules are smaller and more easily attacked by digestive juices. For this reason in the past it was recommended for children and those weakened by illness. Today, however, homogenized cow's milk is as digestible as that of the goat.

  - It is **quite hypoallergenic,** which makes it an alternative in case of intolerance to cow's milk.

Human Milk

Curiously, the milk that nature has provided for the human species is the *poorest* in **protein** and **calcium** of any milk. However, it is the *richest* in **monounsaturated fatty acids** (such as oleic acid) and **polyunsaturated fatty acids** (such as linoleic acid), similar to those found in nuts and seeds (see Vol. 1, pp. 56-57). These fatty acids are necessary for the development of the human brain.

Cow's Milk

Cow's milk contains more than *triple* the **protein** and **calcium** of human milk, although *less* **fats** and **carbohydrates.**

Its fat **globules** are *very large* and tend to float, forming cream. This makes the **digestion** of natural milk *slower* to digest than that of other mammals. Homogenization (see Vol. 1, p. 184) alleviates this inconvenience.

Even though it is the most utilized milk, its composition is ideal for calves, not for humans (see Vol. 1, pp. 190, 215). For this reason, the milk formulas designed for infant feeding are modified to approximate human milk.

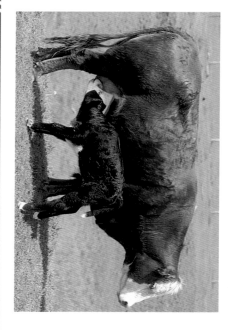

There are 300 million cows, some 25 million buffaloes, about 7.5 million goats, and around 6 million sheep in the world dedicated to producing milk for humans.

Comparative Composition of Various Types of Milk per 100 g

	Human	Cow	Goat	Sheep	Buffalo
Water (g)	87.5	88	87	80.7	83.4
Calories (kcal)	69.6	61.4	68.8	107	96.6
Carbohydrates (g)	6.89	4.66	4.45	5.36	5.18
Proteins (g)	1.03	3.29	3.56	5.98	3.75
Fats (g)	4.38	3.34	4.14	7	6.89
Calcium (mg)	32.2	119	133	193	169
Cholesterol (mg)	13.9	13.6	11.4	27	19

*This chart clearly illustrates that the composition of most used milks in the diet differs considerably from mother's milk. All have from **three to six times** the **protein** and from **four to six times** the **calcium**. On the other hand, all of these milks have a **lower carbohydrate content** than that of humans.*

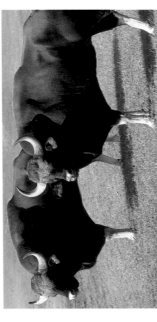

Sheep Milk

Sheep milk stands out as the one *richest* in **protein** (almost 6%), and **fat** (7%), and the *lowest* in **water** (less than 81%).

Its fat **globules** are *very small*. This makes it easy to **digest** and it is well tolerated, even though it is quite concentrated.

Buffalo Milk

In spite of its slightly sour taste, buffalo milk is highly valued in Central Asian countries. It is *noted* for its high **fat** content (nearly 7%) and the **minerals** it contains, which are higher than those in cow's milk.

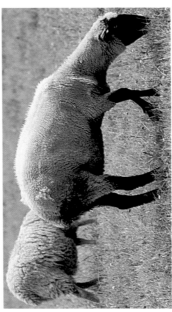

Mare's or Donkey's Milk

These milks are closer to human milk than cow's milk, since their **protein** content is around 2%. In some Asian regions it is given to the ill who have weakened digestive capability. Mare's milk is used in Russia to make **koumiss** (Vol. 1, p. 200).

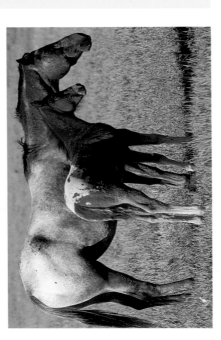

The Enrichment of Milk

Nonfat milk *is usually enriched with the liposoluble vitamins A and D, which are lost when the fat is removed.*

In some countries, such as the United States, enrichment of nonfat or evaporated milk with 10 µg (400 UI) of vitamin D per liter is mandatory. In North America most whole milk is also vitamin D enriched.

*In this way, it is thought that calcium absorption is enhanced, thus avoiding rickets in children. However, systematic enrichment with vitamin D may present serious risk. It can provoke **hypervitaminosis D**.[5] A study has shown that most enriched milks contain much more vitamin D than is permitted.[6]*

*A correct **exposure to sunlight** makes dietary supplemental **vitamin D unnecessary**.[7]*

Nutritional Value

Milk is possibly the most complete and balanced food that exists due to the wide variety of nutrients that it provides. However, it is deficient in vitamin C and iron.

Protein
(3.29%)

Milk proteins are *easily digested and assimilated*. They are of two types (see Vol. 1, p. 190):

- **Casein** (82%): Casein coagulates forming a white curd. It is deficient in the amino acids methionine and cystine.

- **Whey protein** (18%): Whey protein is water soluble and more complete than casein.

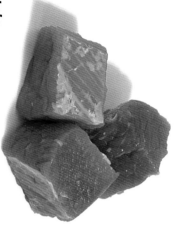

Fats (3.34%)

- **Saturated** fats *predominate*, particularly in cow's milk, in which they represent 65.8% of total fat.

- They are **liquid** at ambient room, as opposed to other animal fats.

- They are well emulsified, in other words, they are mixed finely and thoroughly throughout the aqueous whey. This facilitates the action of gastric juices and makes them *easily* **assimilated.**

Milk contains **cholesterol** (13.6 mg/100 g).

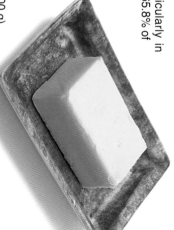

Carbohydrates (4.66%)

The *most important* of these is **lactose**, a disaccharide sugar whose molecule is formed by the union of glucose and galactose. Lactose is six times less sweet than saccharose or common sugar.

Positive effects of lactose

- *Facilitates the absorption of* **calcium.**

- Intestinal bacteria transform it into **lactic acid**, which impedes the growth of intestinal pathogens.

- The **galactose**, which is released along with glucose when lactose is decomposed by the enzyme lactase, is a monosaccharide sugar that is absorbed slowly in the intestine. While this process is being carried out, it exercises a beneficial effect, promoting the development of the intestinal bacterial flora that is responsible for the synthesis of biotin and other B complex vitamins.

Undesirable effects of lactose

- It is **not well tolerated** by *some persons*, in whom it produces intestinal disorders (see Vol. 1, p. 194). This intolerance becomes worse with age.

— Its habitual use is related to higher mortality rates due to **coronary disease** (myocardial infarction).

- **Coronary disease:** According to a study carried out at Nord Middlesex Hospital in London (UK),[8] the **most effective methods** of avoiding it are:

  ✓ *Reduce* **lactose** intake, in other words, drink less milk.

  ✓ *Increase* intake of **polyunsaturated fatty acids** (seed oils) or **fiber** (bran).

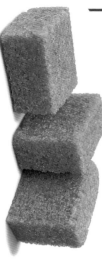

# of Milk

Water (88%)

Milk contains less water, thus more solids, than many **fruits and vegetables.**

Vitamins

Because milk is an emulsion formed by tiny fat particles and water, it contains both fat (liposoluble) and water (hydrosoluble) soluble vitamins. There is **no** food that contains such a **wide variety** of vitamins.

- **Liposoluble vitamins:** Milk contains a certain amount of vitamin A, and very little D, E, and K. Pasteurization and sterilization reduce the content of these vitamins even more. Fat-free milks are usually fortified with vitamins A and D.

- **Hydrosoluble vitamins:** These are all present in moderate amounts; on the other hand, these two are quite abundant in milk:

  - **Vitamin B_2** (one liter provides the RDA).

  - **Vitamin B_{12}** (one-half liter provides 1.78 µg, almost the RDA). Pasteurization and UHT sterilization destroy 10% and 20% of vitamin B_{12}, respectively.

- **Vitamin C:** One would have to consume six liters of milk a day to receive the 60 mg of this vitamin needed daily. Milk is a **very poor** source of vitamin C.

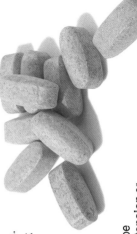

Minerals

Milk contains **all** of the **minerals** and all **known trace elements,** particularly these:

- **Calcium:** This is the most abundant mineral in milk. Three glasses (about 700 ml) provides the 800 mg of calcium needed daily by children up to 10 years of age, or an adult.

- **Iodine:** The concentration of this element varies according to where the animal has fed. Close to the coast, milk contains 37 µg/100 ml. At this level, two glasses of milk provide the RDA. Milk from cows in the inland contains about 13 µg/100 ml. Feeding these cows iodized salt increases the iodine level in the milk.

- **Zinc:** One liter provides 3.8 mg, 30% of RDA.

- **Iron** is the least abundant of minerals in milk (0.05 mg/100 ml). It would take 20 liters of milk to provide the 10 mg RDA of iron.

- **Sodium** is present in rather high concentrations (49 mg/100 ml). A liter of milk provides the 500 mg of sodium considered as the Recommended Daily Allowance. Because of this, milk and dairy products should be used **with caution** in cases of **arterial hypertension** or **low cardiac or renal output.** There are **reduced-sodium** milks available in the market.

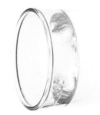

Percentage of Essential Amino Acids Provided by Cow's Milk

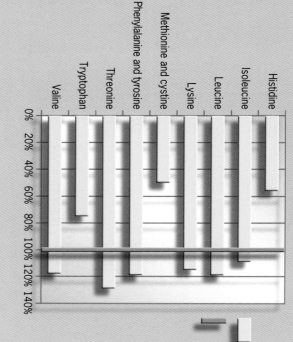

Histidine
Isoleucine
Leucine
Lysine
Methionine and cystine
Phenylalanine and tyrosine
Threonine
Tryptophan
Valine

0% 20% 40% 60% 80% 100% 120% 140%

Cow's milk

Needs for adults[9]

The **protein** found in **cow's milk**, and mammals in general, contain **all of the essential amino acids** that the body requires, but **not** in the **optimal proportion**. This means that if an adult were to hypothetically attempt to gain complete nourishment from milk, he would not gain the necessary proportion of amino acids to synthesize all of the body's necessary proteins.

As this graph shows, an adult drinking only milk would receive only 50% of the methionine and cystine necessary and would suffer a relative deficiency of histidine and tryptophan. It is because of this that milk protein is not given a **biological value** of 100, but rather **84** (see Vol. 1, p. 286). Even though it is of **high quality**, milk protein is **not complete. Ideally**, milk protein should be **combined** with **grains** or **other protein sources** in order to **supplement the milk proteins.**

Continued from page 184

Milk Protein

Quantity

Milk contains between 3% and 3.5% protein, in other words, 3 to 3.5 grams per 100 ml. An adult would have to drink about *two liters* of milk to satisfy the RDA for protein (60-70 g).

Quality

Milk proteins meet most of the amino acid needs for humans. Their **biological value** (see Vol. 1, p. 286) is *84*, which is very similar to the proteins found in legumes, and superior to those in meat or grains. It is second only to the egg.

On the other hand, milk proteins are *highly digestible* (98%); they are surpassed only by those of the egg (99%).

The biological value of cow's milk is not 100%, since it is *relatively poor* in sulfurated amino acids such as methionine (essential) and cystine (nonessential), as well as histidine and tryptophan[10] (see graph on this page).

Curiously, **children** need *less methionine* and *cystine* than adults. Because of this, cow's milk meets the protein requirements of infancy quite well. However, the milk best suited to the needs of nursing babies is, quite logically, mother's milk.

Grain *proteins combine* very well with those found in milk because:

- grain contains *excess* **methionine**, which compensates for the deficit of this amino acid in milk, and,
- grains are *deficient* in **lysine**, which is abundant in milk.

Human milk meets the needs of the nursing infant completely. However, cow's milk does not provide the ideal proportion of amino acids needed by human adults. Therefore, its protein is incomplete.

Protein Equivalents

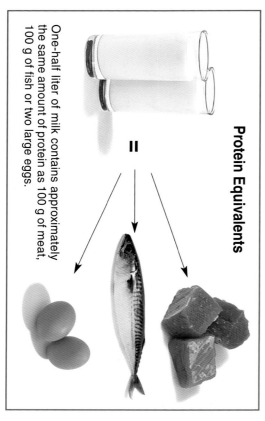

One-half liter of milk contains approximately the same amount of protein as 100 g of meat, 100 g of fish or two large eggs.

Fatty Acid Content of Various Types of Milk
percentage distribution

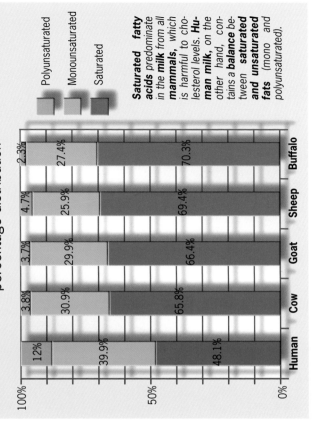

	Human	Cow	Goat	Sheep	Buffalo
Polyunsaturated	12%	3.8%	3.7%	4.7%	2.3%
Monounsaturated	39.9%	30.9%	29.9%	25.9%	27.4%
Saturated	48.1%	65.8%	66.4%	69.4%	70.3%

Polyunsaturated
Monounsaturated
Saturated

Saturated fatty acids predominate in the **milk** from all **mammals**, which is harmful to cholesterol levels. **Human milk**, on the other hand, contains a **balance** between **saturated and unsaturated fats** (mono and polyunsaturated).

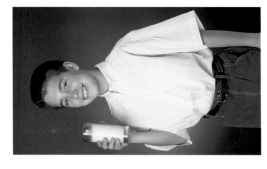

Composition of Milk Protein

The proteins found in milk can be classified in two distinct types:

- **Casein:** This is the *prevalent* protein in milk; making up 82% of the total. It has the following characteristics.

  – It gives milk its **white color.**

  – It *coagulates* or curdles, forming a solid white mass called **curd.**

  – It is deficient in *sulfurated amino acids* (methionine and cystine).

  – It contains **phosphorus.**

  – It *raises* **cholesterol** level when it is eaten in place of vegetable proteins.[11, 12] The fact that *certain* animal *proteins* can *increase cholesterol* levels, even though they are eaten in isolation, without milk fat, has become the object of interesting studies as will be explored in chapter 22.

- **Whey protein:** Whey is the *liquid that remains after the fat and curd have been removed from milk.* In addition to minerals and vitamins, whey contains a complex mix of proteins, among which **beta-lactoglobulin** and **alpha-lactoalbumin** *stand out.* They have the following characteristics:

  – They make up 18% of all milk proteins.

  – They are water-soluble and only coagulate at high temperatures (above 80°C = 176°F).

  – Their biological **quality** is *superior* to that of casein, since they *do not lack sulfurated amino acids.*

  – They are used in the food industry as **emulsifiers** and **gelling** agents, thus improving the physical characteristics of other foods such as soups, buns, and desserts.

It is interesting to note that *whey proteins* are *predominant* in **human milk.** This is the opposite of cow's milk, which contains primarily casein.

Milk Fat

Fat is milk's *most variable component.* Its quantity and quality depend on a variety of factors. For example, in colder climates cows produce more fat, and the more green feed cows eat, the higher the milk's content of monounsaturated oleic acid.

Composition of Milk Fat

Milk fat is formed of around 12.5% glycerin and 87.5% fatty acids that unite chemically to form **triglycerides.** Additionally, it contains a small amount of **cholesterol** (13.6 mg/100 g of cow's milk).

- **Saturated fatty acids:** These are the most prevalent, and most are medium-chain, such as myristic acid (14:0), palmitic acid (16:0), and stearic acid (18:0); and short-chain, such as butyric acid (4:0), which is only found in milk.

- **Unsaturated fatty acids,** such as oleic acid (monounsaturated, 18:1) and linoleic acid (polyunsaturated, 18:2), are scant in milk.

It is precisely **human milk** that contains the *most mono and polyunsaturated fatty acids.* These are **essential** to the development of the **nervous system.**

The color of milk comes from:
- **casein,** which is white, and
- **carotenoids,** which are yellowish

Milk's flavor depends, above all, on
- its **fat content,** and
- its **modifying bacteria** (see Vol. 1, p. 203).

Continued on page 194

Benefits of Milk

Great Variety of Nutrients

Milk is, *without a doubt,* the *most complete* single **food.** It provides practically every necessary nutrient, although some, such as vitamin C or iron, are present in very small amounts (see Vol. 1, pp. 188-189).

Great Concentration of Nutrients

Milk, particularly nonfat milk, provides many nutrients with relatively *few calories.*

Milk is the nutritional opposite of those foods that contain "empty calories," such as snack foods and sweets. These products contain many calories and few minerals and vitamins.

Useful in Tissue-building

Given milk's richness in protein, minerals, and fats, it is a *very important* food during periods of tissue development within the body:

- **growth periods** for children;
- **pregnancy;**
- after **surgery,** bone **fractures, burns,** or **serious injury;**
- during **convalescence** from infectious or debilitating diseases that have produced excessive **weight loss.**

Prevents Osteoporosis

Milk and dairy products are a *good* dietary **source of calcium.**[13] The *regular use of* dairy products during periods of bone development (**adolescence**), contributes to avoid osteoporosis in later years.[14]

In addition, women not eating flesh foods have **higher** bone density and **lower** incidence of **osteoporosis** *than* **omnivorous.**

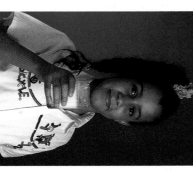

It has been shown that one of the ways to avoid osteoporosis is the abundant consumption of foods rich in calcium, such as dairy products, during periods of bone growth.

The nutrition followed during adolescence will decisively influence the health of the adult.

It Does Not Produce Uric Acid

Milk protein does not produce *any* **uric acid,** as opposed to the proteins found in meat or legumes.

The consumption of milk facilitates the elimination of uric acid through the urine and lowers its level in the blood.[15]

Relieves Acid Stomach

However, *in some cases* a **rebound** action takes place after drinking milk, with an even greater acid level.

MILK, WHOLE Composition
per 100 g of raw edible portion

Energy	61.4 kcal = 257 kj
Protein	3.29 g
Carbohydrates	4.66 g
Fiber	—
Vitamin A	31.0 µg RE
Vitamin B₁	0.038 mg
Vitamin B₂	0.162 mg
Niacin	0.851 mg NE
Vitamin B₆	0.042 mg
Folate	5.00 µg
Vitamin B₁₂	0.357 µg
Vitamin C	0.940 mg
Vitamin E	0.100 mg α-TE
Calcium	119 mg
Phosphorus	93.4 mg
Magnesium	13.4 mg
Iron	0.050 mg
Potassium	152 mg
Zinc	0.380 mg
Total Fat	3.34 g
Saturated Fat	2.08 g
Cholesterol	13.6 mg
Sodium	49.0 mg

% Daily Value (based on a 2,000 calorie diet) provided by 100 g of this food

PROTEIN
CARBOHYDRATE 4.66%

Minerals 0.720%
Carbohydr. 4.66%
Fat 3.34%
Protein 3.29%
Water 88.0%

Monounsat. 0.965 g
Polyunsat. 0.124 g
Saturated 2.08 g

Percentage distribution of **fatty acids**

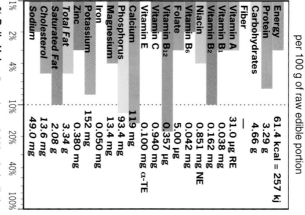

Milk is the **most complete of foods.** It contains **almost all needed nutrients,** except fiber. However, some of them, such as niacin or manganese, are found only in very small amounts. Others, such as vitamin C and iron, are insufficient. Most of the **fat** found in milk is **saturated.**

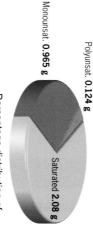

Drawbacks to Milk

Deficient in Some Nutrients

- *vitamin C*
- *iron*
- has absolutely no fiber

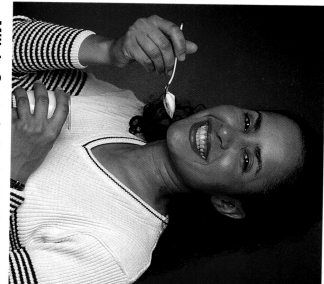

Milk Is Contraindicated in Some Cases

There are **certain situations** in which milk consumption, even in small amounts, may produce more or less serious disorders (see Vol. 1, p. 194).

- lactose intolerance
- allergy to cow's milk
- galactosemia
- stomach surgery

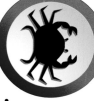

Milk Use Is Related to Cancer

There are epidemiological studies that *relate the regular use* of milk, *especially* **whole milk**, with the following types of cancer (see Vol. 1, p. 197):

- lymphoma
- ovarian cancer
- prostate cancer

Produces or Aggravates Disease

The *regular use* of milk by **adults** is *related with certain diseases* (see Vol. 1, p. 197):

- **digestive disorders** such as irritable bowel, hemorrhages and others;
- **anemia** (iron deficiency), due as much to the lack of iron in milk as to the fact that its consumption may cause tiny intestinal

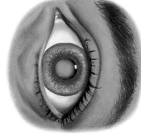

hemorrhages leading to blood (iron) loss through the feces;
- coronary disease (**myocardial infarction**)
- **diabetes;**
- **cataracts,** due to the clouding effect of galactose on the lens of the eye because of galactosemia.

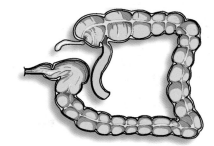

May Be Contaminated

Contamination of milk (see Vol. 1, p. 196) may be:

- **bacterial**
- **chemical** because of:
  - antibiotics
  - pesticides
  - somatotropin (bovine hormone)
- **radioactivity**

Allergy to Cow's Milk

Whey proteins, as well as **casein,** are **very allergenic.** *Some children who have received cow's milk during nursing develop milk allergy . This allergy may persist through adolescence or even into adulthood.*

This allergy manifests by vomiting, diarrhea, skin eruptions, eczema (atopic dermatitis) and asthma.[16] It is possible to have no digestive symptoms leading to the cause of the allergy.

Milk protein allergy is relatively easy to diagnose using tests available today, such as RAST.

Elimination of all dairy products and their replacement with soy derivatives (see Vol. 1, pp. 88-89) tends to lead to great improvement or complete disappearance of the symptoms of milk allergy.

Cow's milk can aggravate autoimmune diseases, such as rheumatoid arthritis.

Africans and Orientals, as well as other darker-skinned peoples, often suffer lactose intolerance. Animal milks make them quite ill. On the other hand, yogurt and cheese are better tolerated since they contain little lactose.

– *Secondary:* This is produced as a consequence of some viral, bacterial, antibiotic, or chemotherapeutic aggression to the mucous lining of the intestine. This is temporary and usually disappears spontaneously.

• **Symptoms:** Between 30 and 90 minutes after drinking milk or lactose, one begins to experience abdominal discomfort, usually accompanied by flatulence, intestinal cramping, and diarrhea. The symptoms tend to disappear after 3 to 6 hours. These symptoms are due to the fact that the lactose is not digested in the small intestine and passes to the large intestine. There it irritates the intestinal wall and is attacked by intestinal bacteria, which transform it into hydrogen and other gases.

• **Solutions**

– Completely **avoid** milk. However, if the lactose deficiency is partial, one may consume small quantities (one glass maximum) of milk without symptoms.[19]

– Use **low lactose** milk or milk **treated with lactase.**

– Use **yogurt or cheese,** which contain less lactose.

Galactosemia

This is a congenital metabolic disorder where the **enzyme** that transforms galactose to glucose in the liver is *missing*. It manifests during the first days of life with vomiting and diarrhea, and occasionally it produces psychomotor retardation and cataracts. Feeding the baby with **soy** derivatives can be effective in treating this disorder.

Stomach Surgery Patients

Patients who have undergone stomach surgery (pyloroplasty or gastrectomy) experience what is known as *dumping syndrome* some 15 to 30 minutes after milk intake.

This is due to the fact that foods, and specifically milk, pass very rapidly through

---

Continued from page 191

Milk: Contraindications

There are various situations where one should not use milk to avoid potentially serious health consequences.

Lactose intolerance

This is due to the *reduction or absence of* **lactase** in the digestive tract. This enzyme is responsible for digesting lactose and converting it into glucose and galactose.

• **Types of lactose intolerance**

– *Congenital:* This is a congenital metabolic malfunction that is quite rare. Lactase is absent from birth.

– *Primary:* This is of unknown cause, and is due to a progressive diminishing of lactase production in the cells of the intestinal mucosa, beginning around two or three years of age. The incidence of adult individuals with lactase deficit varies according to their place of origin. For example:[17]

✓ Swiss: 7%
✓ Mexican:[18] 20-60%
✓ Japanese: 85%
✓ African blacks: 90%.

Diseases Produced or Aggravated by Milk

the intestine, producing nausea, dizziness, cramps, and diarrhea.

Avoiding milk and **sweetened foods** causes symptoms to disappear.

Digestive disorders

In some **sensitive individuals**, cow's milk acts as an irritant to the digestive system, producing a wide variety of disorders, such as:

- **Abdominal pain** and other symptoms similar to those of lactose intolerance, without that being the true cause.[20]

- **Constipation**[21] and *aggravation* of **irritable bowel**[61] (alternating constipation and diarrhea).

- **Gastroduodenal ulcer:** Currently, *liberal use of milk* is *discouraged* in cases of ulcer. It has been shown that, although it momentarily relieves acidity, it stimulates a *rebound* effect resulting in the secretion of even more stomach acid. There are studies that relate milk consumption with stomach and duodenal ulcers.[22,23]

- **Intestinal hemorrhage:** It has been demonstrated that cow's milk can produce inflammation and small intestinal hemorrhages in **nursing infants**,[24,25] which may cause **anemia** due to blood loss.

Anemia

Liberal use of milk *may* cause anemia because, since it satisfies the appetite, there is a tendency *not* to eat **enough** of other **foods** *rich in* **iron**.

Diabetes

Various studies[26,27] demonstrate that **infants** that have been fed cow's milk are at greater *risk* of **insulin-dependent diabetes** from childhood. This type of diabetes,

known as "type 1," requires daily insulin injections.

The **risk** is up to *50% greater* when infants *younger* than *four months* are fed cow's milk.[27] It seems that cow's milk produces an autoimmune allergic reaction in the beta cells of the pancreas where insulin is secreted.[28]

However, *not all studies agree*. A study conducted at the University of Colorado (USA)[29] concluded that no relationship exists between the early consumption of cow's milk and the autoimmune destruction of pancreatic beta cells.

Cataracts

Galactose, one of the simple sugars that make up *lactose* or milk sugar, can cause the lens of the eye to become opaque (cataracts) *in sensitive individuals.*[30]

The *habitual* adult **use** of milk may be one of the causes of cataracts in **certain individuals.**

In addition to cases of true lactose intolerance or milk allergy, milk causes digestive disorders in many adults.

Milk and the Heart

Many studies have shown that milk consumption, **even nonfat milk,** constitutes a risk **factor** for coronary disease (**angina pectoris** and **myocardial infarction**). This is due to negative effects that certain milk components have on cholesterol levels and the cardiovascular system.

- **Saturated fats:** The **predominant fats** in cow's milk are saturated (see Vol. 1, p. 191), which fosters cholesterol production in the body. Using **whole milk and butter** increases mortality rates by myocardial **infarction,** since milk fat also promotes **arteriosclerosis** and arterial **thrombosis.**[31] **Replacing** whole milk with **nonfat milk reduces the risk** of coronary disease.[32]

- **Casein:** This is the prevalent protein in milk, and gives it its white color. When compared with vegetable proteins, casein **increases** cholesterol level 11, 12 (see Vol. 1, p. 191).

- **Lactose:** This is the sugar in milk, which also plays a role in the development of coronary disease[8] (see Vol. 1, p. 188).

There is sufficient data to **discourage** the use of milk, **even nonfat,** in cases of **arteriosclerosis,** myocardial **infarction,** and **heart disease** in general.

Radioactive Contamination of Milk

The nuclear disaster at Chernobyl (Ukraine) in 1986 showed that cattle who feed in areas contaminated by radioactive rain produce milk that is also contaminated by radioactive heavy metals.

*As is the case with pesticides, animals **concentrate** the radioactivity found in contaminated plants many times over. Because of this, the meat and **secretions** of these animals are **much more dangerous** than the plants themselves.*

After a nuclear accident or explosion, the milk or meat from cattle within hundreds or even thousands of kilometers from the site should not be used for various years.

MILK STORAGE

It is extremely important to store milk properly to **avoid the proliferation of microorganisms:**

Temperature: The ideal is between 3° and 4°C (37.4° to 39.2°F).

Packaging: must be opaque to **protect** the milk **from light,** which destroys certain vitamins.

---

tained during antibiotic treatment and up to 48 hours after the last treatment must not be placed on the market. When this is ignored, traces of antibiotic remain in the milk. These are undetectable in the taste of the milk. However, they produce undesirable effects for the consumer, such as:

– **Allergic reactions.**

– **Induced bacteriological resistance:** Ingestion of antibiotics, *even in small amounts*, can habituate the pathogenic bacteria within the body to their presence. When these microbes develop and a physician administers an antibiotic treatment, it is possible that it will not be effective, since bacteria have developed the capability to resist it.

Contamination of Milk

Milk is a food that is prone to various types of contamination. It is best to be aware of them in order to avoid them.

Bacterial Contamination

Despite the cleanliness of the milking process, milk in its *natural* state contains numerous **bacteria**, some of which may be pathogens. It may also be a vehicle for some **viruses** (see Vol. 1, p. 185).

Sanitation methods avoid this problem:

• **Pasteurization** (see Vol. p. 184) only destroys bacterial pathogens, but preserves most of the vitamins and flavor of the milk.

• **Sterilization** (see Vol. 1, p. 184) is safer, since it destroys all bacteria and viruses, although it also causes the loss of some vitamins and flavor.

Chemical Contamination

Many substances hazardous to human health pass through the cow to the milk. Among these are:

• **Antibiotics:** Penicillin is widely used to treat mastitis (mammary inflammation) in cows. Cattle are also given many other antibiotics. Theoretically, milk ob-

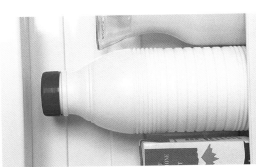

• **Pesticides:** Cattle, like all animals, *concentrate* pesticides that they eat with their feed and *accumulate* it in their body tissue. *Most pesticides* are **fat** soluble, and they combine with the fat fraction of the milk.[33] According to the proponents of so-called "organic farming," even though pesticides in milk do not reach maximum permitted levels, they constitute a hazard to health because of their **carcinogenic effect.**

• **Bovine somatotropin:** Mammals normally produce this hormone in the anterior lobe of the pituitary gland. When it is injected into cows, milk production can be increased 15%-20%, although the animals urinate less.

There is considerable disagreement among scientists concerning the use of this hormone, and according to the latest conclusions:[34]

– *It does not diminish the* **quality** *of the milk.*

– Although a small amount of this hormone is found in milk, there is *no risk* to **humans** that consume it. This is because pasteurization destroys 90% of the somatotropin, as well as the fact that it is not absorbed in the intestine.

In spite of these reassuring reports, the use of somatotropin to increase milk production is rejected by proponents of "organic" foods, since it involves the artificial manipulation of the cow's physiology.

Milk and Cancer

The habitual consumption of milk by adults has been statistically related to the appearance of various types of cancer.

More revealing studies are anxiously awaited that shed light on the disturbing relationship between milk and cancer. Below are some examples of those known to date:

Lymphoma

A longitudinal study was conducted at the University of Bergen (Norway) over eleven and a half years to test the relationship, if any, between milk and lymphoma. It found that those that drank two or more glasses of cow's milk daily had a three to four times greater risk of suffering from lymphoma than those that drank less than a glass a day.[35]

This 340% greater risk of lymphoma (cancer of the lymphatic organs) indicates a strongly positive correlation between milk use and cancer. The fact that cow's milk can transmit the bovine leukemia virus is one of the possible explanations.[36]

Ovarian Cancer

A study conducted at the Roswell Park Institute of Buffalo, New York (USA),[37] confirmed that women that drink more than one glass of whole milk a day, have a three times greater risk of ovarian cancer than those who never drink it.

Curiously, the use of nonfat milk does not present a greater risk of this type of cancer. Because of this, some investigators *speculate* that the substance that promotes this cancer is **milk fat** itself. However, an *in vitro* study demonstrates the opposite;

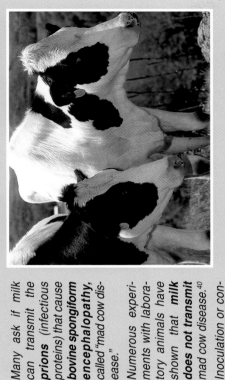

"Mad Cow Disease" and Milk

Many ask if milk can transmit the **prions** *(infectious proteins) that cause* **bovine spongiform encephalopathy,** *called "mad cow disease."*

Numerous experiments with laboratory animals have shown that **milk does not transmit** *mad cow disease.*[40]

Inoculation or consumption of infected nerve or bone tissue do transmit it, however, even though physical (heat) or chemical (formol or alcohol) sterilizing techniques have been employed.

that certain of the fatty acids in milk may prevent the cancerous degeneration of cells.[38]

Prostate Cancer

A study at The Mario Negri Institute of Investigation in Milan (Italy),[39] found that the habitual use of whole or skim milk raises the risk of prostate cancer. However, **cheese** or **butter,** do **not.** Men that drink:

- from one to two glasses of milk a day, have a 20% greater *risk* than men that do not drink milk or that do so only occasionally.

- And for those who drink two or more glasses a day, the *risk* is *multiplied* five-fold (500%).

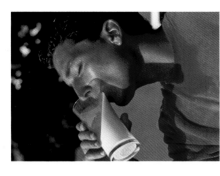

Even though study results are occasionally contradictory, there is ample scientific evidence that regular milk consumption increases risk of certain types of cancer.

Continued on page 201

Dairy Products

Dairy products may be produced by various means:

- **Separation** of milk components
  - *Spontaneously:* When freshly milked and placed to rest, milk spontaneously separates into three parts: **cream**, **whey**, and **curd**.

  - By a variety of **home or industrial methods.**

- By **fermentation** of milk by various microorganisms: **yogurt, biotic yogurt, kefir,** etcetera.
- **By a combination** of both processes (separation and fermentation): **cheeses.**

Cream

This component contains milk's *fatty* material and **cholesterol** (see Vol. 1, p. 191).

Milk Curd

This is the solid mass formed when milk is coagulated. There are two types of milk curd:

- **Spontaneous or natural:** This is formed when fresh milk is placed to rest. It is formed principally of casein (the most abundant protein in milk). It contains virtually no cream or whey, which separate spontaneously.

- **Milk curd coagulated by adding animal rennet to milk.** It contains the cream and part of the whey. It is used:
  - For cheesemaking by removing the whey (see Vol. 1, p. 206).
  - As a dairy product.

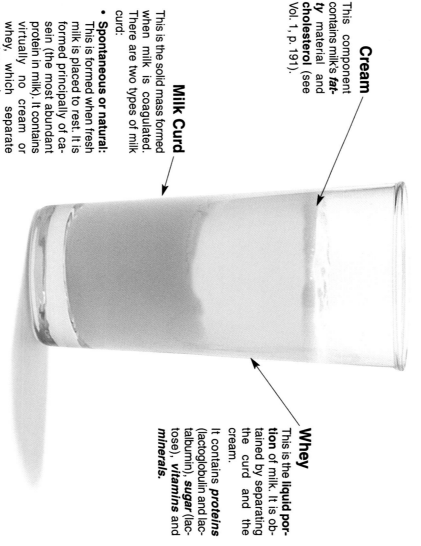

Whey

This is the **liquid portion** of milk. It is obtained by separating the curd and the cream.

It contains *proteins* (lactoglobulin and lactalbumin), *sugar* (lactose), *vitamins* and *minerals.*

A Complex Mixture

From a physicochemical point of view, milk is a heterogeneous blend of numerous substances that form:

- *an **emulsion** (fat),*
- *a **suspension** (casein),*
- *a **solution** (whey proteins, lactose, vitamins, and minerals).*

Derived Through Separation

Whey

Milk whey is a very nutritious liquid that possesses medicinal properties.

- **Composition:** Whey is a solution of diverse substances of great nutritional value in water, which forms 93% of its weight:
  - *Lactose* or milk sugar (see Vol. 1, p. 188).
  - *Proteins* of very *high* biological value, superior to casein (see Vol. 1, p. 190).
  - *Minerals, particularly calcium.*
  - Hydrosoluble *vitamins,* particularly those of the *B group. Vitamin B_{13},* or *orotic acid,* stands out among these. It stimulates the growth and regeneration of cells (see Vol. 1, p. 189).
  - contains *very little* **fat** (1.5% of dry weight) and no cholesterol.
- **Medicinal use:** Whey has a slightly sour taste, but is refreshing and pleasant. It is an *effective blood* **depurative** and **restorative.** In Switzerland there are clinics that specialize in treatments using whey (1-2 liters

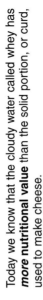

a day). They achieve *positive results* in cases of:

- **rheumatic disease,**
- **hypertension** and **arteriosclerosis,**
- **obesity** and **diabetes.**
- **Industrial uses:**
  Whey has long been considered a by-product of the cheesemaking process, and in many regions it was fed to animals or dumped into rivers.

Today we know that the cloudy water called whey has *more* **nutritional value** than the solid portion, or curd, used to make cheese.

Dehydrated and converted to **powder,** whey is used as an ingredient in many food products such as buns and rolls, milk-based beverages, and preserves.

Whey proteins are coagulated into whey cheese or **ricotta** (see Vol. 1, p. 213).

Milk Curd

Even though it resembles yogurt, its manufacturing process properties are quite different.

- **Manufacture:** milk curd is produced by adding **rennet,** usually animal, to pasteurized cow's or sheep milk at a temperature of 35°C (95°F). The milk is completely *coagulated* about 30 minutes later into a solid that is referred to as **milk curd** or simply **curd.**

This enzymatic coagulation process is the same as that used in the first phase of cheesemaking. If the whey is removed from the curd and it is allowed to mature, it becomes cheese (see Vol. 1, p. 206).

- **Properties:** Milk curd has not been bacterially fermented, and does not contain lactic acid. Therefore it is tasteless and does not have the therapeutic properties of yogurt.
- The **nutritional value** of milk curd is the *same as the* **milk** it is made from. It is somewhat *easier* to **digest** than liquid milk because of its coagulation.

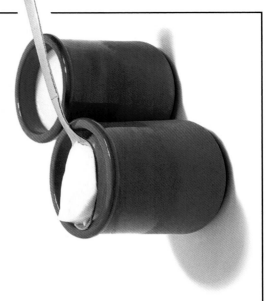

Differences Between Yogurt and Milk Curd

	Yogurt	Milk curd
COAGULATING AGENT	Lactic acid bacteria	Animal rennet
TYPE OF COAGULATION	Acid	Enzymatic
BACTERIAL FERMENTATION	Yes	No
PROBIOTIC FOOD	Yes	No

Dairy Products Derived Through Fermentation

Fresh milk, and even pasteurized milk, **ferments** *spontaneously* at a temperature between 20° and 40°C (between 68° and 104°F). Milk coagulates due to the action of two types of microorganisms:

– the lactic acid bacteria in the milk itself,
– the bacteria in the environment.

From ancient times Eastern Mediterranean and Southeast Asian civilizations developed methods of controlled milk fermentation using the milk's own modifying, particularly lactic acid, bacteria (see Vol. 1, p. 203). Today, the food industry offers a wide variety of fermented dairy products, although many are still produced at home.

Whey Fermentation

- **Acidified whey:** This has the benefits of whey (see Vol. 1, p. 199) and of the fermentation producing lactobacilli.

- **Ricotta** or whey cheese (see Vol. 1, p. 213).

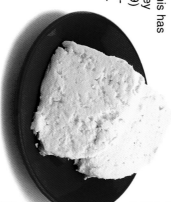

Ricotta

Fermented Dairy Products (From Whole or Nonfat Milk)

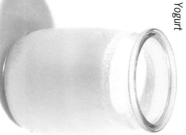

Yogurt

- **Yogurt** (see Vol. 1, pp. 202-203).

- **Acidified or soured milk:** This is made from pasteurized milk, generally nonfat, which is fermented using *Lactobacillus acidophilus* bacteria. Its appearance is similar to that of yogurt, although somewhat more acid and less thick.

  It has the same benefits and uses as biotic yogurt (see Vol. 1, p. 203).

- **Kefir:** This comes from the Caucasus. It is made by fermenting cow's, goat or sheep by means of "kefir balls", about the size of a pea or a hazelnut, made up of:

  – coagulated *casein*;
  – various species of **bacteria** from the genera *Lactobacillus* and *Streptococcus* that produce lactic acid (see Vol. 1, p. 203);
  – *yeasts* that convert lactose (milk sugar) into alcohol.

  In addition to the nutrients found in milk, kefir contains about 5% carbon dioxide (CO_2), 0.6%-0.9% lactic acid, and 1%-2% ethyl alcohol. It is refreshing, nutritious, and easy to digest.

- **Koumiss:** the inhabitants of the Southern Russian steppes make this of **mare's** or **camel's milk.** It is similar to kefir, although more foamy, denser, and richer in alcohol (up to 3%). In Russia it is used as a treatment for pulmonary tuberculosis.

Cream Fermentation

- **Sour cream:** When cream is fermented with *Streptococcus lactis,* it becomes more digestible and acquires a pleasant acid taste.

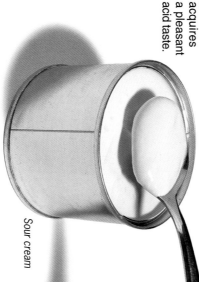

Sour cream

Fermentation and Maturation of Curd

- **Cheese:** This is made by submitting curd to a process of maturation or curing that in reality degrades its nutrients (see Vol. 1, p. 206).

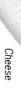

Cheese

Benefits of Fermented Dairy Products

Milk that has been fermented by lactic acid bacteria (see Vol. 1, p. 203):

- contains **less lactose** and is **better tolerated;**
- is of an acidity that **inhibits** the development of **pathogenic microbes;**
- contains beneficial bacteria and lactic acid that **regenerate the intestinal flora;**
- lactic acid coagulates its **casein** (protein), which is **predigested** by the bacteria;
- **combats** intestinal **infection** and **increases resistance** to disease.

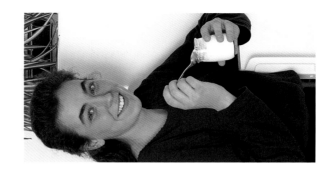

Continued from page 197

Yogurt, the Most Popular Dairy Product

Yogurt is semisolid, white fermented cow's milk, with a somewhat acid or sour flavor. Originally from Southeast Asia, it was introduced in Europe at the beginning of the 20th century from Turkey and Bulgaria.

Production

Processing whole or nonfat milk as follows makes yogurt:

1. Homogenization and pasteurization

2. When the milk is between 40° and 45°C (between 104° and 113°F) it is inoculated at 2% proportion with **bacteria,** which produce lactic acid. Milk is the ideal medium for these bacteria, and they reproduce rapidly.

3. Fermentation during 4-8 hours. The bacteria induce the following compositional changes in the milk:

- **Lactose:** Its level is lowered, since it is partially transformed into lactic acid.
- **Proteins:** These are coagulated and partially digested by the microorganisms, which convert them into peptides (protein fragments) easier to digest.

4. Cooling and packaging

Lactic Acid

Its chemical formula is $C_3H_6O_3$. Bacteria of the genus *Lactobacillus* produce it when fermenting **lactose** (milk sugar).

- **Functions:**

  - In **milk:** It causes the casein to coagulate, and gives yogurt and other fermented dairy products their typical acidic flavor. Additionally, it prevents the development of putrefying or pathogenic bacteria in the milk.

  - In the **cells:** Lactic acid is produced when glucose is burned in the absence of oxygen (anaerobic glycolysis), and can be used as an energy source for the cardiac muscle.

  - In the **intestine:** Lactic acid may reach in the intestine by means of foods such as yogurt, which contains about 1%. Intestinal bacteria may also synthesize it. It contributes to the *balance* of **intestinal flora,** preventing the growth of pathogenic bacteria.

- **Types:** There are two types of **lactic acid** molecules, which are *isomers* (they have the same chemical composition, but a different spatial configuration): **dextrorotatory** and **levorotatory.**

  - **dextrorotatory lactic acid is** *the only one* **utilized** by the body. It is found in the following proportions:
    - ✓ common yogurt: 50% of the total lactic acid;
    - ✓ biotic yogurt: 70% of the total lactic acid.

  - **Levorotatory lactic acid** is **not well tolerated by nursing infants.** As a result, it is preferable to feed them biotic yogurt rather than common yogurt.

Continued on page 204

Yogurt:

Each yogurt contains millions of living things, lactic acid bacteria, that convert it into the most healthful of all dairy products. This is why it is called "probiotic," a term of Greek origin that means "pro life."

Benefits of Yogurt

- **High nutritional value:** Its composition is very *similar* to that of **milk**. Because of this, it provides a wide variety of vitamins and minerals in addition to protein and calcium.

- **Absorption of nutrients:** The nutrients in yogurt are assimilated and absorbed *better* than those in milk because of the fermentation produced by **lactic acid bacteria.** [41]

- **Better tolerated than milk:** The lactic acid bacteria in yogurt transform part of the *lactose* into lactic acid. This improves the digestion of the lactose that remains. [42] Those that suffer digestive disorders with milk, **tolerate yogurt *much better.***

- **Helps prevent intestinal infections:** The lactic acid bacteria in yogurt, together with the **calcium** that it contains, *increases* the digestive system's **resistance** to infections caused by pathogenic microorganisms such as **salmonella.** [43] Yogurt inhibits the growth of bacteria in cases of **gastroenteritis** or **infectious colitis**, and helps stop diarrhea.

- **Increases resistance** against infections, particularly those of the digestive tract. [44]

- **Effective on allergic diseases:** Some studies show that yogurt has a positive effect on atopic dermatitis (a type of allergic eczema), [45] but others find that it produces no benefit in cases of skin [46] or respiratory [47] allergies. When presented with this doubt, the recommendation is that yogurt, as well as milk and other dairy products, be avoided.

- **Increases longevity:** Although there is no statistical proof, inhabitants of the Caucasus region of Southwest Russia attribute their traditional longevity to the consumption of yogurt.

- **Protects against cancer:** Numerous studies demonstrate that yogurt:

  – Inhibits the mutation of cancer-causing cells. [48]

  – Neutralizes the carcinogenic action of certain substances, such as nitrosamine. This is particularly the case with biotic yogurt. [49]

  – Protects against breast cancer (milk, on the other hand does not provide protection, see Vol. 1, p. 197). [50]

The most healthful yogurts are those that contain live, active bacteria, particularly of the genus Lactobacillus. Yogurt is a food that is very much alive.

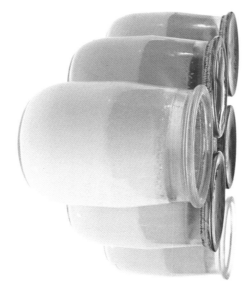

Situations Where Yogurt Is Particularly Recommended

- *Malnutrition.*
- *Infancy, pregnancy, and old age.*
- *Digestive disorders, particularly diarrhea from gastroenteritis or colitis.*
- *Disturbance of the intestinal flora after antibiotic treatments.*
- *Immunodepression (lowered resistance to infection).*
- *Cancer prevention.*

a Probiotic Food

Yogurt's numerous healing properties are not so much the result of its composition, which is very similar to milk, but to its content of certain bacteria.[51]

Very Healthful Bacteria

Milk contains modifying *lactic acid* bacteria (see Vol. 1, p. 201), which produce spontaneous fermentation. Additionally, it is possible to add others to obtain specific products, such as yogurt:

- ***Lactobacillus bulgaricus and Streptococcus thermophilus:*** are used in the preparation of **common yogurt.** These species are not normally found among the human intestinal flora. For this reason, only a few reach the colon alive.

- ***Lactobacillus acidophilus:*** The strain of this bacterium known as "LA1," is normally found in the human intestine. It is used, together with *Streptococcus thermophilus* in the production of **biotic yogurt.**

  Lactobacillus acidophilus provides the following benefits:

  – it reaches the colon alive;

  – it attaches itself to the intestinal mucosa, replacing pathogenic bacteria, such as salmonella, that cause intestinal infections;

  – it increases the resistant capabilities of the intestinal mucosa against aggressive pathogenic bacteria.

- ***Bifidobacterium bifidus*** is another bacterium native to the human intestine. It also arrives in the colon live and active. Its effects are similar to those of *Lactobacillus acidophilus.*

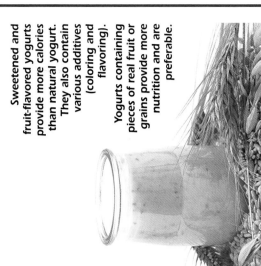

Sweetened and fruit-flavored yogurts provide more calories than natural yogurt. They also contain various additives (coloring and flavoring).

Yogurts containing pieces of real fruit or grains provide more nutrition and are preferable.

Storage of Yogurt

Yogurt is a perishable food that spoils easily through bacterial or fungal action. To avoid this it must be stored:

- *Always refrigerated.*
- In a **closed** container.
- It should *not* be stored for **more than three weeks.**
- Once opened, it should be eaten within **24 hours.**

Drawbacks to Yogurt

- **It is lacking in certain nutrients:** Yogurt, like milk, does not contain fiber, and is deficient in vitamin C and iron.
- **Anemia** results for those whose diet is based on yogurt, since they fail to eat other iron-rich foods.
- **Alcohol:** Yogurt contains small amounts of ethyl alcohol formed during the milk fermentation process. Kefir and koumiss may contain as much as 3% (half the alcohol content of beer).
- Chemical and radioactive **contamination**, if the milk used to make it is contaminated (see Vol. 1, p. 196).

Cream and Butter

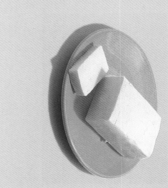

Benefits

- **Easy to digest and assimilate** compared to other animal fats.
- **Good source of vitamin A**, and to a lesser extent, **vitamins D and B₁₂.**
- Advisable when a **greater fat-based energy** source is needed (this should never exceed 30% of caloric intake, see Vol. 1, p. 404), as in the case of:
  – underweight
  – debilitated or malnourished patients
  – children, persons active in sports and those involved in intensive physical labor.

Drawbacks

- They have a **high caloric** content due to their high percentage of fat (whipped cream: 345 kcal/100 g = 1,442 kJ/ 100 g, butter: 717 kcal/ 100 g = 2,997 kJ/100 g).
- **They are not advised** in cases of coronary or cardiovascular disease in general, since they **increase cholesterol** level and **promote arteriosclerosis.**

- a solid called **butter,** formed of solidified fat globules that form a homogenous mass;
- a liquid referred to as **buttermilk.**

Freshly churned sweet butter has little taste or odor. To achieve those characteristics of butter, it is cured with certain lactic bacteria that produce **diacetyl,** a substance that gives butter its characteristics.

Buttermilk

Buttermilk is similar in composition to nonfat milk, but with somewhat more fat. It is **rich** in phospholipids such as **lecithin,** and very nutritious.

Because it is very digestible, it was formerly given to **nursing infants** in place of cow's milk when they suffered digestive disorders or milk intolerance. However, its use has decreased in favor of specially adapted milk formulas.

Continued on page 206

Cream and butter are delicious and easy to digest, but not advisable for the health of the heart and arteries.

Continued from page 201

Cream

Cream is fundamentally an **emulsion of milk fat and water** that can be eaten as it is, or transformed into different products such as whipped cream or butter.

Whipped Cream

Whipped cream is prepared by beating cream to incorporate tiny air or carbon dioxide bubbles into it causing it to double or triple in volume.

Sugar is usually added. A **stabilizer** (usually carrageenan, see Vol. 1, p. 131) may be also added to keep the whipped cream from returning to its liquid state.

Butter

When cream is vigorously beaten for a long period, it separates into two parts:

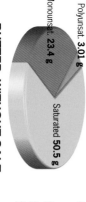

BUTTER, WITHOUT SALT
Percentage distribution of fatty acids
- Polyunsat. 3.01 g
- Monounsat. 23.4 g
- Saturated 50.5 g

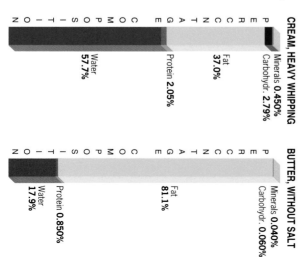

CREAM, HEAVY WHIPPING
- Protein 2.05%
- Water 57.7%
- Fat 37.0%
- Minerals 0.450%
- Carbohydr. 2.79%

BUTTER, WITHOUT SALT
- Protein 0.850%
- Water 17.9%
- Fat 81.1%
- Minerals 0.040%
- Carbohydr. 0.060%

Comparison of Milk Fats and Vegetable Oils

	Milk fats (cream and butter)	Vegetable oils
Flavor	Very pleasant, well accepted by all, even the ill.	There are persons who do not appreciate the flavor of certain oils.
Fluidity	Even though they are solid at room temperature, they are liquid at body temperature. This makes them more digestible than other animal fats.	They are normally liquid at room temperature, thus more fluid than milk fats.
Emulsion	Yes. Their fatty material is already divided into tiny droplets (globules) that are minutely blended with water. This facilitates the action of gastric juices.	No. They must be emulsified by bile in the small intestine.
Digestion	These are the easiest of all animal fats **to digest.** They are even easier to digest than vegetable oils.	Slower to digest than milk fats, since they are not emulsified.
Intestinal assimilation	Milk fats contain a certain amount of medium and short (less than 12 carbon atoms) chain fatty acids, which vegetable oils lack. These fatty acids are incorporated directly into the bloodstream without being circulated through the lymphatic system. Because of this, their assimilation is easier.	Their fatty acids are all long-chain, which complicates their assimilation into the bloodstream.
Saturation	Most of these fatty acids are saturated, which promotes the production of **cholesterol** in the body and arteriosclerosis.	The **fatty acids** in vegetable oils are *predominantly **un-saturated:*** • Monounsaturated, such as oleic acid, which protect against arteriosclerosis. • Polyunsaturated, which reduce cholesterol levels.
Cholesterol	These contain quite elevated levels of cholesterol (cream: 137 mg/100 g, butter 219 mg/100 g), keeping in mind that the maximum daily intake of cholesterol is 300 mg.	Contain little or no cholesterol.
Vitamin A	They are a ***good source*** of this vitamin. • 100 g of cream provides 421 µg RE (42 % of RDA) • 100 g of butter provides 754 µg RE (75% of RDA).	Vegetable oils contain very few carotenoids, the substance that is transformed into vitamin A in the body.
Vitamin E	100 g of cream provides 6% of RDA, 100 g of butter, 16%.	100 g of olive oil provides 126% of RDA (about eight times more than butter).
Vitamin B₁₂	Less than milk, but more than vegetable oils, which contain none. 100 g of cream provides 9% of RDA, while 100 g of butter provides 7%.	Contain none.
Effect on arteries and the heart	***Promote*** arteriosclerosis and coronary disease.	**Help *avoid* arteriosclerosis and *heart disease.***

Percentage of Nutrients Remaining in Cheese
after manufacture

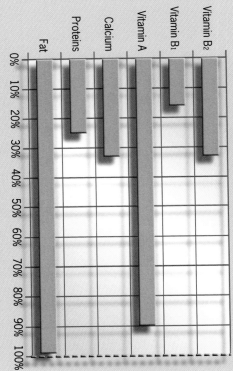

Percentage of nutrients remaining in hard cheese, compared with those in the milk from which the cheese was made, which represents 100%.
If there were no nutrient loss during cheesemaking, this graph would display all nutrients at a value of 100%

Continued from page 204

Cheese

Most cheeses are produced from milk from cows, sheep, or goats.

Cheesemaking is a rather complex process that requires a great deal of experience and art. The secret is in being able to take advantage of the characteristics of various microorganisms empirically, as in antiquity, or scientifically, as in the modern cheese industry.

These are the basic steps in cheese production:

1. Coagulation

Milk must be coagulated in order to form a curd and separate the whey. This process lasts from one to three hours. It may be accomplished in two ways, although there are many cheeses that use both at the same time:

- **Acid coagulation:** This is accomplished by adding a lactic bacterial culture to the milk (see Vol. 1, p. 203). The lactic acid that is produced precipitates the casein. This method is used for **fresh and soft cheeses.**

- **Enzymatic coagulation:** This involves adding a substance called **rennet** (Vol. 1, p. 199), which creates a more compact and elastic curd than that formed by acid coagulation. Emmental and Gruyere are two examples of cheeses made using this method.

2. Draining

This step involves eliminating most of the whey, leaving only the solid curd. Many high quality proteins, water-soluble B group vitamins and minerals *are lost* at this point.

3. Pressing

The curd is placed in perforated molds and placed under pressure, thus removing more whey.

In spite of the draining and pressing processes, the curd always retains a certain amount of whey, thus preserving some amount of vitamins and minerals.

4. Salting

A percentage between 2% and 3% of salt is added to the pressed curd to avoid the development of putrefying bacteria.

5. Maturation or curing

This final step gives the cheese its distinctive aroma, flavor, and consistency. This is accomplished by adding cultures of various microorganisms to the curd. These are known among cheesemakers as **"starters."**

Each type of microbe provides a different aroma and flavor, based on the substances it secretes. The precise microbiotic culture used is the cheesemaker's best-kept secret.

Even though cheese is a **concentrated food, and rich in nutrients as a result, it does not contain all of those found in milk or yogurt.**

During the cheesemaking process most of the whey is discarded, and along with it, a significant portion of protein, minerals and vitamins.

Is There Such a Thing as "Vegetarian" Cheese?

*Few lacto-ovo vegetarians know that animal **rennet** is used to make most cured cheeses. This is obtained from the internal coating or mucosa of the fourth chamber, or abomasum, of ruminants (see Vol. 1, p. 182). **Rennet is** harvested by slaughtering newborn calves or kids after they have first nursed and extracting the appropriate portion of the digestive tract. Therefore, when one eats cheese, one is eating a derivative of animal tissue. The stomachs of pigs are also used as a source of rennet.*

Alternative "rennet" or coagulators

The high cost of animal rennet has led the cheesemaking industry to using alternative "vegetarian" coagulators

- * **Microbial:** Microbes are being used more and more. According to some calculations, a third of the cheeses produced in the world are coagulated in this way (for example, Philadelphia cream cheese). These microbes are obtained from microscopic fungus, such as Mucor miehei.*

- * **Vegetable:** The stamens of the flowers of the cardoon plant have been used since antiquity as a very effective coagulating agent.*

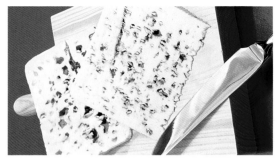

The **maturation** or **curing** of cheese consists in the degradation or decomposition of milk nutrients.

The more mature a cheese is, the less healthful.

- **Microbes used:** There are hundreds of different species, among **bacteria, yeasts,** and **molds** (these are special types of fungi).

- **Duration:** This can be from a few days (soft cheeses) to years (Parmesan cheese).

- **Transformations produced:** During the maturation process the microbes added to the curd proliferate to a very great extent. A mature cheese may contain a million or more bacteria or fungi per gram. Each of these microorganisms is a true chemical factory. Part of the protein, fats and sugars in the curd are degraded or decomposed by the action of their enzymes.

  – *Degradation of proteins* produces free amino acids, hypertensive amines, such as tyramine and histamine, sulfurated amines involved to the processes of putrefaction (cadaverine and putrescine) and ammonia (highly toxic to the liver).

  – *Degradation of fats* releases volatile fatty acids such as butyric acid, acetic acid, and propionic acid (found in Gruyere cheese), that give each cheese its typical aroma. Many other substances such as ketones are also produced.

  – *Degradation of sugars:* Although only a small amount of lactose remains in the curd, this is transformed into ketones and aldehydes that irritate the digestive tract.

Maturation, Uncontrolled Fermentation

Maturation or curing of cheese is a fermentation process during which many new substances are produced at the expense of the decomposition of the nutrients found in the original milk.

The types of substances produced are, to a certain degree, unpredictable and are impossible to control completely. This is due to the huge variety of microorganisms involved, temperature, humidity, and other environmental factors in addition to com-

plex chemical transformations taking place during maturation.

It is certain, however, that *many* of the substances produced during **maturation** are *harmful* to health. For this reason the biological processes at work are compared to the ethylic fermentation of grape juice, where portions of its nutrients are decomposed by microorganisms to form aromatic but toxic substances such as ethylic alcohol.

Natural lactic acid fermentation of milk to produce yogurt and the fermentation that transforms dough into bread do not produce undesirable substances. *To the contrary, they increase the* **nutritional value** *as well as the* **healing** *power of the milk or the flour.*

The Contamination of Cheese Affects Everyone

Outbreaks of salmonellosis, listeriosis and other diseases caused by consumption of contaminated cheese occur, not only in developing countries, but also in developed countries with a high level of hygiene. The following are some recent cases:

- **United States:** In 1985 there was an outbreak that caused 48 deaths, due to a Mexican-style cheese that had been made with poorly pasteurized milk.[52]
- **Canada:** It is calculated that the annual cost of treating diseases caused by Listeria-contaminated cheese reaches 12 million dollars.[53]
- **France:** Four people died in 1995 after eating Listeria-contaminated Brie.[54]
- **Spain:** In 1996 there was an outbreak that included 81 cases of brucellosis caused by eating unpasteurized fresh cheese.[55]
- **Germany:** In 1991 there was an outbreak that included 600 cases of salmonella-produced gastroenteritis among the employees of an important pharmaceutical firm who had eaten contaminated cheese and meat.[56]
- **United Kingdom:** A study conducted in 1993 showed that for every 1,000 samples of raw milk sampled at farms in England and Wales, 3.6 contained Salmonella pathogens, and 51 contained Listeria.[57]

– Although it is normally destroyed by pasteurization, there have been cases of listeriosis in cheese manufactured with pasteurized milk, due to breakdowns in the cheesemaking process.

– It develops above all in soft cured cheeses such as Brie.

Mature Cheeses Are the Most Susceptible

In matured cheeses, particularly those cured using molds, the pH is increased (alkalization), which promotes the proliferation of these and other bacterial pathogens.

On the other hand, the acidity of fresh cheeses and fermented dairy products inhibits the growth of many disease-causing microorganisms.[43]

Contamination of Cheese

Cheese made from unpasteurized milk may contain a wide variety of pathogenic microbes, as does the milk from which it is made. Noted among these pathogens are:

- *Escherichia coli* that causes gastroenteritis and kidney failure.
- Various species of *salmonella* that cause serious gastroenteritis, including septicemia.
- *Brucella melitensis*, which causes brucellosis or Maltese fever.
- *Listeria monocytogenes* which causes listeriosis, possibly the most serious disease of all those transmitted through cheese. Its course includes meningitis and septicemia, and it is fatal in 30% of cases. This bacterium possesses the following characteristics:[58]
  – It comes from the udder of the cow.
  – Resists refrigeration and it may reside in industrial cheese manufacturing facilities.

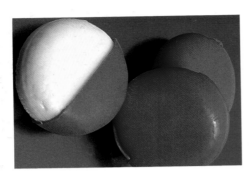

Commercially-produced cheeses are manufactured with pasteurized milk, in accordance with dietary legislation.

However, some private cheesemakers prefer raw milk, since it contains more microbes thus accelerating coagulation and maturation, but with the accompanying health risks to consumers.

Matured Cheeses: When They Should Not Be Eaten

- **Arteriosclerosis and cardiovascular disease,** due to their *high fat* (20%-60%) and *cholesterol* (60-80 mg/ 100 g) content.
- **Arterial hypertension,** due to their *high sodium* (common salt) and hypertensive *amine* contents.
- **Obesity,** due to their very *high caloric and fat* content.
- **Digestive disorders,** due to the irritating action of some of the substances formed during maturation.
- **Renal insufficiency,** due to the excess *protein* they contain.
- **Liver disease,** due to its *protein richness* and the *toxic substances* produced as these proteins are degraded (for example, ammonia).

Nutritional Value of Matured Cheese

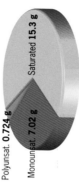

Minerals **3.68%**
Carbohydr. **0.460%**
Fat **24.3%**
Protein **19.8%**
Water **51.8%**

P E R C E N T A G E

C O M P O S I T I O N

CHEESE, CAMEMBERT
Composition
per 100 g of raw edible portion

Energy	**300 kcal = 1254 kj**
Protein	**19.8 g**
Carbohydrates	**0.460 g**
Fiber	**—**
Vitamin A	**252 µg RE**
Vitamin B₁	**0.028 mg**
Vitamin B₂	**0.488 mg**
Niacin	**5.75 mg NE**
Vitamin B₆	**0.227 mg**
Folate	**62.2 µg**
Vitamin B₁₂	**1.30 µg**
Vitamin C	**—**
Vitamin E	**0.655 mg α-TE**
Calcium	**388 mg**
Phosphorus	**347 mg**
Magnesium	**20.0 mg**
Iron	**0.330 mg**
Potassium	**187 mg**
Zinc	**2.38 mg**
Total Fat	**24.3 g**
Saturated Fat	**15.3 g**
Cholesterol	**72.0 mg**
Sodium	**842 mg**

1% 2% 4% 10% 20% 40% 100%

% Daily Value (based on a 2,000 calorie diet)
provided by 100 g of this food

Polyunsat. **0.724 g**
Saturated **15.3 g**
Monounsat. **7.02 g**

Percentage distribution of
fatty acids

Cheese Provides

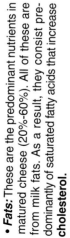

- **Fats:** These are the predominant nutrients in matured cheese (20%-60%). All of these are from milk fats. As a result, they consist predominantly of saturated fatty acids that increase **cholesterol.**

- **Proteins:** from 15% to 30%. These are formed from **casein**, the *least complete* of milk proteins (see Vol. 1, p. 191), since it is deficient in the amino acids methionine and cystine. Whey proteins that are discarded during the cheesemaking process are of *greater* **biological** value than casein.

- **Vitamins:** Cheese contains all except vitamin C. The most abundant are A, la B₂ y la B₁₂.

- **Minerals:** Cheese is a *good source of* **calcium** and **phosphorus**, since 100 g of matured cheese provide about 400 mg of calcium, half of the RDA for an adult.

Drawbacks to Matured Cheese

- **Partial:** Although it is highly concentrated, cheese contains only part of milk. When the whey is eliminated, **proteins, minerals,** and **vitamins** of great biological value *are lost* (see Vol. 1, p.189).

- **Deficient in certain nutrients:** Cheese contains neither vitamin C nor fiber, and it is very poor in carbohydrates and iron.

- **High in salt:** All cheeses except fresh cheeses contain 2% to 3% salt. This way, 100 g of matured cheese contains 2 to 3 grams of salt, which is *half* of the RDA (Recommended Daily Allowance) for an adult.

- **Disadvantageous for the heart and arteries:** Cheese is rich in the substances that are the *most harmful* for the cardiovascular system: fat, cholesterol, sodium (salt), and hypertensive amines such as tyramine and histamine.

- **Additives:** Matured (cured) cheeses usually contain additives such as potassium nitrate to preserve them, in addition to coloring and thickeners.

- **Degradation of nutrients:** The numerous microorganisms in cheese decompose part of its nutrients (particularly proteins and fats), producing substances that are aromatic, but irritant and toxic, as well.

Benefits of Matured Cheese

- **High nutrition concentration:** ten liters of milk will make three liters of fresh cheese or one liter of hard matured cheese. This is a **very concentrated food**, which provides a great deal of nutrients in little volume.

- **Storage:** Cheese lasts the longest of any dairy product and in many cases does not even require refrigeration.

- **Calcium-rich:** The food richest in calcium is cheese, although this calcium is *not the most effective* **mineralizer.**

Matured (Cured) Cheeses:

They are the least healthy cheeses,
and are not recommended particularly in cases of cardiovascular disease.

The manufacture of cured cheeses includes all of the steps described in Vol. 1, pp. 206-207.

- They are produced through **enzymatic coagulation** using **rennet,** usually of animal origin.
- During a variable period (from days to years) they go through a **fermentation** process produced by various non-lactic microorganisms. This process is referred to as **maturation** or **curing.**

Cheese is classified according to its concentration and moisture content as:

- **soft:** contain more than 40% moisture
- **semi hard:** from 35% to 40%
- **hard:** less than 35%

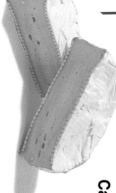

Roquefort

This semi hard cheese of French origin is much appreciated for its flavor.

Maturation takes about two months, and employs, among other microorganisms, the mold *Penicillium roqueforti.* This mold gives the cheese its blue-green color and strong flavor.

Roquefort contains considerable fat (30%) since it is made with **sheep** milk. Its calcium content is among the lowest of any cheese.

The Asturian **Cabrales** (Spain) is another blue cheese matured with mold. It is made with **goat** and **sheep** milks.

Camembert

This is a **soft** cheese made from **cow's milk.** It comes from the Normandy region of France.

The maturation of Camembert is brought about by seeding its surface with spores of the mold *Penicillium cammemberti,* which together with the bacteria *Brevibacterium linens* degrade particularly casein (curd protein).

Maturation takes about 30 days. If it is prolonged, the cheese takes on a strong ammonia odor.

Brie is similar to Camembert, but with more intense, longer maturation.

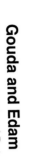

Gruyere and Emmental

These are hard **cow's milk** cheeses from Switzerland. The most significant difference between the two is the size of the "eyes," which are larger in the Emmental.

These cheeses are made using rennet and intense whey removal. Because of this they contain only lower-quality casein protein, and few hydrosoluble B group vitamins.

Their maturation takes from two to three months. The propionic bacteria used to make these cheeses degrade fats, producing carbon dioxide gas, which forms the "eyes."

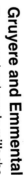

Gouda and Edam

These are **semi hard** Dutch cheeses. They are made from **cow's milk.** The curd is intensively washed to eliminate as much of the whey as possible. Maturation usually takes about a month. They have a rather mild flavor.

Parmesan

This is a **hard** cheese of Italian origin. It is made from **cow's milk,** pressing the curd to remove as much of the whey as possible. Maturation takes a year or more. Its fats and proteins are highly concentrated, and it has an intense flavor.

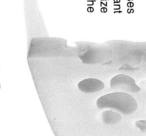

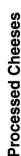

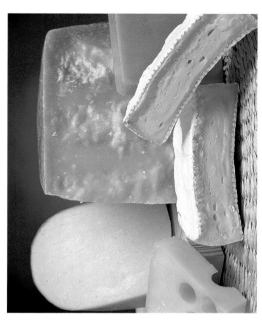

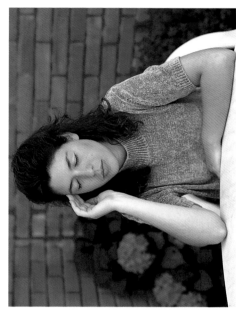

the Most Delicious

Cheddar

This is a **hard** cheese of English origin. It is widely used in the English-speaking world. It is made from whole cow's milk, rennet coagulation, and intense pressing to remove almost all of the whey.

Its maturation takes from three to twelve months. The bacteria employed produce intense decomposition of proteins and fats. They form numerous chemical substances such as amino acids, amines (among these are tyramine and histamine, that are hypertensives), ketones, and sulfurated compounds.

Manchego

This is a Spanish **semi hard** cheese made with **sheep** or **sheep and cow's** milk. There are varieties of this cheese that are less matured, and, as a result, healthier, without losing its delicate flavor.

Processed Cheeses

These are cheeses **recycled**, prepared from other cheeses that are not appropriate for the market. Cheeses with various anomalies, such as defects of shape or flavor, are industrially prepared by melting, blending, and resolidifying them.

The Least Healthful

Cheeses are less healthful, the more:
- ***time** the cheese has **matured** (cured).*
- ***molds** and **yeasts** have been employed.*
- ***pungent** the cheese's **aroma**.*

Matured cheeses contain more than a million microorganisms per gram, which decompose their nutrients into irritating and toxic substances.

Headaches, eczema, allergies, arterial hypertension, and even cardiac arrhythmia can be aggravated by matured cheese.

Fresh Cheeses:

Fresh cheeses without salt are the only ones that are acceptable in the diet of those with cardiovascular disease and those with arteriosclerosis.

Those cheeses that are referred to as **fresh cheeses** are pure white with a soft texture and flavor. They must be refrigerated. They are made from **pasteurized** milk, generally cow's **milk**, although **goat** milk is sometimes used. It is made in the following steps:

- **Acid coagulation:** This is the only microbial transformation used (see Vol. 1, p. 203). Lactic acid bacterial starters, particularly streptococcus, are used. A small amount of rennet is used in some fresh cheeses.

- **Light draining:** Curd is formed after a few hours of incubation at between 25° and 30°C (between 77° and 86°F). This is then allowed to lightly drain for between one-half and one hour.

- These cheeses are *not pressed, nor* are they **matured.**

These are the *healthiest* of cheeses because:
- their *lower* **fat** content,
- they contain *less* **salt,**
- they are *not* **matured.**

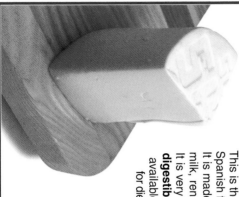

Burgos Cheese

This is the prototypical Spanish fresh cheese. It is made from **sheep** milk, rennet, and salt. It is very **delicate** and **digestible.** Today it is available without salt for dietetic reasons.

Cottage Cheese

This is similar to fresh cheese and is very popular in the United States. It is made from **non-fat or low-fat** milk, to which has been added a starter culture with a lactic streptococcus base and a species of bacteria, called *Leuconostoc citrovarum,* which gives it a very **delicate** flavor.

Ricotta or Whey Cheese

This is made from the whey, which is discarded during most cheese-making processes. After separating the whey with lactic acid, it is heated to 90°C (194°F), to precipitate its protein into a solid white mass, which is ricotta or **whey cheese.**

Ricotta contains **whey protein** of great *biological value,* as well as a small amount of fat and calcium.

the Healthiest

'Petit Suisse'

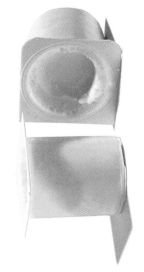

This is a fresh cheese of French origin to which some **cream** and sugar is added, together with coloring and flavoring, to make it more attractive to children. It has had very little whey removed, and is soft and creamy.

It contains more vitamin A, fat (35%), protein (8%), and calories (some 350 kcal/100 g) than other fresh cheeses. For these reasons, it is not particularly healthy.

'Quark' Cheese

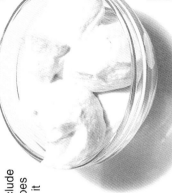

This is Germany's most popular cheese. It represents more than 45% of that country's cheese production. In France it is called **'fromage frais'**(fresh cheese) and in English-speaking countries it is known as **'quark'**. Its characteristics are:

- **Creamy** consistency and *slightly* **acid** flavor.
- It is made from **nonfat** cow's milk.
- Its acid coagulation is done slowly (6-12 hours) using a starter culture based on *Streptococcus lactis and cremoris.*
- Some varieties include **whey** proteins (as does **ricotta**), which gives it a *higher* **nutritional value** than other cheeses.
- This fresh cheese has the *lowest fat* and ***caloric*** content of any.

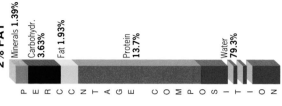

CHEESE, COTTAGE, 2% FAT

Minerals **1.39%**	
Carbohydr. **3.63%**	
Fat **1.93%**	
Protein **13.7%**	
Water **79.3%**	

P E R C C N T A G E   C O M P O S I T I O N

CHEESE, COTTAGE, 2% FAT
Percentage distribution of **fatty acids**

Polyunsat. **0.059 g**
Monounsat. **0.550 g**
Saturated **1.22 g**

CHEESE, COTTAGE, 2% FAT
Composition
per 100 g of raw edible portion

Energy	**89.7 kcal = 375 kj**
Protein	**13.7 g**
Carbohydrates	**3.63 g**
Fiber	—
Vitamin A	**20.0 µg RE**
Vitamin B₁	**0.024 mg**
Vitamin B₂	**0.185 mg**
Niacin	**2.69 mg NE**
Vitamin B₆	**0.076 mg**
Folate	**13.1 µg**
Vitamin B₁₂	**0.712 µg**
Vitamin C	—
Vitamin E	**0.056 mg α-TE**
Calcium	**68.5 mg**
Phosphorus	**151 mg**
Magnesium	**6.00 mg**
Iron	**0.160 mg**
Potassium	**96.2 mg**
Zinc	**0.420 mg**
Total Fat	**1.93 g**
Saturated Fat	**1.22 g**
Cholesterol	**8.40 mg**
Sodium	**406 mg**

% **Daily Value (based on a 2,000 calorie diet)**
provided by 100 g of this food

1% 2% 4% 10% 20% 40% 100%

Ice Cream: the Most Appetizing Dairy Products

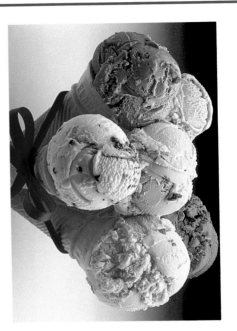

Production

Ice cream manufacture involves the following steps:

1. Mix the following ingredients: milk, cream and milk derivatives, egg, sugar, chocolate or other flavoring. Vegetable fats or proteins may also be used.

2. Whipping, to intermix air with the ingredients.

3. Freezing.

Ice Cream Provides:

- **Water:** 50%-78%.
- **Protein:** 1%-6%. These come from the milk derivatives and egg ingredients.
- **Carbohydrates:** 13%-22% in the form of sugars.
- **Fats:** These are from the milk or from saturated vegetable fats.
- **Vitamins:** Ice cream contains some amount of vitamins A, B, and E, but not vitamin C.
- **Minerals:** Calcium and phosphorous predominate.
- **Additives:** coloring, flavoring, stabilizers, antioxidants, etcetera.

Milk-based Desserts

Milk-based desserts are made from milk **protein and fat** to which **starch** or vegetable flour added.

They are **high** in **protein, fats,** and **carbohydrates,** but **low** in **vitamins.**

Their **advantage** is that they can be stored at **room temperature for months.**

Benefits of Ice cream

- **Refreshing:** They feel very pleasant in the mouth.
- **Nutritious:** Their *primary ingredient* is **milk,** as *opposed to* **sorbet,** which is **water-based.** As a result, ice cream provides a rather balanced proportion of **protein, fat,** and **sugar.** Their caloric content is usually between 170 and 200 kcal/100g.
- **Appetizing:** In summer, children are always ready to eat ice cream. This is not the case with other foods.

Drawbacks to Ice Cream

- They contain **saturated fat** either of animal origin (milk or egg) or industrially hydrogenated vegetable fat.
- They are *not heart healthy,* due to its **saturated fat** and **cholesterol** content.
- **Additives:** The cold temperature of ice cream slightly anesthetizes the taste buds. To compensate for this loss of taste a **wide variety** of **sugars** and other **additives** are used.
- **Headache:** The cold sensation of ice cream on the palate and pharynx can cause or aggravate headache.[59]
- **Contamination:** In spite of its low temperature, ice cream may contain **pathogens** from the milk used in its manufacture. Most of these are *Salmonella* such as in the 1994 outbreak in the United States, in which 224,000 cases of gastroenteritis were reported after consumption of a particular brand of ice cream.[60]

Dairy Products Throughout Life

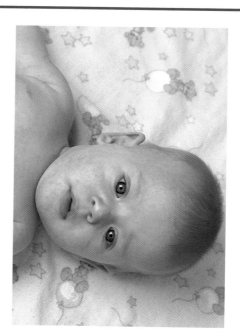

Nursing Infants

Milk is the nursing infant's *best and only* food. The *ideal* milk for the human infant is **mother's milk**. Even though it is deficient in iron and vitamin C, the infant has about six months of reserve of these nutrients left from gestation.

Natural cow's milk should *not* be fed to infants, since it causes allergies and intolerance. Prepared milk-based formulas may be used as an alternative to mother's milk.

Children

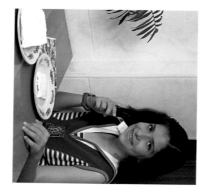

Milk and dairy products provide *essential* materials for building **strong bones: *protein*** and ***calcium*.** They can drink whole milk; however **low-fat (2%)** milk is *preferable* to reduce the high levels of saturated fats that they tend to eat in rolls, sweets, chocolate and meat products.

Children with intolerance or allergies to cow's milk, may tolerate acidified dairy products such as yogurt or fresh cheese.

Children should *avoid* **excessive** use of dairy products, particularly **milk itself,** which may foster **anemia** and **allergic reactions. Two glasses** of milk a day or their equivalent are sufficient (although not indispensable) if the child is eating a balanced diet.

Adolescents

Adolescents can use dairy products with their total *fat* content, such as whole milk, cream or cheeses, assuming that they are involved in *abundant physical* exercise.

Adults

Adults *must* reduce their use of milk, and *in any case* should use **nonfat**, or eliminate it entirely. In its place they may substitute **yogurt**, which provides numerous health benefits, or salt-free **fresh cheeses**.

At this stage of life, dairy products are *less necessary* than ever, and one can enjoy good health without them. The *most beneficial* dairy products for adults are:

Adults should *avoid:*

- **yogurt,**
- **soured** milk and whey (buttermilk),
- **Acidified** dairy products, in general.

- **butter,**
- **cream**
- **matured (cured) cheeses.**

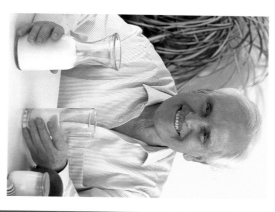

The Calcium in Cheese

Even though **matured** (cured) **cheese** is the food containing the greatest concentration of calcium, ***its mineralizing effect is not as efficient as one might expect.*** This is because its abundant proteins, salt concentration, and acidifying action increase the urinary loss of calcium.

The result is that by eating matured (cured) cheese much of the calcium it contains is lost through the urine. Due to this calcium leaching effect, matured (cured) cheese is not advised for **menopausal** women to others with a tendency to **osteoporosis.**

Alternatives

are available whose nutritional value is very similar to cow's milk.

- **Almond 'milk' or beverage** (see Vol. 2, p. 51): This very pleasant and refreshing beverage provides *proteins, unsaturated fats, and sugars* that are very easy to assimilate. It contains less *calcium* than cow's milk.

- **Oat 'milk' or beverage:** This is very rich in fats and proteins.

- **Tiger nut horchata** (see Vol. 2, p. 160): Horchata contains *less protein* and calcium than milk, but more *carbohydrates, iron, and magnesium.*

Alternatives to Butter

- **Margarine** (see Vol. 1, p. 121): Margarine as a substitute for butter has the *advantage* of containing **less saturated fat,** and *no cholesterol.*

However, it has the disadvantage of containing a great deal of **'trans' fatty acids,** which promote arteriosclerosis (see Chapter 22).

- The healthiest **dietary** fat is neither butter nor margarine, but rather **cold-pressed olive oil** or **seed oils** (see Vol. 1, p. 114).

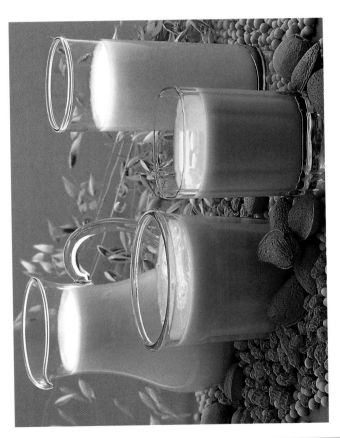

Alternatives to Cow's Milk

The so-called **'vegetable milks'** (see Vol. 1, p. 369) constitute *healthy and healthful* alternatives to milk.

- **Soy 'milk' or beverage** (see Vol. 1, p. 88): This beverage does not naturally contain **vitamin B₁₂,** and has *less calcium* than cow's milk. However, **enriched** soy beverages

Calcium Equivalents

Even though milk and dairy products are good sources of calcium, they are **not essential** in meeting the daily needs for this mineral.

One glass of milk (200 ml) = 100 g of almonds = 100 g of common dry beans = 500 g of broccoli

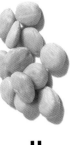 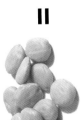 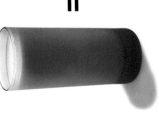 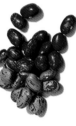

All of these foods provide the same amount of calcium: 240 mg (one third of the RDA: Recommended Daily Allowance).

to Dairy Products

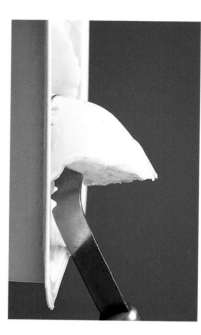

Margarine

Alternatives to Cheese

- **Tofu** (see Vol. 1, p. 88): Tofu is made by coagulating soymilk. Its appearance, texture and nutritional value are similar to that of fresh cheeses; in other words, considerably more than **fresh cheeses** or **cottage cheese**, which contain between 65 and 70 mg/100 g of calcium. and 105 mg/100 g of **calcium**; in other words, considerably more than **fresh cheeses** or **cottage cheese**, which contain between 65 and 70 mg/100 g of calcium.

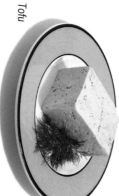

Tofu

Reasons for Avoiding Dairy Products

There are more and more people who, for a variety of reasons that are generally

- **health**-related, or
- based on **ethical** considerations (respect for milk-producing animals, often over-exploited),

prefer not to consume milk and dairy products.

The food industry currently offers a variety of **vegetable products** that can **replace milk** and dairy products, although with lowered amounts of calcium and vitamin B₁₂, but with **various and interesting advantages,** as illustrated in these pages.

Benefits of Alternatives to Dairy Products

- *They produce virtually **no** intolerance or **allergies**.*
- *They do **not** present as high a **risk** of bacterial pathogenic **contamination** as milk, not do they contain antibiotics or **hormones.***
- *Their **fat** is predominantly **mono or polyunsaturated,** which contributes to the reduction of cholesterol and avoiding arteriosclerosis.*
- *They contain **no cholesterol.***
- *They contain **no lactose,** the milk sugar that causes intolerance.*

Milk Beverages

This is an alternative to regular milk that is made by:

- *Eliminating all of the milk **fat** and **cholesterol** from milk.*
- *Adding a **vegetable oil** (usually corn or soy), which is emulsified with the nonfat milk from the previous step.*
- *Enriching with liposoluble **vitamins A** and **D.***

Benefits

- *It retains the **nutritional value** and **flavor** of **whole milk.***
- *It is **rich in** vegetable unsaturated fatty acids. Contrary to the effect of milk's saturated fats, this actually **reduces the cholesterol level.***
- *It contains **no cholesterol.***
- *It is **appropriate** for **patients with heart disease** and those who want to lower their **cholesterol** level; however, it is **not as effective** as **soy or almond milk.***

12 EGGS

O VIPAROUS (egg-laying) animals such as insects, amphibians, fish, and birds are those that, as the name implies, *reproduce by means of eggs.* In contrast to the young of **viviparous** animals, which gestate within the mother's body and are born alive, the offspring of egg-layers form within an egg after it has been expelled from the mother's body. Therefore, everything necessary for life is contained within the egg.

A Nutritionally Complete Food

Each egg consists of two well-differentiated parts:

- **Germinative vitellus** or embryonic disk formed by the **germinal cell,** with its nucleus containing the genetic information. This part of the egg will become the **embryo.**

- **Nutritious vitellus,** formed by the **reserve nutritional substances** used by the embryo as it develops.

Bird eggs are noted for their *very high proportion* of **nutritive reserve,** which includes all of the **egg white** and *most* of the **yolk.** The embryonic disk is simply a small red dot on the surface of the yolk.

During the three weeks that incubation lasts, the yolk and egg white are the only nutrition source for the developing embryo. From them the embryo gains all of the substances needed to form tissues, including bones and feathers.

It is not surprising, then, that bird eggs are among the *most* nutritionally **complete foods** found in nature.

Continued on page 220

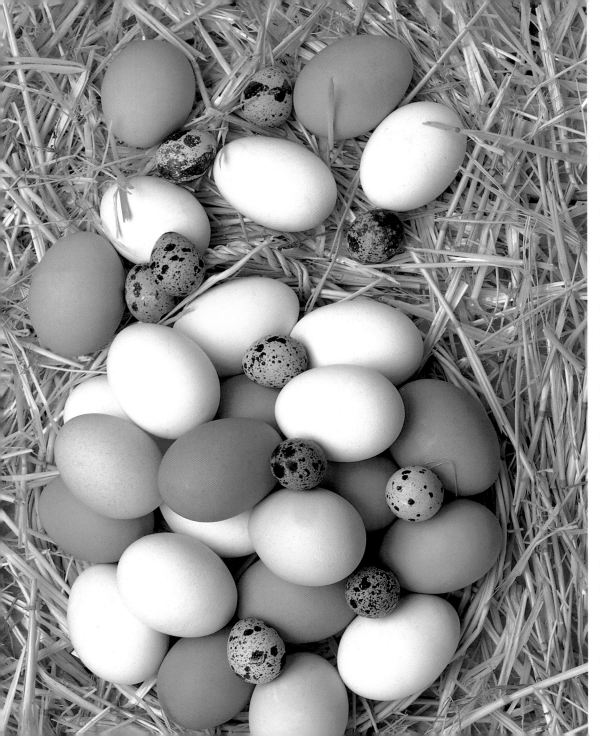

Because of their humble origin and commonness, the egg has always been considered a peasant food. In spite of this, its **nutritional** and **culinary properties** are **outstanding**. Its **protein** complex is of **great biological value** and is **eas-** **ily assimilated**. Eggs are also a very important **vitamin** and **mineral** source. Despite their lowliness, eggs are the basic ingredient in many dishes, from the most popular and traditional to international haute cuisine.

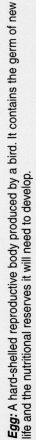

Egg

- ***Egg:*** A hard-shelled reproductive body produced by a bird. It contains the germ of new life and the nutritional reserves it will need to develop.

  When a specific bird is not named, egg refers to that of the **hen**, female of the species *Gallus gallus*.

- ***Fresh egg:*** *One that has not been processed in any way other than refrigeration for a period no longer than 30 days.*

Eggs should be eaten in moderation because of their animal origin and their high concentration of nutrients. It is also important to bear in mind that, as is the case with all animal products, eggs are dispensable either in the kitchen or in a healthy diet.

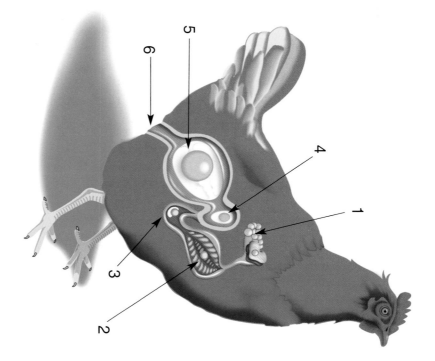

Egg Formation

1. The hen's **ovary** produces the embryonic or germinal disk of the egg, surrounded by a very small yolk.

2. The egg may be **fertilized** in the **oviduct** (equivalent of the Fallopian tubes found in female mammals) if **spermatozoa** from a rooster are present.

3. The walls of the oviduct secrete the **egg white** that accumulates around the yolk.

4. **Membranes** form around the egg white.

5. During 24 hours, the egg remains in a widening of the oviduct (equivalent to the uterus of a woman), while a **shell** is formed around it. After this period, the egg is ready to be expelled through the cloaca.

6. The **cloaca** is the common chamber into which the intestinal, urinary, and genital canals discharge. Because of this, it is not surprising that eggs often come out smudged with feces.

Continued from page 218

Humans can benefit from this great nutritional reserve. However, to better understand its properties, benefits and drawbacks, one must bear in mind that the biological objective of the egg is exclusively the formation of a new bird.

Processing of Eggs: Egg Products

Eggs as food have a very short useful life, since they tend to spoil rapidly and become a breeding-ground for numerous microorganisms.

Eggs, therefore, are *industrially processed* in a variety of ways to *prolong* their useful life and **minimize** microbiological **contamination**. They are thus converted into **"egg products."**

After removing the shell, the egg white and yolk are treated, either together or separately, with one or more of these processes:

- **Pasteurization:** As with milk, eggs are heated long enough to destroy all pathogens. Normally they are heated to a temperature of 60°-65°C (140°-149°F) for two to three minutes,

- **Freezing:** This must be performed only in an industrially controlled setting, since the temperature must be maintained between 0° and –2°C (between 32° and 28.4°F). Deterioration of the egg's properties result at lower temperatures.

- **Dehydration:** this consists of removing the water until the white and yolk are reduced to powder. This is the **safest** way to store eggs.

Egg products *are recommended* for use in food service establishments for preparation of **mayonnaise and sauces.** Egg products help *avoid* **salmonellosis** and other intestinal **infections** produced by microbial contamination of fresh eggs (see Vol. 1, p. 227).

Egg Proteins

Proteins constitute the most important nutrient found in eggs. This is due as much for their amount (about 7.3 g in a 65 g egg), as for their quality, which is the highest of any food.

Egg white proteins (4.2 g per egg):

- **Ovoalbumin** is the most abundant, since it forms **half** of the egg white protein. It is responsible for the foaming action when egg white is beaten, and for its coagulation when heated.

- **Conalbumin** represents 13% of protein in the egg white.

- **Ovomucoid** is a hyperallergenic glucoprotein that is responsible for most egg allergies.[1]

- **Ovomucin** is another glucoprotein found in the membranes and chalaza, giving them viscosity and resistance.

- **Globulins** are present in small quantities, but play an important role by acting as enzymes. The most important is **lysozyme** with its antibacterial action.

- **Avidin** is a protein that was first identified in 1940, and is the least present in egg white. It has the property of **interfere** with the **absorption** of **biotin**, a B complex vitamin found in the yolk. Avidin is rendered inactive by heat when the egg is **cooked.**

Egg yolk proteins (3.1 g per egg):

- **Phosphoproteins** are those linked with phosphoric acid, such as phosvitin.

- **Lipoproteins** are linked to lecithin and other phospholipids such as vitellin.

Egg Substitutes

The food industry has developed products that can be effectively substituted for eggs in culinary applications, but with the following advantages:

- they contain *no cholesterol,*
- they provide about 75 kcal/100 g; in other words, only *half the calories* of an egg,
- they contain *less sodium* than eggs,
- they produce *no allergies* if they are complete substitutes (see below),
- there is *no risk* of **salmonella** contamination.

There are two types of egg substitutes:

- **Complete substitutes** made from a base of **soy** or **milk**, corn oil, and flavorings, but without egg.

- **Partial substitutes** which *include,* in addition to the above ingredients, **egg white,** but not the yolk, which contains all of the egg's cholesterol.

Due to their binding and emulsifying qualities, egg substitutes perform as well as eggs for most culinary applications, including omelets and soufflés.

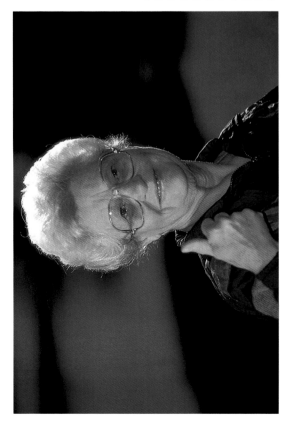

As adults age, they should reduce their consumption of eggs. Egg substitutes, either partial or complete, represent a healthful alternative.

THE EGG

Structure

Each egg contains an embryonic disk with the germinal cell, on the surface of the yolk. The embryonic disk is surrounded by a great amount of reserve nutritive material.

Shell

The eggshell has a protein base (4% of its weight) that contains many calcium carbonate crystals (95% of its weight).

It is **permeable**. The shell of each egg has about 8,000 pores that permit:

- a portion of the water within the egg to evaporate over time, and
- air and microorganisms to enter the egg.

Embryonic Disk

This is a spot on the yolk containing the germinal cell or **ovum** with its nucleus. If the egg has not been fertilized, the nucleus of this cell contains only the hen's chromosomes. If it has been fertilized, it contains the chromosomes of the rooster's sperm as well, with all of the genetic information needed to create a new life.

Air Space

This is formed between the two membranes that protect the egg white. It becomes *larger* with the **passage** of **time**.

Egg White

The egg white is formed almost entirely of water and protein. The white of a 65 g egg contains 4.2 grams of various **proteins**, *predominantly* **albumins**.

Chalaza

This is a thickening of the vitelline membrane that maintains the yolk in the center of the egg. It is formed of a type of **protein** called **ovomucin**.

Membranes

Membranes protect the contents of the egg, even though they are quite porous. There are two membranes surrounding the egg white and one, called the vitelline membrane, surrounding the yolk.

Yolk

The yolk contains the greatest concentration of **nutrients** within the egg. Its principal contents are:

- *proteins*
- *fats*
- *minerals*
- *vitamins* A, D, E, and B.

The typical **yellow color** of the yolk is attributed to **xanthophyll**, a non-nutritive carotenoid. An intense yellow yolk indicates that the hen has been naturally and healthfully fed with corn and other fresh vegetables containing this natural pigment.

Today, however, this may not always be the case. Industrial poultry farms add xanthophyll and other pigments to feed. In this way, the eggs produced all have the desired color in spite of the way they have been fed.

Composition of a 65 g egg

	Eggshell	Egg white	Yolk
Water (g)	0.07	34.27	9.95
Protein (g)	0.26	4.2	3.1
Fats (g)	0	traces	5.85
Sugars (g)	0	0.6	0.2
Minerals (g)	6.2	traces	0.298
Vitamins (g)	0	0	0.002
Total	6.53	39.07	19.4

Nutritional Value

Eggs provide a wide variety of easily digested, high quality nutrients that are of great value for the body's healthy development.

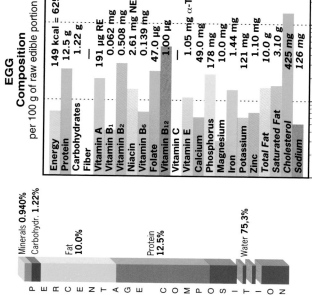

EGG Composition
per 100 g of raw edible portion

Energy	149 kcal = 625 kj
Protein	12.5 g
Carbohydrates	1.22 g
Fiber	—
Vitamin A	191 µg RE
Vitamin B₁	0.062 mg
Vitamin B₂	0.508 mg
Niacin	2.61 mg NE
Vitamin B₆	0.139 mg
Folate	47.0 µg
Vitamin B₁₂	1.00 µg
Vitamin C	—
Vitamin E	1.05 mg α-TE
Calcium	49.0 mg
Phosphorus	178 mg
Magnesium	10.0 mg
Iron	1.44 mg
Potassium	121 mg
Zinc	1.10 mg
Total Fat	*10.0 g*
Saturated Fat	*3.10 g*
Cholesterol	*425 mg*
Sodium	*126 mg*

1% 2% 4% 10% 20% 40% 100% 200% 500%

% Daily Value (based on a 2,000 calorie diet) provided by 100 g of this food

PERCENTAGE COMPOSITION

Minerals 0.940%
Carbohydr. 1.22%
Fat 10.0%
Protein 12.5%
Water 75.3%

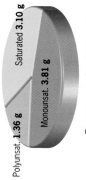

Polyunsat. 1.36 g — Saturated 3.10 g — Monounsat. 3.81 g

Percentage distribution of **fatty acids**

Protein

- **Quantity:** Protein represents 12.5% of the edible portion of the egg, which amounts to about 7.4 grams for a 65 g egg. Various proteins are found in the egg white (albumins) as well as in the yolk (phosphoproteins and lipoproteins).

- **Quality:** The *proportion* of the various *amino acids* that form egg proteins more closely *approximates* the *ideal* for humans than any other food. Because of this, the **biological value** of egg proteins is **94%**, the *highest* of all foods.

- **Digestibility:** Egg proteins are easily digested and assimilated, particularly if they are cooked.

- **Properties:**

  – Egg proteins **coagulate**; in other words, they lose their solubility and become solid or semisolid in the presence of heat, acids, or alkalis.

  – Egg proteins **foam** when beaten, as they incorporate tiny air bubbles. This property allows preparation of lighter foods, such as soufflés, meringues, and omelets.

  – Egg white facilitates **emulsions**, a mixture of two different liquids, such as water and oil. Due to its *lecithin* content, the yolk is an even better emulsifier than the egg white.

Fats

Fats represent 10% of the edible portion of the egg. This represents 5.85 g for a 65 g egg. These fats are of various types:

- ***Triglycerides: mono*** and ***polyunsaturated*** fatty acids surpass saturated fats.

- ***Phospholipids***, such as *lecithin*, act as emulsifiers.

- Other *lipids* (fats) such as **cholesterol** (each 65 g egg contains about 250 mg).

Vitamins

- **Liposoluble:** Eggs are a *good source* of *vitamin A* (retinol) and *vitamin E*. After fish liver oil, the egg is the *most important* natural *source* of *vitamin D*.

- **Hydrosoluble:** All of the *B group vitamins* are found in eggs, including *B₁₂*. One egg provides one-third of the RDA for an adult of this vitamin. Eggs contain no vitamin C.

Minerals

Eggs contain all minerals; however, their percentages of *phosphorous* and *iron* are notable, but one must also bear in mind their relatively high **sodium** content.

- *Iron* found in eggs is *non-heme*, like that of vegetables. As a result, **it is poorly absorbed** (around 10%). The presence of *vitamin C* from other foods improves its availability and absorption.

- *Sodium* is a mineral that is usually consumed in **excess** in the Western diet. The egg is one of the foods **richest** in this mineral. Only one 65 g egg provides about 74 mg of sodium, which represents 15% of the RDA (Recommended Dietary Allowance, which is 500 mg). And, of course, when table salt is added, the amount of sodium is considerably greater.

Trace elements

Eggs contain *zinc* and *selenium*. The former plays an important role as an **antioxidant** in the body's cells.

Benefits of Eggs

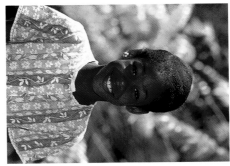

Nutritious

Eggs provide the most **complete *protein*** of any food, together with **fats**, ***vitamins***, and ***minerals***.

Promote Healthy Growth

Even though they are not essential—as is the case with any single food—eggs can contribute significantly to the nutritional needs of **children** and **adolescents** during periods of rapid growth.

Easily Digested

The egg's proteins, fats, minerals, and vitamins are easily digested and **most are assimilated**. The **fats** in the yolk are **emulsified**, thus facilitating their digestion. The exception here is ***iron***, which, as that in vegetable foods, requires ***vitamin C*** to facilitate its absorption.

Soft-boiled eggs are the easiest to digest.

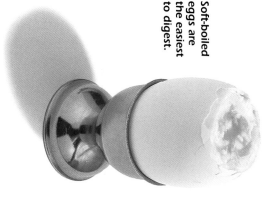

Eggs Do Not Produce Uric Acid

Eggs produce virtually no uric acid in the body, as *opposed* to other protein sources such as **legumes, fish,** or **meat**.

Culinary Possibilities

Eggs (and their substitutes, see Vol. 1, p. 221) are an ingredient in a multitude of culinary creations and other preparations, due to their **emulsifying, binding,** and **coagulating** properties. Additionally, eggs add **nutritional value.**

The Egg, the Liver's Enemy?

There is a popular belief that eggs are harmful to the liver. This **is not the case.** The **amino acids** that compose their proteins and the **vitamins** that they provide are of great value to the hepatic gland.

Eggs in **moderation** are permitted in the diet of liver patients, **taking care**, of course, of the total **fat** intake.

However, the yolk's fats do provoke an intense **draining** of the **gall bladder**, which is located just under the liver. This can produce digestive **disorders** including **colic**, particularly in those suffering from cholelitiasis (gallstones).

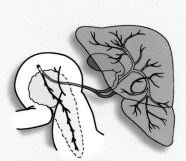

Eggs, specially when they are mixed with oil (fried, mayonnaise, etc.), are particularly indigestible for those suffering from gallbladder disorders.

Drawbacks to Eggs

Deficient in Some Nutrients

Eggs contain little or no:

- carbohydrates
- fiber
- vitamin C.

Allergies

Ovomucoid, a *protein* found in **egg white**, is the genesis of most of the numerous cases of egg allergy found in children and adults. **Yolk** proteins can also produce allergies.[1] It is calculated that *one third* of food allergies in children can be traced to eggs.

Egg allergies manifest the following primary symptoms:[2,3]

- **cutaneous:** skin rash, eczemas, dermatitis, and atopic manifestations;
- **digestive:** abdominal pain, colic, diarrhea;
- **respiratory:** asthma attacks that may be initiated or aggravated by egg consumption.

Eggs produce fewer allergic reactions when they have been thoroughly hard-boiled.

Bacterial Contamination

Birds possess a common chamber into which the intestinal, urinary, and genital canals discharge, called the cloaca (see Vol. 1, p. 220). As it is laid, the egg comes into contact with the hen's feces, which contain numerous microbes, including the feared salmonella.

A study conducted in Hannover (Germany) confirmed that the *principal source* of **salmonella** contamination is the **feed** given to hens and chickens.[4] From the feed, the microbes pass through the intestine of the bird, and on to the egg. On p. 227 of Vol. 1, there is a description of how to avoid infections transmitted by eggs.

Chemical Contamination

Eggs may contain traces of heavy metals (cadmium, lead), pesticides, and the antibiotics administered to the hens.

Cholesterol and Arteriosclerosis

Egg consumption *elevates* blood *cholesterol* levels, but *not by as much* as was once thought (see Vol. 1, p. 226). However, *the worst* is that it *promotes* **arteriosclerosis.**[5]

Sodium Rich

Eggs are one of the natural foods *richest* in **sodium** (see Vol. 1, p. 223). At the same time they are a *poor source of potassium*. For this reason, they must be used with *prudence* in cases of arterial **hypertension.**

Cancer

A team at the University of Minnesota (Minneapolis, USA) studied the relationship between egg consumption and cancer.[6] This study concluded that there is a statistically significant relationship between eating eggs and **colon cancer.** This relationship is more evident in women who eat eggs *daily.* They are at eight times greater risk of suffering cancer of the ascending colon.

Another study carried out in China by the National Cancer Institutes of the United States[7] has found that a positive relationship exists between egg consumption and **stomach cancer.**

Never Before One Year of Age

The egg must not be included in a child's diet before one year of age for two main reasons:

- *To avoid allergic reactions.*
- *To avoid infections [salmonellosis].*

After the first year, *the egg can be given hard-boiled and in small quantities in order to check the child's digestive tolerance.*

Eggs and Cholesterol

The egg has gotten a negative reputation due to its elevated cholesterol content.
Is the egg as harmful to cardiovascular patients as had been thought?

The egg is the *richest* of animal products in **cholesterol** (425 mg/100 g). Only brain tissue is higher (2,200 mg/100 g).

The egg contains so much cholesterol because this lipid is indispensable for the development of the nervous system and endocrine glands of the embryo. However, **humans do not need** to take in cholesterol through their food, since the **liver** is capable of producing even more than the body needs.

One egg contains about 250 mg of cholesterol, an amount close to the 300 mg daily upper limit. This means that eating **one egg a day** and **any other animal product** (milk, meat, fish, etc.) substantially **surpasses** the 300 mg of cholesterol considered the maximum daily allowance.

In addition to an increase in **cholesterol** level, other factors such as **smoking, lack of physical exercise,** or **obesity,** *contribute,* as well, to **lipoprotein oxidation** and to arteriosclerosis. To *the contrary,* **vegetables and fruit** rich in antioxidants *inhibit* this degenerative process.

Eggs Raise Cholesterol Only Slightly...

A study at the Copenhagen Clinic for the Study of Preventive Health (Denmark) demonstrates that eating two hardboiled eggs a day for six weeks produces:[8]

- an *increase* in **HDL** cholesterol (beneficial) of 10%.
- a *slight increase* in **total** cholesterol of 4%.

If this is the case with two eggs a day, it is reasonable to say that **moderate consumption** of two or three eggs a week **does not raise** blood **cholesterol** level.

This and other discoveries confirm that the moderate use of eggs does not increase blood cholesterol level. In fact, cholesterol from food has a relatively limited impact on the blood levels of this lipid. *Saturated fat increases* cholesterol levels *more* than food cholesterol itself (see Chapter 22).

...But Promote Arteriosclerosis

Even though eggs do not raise blood cholesterol levels as much as was once thought, they do *promote* arteriosclerosis **to a greater degree** than was thought.

Cholesterol is only dangerous when it is deposited on the walls of arteries, which become hardened and narrower. Recent investigations have shown that this process, known as arteriosclerosis, is initiated by the oxidation of low-density lipoproteins (LDL), the substances transporting cholesterol in the blood plasma.

Studies conducted at the Rambam Medical Center in Haifa (Israel),[5] have shown that the consumption of two eggs a day for three weeks increases **oxidation of plasma lipoproteins** by 42%. This means that eggs promote the process of arterial deterioration and arteriosclerosis.

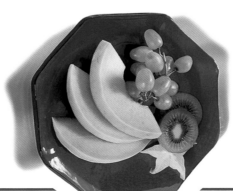

Prevention of Arteriosclerosis and Cardiovascular Disease

Those at **high risk** for arteriosclerosis and cardiovascular disease in general because of high cholesterol levels or other causes, should:

- *Avoid eating eggs,* and use **substitutes** in their place (see Vol. 1, p. 221).
- **Discard the yolk** of the egg. The egg white contains no fats, and as has been shown,[9] its use reduces cholesterol levels.
- *Use eggs enriched* with omega-3 fatty acids (**DHA,** see Vol. 1, p. 228), which do not increase cholesterol and reduce triglyceride levels.[10]
- **Never eat more than two eggs a week.**
- *Avoid fried eggs,* which supply more fat since they retain frying oil, thus promoting an increase in cholesterol.

The Egg and Hygiene

The egg is the ideal medium for the development of microorganisms. Although eggs contain protective membranes and antibacterial proteins such as lysozyme, many commercially available eggs are contaminated, even in developed countries.

A study conducted at the Institute of Social Medicine and Epidemiology in Berlin (Germany) shows that *Salmonella* bacteria in eggs are responsible for 67% of all food-related poisonings.[11]

Avoiding Egg-Transmitted Infections

- **Avoid eating raw eggs:** Sauces, particularly mayonnaise, are excellent media for the development of microorganisms from:
  - the egg itself
  - external contamination from hands, hair, and saliva of those handling the material during preparation.

  Pasteurized egg products should be used in place of raw eggs (see Vol. 1, p. 220).[12]

- **Discard eggs with cracked shells.** Intact eggs may be contaminated with salmo-

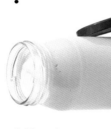

nella[13] because bacteria penetrate the shell through its numerous pores. Those with damaged shells present an even greater risk of contamination.

- **Discard eggs contaminated with feces on the shell.** Washing does not eliminate the possibility of contamination, since the microbes have usually already entered the egg.

- **Store eggs in the refrigerator** and never longer than *three weeks*.

- **Use the freshest (most recently laid) eggs possible.** The longer an egg is stored, the greater the possibility that bacteria have developed in its interior.

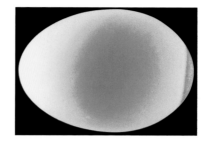

How To Tell if an Egg Is Fresh

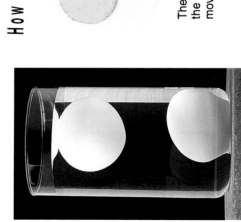

The yolk in recently laid eggs is found in the center. As the egg ages, the yolk moves to the side.

By observing a back-lit egg, one can see the size of the air space and the position of the yolk. As the egg ages, the separation between the yolk and the egg white becomes less distinct.

Recently laid eggs sink in water. As time passes, part of the water within the egg evaporates through the pores in the shell. This enlarges the air space in the egg and causes it to float.

Different Types

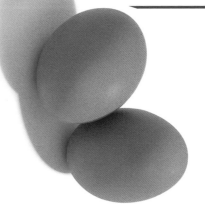

Brown Eggs

There are those who believe that eggs with dark shells are more nutritious than those that are white. This is false. The color of the shell depends only on the breed of hen.

Yellow Yolks

Today, the color of the yolk is no longer a reliable indicator whether or not the hen was naturally fed. The feeds used on high-production industrial farms contain various pigments that give the yolk the desired color.

Fertilized Eggs

These are eggs whose germinal cell has been fertilized by a rooster. When they are incubated, they develop into chicks. They are no more nutritious than unfertilized eggs, and they spoil faster.

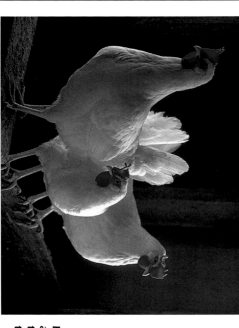

Organic Eggs

So called "organic" eggs come from hens raised in the fresh air (not in industrial settings), fed on grain, vegetables and organic feeds, without antibiotics, sedatives, hormones, or other additives.

Industrial poultry farms place hens in cages, where they have very limited movement and no natural daylight. They are artificially induced to produce various eggs a day. *How can eggs from hens in these conditions be* **equal in nutrition and flavor**, *to those from fowl living well in the fresh air and laying only one egg a day?*

Some consumers prefer organic eggs (from hens raised and fed naturally) because:

- of their superior **flavor and quality**

- they **do not** contribute to the **exploitation** of fowl in such an unnatural way.

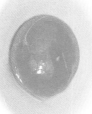

Enriched or DHA Eggs

Enriched eggs come from hens fed with seaweed that contains **omega-3**-type polyunsaturated fatty acids (see Vol. 1, p. 240). Among these, the most important is DHA (docosahexaenoic acid). Because of this, these are referred to simply as DHA eggs, as well.

Docosahexaenoic acid is an omega-3 series polyunsaturated fatty acid, whose molecules are formed by 22 carbon atoms and 6 covalent bonds. It is found in fish oil. Hens that consume it with their feed incorporate it in into their eggs.

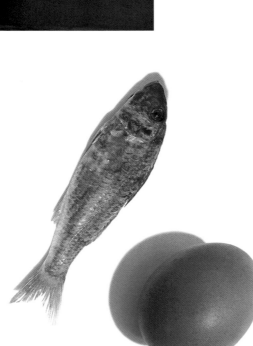

Even though DHA eggs contain cholesterol, as do all, **they do not raise blood cholesterol levels** since they also contain omega-three fatty acids. Additionally, they reduce triglyceride levels.[10]

# of Eggs

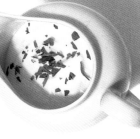

Duck eggs

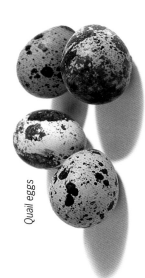

Quail eggs

Eggs of Different Birds

All bird eggs are edible, although those of the following species are preferred:

- **Hen** eggs are the most used throughout the world.

- **Quail** eggs are small, dark, and have a delicate flavor.

- **Duck** eggs are larger and with a thinner shell than those of hens. Their yolks are proportionally larger than those of hen eggs. They are very frequently contaminated with pathogenic microorganisms.

- **Turkey** eggs are somewhat larger and more elongated than hen eggs.

- **Guinea fowl** lay dark eggs that are smaller than those of the hen. They have a very delicate flavor.

- **Goose** eggs are very large, up to 160 g. They have a strong flavor.

Egg Products

These egg derivatives are obtained by pasteurizing the egg white, the yolk or both, with or without dehydration (see Vol. 1, p. 220).

Sauces and other products made with egg products present **no risk** of **salmonella contamination.**

Egg Substitutes

These are a healthy, **beneficial alternative** to eating eggs (see Vol. 1, p. 221).

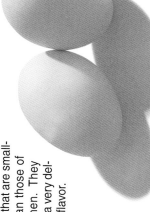

Hen eggs

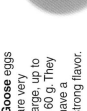
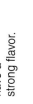

Soy mayonnaise

Raw Eggs

Raw eggs contain **avidin**, a protein that *interferes* with the **absorption** of *vitamin B* or biotin (see Vol. 1, p. 221).

Raw eggs can also transmit pathogenic **bacteria** such as **salmonella.**

For these reasons, eggs must *always* be properly **cooked** before they are eaten.

Egg Size

*In the **European Union** eggs are classified according to the weight of the egg:*

- *small (S):* 43-53 g
- *medium (M):* 53-63 g
- *large (L):* 63-73 g
- *extra large (XL):* more than 73 g

*In the **United States of America** eggs are classified according to minimum weight per dozen:*

- *small:* 18 oz. = 509.4 g per dozen
- *medium:* 21 oz. = 595.6 g per dozen
- *large:* 24 oz. = 680.6 g per dozen
- *extra large:* 27 oz. = 765.7 g per dozen
- *jumbo:* 30 oz. = 850.8 g per dozen

13

FISH AND SHELLFISH

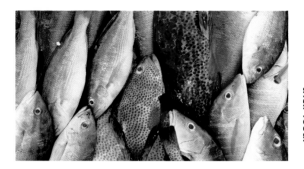

Seas, rivers, and lakes cover most of our planet. Therefore, it is no mystery that many peoples depend on these waters for their livelihood, including their food.

CHAPTER SUMMARY

FROM ANTIQUITY humans have captured aquatic animals for food.

Aquatic creatures used in the human diet are divided into two principal groups: fish and shellfish. These may be from salt or fresh water. Shellfish are sub-divided into mollusks and crustaceans. Other aquatic animals are also eaten such as amphibians (frogs) and chelonians (turtles).

Continued on page 232

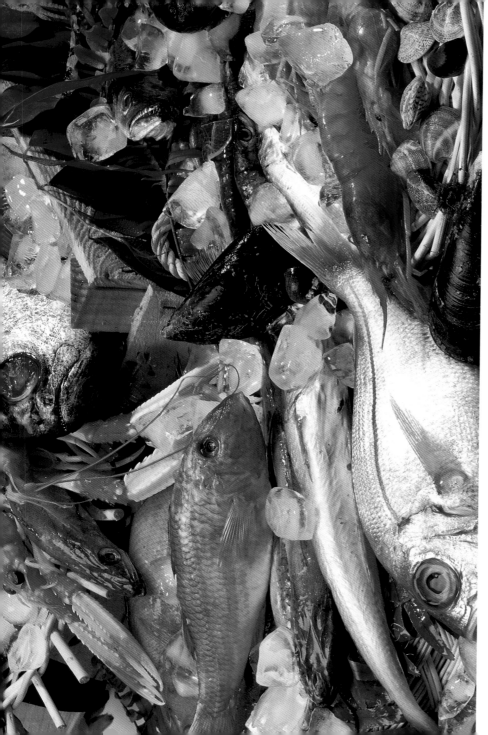

Fish are one of the few foods that still come mostly from the wild. However, **just because a product is "natural" does not in any way mean that it is healthful.** Even though the fish described on the following pages are generally more healthful than meat, one must never forget that they are **dead animals,** and, as such, go through all of the natural processes of decay. There are many marine creatures that are unfit as food, and even toxic. Additionally, seas, above all coastal areas, lakes, and rivers are subject to **appalling and constantly increasing levels of pollution.** This has a serious effect on aquatic creatures, and on those who eat them.

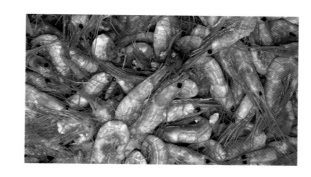

Fish and Other Seafood

- **Fish** are cold-blooded vertebrates living exclusively in fresh or salt water. All fish have **fins,** and most are covered with **scales.**

- **Other seafood** includes, in addition to fish, vertebrates such as **amphibians** (frogs) and **chelonians** (turtles), and invertebrates such as **mollusks and crustaceans,** which are referred to as **shellfish** (see Vol. 1, p. 252).

Although fish have vast reproductive capacity, it is well known that many fishing grounds are nearly depleted. This is because **man is the most voracious predator on Earth. It is imperative that man learns to manage the resources of seas, rivers, and lakes,** as well as the land itself in a way that will allow the world's flora and fauna to maintain or even restore themselves. Human life on the planet depends on it. This does not need to be just a utopian dream. The Creator has provided all of the inhabitants of the earth with ample resources and the intelligence to enjoy them.

Continued from page 230

Fish

Although fish provide *protein, fat, and vitamins* that are of *great nutritional* value, their massive harvesting as it is currently done, requires a huge amount of effort. Commercial deep-sea fishing is one of the *most expensive means* of obtaining food in terms of cost of effort.[1] It has been calculated that for each calorie of fish produced, eleven calories are spent in the form of:

- human effort
- fuel for ships
- energy for the machinery that processes and freezes the fish.

As is the case with raising cattle for meat (see Vol. 1, p. 263), commercial fishing demands enormous resources, and provides *little* **return** in terms of energy. From an **ecological** point of view, it may be said that it is a *veritable* **waste** of resources, the limitations of which we are becoming more and more aware.

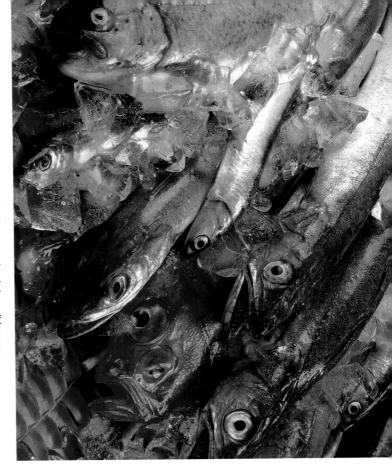

Three Great Threats

Currently, world fishing activity is facing the threats of depletion of resources, marine contamination, and diseases in aquatic life. Each of these threats by itself is sufficient reason not to increase fish consumption, and search for *vegetable* alternatives.

Depletion of Marine Resources

Each year approximately 100 million metric tons of fish and other seafood products are harvested from the seas of the world. This amount is fifty times greater than it was at the beginning of the 20th century, and continues to increase. Even though some governments have taken measures to restrict the numbers harvested, there are marine species that are in danger of extinction.

Fortunately, fish have the greatest reproductive capacity of any animals. Most do not breed except at specific times when the females ovulate into the water at the same time that the males release semen. This produces external fertilization, outside the body of the female. External fertilization allows for thousands or even millions of eggs to be fertilized by one pair of fish.

A female salmon, for example, may lay up to 20,000 eggs; a sardine, 60,000; and hake, eight million.

While it is true that not all of these eggs reach adulthood, the reproductive capacity of fish is very high. However, it is not high enough to resist the constant increase in industrial fishing, which often takes immature specimens.

Processing of Fish

Fish is a very unstable product, and decays very rapidly. To avoid this, two operations must be performed:

• Cleaning

Ideally, this should be done as soon as the fish leaves the water, as is done on modern freezer ships.

• Preservation

This step attempts to inhibit the proliferation of bacteria and other microorganisms that are always present in fish, and which cause rapid decay.

– **Sun-drying:** This is the oldest method known. The process takes various weeks. Its principal **disadvantage** is that the **insects and microorganisms** in the environment may infest the fish during drying.

– **Salting:** The final product of this method contains between 5% and 15% salt. Because of this, it is **harmful** to the **circulatory system.** There is evidence that the high incidence of **cancer of the pharynx** in China is due to feeding salt fish to infants.[5]

– **Smoking:** Today, this method is used to flavor fish rather than preserve it. Therefore, **modern** materials contain **fewer carcinogenic tars than** traditional methods. Still, there are **certain risks** (see Vol. 1, p. 271).

– **Freezing:** This is the **safest and most effective** method of preserving fish. A temperature of –30°C [(30 degrees centigrade below zero) –22°F] is needed to arrest the decay-producing activity of enzymes and microorganisms in fish. Storage times are shorter as temperatures increase. For example:

✓ –25°C [–13°F (4-star freezer)]: two months
✓ –18°C [–0.4°F (3-star freezer)]: one month
✓ –12°C [10.4°F (2-star freezer)]: two weeks

Transport and **distribution** of **fresh fish** must always be conducted at **lower than 0°C (32°F).**

Marine Pollution

The oceans are not limitless, nor are their resources, as some might wish. In the same way, the seas' capacity to absorb and process the wastes of human activity is also limited.

Heavy metals (mercury, cadmium, arsenic, and others), **PCB** (polychlorinated biphenyls), **dioxins,** and **pesticides** are among the *most dangerous* contaminants of the seas.[2,3]

They **accumulate** in animal tissue (both terrestrial and aquatic) and are passed from one to another, until they reach humans. *Many* of these contaminants are **carcinogenic.**

The pollution of the sea and the creatures living in it represents a serious hindrance to the use of seafood products, particularly shellfish, which are the most susceptible (see Vol. 1, p. 256-261).

Diseases of Fish

The increasing numbers of diseased fish caught in their nets alarms fishermen. Some examples are:

• Since 1940, there has been an ever increasing incidence of tumors, particularly of the gonads and liver, in fish from the North American Great Lakes.[4]

• According to studies carried out at the Saint Hyacinthe College of Veterinary Medicine (Quebec, Canada),[6] eels from the Saint Lawrence River in Canada appear with an increasing number of cutaneous ulcers and vertebral deformations.

The hundreds of chemical substances that are continuously dumped into the oceans are the direct cause of these and other fish diseases. Although there is no proof that these are transmitted to humans, they are obviously a cause for concern.

Because of all of this, the Journal of the American Medical Association advises that **increased** fish **consumption** is associated with certain **risks.**[7]

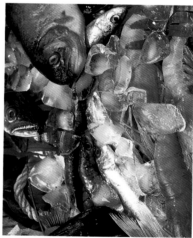

Marine animals increasingly suffer diseases that are a consequence of pollution, just as their land counterparts do.

Continued on page 240

Nutritional Value

Water

Water makes up approximately 80% of the weight of fish.

Protein

- **Quantity:** Fish contains 15% to 20% proteins, an amount similar to meat. However, when *equal raw weights* are compared, lean fish has **more** protein than meat, since meat has a fat content that is missing in fish.

- **Quality:** Fish protein is of high quality, because it contains an almost *ideal* proportion of essential **amino acids.** Additionally, fish protein is easily **digestible.** As a result, the body is able to **utilize** almost the **total amount** present.

- **Types:** The types of proteins present in fish are actin and myosin (proteins that cause contraction in the cytoplasm of muscle cells), nucleoproteins, and collagen (although less than in meat).

Fat

- **Quantity:** The amount of fat in fish varies between 0.64% in hake to 12% in sardines. This number varies depending on many factors.

- **Quality:** The fats in fish are *primarily **unsaturated fatty acids,*** as opposed to the fats found in other animal products (meat, milk, and eggs), in which fats are primarily saturated.

Part of the fatty acids found in fish is *benefit* the **cardiovascular system** (see Vol. 1, p. 240).

Cholesterol

Fish contains between 40 and 130 mg/100 g of cholesterol, an amount *similar* to **meat** and cured **cheese,** but less than that of **eggs** and **butter.**

Vitamins

- ***B group:*** Fish is a **good source** of all of the B vitamins,

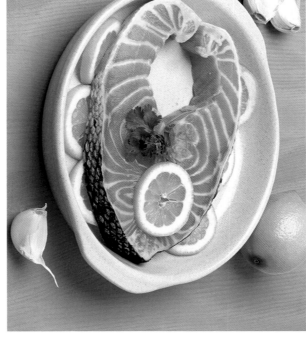

particularly B_{12}. One hundred grams of fish more than covers the RDA (Recommended Daily Amount) for anyone.

- ***Vitamins A and D:*** These vitamins are found particularly in fish liver, but in the meat, as well. One hundred grams of fish provides between 5% and 10% of RDA for vitamin A and about 50% of that for vitamin D. Lean fish provides three to four times less.

- ***Vitamin E:*** This vitamin is also more abundant in fatty fish. One hundred grams provides about 10% of the RDA for an adult. Lean fish contains only small amounts of vitamin E.

Minerals

- ***Phosphorus:*** Fish, like meat, is very rich in this mineral. However, there is no risk of deficiency with a balanced diet.

- ***Calcium:*** Most fish provides *very little* calcium. The anchovy is the exception, providing 147 mg/100 g, somewhat more than milk.

- ***Iron:*** One hundred grams provides from 5% to 10% of RDA; this is less than meat, and much less than legumes, grains, or some vegetables. However, this is heme iron, which is absorbed better than that found in vegetable foods or eggs, which are *non-heme.*

- ***Iodine:*** Saltwater fish are, together with seaweed, the *best source* of this mineral. One hundred grams of saltwater fish provides from 150 to 350 µg, between twice and three times the RDA for an adult. Freshwater fish contains only 0.2 and 0.4 µg/100 g of iodine.

- ***Sodium:*** Regardless of whether the fish is from salt or fresh water, it contains between 40 and 100 mg of sodium per 100 grams. This is 10 to 20 times more than most vegetable-based foods. At the same time, fish contains less potassium than vegetables. Fish must, therefore, be eaten in *moderation,* particularly in cases of **hypertension,** avoiding the fish preserved with salt.

# of Fish

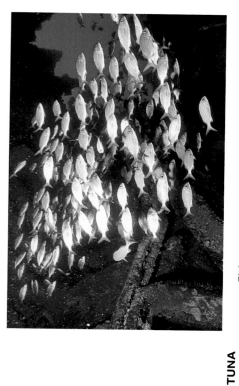

Fish contains as much, and as complete protein, as meat, but with the advantage that it is easier to digest, since it has less collagen fiber. Additionally, fish has many other advantages over meat (see Vol. 1, pp. 300, 301).

TUNA
Composition
per 100 g of raw edible portion

			% Daily Value (based on a 2,000 calorie diet) provided by 100 g of this food
Energy	144 kcal ≙ 602 kj		
Protein	23.3 g		
Carbohydrates	—		
Fiber	—		
Vitamin A	655 µg RE		
Vitamin B₁	0.241 mg		
Vitamin B₂	0.251 mg		
Niacin	13.0 mg NE		
Vitamin B₆	0.455 mg		
Folate	1.90 µg		
Vitamin B₁₂	9.43 µg		
Vitamin C	—		
Vitamin E	1.00 mg α-TE		
Calcium	8.00 mg		
Phosphorus	254 mg		
Magnesium	50.0 mg		
Iron	1.02 mg		
Potassium	252 mg		
Zinc	0.600 mg		
Total Fat	4.90 g		
Saturated Fat	1.26 g		
Cholesterol	38.0 mg		
Sodium	39.0 mg		

1% 2% 4% 10% 20% 40% 100% 200% 500%

TUNA

Minerals **1.18%**
Fat **4.90%**

Protein **23.3%**

Water **68.1%**

P E R C C N T A G E   C O M P O S I T I O N

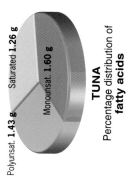

TUNA
Percentage distribution of **fatty acids**

Polyunsat. **1.43 g** Saturated **1.26 g** Monounsat. **1.60 g**

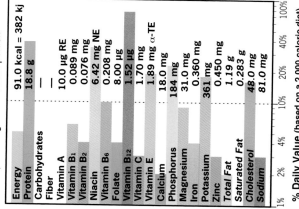

SOLE
Composition
per 100 g of raw edible portion

			% Daily Value (based on a 2,000 calorie diet) provided by 100 g of this food
Energy	91.0 kcal ≙ 382 kj		
Protein	18.8 g		
Carbohydrates	—		
Fiber	—		
Vitamin A	10.0 µg RE		
Vitamin B₁	0.089 mg		
Vitamin B₂	0.076 mg		
Niacin	6.42 mg NE		
Vitamin B₆	0.208 mg		
Folate	8.00 µg		
Vitamin B₁₂	1.52 µg		
Vitamin C	1.70 mg		
Vitamin E	1.89 mg α-TE		
Calcium	18.0 mg		
Phosphorus	184 mg		
Magnesium	31.0 mg		
Iron	0.360 mg		
Potassium	361 mg		
Zinc	0.450 mg		
Total Fat	1.19 g		
Saturated Fat	0.283 g		
Cholesterol	48.0 mg		
Sodium	81.0 mg		

1% 2% 4% 10% 20% 40% 100%

SOLE

Minerals **1.20%**
Fat **1.19%**

Protein **18.8%**

Water **79.1%**

P E R C C N T A G E   C O M P O S I T I O N

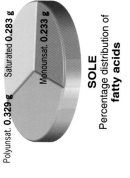

SOLE
Percentage distribution of **fatty acids**

Polyunsat. **0.329 g** Saturated **0.283 g** Monounsat. **0.233 g**

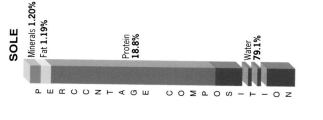

The Pros and Cons of Fish

Fish is generally considered a healthful food. It may well be healthier than meat and its derivatives, but it still presents serious drawbacks to health.

Benefits of Fish Compared With Meat

- **Nutritious**
  - Fish supplies complete *protein*, with a *moderate amount of calories*: 80-100 kcal/100 g for lean fish and 120-200 kcal/100 g for fatty fish. Meat, on the other hand, contains 250-350 kcal/100 g.
  - *Vitamins:* Fish contains liposoluble *vitamins A* and *D*, while meat does not.

- **Ease of digestion:** Fish *protein* and *fat* are more easily digested than those of meat because:
  - Fish muscle is *less* **fibrous** than that of poultry and mammals. This is because fish muscle contains less collagen. Fish collagen is also softer, and tends to break down during cooking.[8]
  - Fish contains *less* **fat** than meat (see Vol. 1, p. 288), and since this fat is *unsaturated*, it is less dense (more fluid, see Vol. 1, p. 240) and more healthy.

- **Fish are typically raised in nature:** With the exception of fish raised on fish farms, most of those used as food live freely in their natural element (seas, rivers, or lakes), as opposed to other animals that are intensively raised in captivity. Their food is that which is provided by nature and it does not contain antibiotics, hormones, or other foreign substances.

- **Heart-healthy:** Even though there are investigations offering contradictory findings (see box on next page), the consumption of fish is associated with lower risk of heart disease.

Fish or fish oils do not reduce cholesterol levels. Their consumption reduces triglycerides (a type of fat that circulates in the blood, see Vol. 1, p. 240).

Drawbacks to Fish

- **Lacking in certain nutrients:** Fish does not contain vitamin C, carbohydrates (sugars or starch), or fiber. It contains little calcium (except anchovies).

- **Constipation:** Since fish contains no vegetable fiber, it is constipating, unless it is eaten with vegetables, whole grains, or fruit.

- **Decalcification:** Eating a great deal of fish, or meat, for that matter, leads to a depletion in bone calcium because:
  - It provides *very little* **calcium** and a *great deal of phosphorous*, leading to an imbalance between these two minerals.
  - *Increases* the **loss** of calcium **through the urine** due to its significant protein content.

  Therefore, fish should be eaten in *moderation* in cases of *osteoporosis*.

- **Allergies:** Fish is the *most allergenic* of all foods (see Vol. 1, p. 249). Its own proteins, the histamine formed during decay, and the anisakis parasite, may provoke allergic reactions.

- **Uric acid:** Fish contains nucleoproteins from the nuclei of their muscle tissue, which become uric acid when metabolized in the body. Because of this, it is *not advised* for those suffering from excess blood levels of **uric acid, gout,** or urate **kidney stones.**

- **Antinutritive factors:** Raw or poorly cooked fish contains **thiaminase,** an enzyme that destroys *vitamin B₁.* Therefore, consumption of raw fish can lead to a lack of this vitamin.

- **Poisoning:** Poisoning resulting from fish occurs because:
  - the fish themselves or some of their body parts are **toxic** (see Vol. 1, p. 246), or
  - they are **contaminated** with bacteria, parasites, or chemical substances such as mercury (see Vol. 1, p. 250).

- **Cancer:** The **chemical pollution** of seas, lakes, and rivers that causes tumors in fish, may have carcinogenic effect on those eating them, as well.[9] **Brine-cured fish**[5] and **sauces,**[10] typical of China and Southeast Asia, contain **nitrosamines,** which exercise a carcinogenic effect on the pharynx and the stomach.

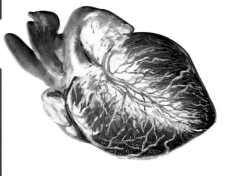

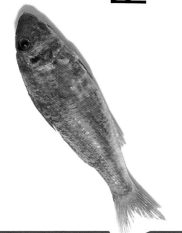

Fish and the Heart

Beneficial Effect

Several epidemiological studies show that *regular con-sumption* of fish, whether lean or fatty, reduces the *risk* of heart attack (*myocardial infarction*). For example:

- A 30-year longitudinal study of 1,822 men in the United States demonstrated that those who ate a kilo of fish per month (one or two servings per week) showed 40% less risk of unexpected death due to heart attack (myocardial infarction).[11]

- Those who habitually eat fish or take fish-oil supplements suffer less arrhythmia and have a lower risk of sudden death due to cardiac arrest, particularly if they have had a previous heart attack (myocardial infarction).[12]

However, not only fish provides this effect. A diet rich in *linolenic acid* from vegetable sources (walnuts, flax-seed or soy products) produces the *same* results.[13]

Neutral or Negative Effect

These studies not withstanding, others find no benefit to fish. For example, a four-year longitudinal study of 44,895 North American male healthcare professionals shows that fish consumption or fish oil supplements have no bearing on heart attack risk.[15]

A study conducted in Finland, a country where fish con-sumption is traditionally high, provided some unexpected results: the more omega-3 fatty acids from fish sources, the greater the risk of death from heart disease such as my-ocardial infarction.[71]

In Summary

How can the apparent contradiction among these studies be explained?

Various facts help explain the effect of fish on the heart:

- If there is no corresponding *reduction* in the consumption of **saturated fats**, fish or fish oil will not protect against cardiovascular disease.[14]

- The **beneficial effects** of fish only become apparent *when it replaces* other foods in the diet which are high in satu-rated fats, such as meat. The idea is not so much to add fish to the diet, but to have fish *replace meat*, whose con-sumption is clearly harmful to the heart.

- The fact that heart attack risk is lowered regardless of whether lean or fatty fish are eaten leads to a conclusion that the beneficial effects are not due so much to fish oil (lean fish has very little), but rather to the fact that fish re-places other foods harmful to the heart.

- Fish, however, can be *harmful* to the cardiovascular sys-tem when:

  – it is **contaminated** with high levels of **mercury** (see Vol. 1, p. 250),

  – it is **contaminated** with **bacteria** that produce histamine and other vasoactive biogenic amines (see Vol. 1, p. 248).

  – It contains a *great* deal of **salt**, as is the case with certain preserving techniques.

Better Than Fish

- **Fish** is *beneficial* to the **heart** if it is accompanied by a *reduction* in **meat.**

- Fish is *not necessary* for a healthy heart.

- **Vegetable** foods such as fruit, whole grains, and legumes provide *more protective* substances to the **heart** than fish, but with *fewer drawbacks.*

Lean and

The nutritional composition of the various species of fish is quite constant, with the exception of fat. Several nutritional characteristics of fish depend on its fat content.

	Lean fish	Fatty fish
FAT CONTENT	Less than 4%-5%	More than 4%-5%
OMEGA-3 FATTY ACID CONTENT	Low	High (approximately 35% of total fat)
DIGESTION	Easy and rapid	Slower and heavier
HISTAMINE FORMATION	Slight	Abundant
ALLERGENIC	Occasional	Frequent
PESTICIDE CONTAMINATION	Occasional	More frequent (these toxic chemicals accumulate in fatty tissue)

Caviar Is Also High in Fat

The sturgeon (Acipenser sturio) is a large fish measuring from three to six meters in length. Its skin is not made up of true scales, but rather a series of large bony plates aligned in five rows.

Authentic caviar is the roe of the female sturgeon, which has been removed from its abdomen, resulting in the fish's death. Other types are obtained from other species of fish.

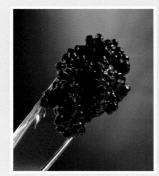

Caviar contains **17.9% fat,** of which almost **half are omega-3 fatty acids,** and 24.6% protein.

There have been cases reported of **hepatitis** transmitted by Russian caviar.[16]

Variations in Fat Content

The fat **proportion** varies **a great deal among** various fish. Even within the same species it can change significantly so that, depending on the time of year the same fish may be either fatty or lean. The most influential factors are:

- **Temperature:** The colder, the more fat.
- **Migration:** Anadromous fish are born in fresh water, spend their adult lives in the sea, and return to their place of birth to spawn. Before they begin the journey back to the rivers, their fat content increases greatly. An eel, for example may contain up to 25% fat during this period.
- **Spawning:** After the females have laid their eggs and the males have fertilized them, the fish contain much less fat.

Fatty Fish

The anchovy, the sardine, and the mackerel are the least contaminated of fatty fish, since they feed on plankton (they are not carnivores, see Vol. 1, p. 248).

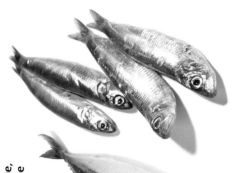

'Surimi': Ground Muscle

Ground muscle is precisely what the word 'surimi' means in Japanese. This name is used to describe the frozen fish sticks found in many supermarkets.

Fish sticks or surimi are made of:

- **ground muscle mass** of various fish, particularly pollock (Pollachius virens), a lean fish;
- **starch:** the most abundant carbohydrate in grains;
- **additives:** generally monosodium glutamate (flavor enhancer) and flavorings extracted from shellfish or elvers.

Composition of Fish per 100 g of Raw Edible Portion

		Calories kcal	Protein g	Fat g	Cholesterol mg	Omega-3 fatty acids* g
LEAN FISH						
SEA BASS	Dicentrarchus labrax	97	17.3	2.33	80	0.77
GROUPER	Epinephelus caninus	92	19.4	1.02	37	0.26
PIKE	Esox lucius	88	19.3	0.69	39	0.13
COD	Gadus morhua	82	17.8	0.67	43	0.19
MONKFISH	Lophius piscatorius	83	14.5	1.52	25	0.20
HAKE	Merluccius merluccius	87	19.0	0.64	40	0.30
POLLACK	Pollachius virens	78	19.4	0.98	71	0.42
TURBOT	Scophthalmus maximus	95	16.0	2.95	48	0.40
FLATFISH (SOLE)	Solea vulgaris	91	18.8	1.19	48	0.21
FATTY FISH						
EEL	Anguilla spp.	184	18.4	11.7	126	0.58
HERRING	Clupea harengus	158	18.0	9.04	60	1.67
CARP	Cyprinus carpio	127	17.8	5.60	66	0.62
ANCHOVY	Engraulis encrasicholus	131	20.4	4.84	60	1.45
RAINBOW TROUT	Salmo gairdneri	138	20.8	5.40	59	0.99
SALMON	Salmo salar	142	19.8	6.34	55	1.73
SARDINE	Sardina pilchardus	178	16.3	12.0	61	1.87
MACKEREL	Scombermorus maculatus	139	19.3	6.30	76	1.38
TUNA	Thunnus thynnus	144	23.3	4.90	38	1.17
SWORDFISH	Xiphias gladius	121	19.8	4.00	39	0.83

* See informative box on the next page.

Omega-3 Fatty Acids

A fatty acid is called **omega-3** (or **n-3**) when the first double bond in the hydrocarbon chain is on the third carbon atom, counted from the terminal methyl group; it is called **omega-6** when it is on the sixth, and so on.

The **omega-3** fatty acids found in fish represent between **30%** and **40%** of their total fatty acids. The most important are these two:

- **eicosapentaenoic acid** (EPA), with 20 carbon atoms and five double bonds;
- **docosahexaenoic acid** (DHA), with 22 carbon atoms and six double bonds. The particular molecular disposition of omega-3 fatty acids found in fish gives them special therapeutic influences not found in other fatty acids.

- They **reduce** blood triglyceride levels.
- They **reduce** the **risk** of a serious heart attack and cardiac arrest.
- They act as **anti-inflammatories**. For example, in cases of **rheumatoid arthritis, ulcerous colitis,** and other **autoimmune diseases.**

this special type of fatty acid, except some shellfish and eggs from hens that have been fed seaweed. In **vegetables,** the unsaturated **omega-3** fatty acid is **linolenic acid,** found particularly in **walnuts, wheat germ,** and evening **primrose** and **canola oils** (see Vol. 1, pp. 124-127, EMP, p. 238).

Beneficial Effects of Fish Oil

Fish oil is used as a *dietary supplement* for the treatment of various diseases.[17] However, in some cases, persons who take it receive **no** real **benefit.** In these instances the effects of fish oil **conflict** with scientific criteria and only serve the **commercial interests** of the producers.

The daily dose of fish oil is 4-10 g, which contains approximately 1-5 g of omega-3 fatty acids. Beneficial effects have been reported in these cases:

- **Alterations in blood plasma lipids:** Even though at one time it was thought that fish oil reduces cholesterol levels, it is well known for years that this is not the case.[18]

  The prestigious journal *The American Journal of Clinical Nutrition* published a supplement in 1997 exclusively dedicated to fish oil. One of these articles concludes, after reviewing all of the reliable studies up to that time, that the **consumption** of 3 to 7 g of fish oil a day for at least two weeks, produces:[19]

  – A 25% to 30% *reduction* in **triglyceride** levels. This is the most consistent effect, although it diminishes with the passage of time.[20] **TRIGLYCERIDES** are a kind of fat circulating in the blood. Their *increased levels* promote **arteriosclerosis** and **coronary disease,** particularly in women.

  – *Maintenance* or *increase* in **cholesterol** levels: Most studies have detected an increase in harmful LDL cholesterol.

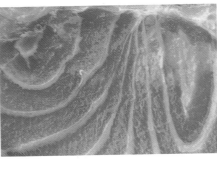

Continued from page 233

The Fat Found in Fish

Characteristics

Fish fat is liquid at room temperature; therefore, it is referred to as **fish oil.** Its *primary components* are **triglycerides** with a small phospholipid (**lecithin**) component.

Fish oil *triglycerides* are composed of *unique* fatty acids that *differ* from those in other foods. Their characteristics are:

- **Long chain:** their molecules contain 20 to 24 carbon atoms. The fatty acids of meat and milk products have no more than 18 carbon atoms; linoleic and oleic acids, which are the most abundant in vegetables, contain 18.

- **Polyunsaturated:** They have up to 6 double bonds. Most other animal fatty acids are saturated.

- *Omega-3:* Some of the fatty acid molecules of fish are of omega-3 configuration. *No other* **animal-based** food contains

The unique constituent of fish, and the one that most differentiates it from other foods, is its fat.

Fish fat, which is liquid at room temperature, gives fish most of its medicinal properties.

The Effect of Omega-3 Fatty Acids From Fish on Triglyceride Levels

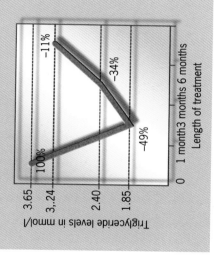

The beneficial effect of fish oil on blood triglyceride levels diminishes over time, even though the use of fish oil is continued.[20]

- **Arteriosclerosis:** The recommended dose of fish oil slows down its progression.[21]

- **Hypertension:** Some studies show that fish oil is effective in reducing arterial hypertension.[22] Others state that it is not.[23]

- **Tendency to thrombosis:** Fish oil lowers the fibrinogen level; this is the blood protein responsible for clotting. **Olive oil** (see Vol. 1, p. 118) has the *same* effect.[24]

- **Ulcerative colitis:** Four months of high doses (6 g daily) of *omega-3 fatty acids*, produces clinical improvement.[25]

- **Crohn's disease:** Avoids or retards relapse.[26]

- **Dysmenorrhea:** Two daily grams of omega-3 fatty acids for two months, reduces the symptoms of dysmenorrhea in adolescents.[27]

- **Rheumatoid arthritis:** Administration of 10 g of fish oil a day for six months, produces a slight anti-inflammatory effect, allowing a reduction in other medications.[28]

- Beneficial effects have also been observed in cases of **migraine, asthma,** and **psoriasis.**[29]

Undesirable Effects of Fish Oil

- **Harmful substances:** fish oil contains *cholesterol* and *traces* of *mercury* (see Vol. 1, p. 250), which impair arterial health.

- **Insufficient *vitamin E*:** When fish oil is taken as a supplement or when a great deal of fatty fish is eaten, supplementary vitamin E is recommended to compensate for the *tendency* of EPA and DHA *omega-3* fatty acids to become *oxidized.*[29]

- **Hypervitaminosis A:** Cases of hypervitaminosis A after prolonged use (more than six months) of fish oil have been reported.[30]

- **Cerebral hemorrhages** are more likely to happen among those who consume *large amounts* of fatty fish or fish oil, as is the case with eskimos.[31]

- **Poor healing of wounds:** After a month of taking fish oil supplements, the healing capability of wounds diminished since collagen tissue in the body is weakened. Because of this, fish oil should be avoided after surgical interventions.[32]

***Even though both fish oil and olive oil protect the heart, the latter has fewer undesirable effects, and is more effective in arteriosclerosis prevention.*[34]**

Fish Oil or Olive Oil?

A study carried out at the University of Leipzig (Germany) demonstrated that, while fish oils play a positive role in the prevention of heart disease, they increase cholesterol levels and are not antioxidants. Salmon oil capsules were less effective than olive oil in preventing the lipid peroxidation that initiates arteriosclerosis.[33]

	Fish oil	Olive oil
Effect on cholesterol	Raises LDL (harmful cholesterol)	Raises HDL (beneficial cholesterol)
Effect on triglycerides	Reduces their level	May increase their level
Propensity to oxidation	Yes, contains little vitamin E	No
Propensity toward thrombosis	Reduces	Reduces

How To Recognize Fresh Fish

Smell: A recently caught fish has little odor. After the first few hours, **trimethylamine** begins to form, creating an increasingly putrid odor.

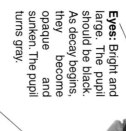

Eyes: Bright and large. The pupil should be black. As decay begins, they become opaque and sunken. The pupil turns gray.

Gills: Red and firm, the gills turn gray and soft as the fish ages.

Scales: Bright and tightly attached to the skin, from which they are difficult to remove.

Belly: Firm and whitish. As decay progresses, it becomes soft and gray.

Flesh: Firm and fixed to the skeleton. It turns brownish and separates from the bones when it no longer fresh.

An **ammonia smell** reveals that the fish's proteins are in a state of advanced decay. Sharks and rays give off this odor even when fresh, due their high content of toxic urea.

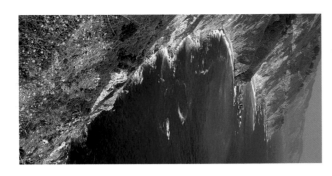

Decay of Fish

Fish is, *together* with **shellfish**, the *most unstable* of foods, since its tissues decay very rapidly.

Some processes taking place during fishing, and even before the fish has been removed from the water, accelerate decay, which continues with the death and further processing of the fish.

Exhaustion of the Fish

If the fish has fought hard as it was caught, it uses up its scarce reserves of muscle glycogen before it dies. This means that it does not form lactic acid after death, thus facilitating the proliferation of bacteria and speeding decay.

Expulsion of Intestinal Content

When fish is caught in a net and rapidly brought to the surface, its swimming bladder fills with water and compresses the stomach and intestines. This internal pressure on the digestive organs, together with that of being piled with other fish, causes the contents of the digestive tract to be disgorged through the mouth or anus. Since this material is highly septic, the whole catch may be quickly contaminated.

Body Rigidity

An hour after capture, fish become rigid, showing signs of *rigor mortis*, as its muscular proteins (actin and myosin) congeal due to the action of the lactic acid formed from glycogen. This rigidity is desirable, since the lactic acid that produces it slows the proliferation of bacteria.

Decay

Six or eight hours after death, body rigidity begins to give way to a softening of the fish's tissues as a consequence of its decay. This may be of two types:

• **Internal:** This begins in the abdomen and head and is caused by:

– The action of **enzymes** from the digestive tract of the animal that have been released as a consequence of death of cells. These enzymes spread throughout the body tissues and degrade them.

– The destruction of tissues caused by **bacteria** from the digestive tract and mouth of the fish.

• **External:** Bacteria and other germs enter through damage to the skin suffered by the fish during catching. In some cases, the ice used to preserve the fish may, itself, damage the skin. The **bacteria** that cause decay come from:

– The **intestines** of the fish itself, either through the mouth or the anus.

– Anti-hygienic **handling** of the fish after capture.

The vast *proliferation* of **bacteria** during the decay of fish produces a variety **of toxic substances:**

– biogenic amines, such as **histamine, putrescine,** and **cadaverine,** which cause scombroid poisoning manifested through allergic symptoms (see Vol. 1, p. 249).

– other **bacterial toxins** causing gastroenteritis and skin symptoms.

Putrefaction

This is the *final phase* of the decay of fish. Bacteria completely degrade protein and fat, producing toxic biogenic amines. *Some of these are* **foul smelling,** which helps determine the state of putrefaction.

How To Slow the Decay of Fish

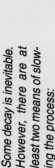

Some decay is inevitable. However, there are at least two means of slowing the process:

• **Cleaning:** *Due to their high content of enzymes and microorganisms, the head and viscera of fish accelerate decay. Both should be removed as soon as possible.*

• **Refrigeration:** *If fish is stored above 0°C (zero degrees centigrade), its bacteria proliferate rapidly, leading to decay of its protein.*

Processed Anchovies: Mediterranean Handicraft

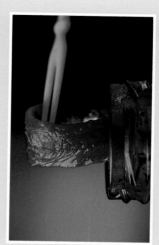

Processing anchovies is a manual process in which anchovy ('Engraulis encrasicholus') fillets are **pressed, salted,** *and* **fermented** *under control.*

This process has been used for centuries in Mediterranean countries to prevent decay and to give the anchovy fillets their typical red color. The anchovy is not a carnivorous fish; therefore, it is less susceptible to contamination.

Fins and scales are the most characteristic features of fish. Ichthyologists (scientists who study fish) use them to identify and classify the various species.

It is interesting that among marine creatures, **those with fins and scales are the more appropriate** for use as food. On the other hand, those creatures lacking these features are unhealthful. In fact, the Law of Moses declares such animals "impure" or contaminated. Once again, science confirms the Biblical classification of animals used for food (see Vol. 1, p. 297).

Shellfish

Shellfish have neither fins nor scales. Their consumption presents many more health issues than fish. They are quite often responsible for various **poisonings.**

Fish

Although all fish have fins, some lack scales. Curiously, those that lack them are the **least healthful** and among them are the most toxic. Of the three zoological classes of fish, the first two never have true scales:

- **Agnatha** (fish without jaws); for example, the lamprey.
- **Chondrichthyes** (fish with a cartilaginous skeleton), also known as **Elasmobranchii** or **Selachii**, such as sharks and rays.
- **Osteichthyes** (bony fish), also called **teleosts**. Most have scales and are those **most often used** as food. However, there are some orders or families of fish covered with a smooth skin; for example, catfish, eels, and swordfish. Osteichthyes lacking scales are precisely the least healthful and most injurious to health.

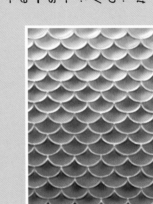

Sharks and Rays

These are the best-known examples of fish of the class Chondrichthyes (see the informational box at left). Their flesh is widely eaten, although it is of low quality.

— **Sharks:** The Great White (*Carcharodon carcharias*) and the Blue (*Prionace glauca*) are voracious predators. There are other sharks that live on plankton, such as the Whale Shark (*Rhincodon typus*), which at fifteen meters in length is the largest fish that exists (whales are not fish, but rather marine mammals).

- **Rays:** the white ray (*Raja alba* or *marginata*) and other species of rays.

Their skin is not covered with true scales, rather with prominences that give it a sandpaper-like feel.

- **Caution:** The **flesh** from all of these fish is **toxic** because of its *high* **urea** content. It gives off a disagreeable ammonia odor that is the result of bacteriological action on the urea. Its consumption often produces headache and malaise.

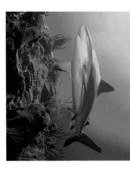

Sharks are covered with tooth-like false scales instead of true scales.

Fish Without Scales: the Most Dangerous to Health

Lampreys

The sea lamprey (*Petromyzon marinus*) and the river lamprey (*Lampetra fluviatilis*) belong to the zoological class Agnatha (fish lacking true jaws). Their skin is smooth and without scales.

- **Caution:** Lampreys feed by sucking blood from other fish through a round mouth that functions as a suction cup. Because of, this many chemical and bacteriological toxins accumulate in their flesh, which, if eaten, may cause digestive disorders.

Catfish

Catfish belong to the zoological order Siluriformes. Its skin is smooth or covered with bony plates. Two species are of dietary interest:

— **North American Catfish** (*Ictalurus punctatus*), and

— **European Catfish** (*Silurus glanis*).

- **Caution:** Their meat is of very poor quality and hard to digest.

Eels and Similar Species

All eels and related species belong to the zoological order Anguilliformes. Their scales are either absent or tiny and barely visible. Eels are also referred to as **apodal,** since they lack ventral fins. The best known are:

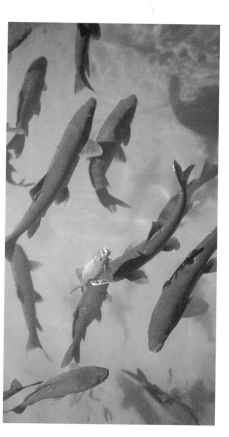

- The **eel** (*Anguilla anguilla* and other species) and the **elver,** which is the immature eel;

- The **conger eel** (*Conger conger*), which measures two to three meters (about 6.6 feet) in length and can weigh as much as 70 kilos (about 155 pounds); and

- The **Moray eel** (*Muraena helena*).

• **Caution:** Although they are much appreciated culinarily by some, their use as food presents at least three health concerns:

- The **blood** of these fish contains a *highly irritating toxin.* It causes vomiting, bloody diarrhea, paralysis, and even death when eaten. Even when the blood is removed before cooking, there are always traces of it left. Persons touching their mouth or eyes with eel blood on their hands suffer serious inflammatory reactions accompanied by itching and pain.

- Eels are the most **indigestible** of fish due to their *elevated fat* content (up to 25% during certain times of the year) and **cholesterol.**

- These are among the fish responsible for the toxic **ciguatera** syndrome (see the following page).

Swordfish

The swordfish (*Xiphias gladius*) has a smooth skin and is very large, reaching 500 kilos (1,111 pounds) and three meters in length.

It is a voracious predator that feeds exclusively on other fish.

• **Caution:** Swordfish flesh is flavorful but unhealthful, as is the case with many carnivorous predatory fish. They are the fish *most responsible* for toxic ciguatera syndrome (see the following page).

Blowfish or Puffer Fish

These members of the zoological order Tetraodontiformes have the peculiar char-

acteristic of inflating their belly with water or air to about twice their size. In Japan, where they are considered a delicacy, they are called **fugu.**

Their skin contains no scales, and in some species it is covered with bony plates or spines.

Blowfish has four rudimentary teeth, hence their zoological name.

• **Caution:** The viscera of these fish contain **tetrodotoxin,** which is the *most potent* toxin found in fish. Its consumption produces a *severe neurological* paralysis known tetrodotoxism (see following page).

Fish raised in commercial fish farms are more susceptible to pollution and epidemics than those raised in the open sea.

Crowding and **artificial feeding** are among the potentially harmful factors that affect them. Constant supervision by technicians is of great importance in guaranteeing the safety of these fish.

Unhealthful or Dangerous Fish

There are some 20,000 different species of fish in the world's seas. Among them there are more or less healthful species. Some are frankly dangerous because of their toxicity.

Two characteristics are useful in recognizing the most unhealthful or dangerous fish in general:

• *Skin appearance: Those with smooth skin (lampreys and eels), those that lack true scales (sharks and rays), and those covered with spines or bony plates (blowfish) are the ones that present the greatest health problems (see the informative box on the preceding page).*

• *Manner of feeding: Carnivorous fish, whose primary or exclusive food is made up of other animals, are generally those that contain the highest concentrations of mercury and other toxins (see the following pages).*

Poisoning From Fish

Fish can cause poisoning for various reasons:

- It may be **unhealthful or toxic in itself.**
- Some **portion** of it may be **toxic.**
- It **may contain** various **toxins** (see this page):
  – ciguatera
  – tetrodotoxism
- **Bacteria** that produce toxins may **contaminate it:**
  – internal bacterial contamination: *scombroid syndrome or histamine poisoning* (see Vol. 1, p. 248)
  – **external** bacterial contamination (Vol. 1, p. 249)
- It may be **infested with parasites** such as anisakis or others (Vol. 1, p. 250).
- It may be contaminated with **mercury** (methyl mercury, Vol. 1, p. 250).

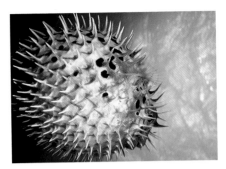

The **blowfish, known in Japan as 'fugu'.**
This fish is covered with bony plates or spines instead of scales. Eating its flesh, which is considered a delicacy in Japan, may lead to **serious poisoning** (see previous page).

Poisoning Caused by Fish Consumption

Poisoning from eating toxic portions of fish

As can be seen on the next page, certain parts or organs of some fish can cause poisoning if eaten.

- **Prevention:** Avoid eating.

Ciguatera Poisoning

This toxic syndrome is produced from eating certain tropical and subtropical fish, usually predatory carnivores. More cases of ciguatera are seen in nontropical regions as a result of climatic change.[35]

- **Fish that produce ciguatera:** There are about 300 known species of **ciguatic** species, so called because they can cause ciguatera poisoning. A substantial number of these lack scales and/or are carnivorous predators that feed on other fish. Among these are the **conger eel** (*Conger conger*), the **moray eel,** (*Muraena helena*), the **swordfish** (*Xiphias gladius*), the **barracuda** (*Sphiraena barracuda*), the **sea bass** (*Dicentrarchus labrax*) and the **grouper** (*Epinephelus caninus*).

- **Causes:** Various toxic substances have been isolated in the flesh of these fish. The most significant is **ciguatoxin.** It is produced by *Gambierdiscus toxicus* and other microscopic dinoflagellate algae (see Vol. 1, p. 259). These algae form part of the plankton living in warm seas, generally in the vicinity of coral atolls. These **toxins** *are passed* from smaller fish feeding on **plankton,** to **larger** fish feeding on the smaller ones, and so on up the food chain becoming more and more *concentrated.* The more carnivorous a fish, the greater the possibility of storing dangerous amounts of ciguatoxin.

- **Symptoms:** From thirty minutes to several hours after eating ciguatic fish, two types of symptoms appear:
  – **Digestive:** nausea, vomiting, diarrhea.
  – **Neurological:** These symptoms appear in the most severe cases. There is a paresthesia (tingling) in the mouth, throat and limbs, general weakness, and paralysis. If death does not result, these symptoms may last for several weeks.

- **Prevention:** The **appearance and flavor** of a contaminated fish is *absolutely* **normal.** On some islands suspicious fish is first given to cats, because there is no other way to detect these toxins, which are not destroyed by cooking.
Because of all of this, the *best and safest* preventive measure is to **avoid** *potentially* **contaminated** species.

Tetrodotoxism

This poisoning is *severe,* even fatal in many cases. It is produced by eating the **viscera** (particularly the ovaries) or the **flesh** of various species of fish without scales known as blowfish or puffer fish.

- **Causes:** The viscera of these fish, particularly the ovaries, contain a potent paralytic toxin called **tetrodotoxin.**[36] When these fish are eviscerated (cleaned) their flesh also becomes contaminated, although in Japan there are true specialists in cleaning these fish without contaminating them.

Continued on page 248

Potentially Toxic Portions of Fish

Blood: A **severe irritation** results from touching the **mouth** or **eyes** with hands contaminated with **eel, conger eel,** or **moray** blood. This often occurs while they are being cleaned (see Vol. 1, p. 245).

Fins: Some species have spines in their dorsal fin that **inject poison** when touched.

Swim Bladder: This in itself is not toxic. However, it promotes bacterial contamination in fish. As it swells during the net-fishing process, it **compresses** the **stomach** and **intestine,** expelling their contaminated contents.

Skin: When it does **not** have **scales** and is **smooth,** it may contain **irritants;** in this case it *should be* handled with caution and **discarded** (lampreys, for example).

Liver: Fish liver contains *large amounts* of **vitamin A** in the form of retinol, which can cause **hypervitaminosis,** as opposed to provitamin A from plants. **Shark** and **ray** livers are *particularly* toxic.

Stomach and Intestines: These organs harbor the larvae of the **anisakis** parasite, which perforates the walls of the digestive tract and enters the fish's flesh causing parasitosis and serious allergic reactions (see Vol. 1, p. 250).

Roe: These are the **ovaries** of female fish at the time of egg-laying. They are *rich in fat* and *vitamins B₁* and *B₂*.

About **40 species** of fish have been found to have **poisonous roe** without affecting the rest of the fish. These are primarily anadromous species (those that have marine and fluvial cycles), such as the **mullet** and the **salmon.**

Roe **poisoning** presents the following **symptoms:**

- **Digestive:** nausea, vomiting, diarrhea, dryness of the mouth;
- **General:** headache, fever, sweating, dizziness.

These symptoms tend to disappear after a few days. There is no specific treatment. The **fish eggs** themselves are *not* **toxic.**

The Food Pyramid

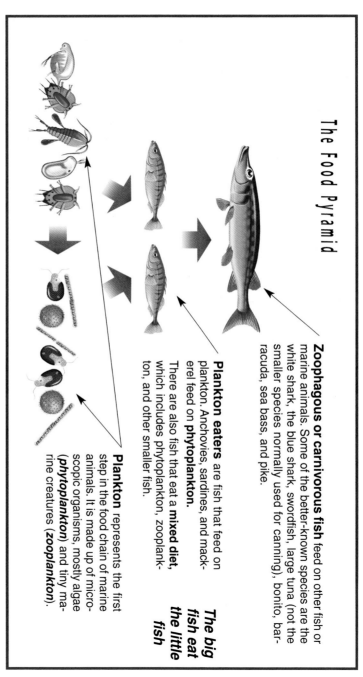

Zoophagous or carnivorous fish feed on other fish or marine animals. Some of the better-known species are the white shark, the blue shark, swordfish, large tuna (not the smaller species normally used for canning), bonito, barracuda, sea bass, and pike.

Plankton eaters are fish that feed on plankton. Anchovies, sardines, and mackerel feed on **phytoplankton.** There are also fish that eat a **mixed diet,** which includes phytoplankton, zooplankton, and other smaller fish.

Plankton represents the first step in the food chain of marine animals. It is made up of microscopic organisms, mostly algae (**phytoplankton**) and tiny marine creatures (**zooplankton**).

The big fish eat the little fish

Zoophagous or **carnivorous fish,** and particularly the great marine predators, are at the **top of the food chain.** These fish eat all others, but are not eaten themselves.

Mercury, pollutants such as **pesticides,** and **toxins** such as ciguatera pass from plankton to zoophagous fish. Since these harmful substances are not eliminated from animal tissue, they go through a process of **bioconcentration:** The more carnivorous the fish —just the same as with land animals—the more toxins accumulate.[2]

Continued from page 246

- **Symptoms** appear about half-hour after eating the viscera or contaminated flesh of these fish, depending on the severity of the poisoning. They progress from paresthesia (tingling), euphoria, and dizziness, and finally muscular paralysis similar to that produced by curare. Death results after six hours due to paralytic asphyxiation.

- **Prevention:** Cooking does not destroy this toxin. In Japan and other oriental countries, these fish are considered a delicacy and are eaten in spite of the risks. Some feel that this is because of the euphoric effect produced by the small amount of toxin that is always present in their flesh.

Poisoning Caused by Internal Bacteriological Contamination

This **scombroid** or **histamine** type of poisoning is one of *the most common.* It is produced by eating fish **in a certain state of decay,** but before it reaches putrefaction, which would render it inedible. This is found in the fish of the Scombroid family such as tuna, bonito, mackerel, sardine, and **fatty fish** in general.

- **Causes:** The bacteria that decay the fish and come from its own digestive tract (internal contamination) produces various toxic substances:

  - **histamine,** from the amino acid histidine, found free in the flesh of many fish.

Fish Allergies

Fish, **together with eggs** and **milk**, is the **most allergenic** of foods.[39] These allergies fall into various classifications:

- **Allergy to the fish itself:** This is caused by certain special proteins found in the fish, which pass directly to the bloodstream without being digested in the intestine.[40]

- **Internal bacterial contamination** fosters scombroid syndrome and histamine poisoning. It comes from eating poorly preserved fish. It presents the same symptoms as an allergy (see accompanying text).

- **Anisakis allergy:** Anisakis is a parasitic worm that infests fish and produces allergic reactions in persons who eat them (see following page).

Fish that Produce Allergies

There is usually a crossover allergic reaction to these two groups of fish:[41]

- cod, haddock, salmon, trout, and tuna;
- anchovies and mackerel.

This means that if one is allergic to a fish in one group, he is usually allergic to the rest.

Symptoms

The most common symptoms are itching skin rash and respiratory difficulty.[41] The symptoms in **children** that suffer from **atopic dermatitis** and **asthma** get significantly worse when they eat fish.[42]

Prevention

Cooking fish does not reduce their allergenic properties. **The only possible prevention** is a proper diagnosis by an allergist physician and **refraining** from eating fish or, at least those fish causing allergies.

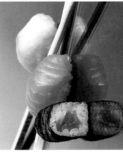

Dishes based on raw fish (such as Peruvian cevichi or Japanese sushi)[43] are the cause of various parasitic infestations such as anisakis.

hours after eating bacterially contaminated fish:

- **digestive:** symptoms of gastroenteritis including nausea, vomiting, and diarrhea.

- **cutaneous:** rash and itching typical of urticaria.

All of these symptoms tend to subside spontaneously within two or three days.

- **Prevention:** Less aggressive fishing technology and scrupulous hygiene during

— other toxic biogenic amines such as **putrescine** and **cadaverine**, which *foster* the activity of histamine.

Most fish contain *some amount of* **histamine** in their muscle tissue. The formerly named species produce a great deal of it as the decay process advances. When it reaches 50 mg/100 g it produces toxic symptoms.[37] **Histamine** is also present in certain fermented cheeses (see Vol. 1, p. 207).[38]

- **Symptoms:** Consuming histamine produces the same symptoms as an **allergic reaction.** A few minutes after eating affected fish, one feels an itching in the mouth and throat, stomach pain, nausea, diarrhea, and itching skin rash. In severe cases arterial hypotension may be included. All of these symptoms tend to disappear spontaneously within 24 hours.[38]

- **Prevention:** Clean the fish as soon as it is caught and store it at least at 0°C (32°F) and out of the sun. Discard any fish whose flesh has turned soft, or which smells or tastes strongly. **Cooking** *does not destroy* **histamine.**

Poisoning Caused by External Bacterial Contamination

Contrary to those of shellfish, fish tissues do not usually harbor pathogenic microorganisms. However, bacterial contamination occurs *easily* during **handling, transportation,** and **storage** of the fish.

- **Cause:** The bacteria involved in this type of contamination of fish tend to be *Staphylococcus pyogenes* and various species of streptococci. External bacterial contamination is promoted by two factors:

  - The **exhaustion** suffered by the fish while being *caught.*

  - **Skin damage** suffered during *handling* (see Vol. 1, p. 243).

- **Symptoms:** Two types of symptoms appear between thirty minutes and three

Mercury and the Heart

Investigators at the University of Kuopio (Finland) noted that men who ate more freshwater fish, compared with those who ate less,[44] were at:

- **double** the risk of suffering a heart attack (myocardial **infarction**) and
- **triple** the risk of dying of a **heart attack.**

The species in question contained more than the 0.5 ppm* of **methyl mercury**, considered the daily allowable intake.

The greater the consumption of fish containing high levels of mercury, the greater the risk of coronary disease or heart attack.

These findings led the Finnish scientists to conclude that high-level **mercury** contamination in fish can **offset** the **beneficial effects** of fish oils on the cardiovascular system.

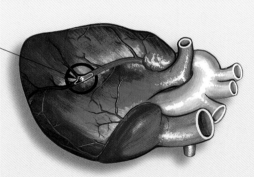

Obstruction of a coronary artery, the cause of infarction.

---

* ppm = parts per million. 1 ppm = 0.1 mg/100 g = 1mg/kg When it is said that a fish contains 1 ppm of mercury, it means that it contains one part of mercury by weight for each million edible parts.

The **parasite** that *most* affects the fish consumed in *Western countries* is **anisakis** (*Anisakis simplex*). This is a nematode (roundworm) approximately two centimeters in length, whose larvae live in the digestive tracts of many species such as hake, tuna, cod, cephalopods (octopus and squid), and crustaceans (lobster, crab, etc.). When the fish or shellfish dies, the parasite passes through the wall of the digestive tract into the muscle tissue.

Consumption of anisakis infested fish can produce two clinical scenarios:

- **Anisakiasis:** This is an infestation (parasitic disease) that results from eating fish or shellfish infested with live or dead anisakis. These develop in the human stomach and intestines, causing pain similar to that of a gastroduodenal ulcer. It is difficult to diagnose, and requires a specialized treatment in order to destroy the parasite.

- **Anisakis allergy:** This allergic reaction is the result of eating fish or shellfish infested with live anisakis. *Even though* **cooking** the fish has *killed* the parasite itself, its **antigen** remains in the flesh. This antigen is a special type of protein that provokes an intense allergic reaction similar to histamine poisoning: digestive distress, skin rash, and itching.[46]

- **Prevention:** Protection against anisakis consists of:

  - **Cleaning** the fish as soon as they are caught.
  - *Avoiding* eating **raw** fish and seafood, since these may contain live anisakis.
  - **Cooking** fish suspected of parasite infestation for at least ten minutes to deactivate the protein antigens.

Mercury Poisoning

Between 2,000 and 3,000 metric tons of mercury are emitted into the air each year as a result of industrial activities. This mercury vapor settles on land, rivers, and the

---

the handling, processing and storage of the fish can minimize bacterial contamination from external sources.

Parasitic Infestation: Anisakis

While fish does not typically harbor pathogenic microbes, they do transmit various parasites such as the liver fluke (*Metorchis conjunctus*), a trematode that develops within the human liver from eggs taken in with raw fish. It causes fever, pain in the right side, and liver damage.[45]

Mercury in Different Fish

All fish and shellfish contain a certain amount of mercury. Most Western nations prohibit the sale of any fish with more than 1 ppm.

Proportion of methyl mercury	Fish	Amount of fish that may be eaten* per week
		Pregnant women: 30 g (about 1 ounce) (the fetus is particularly sensitive to methyl mercury).
		General population: a 200 g (about 7 ounces) portion
More than 1 ppm	Large carnivorous predators such as white and blue **sharks, swordfish,** and the large **tuna** (not those commonly used for canning)	
From 0.5 to 1 ppm	Other carnivorous fish such as **sea bass, pike,** and **barracuda**	Two 200 g (about 7 ounces) portions
Less than 0.5 ppm	Most **fish** taken in the **open ocean,** including **tuna** used for canning (fish from **close to shore** may contain **more** mercury if there is industrial effluent)	Five 200 g (about 7 ounces) portions

* *These amounts are for orientation purposes. The reality is that the intake of small amounts of mercury, even though accepted by health authorities, may have a long-term toxic effect.*

seas. Polluters dump more directly into coastal waters where it mixes with the particles in the sea. This explains that, while there is more mercury present near the coasts, it is also present in the open ocean.

- **Causes:** Certain marine microorganisms *transform* the soluble mercury in the water into **methyl mercury,** which is *much more toxic.* Methyl mercury permanently binds with the proteins of marine animals. Once this has taken place, it *cannot be eliminated,* and is passed up the food chain through a process of **bioaccumulation.**[2] (The mercury referred to here is **methyl mercury,** the form in which it accumulates in living things).

Mercury poisoning produces two types of symptoms:

- **Neurological symptoms** that appear when the fish that has been eaten contains relatively high amounts of mercury: more than 10 ppm (the maximum permissible limit is 0.5-1.0 ppm). The first symptoms are those of paresthesia (tingling sensations and numbness) in the mouth, hands, and feet. In advanced cases symptoms include:
  - muscular weakness, fatigue, and impaired mental concentration
  - trouble with gait and dysarthria (impaired speech and articulation).

Mercury poisoning can lead to coma and death, as happened in Minamata Bay in Japan between 1950 and 1960.

- **Cardiac symptoms** may appear at relatively low doses of mercury, much lower than that necessary to provoke neurological symptoms. Coronary **arteriosclerosis** and myocardial **infarction** (heart attack) stand out. The explanation for this is that methyl mercury creates the following harmful situations in the cardiovascular system:
  - generates oxidizing free radicals,
  - deactivates glutathione and other naturally occurring antioxidants within the body,

- blocks antioxidant action of selenium. This all *facilitates* the **peroxidation** of the lipoproteins in the blood plasma, leading to **arteriosclerosis.**

- **Prevention:** Avoid eating fish that is potentially contaminated with methyl mercury:
  - those caught in **coastal areas** where mercury-bearing waste is dumped;
  - **carnivorous fish** are the ones with the highest accumulations of methyl mercury, *particularly* **sharks** and **swordfish.**
  Supplemental doses of **selenium** *may neutralize some* of the negative effects of mercury on the heart.

Fish constitutes the **primary food source of mercury.** A study conducted at the Heinrich-Heine University of Dusseldorf (Germany) demonstrated that on days when the children in the study ate fish they took in 16.6% of the Acceptable Daily Intake of methyl mercury. On days when their diet did not include fish, they only took in 5.2%.[47]

The problem is that although the maximum Acceptable Daily Intake is not reached, mercury **accumulates** in the body. Its **toxic effects** on the nervous system and the heart are **based** on the **total amount** of mercury **accumulated** in the body, and not on the daily intake.

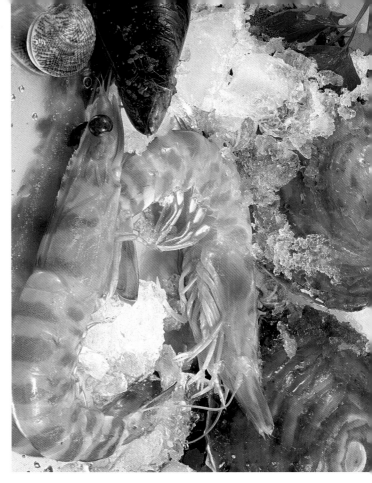

Shellfish

Shellfish: are any marine invertebrate, particularly crustaceans and mollusks. They are different from fish in that they **lack an internal skeleton and fins,** nor do they have scales, which are present on most fish.

Shellfish are classified zoologically in two main groups:

• **Crustaceans,** which form a zoological class that belongs to the phylum of **arthropods,** and includes some 25,000 species.

• **Mollusks,** which form a zoological phylum that includes 7 classes, only three of which are of dietary interest (**bivalves, cephalopods, and gastropods**). Altogether there are about 100,000 species of mollusks.

Shellfish, bivalve mollusks in particular, are usually so contaminated that it is best to decontaminate them before they are placed for sale.

Placing the live shellfish in fresh water with chlorine for at least 48 hours decontaminates them.

Shellfish

Devotees of shellfish hold *no other food* in such high esteem. However, no other food tends to be as **contaminated** by bacteria, viruses, and toxins. Unfortunately for shellfish lovers, it is technically **difficult, if not impossible, to determine** which shellfish are **contaminated.**

The high health risk associated with crustaceans and mollusks has to do with how and where these creatures live and, particularly, what they eat. If one understands these things, it is easier to understand the drawbacks to shellfish.

Crustaceans

Crustaceans can be classified by their dietary habits as:

• **Carrion eaters** that feed primarily on dead and decaying animals. They act as sea *vultures,* moving across the sea bottom cleansing the sea of remains and organic waste.

• **Carnivores:** Crustaceans can tear up other aquatic animals with their powerful pincers. They typically choose those that are sick or weak, and, as a result, usually contain *more germs.*

• **Cannibals:** These creatures devour their own young, or others of their own kind, that have lost their protective shell due to molting.

The particular means that these animals feed themselves explains why they are, together with mollusks:

– The sea creatures that *harbor the most germs.*

– The ones that *accumulate the most* **contaminants** and **toxins,** since they *concentrate* everything present in their food sources.

Bivalve Mollusks

These creatures feed by filtering large amounts of water (up to 9 liters per hour), and retaining the solid particles it contains. In this way their tissues **accumulate:**

– pathogenic **microbes** found in the water, particularly in coastal waters near large urban areas;

– toxic dinoflagellate **algae** that thrive in polluted water (see Vol. 1, p. 259);

– **chemical pollutants,** some of which are carcinogenic.

Continued on page 256

Crustaceans and Mollusks

Crustaceans

The lobster, the large-clawed lobster, the crab, the spiny lobster, and the shrimp are some of the best known.

The **external skeleton** is formed of a **chitin** shell.

They have **five pairs of extremities.** The first pair is usually powerful pincers with which they tear the bodies—living or dead—of other marine creatures.

The body is segmented in various rings. Its flesh is rich in free amino acids, which gives them a particular flavor, but also *promotes* the development of a **wide variety of microbes.**

They usually live in **coastal** areas, particularly in the **mouths** of rivers where **pollution** levels are *the highest.*

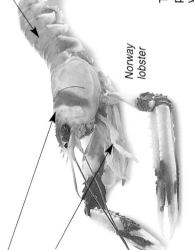

Norway lobster

Mollusks

Those considered edible belong to one of these three classes:

Gastropods

These are both land and water varieties of **snails.** Their flesh is **indigestible,** produces allergic reactions, and *may* contain **toxins.**

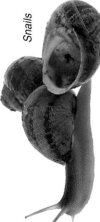

Snails

Cephalopods

These are fleshy mollusks such as the **cuttlefish,** the **squid,** and the **octopus.** The shell is internal and is either small or nonexistent. Its flesh is rich in fibrous connective tissue, making it **difficult to digest.**

They have eight or ten extremities, which branch from the head. These are used to swim and capture their prey.

They are *major* **carnivorous predators,** and they feed on **carrion,** as well.

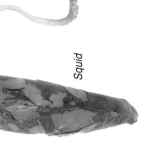

Squid

Bivalves

These are **mussels, oysters, clams,** and others whose bodies are enclosed within a shell composed of two valves. They are also called **Lamellibranchia,** as their gills are laminar.

They live in coastal waters where there is an abundance of organic material. Since they are immobile, they feed by **filtering seawater.**

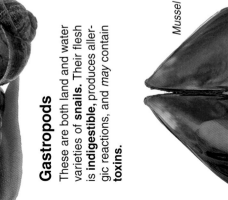

Mussel

Nutritional Value

of fish. However, those of **mollusks** (octopus, mussel, oyster, etc.) **lack** methionine and lysine and other essential *amino acids.*

- **Free amino acids:** Shellfish are the animal product *richest* in free amino acids. Amino acids are released when protein is digested in the intestine, and it is unusual that foods contain free amino acids. The free amino acids in shellfish are responsible for
  - Their particular **flavor**, along with the fatty acids.
  - The rapidity with which **bacteria** attack them. When the animal dies, the numerous bacteria that it harbors find predigested proteins in the free amino acids. These are very nourishing for the bacteria, which **proliferate rapidly**, decomposing the flesh.

- **Fat:** Shellfish contain between 1% and 8% fat, somewhat less than fish. Although part of their fatty acids are of *omega-3* configuration (see Vol. 1, p. 240), any beneficial action that these fatty acids may have on the arteries is *neutralized by abundant cholesterol*, which is also present in shellfish.

- **Glycogen:** Mollusks contain a small amount (1%–2%) of this starch-like carbohydrate found only in animals.

- **Vitamins:** Mollusks contain A, B, C, and D. Oysters and clams contain abundant **vitamin B₁₂**. For example, 100 g of oysters provides eight times the RDA of vitamin B₁₂.

- **Minerals:** Mollusks are *particularly rich* in **heme iron** (easily absorbed) and **zinc.** One hundred grams of oysters provide more than half the RDA for iron and more than double that of zinc.

Shellfish provides:

- **Protein,** which makes up between 5% and 20% of the edible portion. Shellfish muscle contains *more* **connective tissue** than that of fish, and as a result, more collagen. This makes it more **difficult to digest. Crustacean** (shrimp, lobster, etc.) proteins are **complete,** as are those

Positive Aspects of Shellfish

- **Flavorful:** Many consider shellfish an exquisite dish. However, shellfish's appeal is not universal and many find them repulsive.

- **Nutritious:** Crustaceans (not mollusks) provide very high quality *protein similar to that of fish.*

- **Rich in *vitamin B₁₂* and *iron*:** Among foods of animal origin, *only* the liver of mammals exceeds oysters in vitamin B₁₂ and iron.

SHRIMP Composition
per 100 g of raw edible portion

Energy	**106 kcal = 444 kJ**
Protein	**20.3 g**
Carbohydrates	**0.910 g**
Fiber	—
Vitamin A	54.0 µg RE
Vitamin B₁	0.028 mg
Vitamin B₂	0.034 mg
Niacin	7.27 mg NE
Vitamin B₆	0.104 mg
Folate	3.00 µg
Vitamin B₁₂	1.16 µg
Vitamin C	2.00 mg
Vitamin E	0.820 mg α-TE
Calcium	52.0 mg
Phosphorus	205 mg
Magnesium	37.0 mg
Iron	2.41 mg
Zinc	1.11 mg
Potassium	185 mg
Total Fat	1.73 g
Saturated Fat	0.328 g
Cholesterol	*152 mg*
Sodium	148 mg

% Daily Value (based on a 2,000 calorie diet) provided by 100 g of this food

Water 75.9% · Protein 20.3% · Fat 1.73% · Carbohydr. 0.910% · Minerals 1.20%

OYSTER Composition
per 100 g of raw edible portion

Energy	**59.0 kcal = 247 kJ**
Protein	**5.22 g**
Carbohydrates	**5.53 g**
Fiber	—
Vitamin A	8.00 µg RE
Vitamin B₁	0.105 mg
Vitamin B₂	0.065 mg
Niacin	2.25 mg NE
Vitamin B₆	0.060 mg
Folate	18.0 µg
Vitamin B₁₂	16.2 µg
Vitamin C	4.70 mg
Vitamin E	—
Calcium	44.0 mg
Phosphorus	93.0 mg
Magnesium	33.0 mg
Iron	5.78 mg
Potassium	124 mg
Zinc	37.9 mg
Total Fat	1.55 g
Saturated Fat	0.443 g
Cholesterol	*25.0 mg*
Sodium	178 mg

% Daily Value (based on a 2,000 calorie diet) provided by 100 g of this food

Water 86.2% · Protein 5.22% · Fat 1.55% · Carbohydr. 5.53% · Minerals 1.50%

# of Shellfish

Signs of Decay in Shellfish

- *Ammonia smell*
- *A viscous substance appears under the shell*
- *In the case of **crustaceans** the part that joins the head to the body turns black, and the head is easily removed.*

The Role of Shellfish in the Diet

- *Shellfish are in **no way necessary** in the human diet.*
- *All of the **nutrients** that shellfish provide are available from **other, more healthful foods.***
- *Their few positive aspects **do not compensate** for the **numerous risks** associated with eating shellfish.*
- *Shellfish are an **especially dangerous** product and they should not form part of a healthy diet.*

Drawbacks to Shellfish

- **Rapid decay:** Shellfish are possibly the *most perishable food product* that exists. As soon as the animal dies, a very rapid decay process begins, facilitated by:

  - The **huge quantity and variety of bacteria and viruses** it harbors, many of which are pathogenic.
  - The presence of **free amino acids** in its tissues, which nourish the bacteria.

  The shellfish that has decayed to some degree is all the more dangerous because it contains more germs. Additionally, it may cause more allergic reactions.

- **Difficult to digest:** Their flesh contains abundant connective tissue rich in *collagen* (animal fiber), particularly mollusks. This slows the action of the digestive juices.

- **Cholesterol:** Crustaceans contain around 150 mg/100 g, more than double that of lean beef. It should be avoided by all who need to control their cholesterol level.

- **Uric acid:** Shellfish proteins are *substantial generators* of uric acid in the body. Lobsters and prawns are possibly the species that produce the most uric acid.

- **Allergies:** Eating shellfish, particularly shrimp and squid, is one of the most common causes of food allergy. The most frequent manifestations are urticaria, asthma, and rhinitis.[48]

- **Contraindicated in *many cases*** (see Vol. 1, p. 257).

- **Infections** (see the following pages): Shellfish harbor numerous pathogens, such as:

  - salmonella, which causes serious gastroenteritis
  - cholera-producing vibrios
  - hepatitis A and C virus.

- Shellfish is responsible for *most* foodborne infections.

- **Parasitosis** (see Vol. 1, p. 258): Anisakis is a worm that infests cephalopods (octopus, squid, and cuttlefish), causing serious allergic reactions.

- **Poisoning** (see Vol. 1, p. 258): Shellfish can carry various types of toxins that cause serious paralysis, diarrhea, or neurological disorders such as amnesia (loss of memory).

- **Contamination:** Shellfish *concentrate germs, toxins,* and **industrial chemical pollutants** dumped into the sea, such as mercury, cadmium, and others.

  Additionally, **boric acid** (prohibited by health authorities) used to maintain shellfish's rosy color and retard decay, is toxic.

- **Cancer:** Some of the chemical substances dumped into the sea and accumulated in shellfish, are carcinogens; for example, PCB (polychlorinated biphenyl),[49] dioxins, and pesticides. Because of this, *regular consumption* of shellfish *increases* the **risk** of suffering from cancer caused by chemical contaminants.

Even though shellfish is contaminated with virus such as hepatitis or it contains toxins, its appearance and flavor are usually absolutely normal. Furthermore, most of the pathogenic viruses and toxins that shellfish harbor are resistant to the heat of cooking.

Continued from page 252

Shellfish-transmitted Disease

There are many germs, both viral and bacterial, living in both salt and fresh water. Because of the way shellfish feed, they are *particularly* **prone** to contamination by these microorganisms.

Shellfish **consumption** is responsible *for the bulk* of **food-related disease.** Japan, where consumption of raw fish and shellfish is the greatest, is precisely the country with the highest incidence of these diseases.

Great efforts are made the world over to assure pathogen-free shellfish gets to the market. In spite of these efforts, however, disease related to eating contaminated shellfish continues unabated. These are even fatal in some cases.[50]

Bacteria

Shellfish may be bacterially contaminated in two ways:

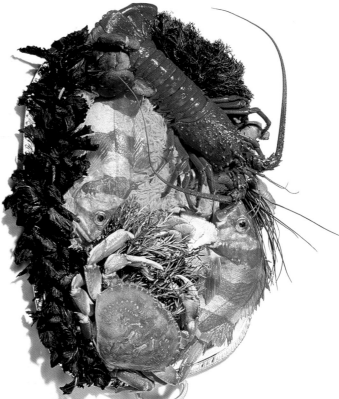

— While living **in the sea**, which is the most frequent mechanism.

— **After capture**, by microbes from those handling them or the containers or other utensils used to store them.

Shellfish are *particular susceptible* to **contamination from external sources**, since their tissues contain *many* **free amino acids**, which provide an ideal media for bacteria (see Vol. 1, p. 254).

These are the **pathogenic bacteria** most often associated with shellfish:

- **Vibrios:** Shellfish are carriers of six of the eleven known pathogens of the genus *Vibrio*.[51] Among these the **cholera**-causing *Vibrio cholerae* is the most feared, although there are other species that produce infectious **diarrhea**, which is less severe. The main cause of cholera in developed countries is the consumption of raw oysters.

- *Vibrio vulnificus:* This is a highly pathogenic vibrio that is becoming more and more common in the Atlantic and Pacific oceans. It produces two distinct clinical scenarios:

  — **Ingestion** of contaminated shellfish produces severe **gastroenteritis** accompanied by **septicemia** (blood poisoning). This proves fatal in half of the cases.[52]

  — **By contact**, through a wound produced by an infected shellfish, which produces a **severe infection** that may require amputation. There have been cases of this among fishermen and other workers in the shellfish industry.

- *Aeromonas hydrophyla* is responsible for many cases of **gastroenteritis.** Its primary dietary source is oysters and other bivalve mollusks. It has the peculiar characteristic of being resistant to freezing.

- *Clostridium botulinum* is the cause of **botulism**, most commonly associated with canned or preserved foods, may also be

Contraindications to Eating Shellfish

When eating shellfish poses particular danger

Shellfish consumption is always a risk to health. But there are situations in which the risk is extremely high, and shellfish are formally contraindicated:

- **Immunodepression** (lowered resistance) due to:
  - AIDS,
  - eukemia and lymphoma,
  - malignant tumors in general,
  - chemotherapy cancer treatment,
  - immunosuppression treatment to prevent transplanted organ tissue rejection.

- **Chronic kidney failure:** renal dialysis

- **Diabetes**

- **Liver disease:** hepatitis, cirrhosis, and others

- **Alcoholism**

- **Lack of gastric acid due to:**
  - chronic gastritis (with scant gastric juice production).
  - treatment with antacids or ulcer medications that reduce stomach acidity.

In all of these cases, it has been proven that there is a greater susceptibility to the pathogens and/or the toxins found in shellfish.

transmitted by raw or poorly cooked shellfish.

- *Salmonella* and *shigella* **bacteria:** Shellfish, particularly bivalve mollusks (**oysters, mussels, etc.**), *together* with **poultry, are** the *primary* vectors of **salmonella.** These bacteria cause severe gastroenteritis, such as the much-feared typhoid fever.

- *Staphylococcus aureus* is the cause of *most* **external infections** resulting from handling and processing shellfish. Eating shellfish containing this bacterium results in **gastroenteritis,** accompanied by general symptoms of **food poisoning.**

Viruses

Viruses reach the sea through wastewater dumped from the coast. *Most of* these are enteroviruses, in other words, viruses that normally live in the human digestive tract and are eliminated through the feces.

Enteroviruses have two characteristics that make them *extremely dangerous*

- *They usually* **survive** processing at **wastewater treatment plants.** Even if all of the wastewater dumped into the world's seas was properly processed, something that is far from the fact, even in developed countries, enteroviruses would still reach the sea alive.

- **They survive** in the marine aquatic environment for *long periods of time.* It has been proven that the hepatitis A virus, for example, can remain alive in the sea for more than a year.[53]

- These viruses *very commonly* **infect shellfish,** crustaceans and mollusks alike. While it is extremely *rare* to find fish *infected by viruses,* shellfish *usually* **are,** due to their unique physiology:
  - They feed on decaying organic matter.
  - They filter great quantities of water, retaining any microorganisms present in it.

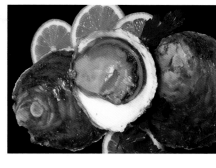

The **viruses** *most frequently* found in **shellfish** are:[54]

- **Hepatitis A virus:** This virus is quite common in shellfish. A British study attributes 25% of all hepatitis A outbreaks in the United Kingdom to **bivalve mollusks.**[55] Along the French coast, 1.7% of **oysters, mussels, and cockles** are contaminated with hepatitis A virus.[56]
  Hepatitis A follows a relatively benign course, and usually disappears without aftereffects within two to three months. Boiling the shellfish for 20 minutes can destroy the hepatitis A virus.

- **Hepatitis non-A, non-B** also known as **hepatitis C:** This virus is more severe than hepatitis A. *Many cases are* never fully cured, but persist in a **chronic** state, which may result in cirrhosis. A study conducted at the Health Institute of Rome (Italy), demonstrated that the con-

Although some viruses and toxins resist cooking, bacteria are usually destroyed with heat. Therefore, the custom of eating oysters or other shellfish raw exposes the consumer to even greater risk of contracting infectious diseases.

Wastewater: the Never-ending Effluent

All the cities of the world dump thousands of liters of wastewater a day into the sea that is contaminated with numerous microorganisms.

A study conducted by the University of Nancy (France), showed that any mid-sized coastal city dumps wastewater into the sea that contains

- **Tens of millions of viruses.** These viruses can be found in the open sea as much as five kilometers from the point where they were dumped.[56]

- **Billions** of pathogenic **bacteria** (coliforms, salmonella, etc.).

The concentration of microorganisms within shellfish is from 100 to 1,000 times greater than that of their marine environment. Anyone eating shellfish is taking in seawater concentrated with all of its pollutants.

Wastewater treatments are not enough

Many viruses and pathogenic bacteria found in feces, such as salmonella, **resist the action of wastewater treatment plants.**[57] Since they travel alive to the sea with the treated wastewater, these germs **contaminate the shellfish** living along the coast. **Bivalve mollusks are particularly** vulnerable since they filter several liters of water per hour.

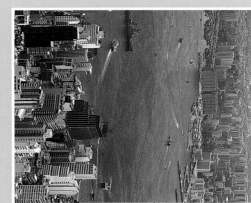

sumption of **raw oysters** is associated with this type of hepatitis, as are blood transfusions and intravenous drug use.[58]

- **Gastroenteritis-producing viruses:** Shellfish may contain various viruses that cause gastroenteritis. The best known of these is the Norwalk virus. All of these viruses have caused numerous gastroenteritis outbreaks among shellfish lovers throughout the world.

The most conspicuous and dangerous **characteristics** of these **viruses** are:

– There are no detectable signs in contaminated shellfish. Contaminated crustaceans or mollusks appear *completely* normal both **visually and to the taste.** It is extremely difficult, even for trained microbiologists, to detect the presence of these viruses in shellfish.[59,60]

– **They are** *not* **destroyed** during **cooking.** According to the Center for Disease Control in Atlanta (Georgia, USA), cooking shellfish, whether steamed, roasted, or fried provides no protection from these viruses nor from the gastroenteritis they cause.[61,62]

– The **gastroenteritis** caused by these viruses is *more severe* than the diarrhea produced by diarrheic shellfish toxins (see Vol. 1, p. 260).

Shellfish Parasitosis

Cephalopods (octopus, squid, cuttlefish), and less often crustaceans, may contain larvae of the *Anisakis simplex* parasite, which also infests fish (see Vol. 1, p. 250).

Eating anisakis-infested shellfish or fish produces *severe* **allergic reactions,** even though the parasite is dead.[63]

When ingested alive, the parasite develops in the human intestine, resulting in parasitosis or infestation. This usually occurs when shellfish is eaten raw or poorly cooked.

Shellfish Toxins

Since antiquity it has been well known that more or less severe pathological symptoms, which may even end up causing death may occur after eating shellfish.

It has only been within the last few decades, however, that the causes of these shellfish poisonings have been discovered. There is a range of toxins that can be classified according to their pathological effects.

Toxic Dinoflagellate Algae

Dinoflagellates are a type of microscopic alga found in the sea. *Together* with **diatoms**, they form **phytoplankton.** This is the name given to all microscopic marine plants. They serve as *basic food* for the tiny animals that make up **zooplankton**, as well as for mollusks, crustaceans, fish, and other sea creatures.

Dinoflagellate algae have the following characteristics:

- **Unicellular:** They are formed of a single cell, with two flagella or tails that are whipped about, allowing it to move.

- **Red:** They are brown or reddish in color, and cause the so-called **red tides**, which are frequent along America's tropical coasts. Some species are also phosphorescent, and when they are abundant, they cause the sea to glow at night.

- **Numerous:** Dinoflagellates are the *most plentiful inhabitants of the sea.* Each liter of seawater contains between 100,000 and 36,000,000 of them. Some decades ago these algae were confined almost exclusively to certain tropical locations. Today, however, they are spreading to other waters. In Mexico, for example, red tides are appearing in places where they have never been, such as Acapulco Bay.[64] At least two causes promote the excessive proliferation and extension of dinoflagellate algae:

  - *Increase* in marine **pollution:** Organic waste dumped into the sea fosters the growth of these algae.

  - **Climatic change:** The *progressive warming* of the water of the oceans permits the extension of these algae to nontropical waters, such as the coasts of Europe.

- **Toxic:** There are around 1,000 known species of dinoflagellate algae, grouped in 120 genera. Unfortunately, some of them produce various toxins. The marine animals eating these algae incorporate toxins in their tissues. In this manner the poison is passed from one creature to another, *concentrating more and more* as it moves up the food chain. The *maximum concentration* of toxins is reached in two groups of marine animals:

  - **Shellfish,** which accumulate paralytic toxins, diarrheic toxins, and neurotoxins produced by dinoflagellate algae.

  - **Carnivorous fish** accumulate the toxins of certain species of dinoflagellates that cause **ciguatera syndrome** (see Vol. 1, p. 246).

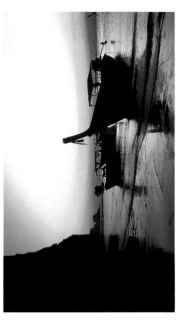

Paralyzing Toxins

These toxins are also known by the acronym PSP (*Paralytic Shellfish Poisons*). The most notorious is **saxitoxin** (mussel toxin). Its chemical formula is $C_{10}H_{17}N_7O_4 \cdot 2HCl$.

This is one of the *most potent poisons* known. One to four mg is sufficient to kill an adult human.[65]

- **Source:** These paralyzing toxins come primarily from three species of dinoflagellate:[57]

  - *Gonyaulax catenella*, which is found along the Pacific coast of North America and the seas around Japan.

  - *Gonyaulax tamarensis*, which proliferates in the North Atlantic along the North American and European coasts.

  - *Pyrodinium bahamense*, which is found in the warm seas of South America and Southeast Asia.

Mollusks, particularly mussels, have the particular property of concentrating the toxins of these algae in their tissues.

- **Symptoms of paralytic shellfish poisoning** are similar to those of ciguatera syndrome that affects fish (see Vol. 1, p. 246). The following symptoms progressively appear beginning about half an hour after eating contaminated shellfish.[66]

Red Tide: Danger Signal

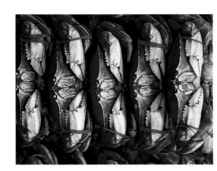

*Periodically, and quite unpredictably, there is an excessive proliferation of toxin-producing **dinoflagellates** along some tropical coasts, and even along the coasts of Europe. This proliferation gives the surface of the water a reddish appearance.*

*Those that cultivate **shellfish** fear red tides, since **harvests** made during the tide and several months thereafter **may be toxic** to consumers.*

The **only** effective **prevention is to refrain** from eating shellfish, particularly if a red tide has been sighted in the area from which it has been harvested.

- **Treatment:** If symptoms of paralytic shellfish poisoning appear soon after eating seafood, particularly mussels, rapid action is required. The affected individual must be taken to a hospital equipped with an intensive care unit. The most important therapeutic measures are:
  - gastric lavage,
  - administration of cardiorespiratory analeptics,
  - oxygen therapy and respiratory support.

Diarrheic Toxins

These toxins are known by the acronym DSP (*Diarrheic Shellfish Poisons*).

- **Source:** Dinoflagellate algae of the genera *Dinophysis* and *Prorocentrum* produce diarrheic toxins. These are found particularly in the North Atlantic, the Mediterranean, and the seas of Japan. There have been toxic outbreaks in the Netherlands, France, Spain (in the Galician estuaries), and Italy, due to consumption of various shellfish, particularly mussels and other mollusks.[57]

- **Symptoms of diarrheic shellfish poisoning:** One to two hours after eating contaminated shellfish, one experiences nausea, vomiting, diarrhea, and abdominal pain. These symptoms tend to last two or three days. Recovery tends to be spontaneous with no lasting effects. This is in contrast to gastroenteritis caused by bacteria or viruses, which tend to be more severe and from which it takes longer to recuperate.

- **Prevention:** There is **no way to detect** the presence of these toxins in shellfish. Additionally, diarrheic toxins are resistant to heat; therefore, cooking will not mitigate their effects.

Shellfish-produced paralytic poisoning causes symptoms similar to those of ciguatera poisoning (see Vol. 1, p. 246) produced by eating certain fish.

- Tingling sensation in the lips, tongue, and face.
- Headache, nausea, and vomiting.
- Severe cases may result in numbness and paralysis of the extremities. Death occurs within two and twelve hours, due to the paralysis of the respiratory muscles.

- **Prevention:** It is *impossible* to **detect** contaminated mussels or other shellfish, since their appearance and flavor are completely normal. It is extremely difficult to detect these toxins using chemical tests. The method currently used for this purpose is to inject tissue extracted from the suspected shellfish into laboratory mice, and see whether they die. Normal cooking destroys approximately 70% of paralytic toxins.

Land and Marine Snails

*Snails, both land and marine, are **mollusks** that belong to zoological class of the **gastropods**. Both types of snails are considered a delicacy by some persons in Europe and America, in spite of the natural repugnance that they provoke.*

Drawbacks

- *Indigestible: Their flesh is very rich in collagen, and very difficult to digest, causing dyspepsia and intestinal disorders.*
- *Allergenic: Land snails cause allergies with some regularity, which usually manifest as asthma-like respiratory symptoms.[70]*
- *Toxic: Many marine snails, such as the species Neptunea antiqua eaten in the United Kingdom, may contain paralytic toxins that appear clinically similar to paralytic shellfish poisoning (see Vol. 1, p. 259), but less serious.[57]*

*Snails, along with the remaining mollusks, are **unfit for human consumption and cannot** be part of a **healthy diet.***

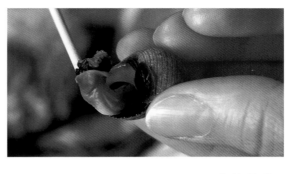

Neurotoxic Toxins

These are also called NSP (*Neurotoxic Shellfish Poisons*).

- **Source:** Neurotoxic toxins are produced by the *Ptychodiscus brevis* dinoflagellate seaweed, which is found along the coasts of Florida, the Indian Ocean, and in Europe in the Cantabrian Sea. It is present especially in **oysters** and **clams**.
- **Symptoms of Neurotoxic Shellfish Poisoning:** Three days after eating contaminated shellfish, paresthesia (tingling), lack of motor coordination, nausea, and vomiting; there is no paralysis and symptoms tend to disappear spontaneously within a few days.
- **Prevention:** The *only* possible way to prevent NSP is by *avoiding* shellfish, since there is no way to detect the presence of these poisons. Neurotoxins are heat-resistant.

Amnesic Toxins

These are known as ASP (*Amnesic Shellfish Poisons*). The first recorded occurrence of this type of poisoning was in 1987 in Canada in which 107 were affected with three deaths after eating mussels.[67] Since then, there have been various outbreaks on the west coast of North America.

- **Source:** Amnesic toxins are chemically composed of domoic acid, an amino acid toxic to the nervous system. It is produced by the diatomaceous alga *Nitzschia pungens*, and concentrates in bivalve mollusks. There have been cases involving crabs and clams.[68]
- **Symptoms of Amnesic Shellfish Poisoning** appear between 24 and 48 hours after eating contaminated shellfish:[69]
    - Nausea, vomiting, diarrhea, which tend to desist spontaneously within a few days.
    - Amnesia (loss of memory) and progressive mental disorientation. Memory loss may last as long as five years.

A 1 mg per kilo of body weight dose of domoic acid causes a slight poisoning effect primarily gastrointestinal in nature. Two to four mg per kilo of body weight produces severe neurological deterioration.[68]

- **Prevention:** The domoic acid responsible for amnesic poisoning can be detected chemically, thus contaminated shellfish can be discarded. Canadian health authorities have established a maximum limit of 20 µg (micrograms) of domoic acid per gram of mussel, requiring disposal of any that contain more than that amount.

14

MEAT

Meat has a certain value from a nutritional standpoint, but when contrasted with plant-based foods, it lacks healing power, except in certain cases of anemia. In addition, it has many drawbacks.

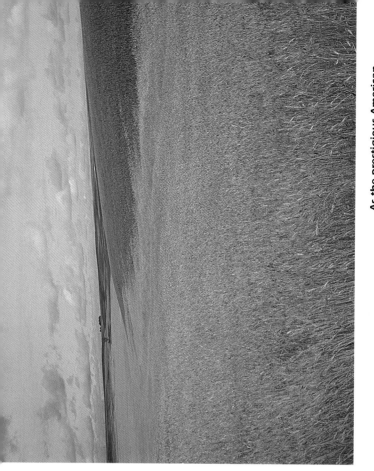

MEAT IS possibly the most controversial of all food products. For some it is such an important part of their diet that they cannot imagine living without it. For others it provokes revulsion to such a degree that they would never think of placing it on the table.

Both groups have their reasons for feeling the way they do. It is necessary to understand and respect both points of view. This debate could be said to be simply a question of personal taste if it were not for the fact that the massive and growing meat consumption by Western societies is having serious repercussions, both on humans and the planet on which we live.

Until the industrial revolution in the 19th century, meat consumption was quite limited in Western countries, except in extremely cold regions with little vegetation. Currently, however, meat has become the daily staple of the diet. This change in dietary habit has brought these consequences:

- **Consumers** exhibit a *noticeable increase* in the incidence of various **diseases,** particularly cardiac, cardiovascular, and rheumatic. There is also an *unprecedented incidence* in various types of **cancer.**[1]
- The **animals** themselves suffer *more dis-ease* due to the poor conditions in which they are raised and live. Some of these diseases may be *transmitted* to humans.
- The **environment** is affected by the need to satisfy the ever-increasing demand for meat in rich countries. This impact is being felt in poor countries and has repercussions for the entire planet:

  - Tropical **forests** are being burned to clear land for cattle grazing.

  - A large portion of the **soy** and **grains** produced in the non-industrialized world is used to feed livestock for the market rather than going directly to feed the human population. The same is happening with water resources in the developing world.

The pages that follow will describe the impact of meat consumption today, particularly on consumers.

As the prestigious American Journal of Clinical Nutrition states "Consumption of meat represents a tax on the consumer, as well as on the health of the poorest of the world."[2]

This is in contrast to the use of grains and legumes as protein sources, which is much more respectful of the environment and health.

Meat and Meat By-products

- ***Meat*** *is the **muscles** (see box Vol. 1, p. 266) of animals used as human food. By extension, it includes all of the structures that form the animal's* ***carcass:***

  - *the tissues that surround the muscle, such as bone, cartilage, skin, fat, tendons, and aponeurosis (conjunctive tissue membranes).*

  - *the nerves, arteries, veins, and lymphatic vessels that always accompany the muscles.*

- ***Offal*** *are the **viscera and glands** of the animal destined for the human table that are not part of the carcass. The most commonly used are the brains, the liver, and the kidneys (see Vol. 1, p. 317).*

Meat Production

From the time an animal is ready for slaughter until the meat is ready to eat, there is a series of rather complex processes that affect the product's quality and the consumers' health. It is important to understand such processes, which consist of three basic phases:

1. slaughter,
2. rigor mortis, and
3. aging.

1. Slaughter

The way an animal is slaughtered has an important effect on the subsequent quality of the meat. It is *important* that animals reach the slaughterhouse **rested**, and that they experience as *little* **stress** as possible just before slaughter.

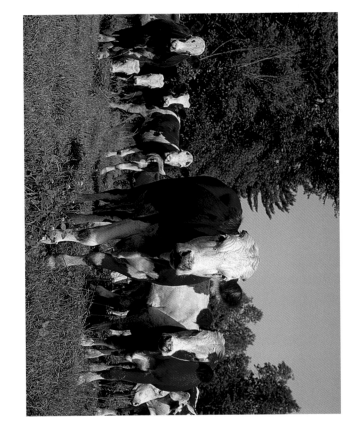

Meat from stressed animals is much more easily affected by bacteria, and as a result, is much more likely to change in ways that are harmful to health (see Vol. 1, p. 269).

Most of the meat eaten in industrialized countries comes from **slaughterhouses.** There, the slaughtering process must be done under carefully controlled hygienic conditions under the supervision of veterinarians. The slaughter phase takes place, in turn, in a series of phases:

a. Anesthesia
b. Slaughter
c. Skinning and evisceration
d. Inspection

a. Anesthesia

Anesthesia of animals before slaughter is *required* **by legislation** in advanced countries. While this is not always done, the most common means are:

- **Hammer blow** to the head.

- **Electric shock** to the head, which stuns the animal.

- Gun firing short-range **plastic bullet** used on cattle and designed to cause brain damage, which causes strong muscular contractions throughout the animal, while leaving it unconscious.

- Forced breathing of **carbon dioxide** (CO_2) stuns the animal through lack of oxygen. The meat from animals anesthetized in this manner is of lower quality than when the other methods are used due to the level of asphyxiation.

b. Slaughter

Once the animal has been anesthetized, the **jugular** vein is cut and it is suspended head down, bleeding it to death. In some cases the head is removed to speed the bleeding process. But even doing so, **bleeding** is *not complete* since the heart stops beating early due to brain damage.

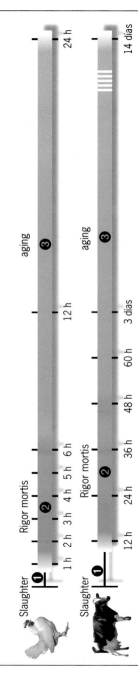

Quality of Meat Based on the Time of Consumption

Slaughter
❶
1 h 2 h 3 h 4 h 5 h 6 h   12 h   24 h
Rigor mortis ❷   aging ❸

Slaughter
❶
12 h 24 h 36 h 48 h 60 h   3 dias   14 dias
Rigor mortis ❷   aging ❸

❶ *Recently slaughtered fresh meat contains less proliferation of bacteria than aged meat, and as a result, less flavor and also fewer toxic substances. It also contains less hypoxanthine (stimulant) than aged meat. However it has the drawback that its soft elastic texture makes it rather unappetizing. It is not generally available to the public since it cannot be marketed.*

❷ *Meat in the rigor mortis phase is tough and stringy, inappropriate for consumption.*

❸ *Aged meat if prepared at its optimal point, is the most tender and flavorful. However more bacteria and toxic substances have developed in it than in the earlier phases (see Vol. 1, p. 268).*

When the optimal aging point is passed (24 hours for poultry and 14 days for red meat), there is excessive bacterial proliferation and a greater possibility that it may transmit infectious diseases (see Vol. 1, p. 302).

In order for the blood to be drained completely from the tissues, the heart must continue beating during hemorrhage. This requires not damaging the brain stem—with a projectile, electric shock, or other means—since the activities of the heart are controlled there.

c. Skinning and evisceration

• **Skinning,** as the word implies, is the *removal of the hide from the animal.* This must be done with *care* so as not to leave blood on the carcass that may be a culture medium for microorganisms.

• **Evisceration** involves removing the *internal organs* from the carcass. This must be done with *extreme care,* particularly with digestive organs, to assure that they do not open, spilling their contents and contaminating the meat.

d. Inspection

Animals with tumors, cysts, or others signs of **disease** must *not be used* for food.

Pork must be **microscopically** examined to assure the absence of trichina parasites (see Vol. 1, pp. 322, 323).

The remainder of the animal, after the skin, viscera, and other by-products have been removed is the **carcass.** This is made up *primarily* of **muscle** and **bone,** and is the portion of the animal sold as meat.

2. Rigor mortis

Some hours after death, the flesh of all vertebrate animals becomes hard and inflexible through a process known as *rigor mortis.* Meat in this condition is rigid and inextensible, and, therefore, inappropriate as food. It is after some hours or days have passed and this hardness has attenuated that the aging phase begins.

If meat were cooked immediately after the death of the animal, before rigor mortis had begun, it would be very soft, but fibrous and elastic. If, on the other hand, it were cooked

The meat of a slaughtered animal does not remain stable, but goes through a series of modifications in the hours and days that follow.

The quality of the meat can vary significantly depending on when the meat is consumed.

Microstructure of Muscle Tissue

Meat is formed from the skeletal muscles of the animal together with the tissues that accompany them.

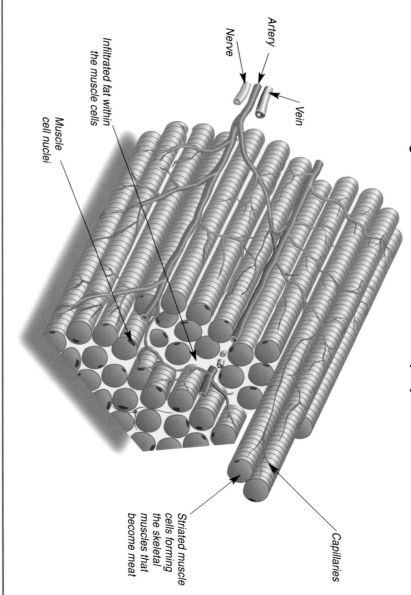

Artery

Nerve

Vein

Infiltrated fat within the muscle cells

Muscle cell nuclei

Capillaries

Striated muscle cells forming the skeletal muscles that become meat

during the rigor mortis phase, its texture would be tough and stringy. In either case, it would be unfit to eat.

Slaughterhouses place the cleaned carcasses in special chambers at an optimal temperature of 15°C (59°F) to facilitate rigor mortis. This process is called **airing**.

'Post mortem' Chemical Reactions

After death, blood and oxygen supplies to the tissue cease, but the muscle cells continue to experience chemical changes for some time. Two of the most important of these, produced by some 20 enzymes that remain active after death, are:

• The breaking down of glucogen into glucose (**glucogenolisis**). Glucogen is the most energy reserve for muscle cells, the same as starch is for vegetable cells.

• The decay of glucose in the absence of oxygen (**anaerobic glucolysis**) creates lactic acid. This **lactic acid** produced in the muscle cells after death changes the pH (*acidity level*) of meat from its normal level of 7.3 (slightly alkaline) in a live animal, to 5.5 (quite acid).

Causes of Rigor Mortis

The muscle contractions that begin some hours after the animal's death are caused, as in any muscle contraction, by the interaction of two types of proteins found in the muscle cells: actin and myosin. Two biochemical mechanisms result in the union of **actin** and **myosin**, with the resultant muscle rigidity:

During aging the rigidity of the meat disappears and it becomes juicier and more flavorful. But the degradation of its amino acids gives rise to many substances, some of which are toxic.

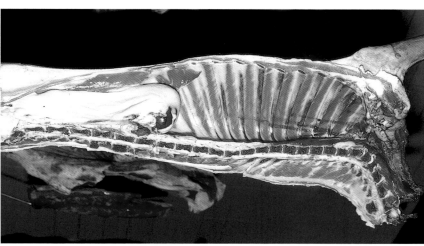

- The **acidification** produced in the muscle cells produced by the presence of **lactic acid.**

- *Lowered* levels of **ATP** (adenosine triphosphate), a substance that results from glucose and oxygen and serves as an energy source for cells.

Positive Effect of Rigor Mortis

Meat considered top-quality has gone through an adequate process of rigor mortis.

The acidity produced in the meat after the animal's death, and which causes rigor mortis, also prevents the proliferation of bacteria that are always present in the carcass. The **lactic acid** that forms in the meat is a *good* **antiseptic.**

Stopping bacterial proliferation that accompanies rigor mortis reduces the possibility that the meat will transmit infectious disease and that it will experience bacterial decay with the accompanying appearance of toxic substances.

Necessary Conditions for Rigor Mortis

There must be a certain amount of glucogen in the muscle cells, which is transformed by enzymes into **glucose** and then into lactic acid. **Lactic acid,** in turn, causes rigor mortis.

Only animals slaughtered under favorable conditions retain sufficient glycogen reserves in their muscle cells to produce the desirable level of acidification and rigor mortis.

On the other hand, animals exposed to stress or exhaustion during the hours before slaughter produce meat of low quality, since the acidity and accompanying rigor mortis are inadequate.

3. Aging

Several hours or days after the onset of rigor mortis, it begins to disappear. The optimal point for consumption of the meat varies with the animal species and the temperature of the environment. For example:

- **Beef:** between *10* and *14 days* after slaughter.

- **Chicken:** from *12* to *24 hours* after slaughter (see chart Vol. 1, p. 265).

Objectives of Aging

Two objectives are met during aging:

- The meat is **tenderized** by proteolytic enzymes that break down protein from the muscle cells.

- The meat acquires its particular **flavor** due to the controlled proliferation of bacteria that degrade amino acids.

Assuring Meat Tenderness

Meat is almost inedible if it is not processed correctly. Since consumers demand tender meat above all, it is necessary to prepare it using some of these methods:

- **Hanging the carcass** either in fresh air or in refrigerated chambers. During this process the meat goes from the **rigor mortis** phase to that of **aging**. In this phase the meat becomes tender and more flavorful, with an optimal point for beef of 14 days (see preceding page). Only meat from animals slaughtered under appropriate conditions and handled hygienically to avoid bacterial proliferation lends itself to proper aging from the point of view of health. Unfortunately these conditions are not always met.

- **Treatment with vegetable enzymes** such as papain from the papaya and bromaline from pineapple partially dissolves the muscle fibers, collagen, and elastin that make meat tough.

- **Electrical stimulation** consists of submitting the carcass to electric discharges that artificially rupture the contracting muscle fiber.

Substances Produced

A series of chemical reactions take place in the meat during aging. Some of these reactions are produced by germs the meat contains, while others are caused by enzymes from the muscle cells. The new substances produced as a result are unpredictable and uncontrollable due to the variety of enzymes and germs at work.

New Substances Resulting From the Degradation of Amino Acids

There is always a certain amount of enzymatic and bacterial activity during the aging process in spite of the acidity and refrigeration.

Some proteins are decomposed into their constituent amino acids by enzymes. The bacteria transform the amino acids into other substances that give the meat its particular flavor: hydrocarbons, aldehydes, ketones, sulfides, mercaptans, ammonia, and amines (such as histamine and tyramine).[3]

Some of these substances that result from normal **bacterial degradation** produce undesirable, even toxic, effects. For example:

- Aldehydes, ketones, and sulfides can produce **migraines;**

- Histamine, present particularly in pork, *fosters* **allergic** and inflammatory reactions;

- Tyramine produces vasoconstriction leading to an *increase* in **arterial pressure.**

Other Substances Produced During Aging

The most important, due to their flavor contribution and simulative effects are **hypoxanthine** and its derivatives (see box **"Is meat addictive?"** Vol. 1, p. 283).

Risks of Aging

The principal risk during the aging of meat is the possibility of *excessive* **bacterial proliferation** with its accompanying **decay.** This risk is *minimized* by:

- The **lactic acid** produced during rigor mortis, which acts as an antiseptic. For this reason adequate **acidification** manifest by rigor mortis is *very important* in reducing harmful substances in meat.

- **Refrigeration** between 2° and 4°C (between 35.6° and 39.2°F) under strict hygiene controls.

Continued on page 270

Stress in Animals

affects meat quality

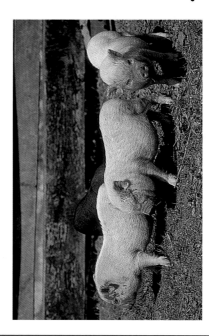

Swine are the farm animals with the lowest stress tolerance. Light exercise or a few hours without food is enough to deplete their glycogen reserves.[5] Meat from animals slaughtered under these conditions is not acid and presents a high risk of bacterial contamination.

To a significant degree, the **detrimental effects** of meat depend on the **diet** and **living conditions** of the animal throughout its life. Even its **final days or hours** are of a **much greater** influence than it would seem.

Animals raised for meat are sensitive to stress, which is particularly intense during transport to the slaughterhouse and in the moments before slaughter.

Causes of Stress in Animals

The **most stressful** situations for livestock prior to slaughter are:

- Hunger or thirst,
- Heat and cold,
- Physical exhaustion,
- Overcrowding,
- Fear.

Undesirable Changes in Meat According to theTtype of Stress

Just as happens with humans, stress in animals causes a very complex series of hormonal and nervous reactions. Experts have observed that two types of change take place in meat depending on which type of stress, physical or psychological, predominates:[4]

- **Predominantly physical stress:** extended food deprivation or excessive physical exercise prior to slaughter causes the *depletion* of the animal's muscle tissue **glycogen** reserves. As a result, *little* **lactic acid** is formed and the char-

acteristics of **rigor mortis** are virtually *absent*. The meat presents these characteristics:

- **Deep red** in color.
- Dry consistency when cut.
- Releases little moisture.
- It is *not* acidic (its pH stays around 7), and as a result it is highly susceptible to bacterial proliferation.

The meat of **bulls** killed in the ring is of this type, which is considered among the most unhealthful. Similar things occur with livestock that has been improperly transported.

- **Predominantly psychological stress:** overcrowding and the fear of imminent death that the animal senses are causes of psychological stress, even though the animal is rested and well fed. Glycogen remains within cells and will produce lactic acid after death.

However, due possibly to excess adrenaline or other hormones produced by fear, the meat of these animals has the following characteristics:

- **Pale** in color
- **Soft**, almost pasty consistency
- Watery
- Its **pH drops** *rapidly* after slaughter, while the carcass is still warm. This rapid acidification also reverses itself rapidly, which prevents proper rigor mortis.

The result is soft, moist meat of poor quality that decays easily from bacterial action.

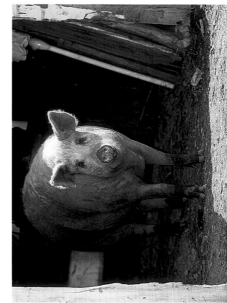

Some strains of swine such as the Danish Landrace and the Belgian Pietrain are very sensitive to the psychological stresses of slaughter.[4]

Continued from page 268

Meat Preservation

Meat is a *highly perishable* product in which bacteria and viruses proliferate very easily. Therefore, it is necessary to preserve it in some way. Although it may seem a paradox, these processes are not free from health risks.

Curing

Traditionally the term "cured" referred to various processes that dried and toughened meat, such as sun **drying, smoking,** and **salting.** This applied particularly to ham, *bacon,* and certain sausages.

Today, **cured meat** *is that which has been treated with common salt (sodium chloride) mixed with sodium nitrite and potassium nitrite.* **The curing salt** used currently in the European Union contains between 4 and 6 grams of sodium nitrite per kilo (0.4%–0.6%).

Advantages of Curing With Nitrites

- **Antisepsis:** common salt *stops* **bacterial proliferation.** However, it does *not* destroy the **spores** of certain very dangerous bacteria usually found in meat. Such as Clostridium botulinum, which causes the deadly disease known as **botulism.** That is why nitrates began to be used, and currently **nitrites,** the latter of which are very effective against the most dangerous and tenacious germs found in meat.

- **Color:** Nitrites react with the myoglobin in the meat to form an **intense red** pigment. Many mistake this color as a sign of quality.

- **Flavor:** Nitrites give cured meats their typical strong flavor.

Drawbacks to Nitrites

- **Toxicity:** *Nitrites are toxic salts, even in moderate doses.* They react with the hemoglobin in the blood to form metahemoglobin, which is incapable of transporting oxygen. The *lethal dose* of nitrite for an *adult* is approximately *one gram,* which is the amount in about *five kilos of* **cured ham.** The amount of nitrite ingested with a serving of ham is obviously much less than a lethal dose. The body is capable of neutralizing the powerful toxic effects of small amounts of nitrites. However, its mid and long-term carcinogenic effect remains.

- **Carcinogenic effect:** An interesting study was conducted at the University Hospital of Darmstadt (Germany) that reviewed old cookbooks from Germany and Austria.[6] Its findings were:

If nitrites were not used in curing sausages and ham, the risk of botulism (a deadly foodborne disease) would rise dangerously.

On the other hand, the use of nitrites multiplies the risk of forming carcinogenic nitrosamines.

The dilemma, then, with cured meats (ham, bacon, and sausages), is choosing between the risk of botulism and the risk of cancer.

Additives Used in the Preparation of Cured Meats and Sausages

- ***Nitrites** prevent the **putrefaction** of cured meats and sausages. They also destroy the spores that cause **botulism** (a deadly foodborne disease). On the other hand, they foster the formation of **carcinogenic** substances such as **nitrosamines.***

- ***Nitrates** are used to **complement nitrites**, even though their effectiveness as antiseptics and color and **flavor enhancers** is lower. Their **risk** to health **rises** when they are used in **conjunction** with reducing agents such as **sugar** (as is the case with certain types of ham). The following reactions take place in meats thus cured*

  – *Sugar fosters the transformation of nitrates to nitrites*

  – *Nitrites react with amino acids to form carcinogenic nitrosamines*

- ***Sodium ascorbate** accelerates the curing process*

- ***Sodium polyphosphate** causes the meat to retain more moisture, making it tenderer and juicier. It is used primarily with cooked ham and sausages. Its possible toxic effects are not well known.*

– **Saltpeter** (potassium nitrate, NO_3K) mixed with common salt began to be used in central Europe to improve the color of meat in the 18th century. Until then only common salt had been used.

– In the 19th century **sugar** was added, along with saltpeter, to improve preservation. The presence of the sugar converted the nitrates into nitrites, which are much more active and effective in improving color and preservation. However, nitrites are more toxic than nitrates.

It was precisely then (the 19th century), and coinciding with this practice, that a significantly *increasing* number of instances of **colon cancer, multiple sclerosis,** and **rheumatoid arthritis** began appearing in the medical literature. All of this indicates the existence of a cause and effect relationship.

Today it is well known that sodium **nitrite** and potassium **nitrite** as used in the meat curing process, or that form from nitrates, react with amino acids in the digestive system to form **nitrosamines.** These substances act to *induce* **cancer** or to *foster* in its development.

There have been numerous epidemiological and experimental studies conducted that relate cured meats, particularly ham and sausages, with various types of cancer (see Vol. 1, p. 324).

Thanks to advances in hygiene and the use of cold storage as means of meat preservation, the meat industry is *attempting* to use **fewer nitrites.** However, nitrites are **essential** to *avoid* **botulism**[7] transmission through cured meats, an infection that is usually fatal.

Smoking

Smoke, with heat and drying have been used since antiquity to preserve meat. Today it is used primarily for the intense flavor it imparts.

Advantages of Smoking

Smoke is a *good* meat *preservative* due to its formaldehyde and phenol content, which have **antiseptic** and **antioxidant** properties.

Drawbacks to Smoking

However, suspended substances in smoke such as **benzopyrene** and other polycyclic aromatic hydrocarbons, which are *proven* **carcinogens,** are deposited in the smoked meat.

Modern smoking systems eliminate most of the carcinogenic aromatic hydrocarbon particles so meat that is smoked using these newer techniques is *not as dangerous*. How-

Sodium Nitrite
maximum permitted amount for various meats

Type of meat	mg of nitrite/kg of meat*
Cooked meat in sterile container	50
Acidified or fermented cured meat	50
Bacon or ham without sterile container	200
Other cured meats	150

* These maximum limits are those applied in the United Kingdom.[8] Other countries are similar.

ever, meat as well as fish and sauces with smoke flavor always retain some amount of carcinogenic substances. According to analyses conducted by the Department of Food Science and Human Nutrition of the University of Michigan (USA), these amounts vary among the following values:[9]

- **Meat:** from undetectable amounts up to 7.4 µg/kg in smoked pork.
- **Fish:** from 0.2 µg/kg in smoked trout to 16 µg/kg in smoked salmon.
- **Smoked-flavored sauces:** from 0.3 to 10.2 µg/kg.

Canning

Canned meat such as *corned beef* is traditionally prepared with boiled meat to obtain an extract of the meat. Today other types of meat are also canned, a process that includes one of these two sanitizing procedures:

- **Pasteurization** by applying just enough heat to destroy only pathogenic bacteria.
- **Sterilization** by heating to more than 100°C (212°F) to destroy all microorganisms.

Advantages of Canned Meat

- It usually contains little **fat** (around 5%).
- **Bacterial** contamination is *controlled* or *eliminated* by pasteurization or sterilization.

Drawbacks to Canned Meat

The meat used for canning is usually the *worst* **quality.** Also, **additives** such as nitrites and polyphosphates are added.

If, as is often the case, the meat has only been pasteurized, it still contains germs that can cause decay. Therefore, it must be refrigerated.

Freezing

The ideal temperature for freezing meat products is between –18° and –20°C (between –0.4° and –4°F).

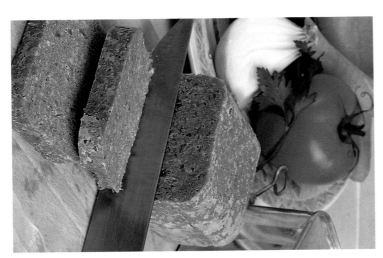

Canned meat contains fewer bacteria, and, as a result, presents less risk of infectious disease. However, it contains significant amounts of potentially toxic additives.

A temperature of −10°C (14°F) was used at first, but at that temperature certain molds survived, causing black spots on the frozen meat.

Advantages of Frozen Meat

- **Long-term storage:** If the freezing process has been correctly carried out in optimal hygienic conditions, the meat may be stored in good condition for one to two years. Ground meat can be stored for shorter periods, since germs can more readily attack it.

- **Parasite free:** freezing usually kills taenia (tapeworm) and other parasites.

Drawbacks to Freezing

The primary drawback to frozen meat is that it **decays rapidly** *after* it has been *thawed*.

Most of the germs in the meat at the time it is frozen survive the low temperatures, but are unable to reproduce. When the meat is thawed these germs and spores develop rapidly.

Thawed meat must be refrigerated and eaten the *same day* to avoid rapid decay.

Irradiation

Application of high doses of **X-rays or gamma rays** *destroys all* of the **microorganisms** found in meat. For this reason, this procedure is also referred to as **cold sterilization.**

Irradiation of foods does *not* make them **radioactive,** as some consumers fear. However, there are *still* **doubts** regarding the unpredictable long-range effects it may have on meat and other foods.

Advantages of Irradiated Meat

- It permits a *reduction* in the dose of **nitrites** and other chemical **preservatives** with known side effects.

- It *destroys* **parasites** that may be in the meat, such as trichina and tapeworm in swine.

Drawbacks to Irradiated Meat

- **Chemical changes** take place in meat that has been submitted to *high doses* of radiation. The high dose of ionizing radiation (5×10^4 Gray) sterilizes meat and other foods, but it causes significant changes in their chemical makeup. Irradiated meat can be stored for certain periods; however, over time it develops a *foul* **smell and taste.** This is because the proteolytic enzymes that degrade meat protein are not destroyed by the radiation.

- *Lower doses* of radiation **do not eliminate pathogens.** The WHO (World Health Organization) recommends that the dose not exceed 10^4 Gray.[4] This low level radiation only eliminates the pathogens, the same as pasteurization, and not those normally found in meat. This type of irradiation does not permit long storage periods. In practice it only serves to *prolong* the preservative action of other methods such as **curing** or **refrigeration.**

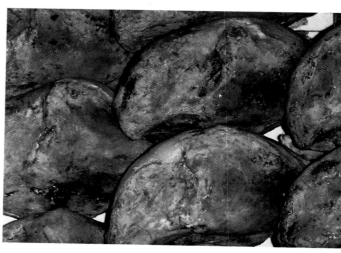

The meat containing the most nitrites is cured ham. Without these additives, cured ham would be an unattractive gray in color, besides the botulism risk.

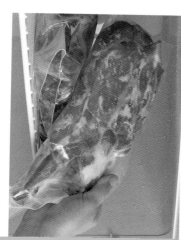

When done properly, freezing is the safest way to preserve meat. Unfortunately, neither producers nor consumers maintain this chain of cold.

Cooking Meat

It might seem that the least harmful way to eat meat for those that wish to include it in their diet is to eat it raw, just as carnivorous animals do. In this way all of the nutrients would be used and the cancer risk would be lowered.

However, the bacterial, viral, and parasitic contamination that often affects meat makes its **cooking** *necessary* to avoid infections.

The paradox is that the action of heat on meat that protects the consumer also creates serious drawbacks.

Benefits of Cooking Meat

- *Most* bacteria and *all* parasites are **destroyed**, but *not* the **spores** of microbes. The effect of heat is similar to that produced in the pasteurization of dairy products.

- Muscle proteins are coagulated, making them *easier* to **digest.**

- The **collagen** forming the connective tissue that makes meat tough is tenderized as it is *converted* to **gelatin** by the heat.

- The formation of aromatic substances due to the heat and the addition of **salt** and **seasoning** *intensify* **flavor.**

Drawbacks to Cooking Meat

Loss of Nutritional Value

Protein and vitamins are the nutrients most affected by heat:[10]

- *Protein:* Some amino acids in meat are destroyed by heat, which causes a proportional loss in the **biological value** of its protein. The loss of amino acids comes about by two mechanisms:

  – **Maillard reaction** produced by high temperature cooking: Lysine, one of the essential amino acids found in meat,

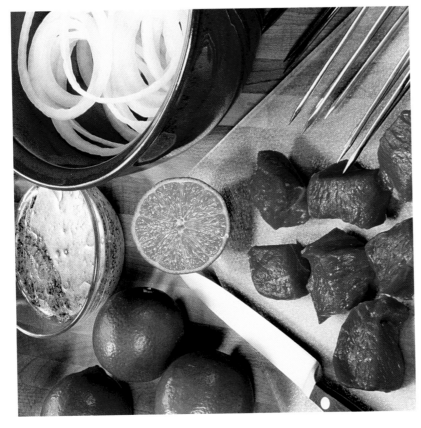

Cooked meat protein is easily digested, but its nutritional value is lower, due to the destruction of some amino acids.

Characteristics of Meat
according to degree of cooking

	Nutritional	Contamination	Carcinogenic
Rare or raw	+	+	–
Well-done	–	–	+

Raw or Well-Done?

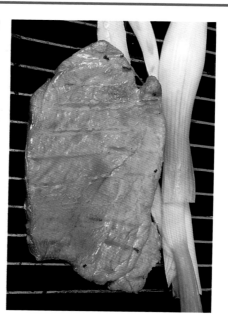

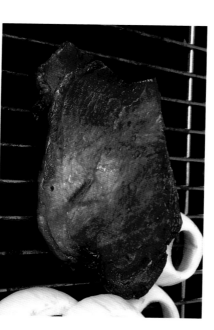

Rare or raw meat does *not* contain **carcinogenic heterocyclic amines** and **benzopyrene**. But, on the other hand, **pathogenic bacteria** such as salmonella and the feared *Escherichia coli* O 157:H7 commonly develop on it.

Pathogenic **germs** are eliminated from well-done meat. But other substances are formed that are possibly carcinogenic:

- **Heterocyclic amines;**
- **Aromatic hydrocarbons** such as **benzopyrene** that is also found in tobacco smoke; and
- **Nitrosamines** formed spontaneously by the action of heat on the meats that have been previously treated with nitrites, such as ham, sausage, and others.

reacts with carbohydrates to form an insoluble compound that the body cannot use.

This reaction results in *the loss* of up to *20%* of the *lysine* content of meat.

- **Destruction of amino acids:** Several of these such as **cystine, lysine,** and **leucine** are thermolabile, and are destroyed by heat. The loss varies from *6%* from a 30-minute cooking period to *25%* for longer cooking times.

- *Vitamins:* When meat is cooked it loses part of its vitamins. This can be by as much as *50%* of its content when raw. This is caused by:

- Destruction by **heat:** This affects all vitamins, but particularly the most thermolabile such as B_1, B_2, B_6, niacin, and folates.

- Loss in **solution:** The muscle juices released during roasting draw part of the vitamins out of the meat. In the case of stewing they remain in the broth in which the meat is cooked. But care must be exercised. Meat stews, though rich in vitamins, are also high in

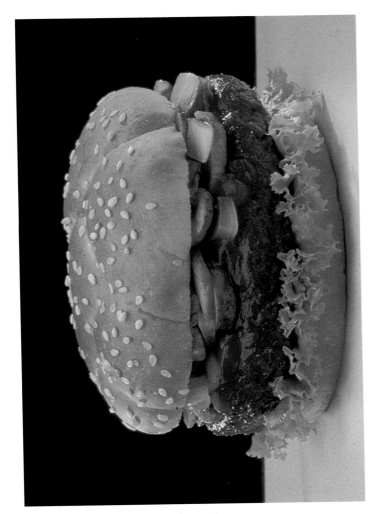

A grilled hamburger contains a few millionths of a gram of carcinogenic polycyclic aromatic hydrocarbons (8.6 μg/kg of benzopyrene and 26.5 of pyrene).

Even though this is a miniscule amount, consumption of two hamburgers a day for five days provides enough to cause changes in the DNA (Deoxyribonucleic acid) of mononuclear blood cells.

This study *was* carried out at the University of Limburg (Maastricht, the Netherlands).[11]

cially when the flame or coals come into contact with the meat. This occurs particularly with **grilling** and **barbecue.**

- **Nitrosamines** are formed when the **nitrites** used to cure the meat *react* with the *amino acids* in it (see Vol. 1, p. 268). **Heat** *enhances* the formation of carcinogens. For this reason, **bacon, ham, and sausages,** which are normally prepared with nitrites, are *particularly* **mutagenic** (causing genetic mutations) when they are **fried** or **grilled.**[14,15]

Cancer and Cooking Meat

A great number of **scientific experiments** have demonstrated the capacity of **amines, hydrocarbons,** and **nitrosamines** formed during the cooking of meat to produce:

- **Cellular mutations,** that is, alterations in the genes (mutagenic action). Cells that

purines, which form uric acid and carcinogens in the body (see Vol. p. 306).

Formation of Carcinogens

Since the middle of the 20th century it has been known that various carcinogens are produced during the *normal cooking* of meat:

- **HCA's** (*Heterocyclic amines*) are formed by the reaction of creatine with the amino acids in meat.[12] **Creatine** is a nitrogenous substance ($C_4H_9N_3O_2$) that provides energy for muscle contraction.

The *higher* the **temperature** the *more* **HCA's** are formed. **Grilling** and **frying** are the cooking methods that produce the most HCA's, particularly when the meat is well-done.[13]

- **PAH's** (*Polycyclic aromatic hydrocarbons*) such as **benzopyrene** are formed espe-

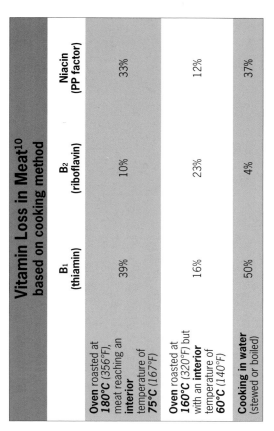

Vitamin Loss in Meat[10] based on cooking method		
B₁ (thiamin)	B₂ (riboflavin)	Niacin (PP factor)
Oven roasted at **180°C** (356°F), meat reaching an **interior** temperature of **75°C** (167°F) 39%	10%	33%
Oven roasted at **160°C** (320°F) but with an **interior** temperature of **60°C** (140°F) 16%	23%	12%
Cooking in water (stewed or boiled) 50%	4%	37%

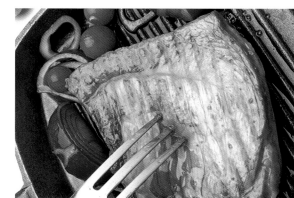

The more "well-done" meat is, the fewer germs it contains, but the higher its cancer risk. When well-done meat is punctured, its juice is no longer pink but turns grayish.

have experienced genetic mutation are not yet cancerous, but have a great possibility of becoming so. It has been proven that a short time after eating fried pork, HCA's and other mutagens can be detected in the urine.[14] This means that these harmful substances are circulating in the blood and can reach all of the body's cells.

- Cancerous **tumors** in every organ of experimental animals such as rats and monkeys. This is the experimental proof of the carcinogenic action of these substances.[12,13]

- **Cancer** in humans that eat meat "well-done."

Recent Studies

The following are *epidemiological* examples demonstrating the **carcinogenic effect** of the substances formed during the cooking of meat:

- An investigation carried out in Los Angeles (California, USA) demonstrated that those who ate meat cooked "well-done" more than once a week presented more than double the incidence of adenoma of the colon than those who ate meat cooked "rare" once a week or less. Adenoma of the colon is a benign tumor that frequently degenerates into cancer.[16]

- A study carried out by the National Cancer Institute of the United States showed that the consumption of large amounts of red meat is directly related to an increased risk of stomach or esophageal cancer. This risk is even higher for those who eat meat grilled "well-done."[17]

- In Uruguay, a country known for high meat consumption, it has been proven that women that ingest more HCA's by eating meat fried or grilled, present more than triple the risk of breast cancer.[18]

Continued on page 284

*According to the numerous scientific studies described in this chapter,
the healthiest choice is to eliminate meat from the diet.
However, those who are not aware of how to or cannot do this should prepare meat
in ways that present the least risk to their health.*

Roasting

Roasting consists of the *application* of *dry heat*: it is used for the tenderest least fibrous cuts of meat; those with the least connective tissue. A roast may be prepared in the **oven, grill,** or **casserole.**

In order to *reduce* production of **mutagenic** and **carcinogenic** heterocyclic amines the meat's interior should reach *no more than* **70°C** (*158°F*). This is the temperature used for pasteurization and is sufficient to destroy most pathogens and parasites. The internal temperature of meat can be measured with a special thermometer.

To maintain an interior temperature of 70°C (158°F), the **oven** should be set between **180°** and **190°C** (between **356°** and **374°F**). When it rises *above* **200°C** (*392°F*), which happens with many ovens or when roasting chicken on a *grill*, there is a *considerable increase* in the formation of **heterocyclic amines** (see Vol. 1, p. 276). These substances are much more abundant in meat cooked "well-done."[19]

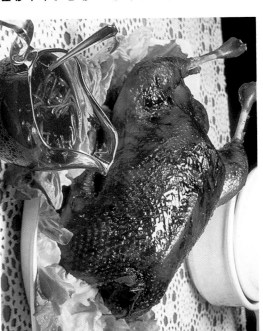

The higher the oven temperature during roasting, the greater number of carcinogenic substances forms in the meat.

Grilled or Barbecued

When meat is barbecued, it is in direct contact with the flame. This gives it its unique flavor and texture, which are very much enjoyed. At the same time, however, this cooking method produces an *elevated amount of aromatic* polycyclic **hydrocarbons** (see Vol. 1, p. 276). This happens when the melted fat drips onto the hot coals.

It is possible to *mitigate* the **carcinogenic effect** of barbecued meats by following these recommendations:

- *Remove* as much **fat** as possible from the meat before placing it on the grill.

- **Precook** the meat in the oven or microwave to reduce the time it must be on the grill.

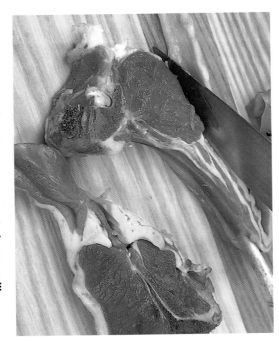

Fire acts directly on meat roasted on a grill, producing many carcinogenic substances.

Cooking Meat

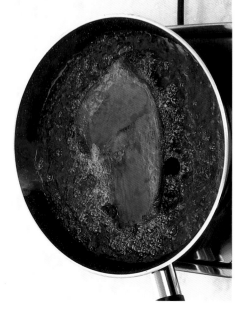

According to studies carried out at the Karolinska Institute of Sweden, cancer-causing mutagens begin forming during the first moments of cooking pork.[15]

Frying

Due to the high temperatures used in this method [above 200°C (392°F)], considerable amounts of mutagens and carcinogens are formed. *Fried pork* contains numerous heterocyclic amines, possibly *more* than *any other type* of meat.[20]

An experiment conducted with laboratory rats at the Karolinska Institute of the University of Huddinge (Sweden) proved that fried meat has significant mutagenic power.

Wheat **bran, pectin,** and **vegetable fiber** (see Vol. 1, p. 388), in general, reduce this mutagenic power of fried meat when they are eaten together with it.[21]

Stewing

Meat may be cooked **in liquid** or it may be **steamed.** Since the temperature remains at 100°C (212°F) while the water is boiling, this method does not reach such high temperatures as other methods.

However, cooking in water takes considerable longer than roasting or frying thus the meat is in contact with heat for a longer period. This results in the formation of mutagenic and carcinogens, as well.

The **pork** juices that result *from stewing* have attracted the attention of researchers because of their *high concentration* of heterocyclic **amines.** These substances, which are dissolved in the broth created by boiling the meat, cause genetic **mutations** in cells, thus promoting the development of cancer.

There are two facts of special interests for scientists:

- The broth that results from boiling **pork** contains *four times more* heterocyclic **amines** than roast beef.[22]

- The amount of heterocyclic **amines** in the broth is *significantly reduced* when pork is cooked with **onions and garlic.** The sulfurated essences found in onions and garlic are capable of arresting, at least partially, the production of heterocyclic amines during cooking.[23]

This study clearly illustrates that meats, particularly pork, contain carcinogenic substances, while plant foods, in this case garlic and onions, protect against cancer (see *EMP* p. 233; Vol. 2, p. 144).

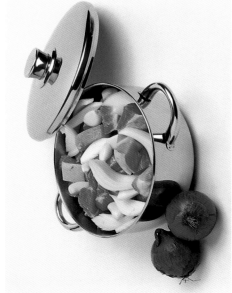

Studies conducted at the Institute of Food Science of Taichung (China) demonstrated that meat cooked with onions and garlic is less carcinogenic than when it is cooked alone.[23] This is because garlic and onions protect against cancer even before they are eaten.

Nutritional Value

Water

The muscle tissue of livestock and poultry contains between 70% and 80% water by weight. There are specific circumstances in which the water in meat increases:

- **Age** of the animal: the younger the animal, the more water its meat contains.

- **Stress** before slaughter: animals that suffer psychological stress before slaughter produce soft, pale meat that oozes water (see Vol. 1, p. 269).

Hormone treatment in the days leading up to slaughter causes the animal to urinate less and retain water in its tissues. The animal weighs more and the farmer is paid more.

This practice is prohibited since it constitutes **fraud** for two reasons: In addition to a *higher percentage of water* than normal, this meat also contains *more* **urea** and other **toxic substances.**

Fiber

Collagen represents 1% to 2% of any fiber that meat contains, which consists of tendons and the fibrous network of the muscles. This fiber is formed from **protein,** and bears no similarity in composition or properties to vegetable cellulose fiber. Collagen turns to **gelatin** when heated.

Collagen fiber from meat digests poorly, does not have laxative properties, nor does it protect against colon cancer, as does the cellulose fiber of plant foods (see Vol. 1, p. 388).

Fats

Fats are the nutrients whose proportion in the meat varies the most depending on the zoological species of the animal, its food, and its living conditions.

- The **carcass** as a whole contains between 20% and 40% fat, most of which is visible.

- The **muscle,** which is **lean meat,** has very little visible fat. But it contains between 4% and 11% invisible intramuscular **fat. Pork** contains the most invisible fat, between 9% and 11%.

About 100 g (about 3.5 ounces) of meat provide between 10% and 50% of the Daily Value of total fat (about 65 g), and between 15% and 60% of the Daily Value of saturated fat (about 20 g).

Carbohydrates

The muscle cells of live animals contain a small percentage of **glycogen** (0.1%), a substance similar to starch in plants. After death, however, the glycogen is transformed into lactic acid. The meat, then, *contains no* significant amounts of carbohydrates.

Protein

Protein represents one of the most valuable components of meat.

- **Quantity:** between 15% and 20% by weight, a higher percentage than **grains,** but lower than **legumes.**

- **Digestibility:** meat protein is digested and absorbed very well; its digestibility reaches 97%. Legume and grain proteins are between 80% and 95% digestible.

- **Quality:** the biological value of meat protein is not 100%, as some believe, but **75%.** This is due to a deficiency in three essential amino acids: methionine, tryptophan, and histidine.

Minerals

The most important minerals provided by meat are iron and zinc.

- *Iron:* although the iron in meat is absorbed better than that of vegetables, dairy products, or eggs, it is found in relatively small quantities. One hundred grams of beef or pork provide only between 7% and 8% of the RDA (Recommended Dietary Allowance). Meats richest in iron are:

  – **Lamb:** It provides between 16% and 18% of the RDA of iron;

  – **Offal:** One hundred grams of **variety meats** provide 40% to 50% of the RDA of iron.

- *Zinc:* One hundred grams of meat covers between 20% and 30% of the RDA. Vegetables also contain zinc, even though its absorption is somewhat more difficult.

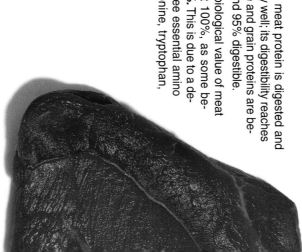

# of Meat

Vitamins

The *only* vitamins that meat provides in any significant amounts are those of the **B complex**, excluding folates, which form part of the B group but are present in very small amounts. Offal or variety meats are richer in B vitamins than the muscle or meat itself. These are salient:

- *Vitamin B₁* is found particularly in pork. One hundred grams provides 40% of the RDA (Recommended Dietary Allowance) of this vitamin.

- *Vitamins B₂, B₆ and, niacin:* meat overall contains between 10% and 30% the RDA of these vitamins. It also contains other B complex vitamins such as biotin and pantothenic acid.

- *Vitamin B₁₂:* meat in general is a good source of this vitamin, which is absent from most plant-based foods (see Vol. 1, p. 395). **Lamb** is the meat richest in vitamin B₁₂; 100 g more than covers the RDA (2μg). **Chicken** and **poultry** in general are *less rich:* 100 grams provides from 10% to 20% of the RDA. One hundred grams of **variety meats**, particularly liver, provide up to *23 times* the RDA for this vitamin.

Meat is incomplete from a nutritional standpoint, since it lacks or contains very low percentages of fundamental nutrients such as carbohydrates, antioxidant vitamins (A, C, and E), and calcium (see Vol. 1, p. 281).

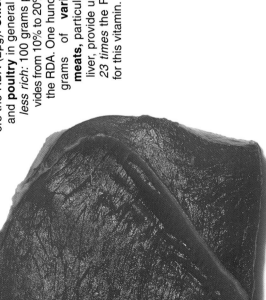

Cholesterol

Meat is quite rich in cholesterol, even when lean. The more fat meat contains, the more cholesterol it provides. There is between 70 and 80 mg of cholesterol in 100 g (about 3.5 ounces) of lean meat, which represents approximately 25% of the Daily Value (300 mg).

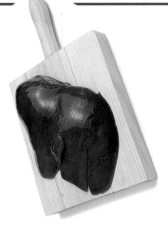

Liver and other viscera contain much more nutrients than meat itself, but its use presents more health drawbacks (see Vol. 1, p. 317).

Nonprotein Nitrogen Compounds

Non-protein nitrogen compounds are substances containing nitrogen in their molecules, but are not proteins. Although present in small quantities, they are important because of their high physiological activity. Non-protein nitrogen compounds produce some undesirable effects. Some examples are:

- **Creatine** provides energy for muscle contraction. It reacts with the *amino acids* in meat and with **nitrites** added as preservatives to form carcinogenic **nitrosamines** (see Vol. 1, p. 276).

- **Urea, uric acid, purines, and creatinine** are waste substances from the animal, which the human body cannot use. Because of this it requires metabolic effort to eliminate them (see Vol. 1, p. 300). Purines contribute to the typical aroma and flavor of meat, but they convert to uric acid in the body and become toxic.

- **Hypoxanthine** is a purine that acts as a stimulant, whose chemical composition and effect are similar to the caffeine in coffee. It is responsible for the euphoric effect experienced after eating meat (see Vol. 1, p. 283), and can be addictive.

- **Vasoactive amines** such as **histamine** and **tyramine** act on the blood vessels, particularly the arteries, producing arterial hypertension. These are found primarily in:
  - pork;
  - very aged meat or meat poorly preserved. In both cases there is a proliferation of bacteria that produce vasoactive amines (see Vol. 1, p. 268).

Nutritious But Not Necessary

Meat is not an indispensable food, nor is it necessary for humans.
This is clearly stated in the World Health Organization's journal World Health Forum.[24]

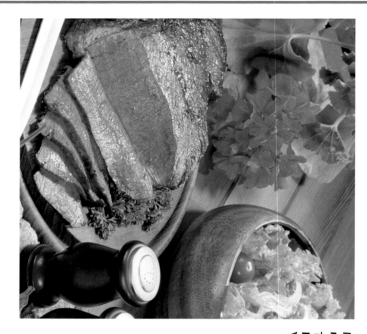

Meat: the Facts

- Meat is *not* a **necessary** food in the human diet.

- According to available scientific information, meat consumption presents so *many* **health risks** that any **benefit** derived **does not** *offset* them (see Vol. 1, p. 300).

- *Habitual* consumption of meat and its derivatives is associated with a variety of diseases, particularly **cardiac** disease (see Vol. 1, p. 304), as well as certain types of **cancer** (see Vol. 1, p. 306).

- The best course is to *progressively reduce* meat in the diet, replacing it with foods of plant origin (see Vol. 1, p. 332).

- The meats that present the *least risk*:
  - Are from healthy animals,
  - Contain little fat (see Vol. 1, p. 294),
  - Are properly cooked (see Vol. 1, p. 274), and
  - Are not cured (see Vol. 1, p. 270).

- **Pork** and its derivatives present the *highest risks* of any meat products (see Vol. 1, p. 319).

Positive Aspects of Meat

- **Nutritious:** Meat is a good source of protein, vitamin B$_{12}$, iron, and zinc.

- **Easy to digest:** meat proteins are better digested and absorbed than vegetable proteins. For this reason, meat, cooked simply, is useful for persons with weak digestive systems due to
  - debilitating illness;
  - serious infections;
  - extensive trauma or burns;
  - recovery from major surgery.

- **Nutritional complement:** meat nutritionally enriches poor or monotonous diets, such as those followed by the poorest inhabitants of developing countries. The addition of small portions of meat can enhance the value of grain proteins, as well as providing iron and vitamin B$_{12}$. However, diets consisting of plant-based foods are nutritionally completely satisfactory if they offer variety and balance, including occasional **dairy products** and **eggs.** There is absolutely no nutritional risk with this type of diet and *no need* for meat.

- **Dietetic treatment** of certain nutritional deficiencies: Meat, and particularly liver are traditional dietetic remedies for anemia due to lack of iron or lack of vitamin B$_{12}$. However, even though it can be useful in these cases, it is in no way indispensable. There are other non-meat sources of these essential nutrients.

Is Meat Addictive?

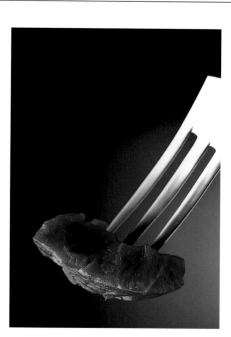

The stimulant hypoxanthine, not any special properties of its protein, vitamins, or minerals, is responsible for the satisfying and stimulating effects of meat. It is similar in chemical formula and effect to caffeine.

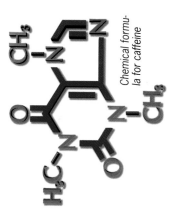

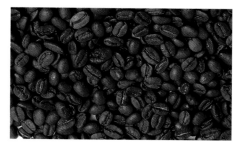

Chemical formula for caffeine

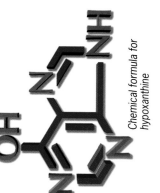

It has been known since antiquity that those who regularly eat meat experience some degree of enervation when they are deprived of this food for some time.

This sensation that "something is missing" always results from abruptly removing meat from the diet, even when it is replaced with plant foods and dietary supplements providing as much or even more protein and nutrients as meat.

A Stimulant in Meat

The enervation that some persons experience when they stop eating meat products is not due to lack of its protein or other nutrients that some consider irreplaceable. It is due to a type of stimulant found in meat.

Today it is known that the muscle cells of meat contain **hypoxanthine,** which increases in concentration as the meat ages. Hypoxanthine is formed by:

- The degradation of ATP (adenosine triphosphate),
- The decomposition of the nucleotides that form DNA and RNA in the nuclei of the cells.

Chemical formula for hypoxanthine

Continued from page 277

Meat Proteins

All living things, whether vegetable or animal, have protein in their cells. However, the *only* living things capable of **producing** protein *by themselves* from the inorganic compounds such as minerals found in the soil and the gases in the air are **plants** and some types of **bacteria**.

Protein Sources

Animals, including those used to produce meat, create their own protein from:

- Proteins and nitrogen compounds found in legumes, grains, grasses, or other

- Proteins from **other animals** in the case of *carnivores* or *omnivores* (those that eat everything) such as swine.

In sum, *all* of the *amino acids* that form meat protein come *directly from* **plant *protein***. Animals used for meat are not the true "protein factories" that some believe they are. In reality they are "processing plants" that use protein from plants or other animals as raw material.

Efficiency With Which Animals Transform Protein

Animals are *very inefficient* transformers of the protein they take in. The accompanying graph shows that for each 100 g of vegetable protein invested in feeding cattle, only 10 g of protein is returned in the case of beef. This shows that the production of animal protein is a true squandering of resources, incompatible with sustaining the growth of the world's population.

Types of Meat Protein

Meat is formed primarily of muscle tissues wrapped in a web of collagen fiber. Each type of protein has a specific location.

Contractile Protein

These proteins are *actin* and *myosin*. They are found in the cytoplasm of muscle cells forming a dense web of fibrils capable of contracting. These two constitute approximately 50% of the total protein found in meat.

Sarcoplasmic Protein:

These are dissolved in the cytoplasm of muscle cells and constitute 40% of meat protein. Since these are water-soluble, a portion remains in the cooking broth. *Contractile* and *sarcoplasmic* proteins are

plants, in the case of *herbivores* such as the cow or lamb.

Efficiency With Which Animals Transform Protein

For each 100 g of soy protein, for example, used as animal feed the return is

Meat proteins are actually second-hand. They are formed from those of plant origin.

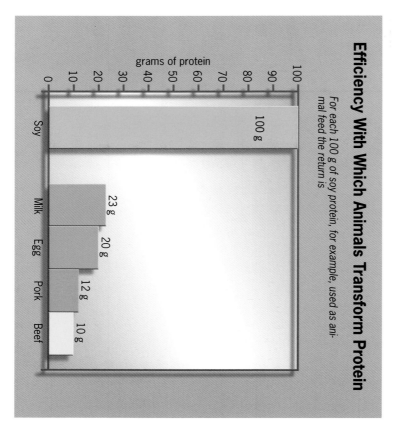

grams of protein

- Soy — 100 g
- Milk — 23 g
- Egg — 20 g
- Pork — 12 g
- Beef — 10 g

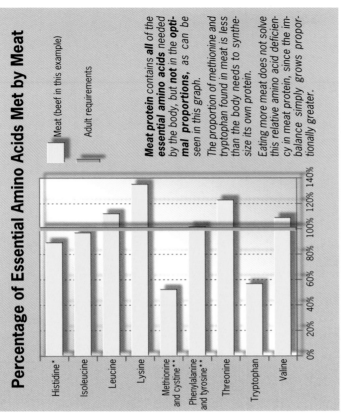

Percentage of Essential Amino Acids Met by Meat

Meat (beef in this example)

Adult requirements

Histidine*
Isoleucine
Leucine
Lysine
Methionine and cystine**
Phenylalanine and tyrosine**
Threonine
Tryptophan
Valine

0% 20% 40% 60% 80% 100% 120% 140%

Meat protein contains **all** of the **essential amino acids** needed by the body, but **not** in the **optimal proportions,** as can be seen in this graph.

The proportion of methionine and tryptophan found in meat is less than the body needs to synthesize its own protein.

Eating more meat does not solve this relative amino acid deficiency in meat protein, since the imbalance simply grows proportionally greater.

Meat alone is not as nutritious as some believe. The biological value of its protein is not 100%, but rather 75% (see Vol. 1, p. 286).

Meat proteins com**plement** those of **grains** (bread, pasta, semolina, and cuscus), and **legumes.**

* Histidine is not essential for adults.

** Cystine and tyrosine are not essential amino acids, but they are included because a part of them serves the purpose of meeting the requirements of methionine and phenylalanine, respectively.

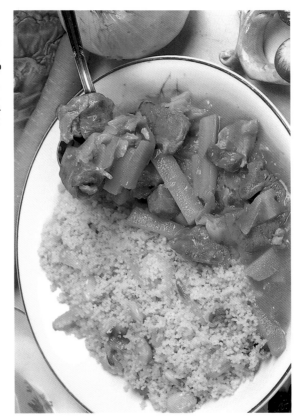

those considered of the *greatest* biological quality.

Myoglobin is one of the sarcoplasmic proteins that, although present in very small quantities (1-5 mg/100 g of meat), is important since it gives meat its typical red color.

Nuclear Proteins or Nucleoproteins

These proteins are found in the nuclei of muscle cells and form part of their genetic material (genes and chromosomes).

Nucleoproteins are bonded with nucleic acids: ribonucleic acid (RNA) and deoxyribonucleic acid (DNA).

These nucleic acids that accompany the nucleoproteins of meat contain purines, which transform to uric acid when consumed.

Collagen

Collagen is the protein that forms the connective tissue in meat. This is a form of fibrous netting that surrounds muscle cells. Collagen, together with *elastin*, also forms tendons and aponeuroses or membranes that cover the muscles. Collagen makes up about 10% of meat protein or about 2% of the animal's total weight.

Collagen, as well as *elastin*, is difficult to digest, and are of *low* biological **value** since they lack various essential amino acids.

When collagen is heated during cooking, it transforms into **gelatin.**

Protein Quality

Means of Evaluating Protein

There are several ways to evaluate the nutritive quality of a protein. The most common are:

• **Digestibility** reflects the percentage of the protein that is absorbed and passes to the blood in the form of amino acids. The portion of the protein that is not absorbed is eliminated through the feces.

Nutritional Value of the Proteins of Various Foods

The **digestibility** and **biological value** of the proteins found in foods varies a great deal according to researchers. This is possibly due to the inherent difficulty in quantifying them. Additionally, in many cases the calculations are based on laboratory guinea pigs, so the data are not completely applicable to humans. This table is a summary of values proposed by various authors. [5, 10, 25, 26, 27]

Foods of ANIMAL ORIGIN	Digestibility (D)	Biological value (BV)	Net protein utilization (NPU)
Meat	97	75	73
Eggs	99	94	93
Milk	98	84	81
Cheese	98	71	70
Foods of PLANT ORIGIN			
Legumes	83	85	71
Refined grains	95	60	57
Whole grains	85	65	55

Meat proteins are quite complete, but not to the point that they should be considered ideal or perfect. By themselves they do not completely meet the needs of the body, whether of a child or an adult (its biological value is about 75%).

- **Biological value** reflects the percentage of total amino acids present in a protein that are retained and used by the body once they have been absorbed. The higher the biological value of a food protein, the better it is utilized by the body, and the greater number of new proteins can be produced from it.

- **Net Protein Utilization** (NPU) is an index derived by combining the two previous measures and is the most accurate measure of protein quality. The formula for this calculation is:

$$NPU = \frac{DIGESTIBILITY \times BIOLOGICAL\ VALUE}{100}$$

Quality of Meat Protein

- The **digestibility** of tender meat is 97%, which is superior to all vegetable protein and can only be compared with milk and egg protein. When the meat is very fibrous, its digestibility is reduced to 95% or less.

- The average **biological value** of meat protein is around 75%. This is relatively high compared with other foods, but it is *not ideal*; indeed, the biological value of meat protein is lower than the **egg's** (see Vol. 1, p. 221). This means that the human body is incapable of completely using the **amino acids** in meat to form its own proteins. Some are present in excessive amounts, such as *lysine* or *threonine*, while others *are deficient*, such as *methionine* and *tryptophan*.

In other words, if a human adult or child ate only meat, he or she would not receive the necessary proportions of essential amino acids needed to form its own protein.

The **limiting amino acid**, or the one found in the lowest proportion, is *methionine*, followed by *tryptophan*. Grain protein contains excess *methionine* and *complements* meat well.

- The **NUP** (Net Protein Utilization) index of meat is quite high, combining excellent digestibility (97%) with a rather high biological value or utilization (75%).

Meat protein quality has been praised, at times to the point of exaggeration, without taking into account that its **biological value, while good, is *not ideal.***

However, thanks to its *high digestibility*, it achieves a net protein utilization of 73%, which is positive; somewhat superior to **legumes** (71%), but quite inferior to that of **eggs** (93%) and **milk** (81%).

Continued on page 288

Nutritional Value of Various Proteins

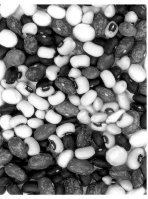

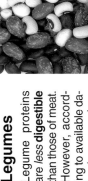

Legumes

Legume proteins are *less* **digestible** than those of meat. However, according to available data (see previous page), their **biological value** is *greater* than that of meat. The combination of factors gives an **NPU** (net protein utilization) of 71, *slightly* **less** than meat, which is 73.

Soy is the legume whose protein has the highest biological value. Any legume combined with a grain provides a very complete protein, endowed with high biological value.

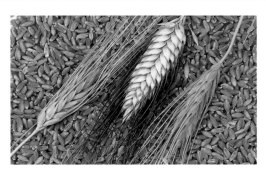

Grains (Cereals)

Grain proteins have the *lowest* **biological value** of any. However, it *increases* greatly when grains are *combined* with **legumes** and **dairy products.**

The **biological value** of **whole** grains is *greater.* However, their **digestibility** is *lower* due to the fiber they contain.

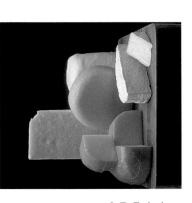

Meat

As the preceding page shows, meat proteins are *very* **digestible** (97%) and have a *rather high* **biological value** (75%). However, meat proteins are *inferior* to those of **eggs, milk,** and even **legumes.** When the indexes are combined, the resulting **NPU** (net protein utilization) of meat is 73%, slightly higher than legumes (71%).

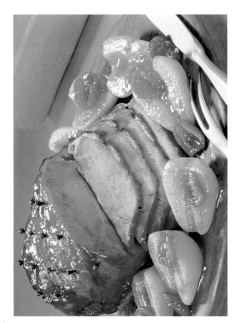

Eggs and Milk

The **digestibility** and **biological value** of the proteins of eggs and milk are *superior* to those of meat.

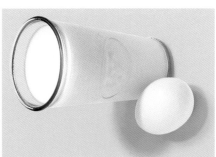

Cheese

Cheese proteins are *highly digestible,* but their **biological value** is *less* than that of milk because the whey, which contains the most complete milk proteins, is discarded during the cheese-making process.

Types of Fat in Meat

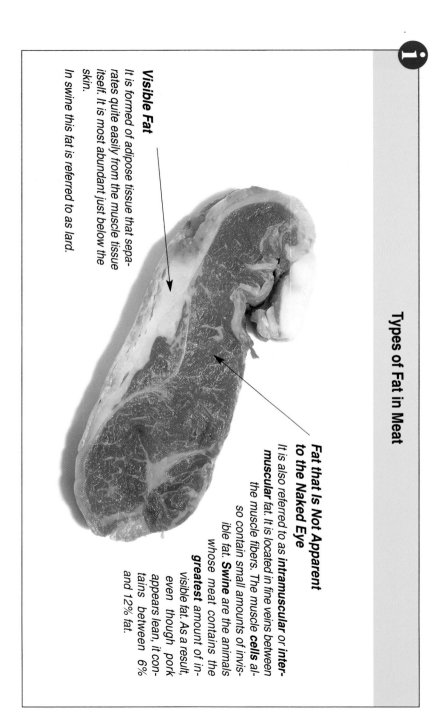

Visible Fat

It is formed of adipose tissue that separates quite easily from the muscle tissue itself. It is most abundant just below the skin.

In swine this fat is referred to as lard.

Fat that Is Not Apparent to the Naked Eye

It is also referred to as **intramuscular** or **inter- muscular** fat. It is located in fine veins between the muscle fibers. The muscle **cells** also contain small amounts of invisible fat. **Swine** are the animals whose meat contains the **greatest** amount of invisible fat. As a result, even though pork appears lean, it contains between 6% and 12% fat.

Continued from page 286

Meat and Fat

Many ancient cultures, and even some modern ones, consider the fat from animals used for food as a symbol of abundance and food quality. The fatter an animal was, the greater the value that was placed on its meat.

However, there was a notable exception to this constant in food history. About 3,500 years ago, when there could be no understanding of saturated and unsaturated fat or cholesterol, Moses had already directed the Hebrew people regarding meat: *"This is a lasting ordinance for the generations to come, wherever you live. You must not eat **any** fat or any blood."*[28]

It was not until well into the 20th century that the harmful effects of animal fat were discovered. The Biblical injunction, however, has withstood the test of time, and is just as valid today in the Western world. In fact, today there are many who are trying to produce or find foods that are low in animal fat, or are completely without it: nonfat milk and yogurt, sauces without eggs, cookies and pastry without animal fat, lean meat, etcetera.

Meat as a Source of Dietary Fat

Meat and its derivatives provide most of the fat in the typical Western diet. For example, in the United States meat alone (red meat and poultry) and fish contribute 53.3 g of fat per person per day.[26] And this in spite of all the campaigns conducted by health authorities to reduce fat consumption. If this amount is combined with the fat from dairy products, eggs, oils, and other products that normally form part of the di-

Daily Fat Consumption and the Average North American Diet

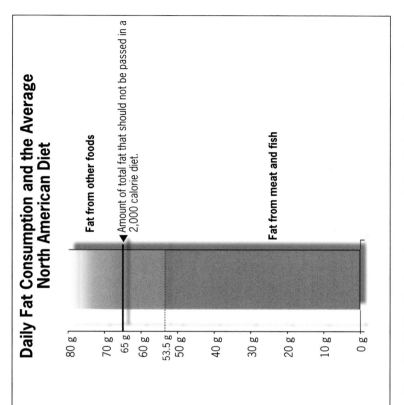

Fat from other foods

Amount of total fat that should not be passed in a 2,000 calorie diet.

Fat from meat and fish

80 g
70 g
65 g
60 g
53.5 g
50 g
40 g
30 g
20 g
10 g
0 g

...et, it is well in excess of the 65 g of total fat considered acceptable for a 2,000 calorie diet (see Vol. 1, p. 404-405).

Diets based on foods of animal origin generally furnish fat amounts well above those recommended.

Factors that Determine the Fat Content of Meat

Fat is meat's *most* **variable** component in terms of percentage of the total weight it represents and its chemical composition. Probably fat produces the *most* **undesirable** health effects of any meat component.

Because of this, it is important to understand the factors involved in the quantity and composition of meat fat.

Species

The quality and composition of fat, together with the meat, vary with the species (see Vol. 1, p. 296).

The animal producing the *highest* proportion of *fat* is the **swine**, followed by lamb, cattle, and poultry.

The Animal's Age

The fat proportion is usually less in very young animals and in older ones.

The Animal's Living Conditions

The more sedentary the animal or poultry, the more fat its meat contains.

Type of Diet

The influence of an animal's diet on fat composition depends on the anatomy and physiology of the animal:

- **Ruminants:** (cattle, lamb, etc.): The quantity and composition of fat are *quite* **constant** and depend little on the diet of the animal. This is due to the peculiar stomach of these animals, which is divided into four chambers (see Vol. 1, p. 297) where various bacteria and protozoans

The World Health Organization and the National Academy of Sciences (USA) recommend that fat make up no more than 30% of total calories in the diet (see Vol. 1, p. 404-405).

This represents 65 grams of total fat a day for a 2,000 calorie diet.

In the average North American diet, only meat and fish provide 53.3 grams of fat a day.[26] This easily exceeds the 30% of total daily calories in the form of fat.

digest and transform food. This way, the same types of fatty acids and other nutrients are produced independent of what the animal has eaten. Even though a cow or lamb has been inappropriately fed, the composition of its fat varies little.

- **Monogastric animals:** (swine, horse, etc.): The composition of the fat of these meats *depends* a **great** deal on the diet of the animal. If a swine lives on a diet of acorns and other plants, its meat has a higher proportion of unsaturated fatty acids. However, if it is fed commercial feeds, which is the most common, the percentage of saturated fatty acids is proportionally higher as will be the total fat content.

Fat and Cholesterol in Various Meats
per 100 g of edible portion

	LEAN MEAT		MEAT WITH COMPLETE FAT	
	Fat (g)	Cholesterol (mg)	Fat (g)	Cholesterol (mg)
CHICKEN	3	70	15.1	75
BEEF	2.87 - 4.5	83	6.77 - 11	82
LAMB	5.25	65	17.1 - 21.6	72
PORK	5.9 - 12	61	12 - 35.1	74

Lean meats are not lower in cholesterol than meats containing more fat.

The fundamental difference between lean and fatty meats is the quantity of total fat and not their proportion of cholesterol.

The meat of inappropriately fed monogastric animals contains more fat and adversely affects cholesterol levels.

Drugs Given to Livestock

Intense factory farming techniques force animals into a **sedentary life** that *fosters high-fat* meat. On the other hand, the production of leaner meat has become a priority for the livestock industry in its efforts to meet the demands of consumers. To do this they resort to the administration of various drugs to animals, such as:[29]

- **Anabolic steroids,** which are hormones similar to what athletes use to dope themselves. These drugs cause an increase of muscle mass with little fat. One of the most common is **clembuterol** (see Vol. 1, p. 303).

- **Growth hormones** produce greater muscle development. These are also used to increase milk production in cows (see Vol. 1, p. 196).

- **Beta-adrenergic agonists** are extremely potent drugs that stimulate the animal's autonomic nervous system, causing it to use up fat reserves.

Not enough is known about the repercussions that these drugs may have on the quality of the meat or on the health

Livestock raisers administer hormones and other drugs to sedentary animals in an effort to reduce fat levels in their meat.

The meat consumer lacks a healthful choice: eat excessive fat or hormones and drugs.

of humans that eat it. The question remains as to whether the fat reduction achieved outweighs the health risks of the use of hormones and other drugs on livestock. Is it more desirable to eat meat with more fat but without hormones or less fat with hormones? The former is unhealthful, while the latter is risky.

Composition of Meat Fat

Meat fat is made up *primarily* of *triglycerides*. Additionally, there are *small amounts* of *phospholipids* and *cholesterol*.

Each triglyceride molecule is made up chemically of a glycerin molecule bonded with three other fatty acid molecules, which may be saturated, monounsaturated, or polyunsaturated. Each of these three types has its own characteristics, as will be seen.

Saturated Fatty Acids

Saturated fatty acids predominate in **beef** and **lamb** (around 47%). **Chicken** contains as much as 31.3% and **pork,** 38.7%. These saturated fatty acids cause the fat to be **solid** at room temperature, and are the *most harmful* to health. It has been shown that consumption of saturated fats:

- *Increases* **cholesterol** production in the body and *promotes* **arteriosclerosis,** and
- *Increases* the **risk** of suffering from breast, colon, or prostate **cancers.**

Monounsaturated Fatty Acids

The *most abundant* fatty acids in **pork** are monounsaturated, reaching 49.5% of all fatty acids. Most of these are formed by *oleic acid,* the same as is found in olive oil. This fatty acid alone makes up 42% of **pork** fat and 38% of that of **beef.**

It is true that a diet rich in oleic acid reduces the risk of heart disease, arteriosclerosis, and cancer (see Vol. 1, p. 119). How-

Calories From Saturated Fat of Some Foods

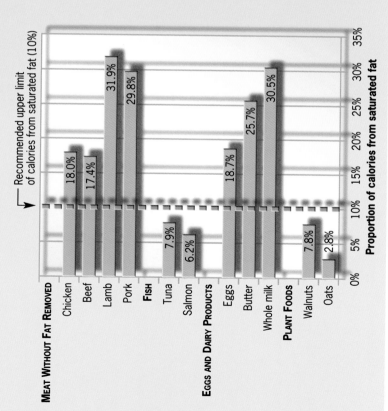

Recommended upper limit of calories from saturated fat (10%)

Proportion of calories from saturated fat

MEAT WITHOUT FAT REMOVED
Chicken — 18.0%
Beef — 17.4%
Lamb — 31.9%
Pork — 29.8%

FISH
Tuna — 7.9%
Salmon — 6.2%

EGGS AND DAIRY PRODUCTS
Eggs — 18.7%
Butter — 25.7%
Whole milk — 30.5%

PLANT FOODS
Walnuts — 7.8%
Oats — 2.8%

(0% — 5% — 10% — 15% — 20% — 25% — 30% — 35%)

Saturated fat is **unnecessary** in the diet, and is **harmful** above a certain quantity since it **promotes cholesterol** production within the body and **arteriosclerosis.**

Consequently, the World Health Organization and the National Academy of Sciences (USA) recommend that a healthy diet include 10% or less of its calories from saturated fats.

In fact, **saturated fats** make up **more than 10% of total calories** of all meats, including lean meats, as well as eggs and dairy products (vertical broken line).

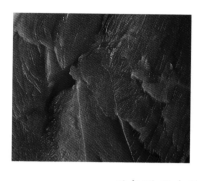

Plant foods do not contain cholesterol; nor is there any meat, no matter how lean, that does not (see following page). Even though it may not be visible, meat always contains fat (see Vol. 1, p. 288).

ever, this has only been proven with olive oil and other vegetable oils rich in oleic acid, but not with pork fat.

There have been campaigns promoting pork based on its benign appearance and the fact that it contains the same oleic acid as olive oil. Be that as it may, there is no reason to believe that pork or beef fat is in any way beneficial simply because it contains oleic acid. Quite the contrary; there is a great deal of evidence that they are harmful.

Polyunsaturated Fatty Acids

Poultry and **pork** are the richest of all meats in polyunsaturated fatty acids (23.4% of the total fat in chicken and 11.8% in pork). Vegetable foods rich in these fatty acids such as walnuts (see Vol. 2, p. 64) and seed oils (see Vol. 1, pp. 124-127) *reduce* the level of LDL (harmful) cholesterol. Nevertheless, neither pork fat nor chicken fat does this.

Is Meat Fat Truly Harmful?

Meat fat, particularly pork fat and chicken fat, does not seem particularly harmful upon a quick review of the data. Meat fat, particularly that of pork and chicken, truly does contain some percentage of mono and polyunsaturated fatty acids, which are healthful in principle.

Fat Composition of Various Foods

	% saturated	% monounsated	% polyunsated	P/S
MEAT WITHOUT				
Chicken	31.3	45.3	23.4	0.75
Beef	47.8	44	8.2	0.17
Lamb	47.3	44.2	8.5	0.18
Pork	38.7	49.5	11.8	0.31
FISH				
Tuna	29.3	37.3	33.4	1.14
Salmon	17.4	37.4	45.2	2.59
EGGS AND DAIRY PRODUCTS				
Eggs	37.5	46	16.5	0.44
Butter	43.7	49.9	6.4	0.15
Whole milk	65.6	30.5	3.9	0.06
PLANT FOODS				
Walnuts	14.4	36.5	49.2	3.42
Oats	20.5	36.7	42.7	2.08

The fewer polyunsaturated fatty acids and more saturated fatty acids the fat of a food contains, the lower its P/S (polyunsaturated/saturated) index and the more detrimental it is in terms of cholesterol and arteriosclerosis.

Meat fats, eggs and, dairy products have an index below one; fish and plant foods have a higher index (greater than one).

Cholesterol

Foods of animal origin always contain cholesterol (between 50 and 90 mg/100 g). While this appears to be a very small quantity in absolute terms, it affects health a great deal. Meat cholesterol is harmful for two reasons:

- It, by itself, *promotes* **arteriosclerosis.**
- It *exacerbates* the negative effects of *saturated fats.* The combination of saturated fat and cholesterol in meat is more harmful to the arteries than saturated fat alone, as it is found in lower amounts in plant foods.[30]

In spite of this, these fatty acids are only beneficial when they come from plant sources. Scientific investigation demonstrates that, while pork and chicken fat might have seemingly positive qualities, there are many reasons to consider them just as unhealthful as other animal fats.

Low P/S Index

The P/S index (polyunsaturated/saturated) measures the relation between polyunsaturated and saturated fatty acids. It normally varies between 0.2 and 0.3 in the meat from mammals, including swine, and around 0.7 in poultry. The index for most plant foods and fish is higher than 1.2. The *lower* this index, the *greater* the processes of arteriosclerosis) of a fat, and the more negative its effect on cholesterol levels.

Meat fat contains polyunsaturated fatty acids that, in theory, should offset the negative effects of the saturated fatty acids. Yet they are available in insufficient amounts to have any beneficial effect:

- *Five times less* polyunsaturated than saturated in **beef** and **lamb** (P/S index = 0.2 approximately),
- *Three times less* in **pork** (P/S index = 0.31), and
- *30% less* in **chicken** (P/S index = 0.75).

It has been proven with laboratory animals that **saturated fatty acids** are *twice* as "effective" at *raising blood cholesterol levels* as **polyunsaturated** fatty acids are in *lowering* them.[31]

This explains the adverse effects of the fat found in beef, lamb, and pork on cholesterol, in which saturated fatty acids clearly outbalance polyunsaturated.

Lacking in Antioxidants

Meat and its fat are **extremely deficient** in vitamins and antioxidants such as A, C, and E, which neutralize the negative effects of cholesterol by keeping it from oxidizing and being deposited in the arteries. This is just the opposite of the case with plant foods. As a result, a meat-based diet, particularly one that is high in fat, promotes arteriosclerosis and increases the risk of heart disease such as myocardial infarction.

Lose Weight With Meat?

*It is well known that **no food causes weight loss**. Therefore, the real question is: Is meat adequate in a weight-loss diet?*

*In spite of what some suggest, meat-based diets are a method that is **not always effective** for weight loss and are **unhealthful** for various reasons:*

- *It is **very important** that weight-loss diets be balanced in terms of calorie sources:*

  *– **10% - 15%** from **protein**;*
  *– less than **30%** from **fats**;*
  *– and **55% - 60%** from **carbohydrates**.*

A diet based on meat, even though it is lean meat, tends to be unbalanced in terms of calorie sources (see Vol. 1, p. 305). This imbalance causes metabolic disorders that are incompatible with healthy weight loss.

- *The **excess protein** taken in with a meat-based diet adversely affects liver and kidney function. These eliminatory organs are particularly important in the detoxification process involved in weight loss.*

- *Meat-based diets tend to be **poor** in necessary components such as **vegetable fiber** and **antioxidant vitamins** (A, C, and E), since meat lacks both.*

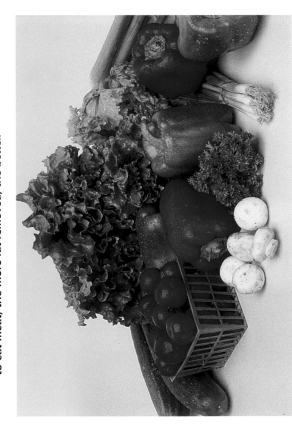

Meat fat offers some positive features, such as the presence of oleic acid. However, epidemiological research and tests demonstrate that, on balance, it is detrimental. If one wishes to eat meat, the more fat removed, the better.

Promotes Cancer

A number of studies, both with laboratory animals and epidemiological, show that eating animal fat *increases the risk* of suffering from certain types of **cancer**. In reality animal fat *does not* cause cancer, but it does *foster its development* once it has begun. Some examples are:

- Hamsters that had been fed beef fat developed more tumors of the pancreas when they were given a carcinogenic substance than those that were fed corn oil.[32]

- A very broad study of 88,751 women conducted by Harvard University (USA) showed that *high* animal *fat consumption doubled* the **risk** of **colon cancer.** High-fat beef, lamb, and pork raised the risk a great deal more than skinless chicken or fish.[33]

- The *higher* the **intake** of *saturated* animal *fat,* the *higher* the **risk** of ovarian,[34] prostate,[35] and breast **cancers.**[36]

Continued on page 296

Meat and Cholesterol

Meat always contains some amount of cholesterol, even though it appears very lean (see Vol. 1, p. 290).

The ideal way to reduce cholesterol levels is to give up meat and its derivatives. Nevertheless, if this is impractical, then one should, at least, follow this simple advice.

1. Chose meat with as little fat as possible

Skinless poultry (chicken, turkey, and partridge) contains less saturated fat than meat of mammals (cattle, sheep, or swine), in addition to being among the leanest. This means that poultry fat has less negative effect on cholesterol than that of mammals.

Sausage-like meat products cannot be recommended because they are very high in fat, which produces high cholesterol levels.

2. Remove as much fat as possible

Visible fat is adipose tissue that can be removed rather easily from the muscle tissue to which it is connected (see Vol. 1, p. 288).

- **Poultry meat:** most of the visible fat is just below the skin and is removed with it.

- **Mammal meat:** The visible fat is more widely distributed than that of poultry. It is located primarily under the skin and between the muscles.

Even though all visible fat is removed, meat always contains a certain amount of invisible fat. This is particularly true of pork. This type of fat can only be partially removed through prolonged cooking in water and, of course, disposing of the broth.

3. Avoid fried meats

The more total fats one eats, the greater the risk of raising the cholesterol level. Frying meat adds poor quality fat (frying oil is modified; see Vol. 1, p.122) to the fat already in the meat, making it doubly harmful.

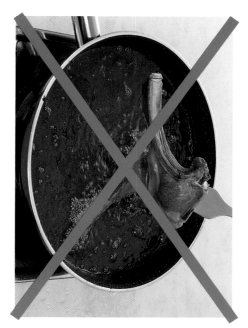

4. Serve meat with vegetables and/or fruit

Ideally this should be done in the **same meal** so antioxidant vitamins can partially compensate for the negative effects of fat and meat.

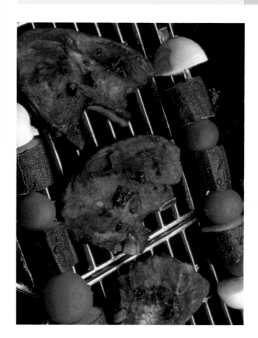

No Meat Lowers Cholesterol

No meat lowers cholesterol. Normally, the more meat in one's diet, the higher the cholesterol. Meat fat **raises** cholesterol levels by two mechanisms:

- **Because it contains cholesterol**, which is absorbed in the intestine and is passed to the blood.

- **Because it contains large quantities of saturated fatty acids**, which foster production of cholesterol in the body (see Vol. 1, p. 292).

Protein Is Not Everything

Comparison between two dishes, one with meat and the other without

These are the ingredients for two standard luncheons, one based on meat and the other on vegetables.

They both provide the same amount of protein, but the one based on meat contains much more fat and cholesterol and very little fiber.

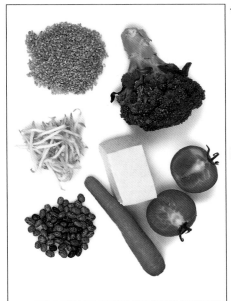

MEAT-BASED MEAL*

French-fried potatoes (150 g)
Beefsteak (150 g)
Lettuce (20 g)
Onion (20 g)
Tomato (50 g)

* All quantities refer to the raw food. See measuremet conversions in Vol. 3, p. 389).

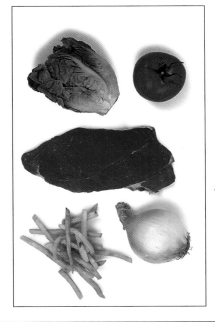

VEGETABLE-BASED MEAL*

Common beans (100 g)
Soy sprouts (30 g)
Whole-grain rice (50 g)
Carrot (100 g)
Tofu (50 g)
Broccoli (50 g)
Tomato (100 g)

	Meat-based meal	Vegetable-based meal
Protein (g)	35.3	35.6
Carbohydrates (g)	38.6	94.9
Total fat (mg)	20.6	5.34
Saturated fat (mg)	6.29	0.92
Fiber (g)	4.43	13.5
Cholesterol (mg)	129	0
Calories (kcal)	498	540

Nutritional Analysis of Both Meals

- ***Proteins:*** both meals provide a very similar amount. The proteins in the vegetable-based meal are as complete as those of the meat. This is the result of the combination of the legumes (beans and tofu) with the grain (rice). Vegetable foods provide the same quality and quantity of proteins as meat, but with many added benefits.

  If one does not wish to eat so many vegetables, tofu or fat-free dairy products may be substituted for some of them.

- ***Carbohydrates:*** the vegetable-based meal provides more than double that of the meat, thus providing better balance. This agrees with the recommendation that

carbohydrates should provide most of total daily calories (60%; see Vol. 1, p. 387).

- ***Fat:*** the meat-based meal contains much more total and saturated fats, which has many drawbacks (see Vol. 1, p. 291).

- ***Fiber:*** much more abundant in the vegetable-based meal, which helps reduce cholesterol.

- ***Colesterol:*** vegetables contain no cholesterol.

- ***Calories:*** somewhat higher for the vegetable-based meal, which does not mean that it is more fattening than the meat-based meal, since these calories are primarily from complex carbohydrates that are absorbed slowly.

Continued from page 293

Factors That Influence Meat Quality

Meat is possibly unique as a food because its nutritional value and possible adverse health effects depend on so many elements both the unique characteristics of each animal and external factors.

The fact that the substantial differences existing among the various species makes some less healthful than others has been known since antiquity. Noah meticulously classified the animals as clean and unclean.

Species

Since antiquity it has been known that each living organism has its own characteristics. Aristotle, the epitome of the philosopher, spoke of this in the fourth century before Christ in his treatises on natural history. In the first century of the Christian era Paul of Tarsus said "All flesh is not the same: Men have one kind of flesh, animals have another, birds another, and fish another."[37]

An Ancient Classification

Some believe that these classifications are purely religious, pertaining only to Jews and Moslems. The fact is that they existed in Noah's time, about 1,500 years before Moses and the organization of the Israelite nation as it left Egypt.

In reality, the classification of clean and unclean animals assembled by Moses in the 11th chapter of the book of Leviticus does no more than repeat and update what had been known from the dawn of history. Many contemporary Jews, Moslems, and some Christians continue to bear these distinctions in mind, in part or in whole, considering them an expression of Divine wisdom to protect human health.

Continued on page 298

Though meat provides nutrients of very high biological quality, it presents more risks than any other food due to the many factors that can alter its quality.

Moses' Dietary Laws

	Mammals classified as clean and fit for human consumption	Mammals classified as unclean and unfit for human consumption
HOOF	Split (artiodactylous ungulates)	Not split or without hoof
DIET	Herbivore	Omnivore such as swine or carnivores such as dogs and cats
STOMACH	Divided into four sacs or compartments for fermentation plant foods consumed	Formed of a single sac (monogastric) in which no fermentation takes place

The First Classification
of animal species appropriate for consumption

Although a diet based on plant foods is presented as the ideal for humans,[40] the possibility of eating meat is also noted in the early Judeo-Christian holy writings just after the universal Deluge. In the eleventh chapter of the third book of Moses, called Leviticus, we find the first classification of species that are fit for human consumption, even though the origin of the classification was much earlier.

Anyone who wishes to eat meat can easily identify the least harmful species by following these simple norms.

Aquatic Animals

Eliminate those *not having* **fins** and **scales** such as the blowfish (some of the most toxic) shellfish (crustaceans and mollusks). Curiously, these aquatic animals are precisely those that represent the highest health risks (see Vol. 1, p. 252).

Shellfish are eliminated along with birds of prey: both are carnivores and/or carrion eaters that feed on decaying organic matter.

Fowl

Eliminate all **carnivores** or those who feed on **carrion**, such as the eagle or the crow, which provide the poorest quality meat.

Mammals

Ruminants having a **split hoof** are acceptable. All of these belong to the zoological order Artiodactyla (ungulates with split hooves with an even number of toes) and chew the cud.

THE STOMACH OF A RUMINANT with its four fermentation sacs (rumen, reticulum, omasum, and abomasum, see Vol. 1, p. 182).

Non-ruminants such as the horse, the swine, or the rabbit have monogastric stomachs. This is also the case in humans.

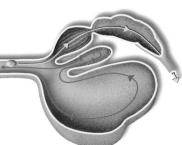

- *Included* animals: **cattle, sheep, goats,** and **deer.**
- *Excluded* animals: **swine** (split hoof, but does not chew the cud), the **horse** (has an only toe and does not have a split hoof), the **hare** and the **rabbit** (these are not ungulates).

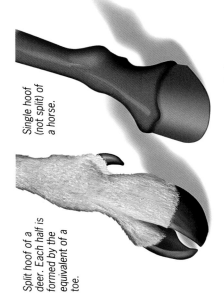

Split hoof of a deer. Each half is formed by the equivalent of a toe.

Single hoof (not split) of a horse.

The classification of species that appears in the book of Leviticus might seem unscientific on the surface. However, it is based on physiological and health criteria that are just as valid today.

A variety of interpretations have been suggested as to why these animals in particular—those that have a split hoof and chew the cud—are the only ones considered fit for human consumption. The two most convincing ones are based on the unique physiology of these species:

- They are all **herbivores**, whose diet is exclusively plant food. This places them on a lower position on the food chain and means that their meat contains less toxic residue and contaminants. These substances, whose presence in the biosphere has increased dangerously since the Industrial Revolution of the 19th century, are concentrated in animal tissue. The *more carnivorous* the animal, the *greater* this concentration is. The same is true for aquatic animals (see Vol. 1, p. 248).

- They have a *complex gastric system* consisting of four sacs in which everything they eat is fermented and chemically *disinfected* to some degree before it passes to the intestine and into the bloodstream. In monogastric animals such as the horse, the swine, the rabbit, and humans, fermentation normally takes place in the final section of the digestive tract (the large intestine), and not in the stomach.[38]

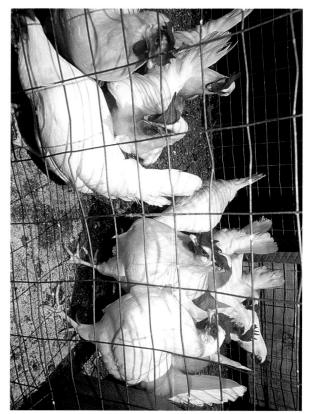

The diet and living conditions of animals have a great deal of influence on the quality of their meat.

- Sheep,
- Goats,
- Poultry (chicken, turkey, and partridge),
- Bony fish (Osteichthyes).

Of course, not all animal species are equally appropriate for human consumption. If it were necessary to enumerate those that provide the highest quality meat with the lowest accompanying risks to health, that list would duplicate the one Moses created 3,500 years ago.

Many health researchers are surprised to find that the scientific data of healthful meats validates the Biblical dietary and lifestyle norms.

The Original Diet Is the Best

Going even further back, exploring the origins of the human species, many anthropologists and nutrition specialists find that the original human diet, and the ideal for maintenance of good health, is plant based. Again, it is surprising that the first chapter of Genesis states that the original diet of mankind consisted of fruit and grains, that is, foods of plant origin.[40]

As the Bible itself declares, this is the same type of diet that will be eaten by humans and animals in the New Earth that Jesus Christ promised to reestablish,[41] in which there will be no death or disease.

The Animal's Diet

Even though an animal is of a species appropriate for the human diet, it will provide poor quality meat if it has been improperly fed.

Unfortunately there is so much fraud where livestock feed is concerned that the community has a right to be concerned. But this is nothing new. Many generations of animals have been poorly raised.

Poorly Fed Animals Become Diseased

At the beginning of the 20th century a respected North American author spoke of

Continued from page 296

Health regulations in the developed world today also classify various species of animals as fit or unfit for human consumption according to sanitation norms. Generally, the meat of only about twenty species of mammals, among the 2,000 known, is considered acceptable. The World Health Organization's journal *World Health Forum* also recognizes the significant difference between the meats of various animals.[39]

Just as Valid Today

It is interesting that all of the animals classified as clean by *Moses*—and *Noah* before him—are still those considered as the fittest for food by the health authorities of modern countries:

- Cattle,

Factors Influencing Meat Quality

Means of Processing

Cured meat and **sausages** present **greater** health **risks** than fresh meat due to:

- The **additives** used in their preparation, some of which, such as **nitrites,** can be carcinogenic (see Vol. 1, p. 270).
- Greater bacterial contamination (see Vol. 1, p. 320).

Cooking Method

The **more heat** used during the meat-cooking process, the **greater** the risks of forming **carcinogenic** substances (see Vol. 1, p. 276).

Portions of the Animal Used

Variety meats (offal) present **greater** health **risks** than lean meat (see Vol. 1, p. 317). The brain tissue of cows, sheep, and goats is considered Specified Risk Material (SRM) for spongiform encephalopathy (mad cow disease, see Vol. 1, p. 310).

---

livestock stating "some of the processes of fattening them for market produce disease."[110] One of the most pathetic examples that demonstrates the truth of this statement is the case of bovine spongiform encephalopathy, the so-called *"mad cow disease"* (see Vol. 1, p. 310).

Affected cattle in the United Kingdom and other European countries were given feed prepared with animal byproducts. These herbivores were thus forced to be carnivores. The consequence was the greatest cattle bovine epidemic in recent years.

Healthy Foods for Animals, As Well

The more healthful and natural the animal's diet, the better its meat. Grain, legumes, and green grass produce better quality meat than that of commercial feeds usually made with animal byproducts.

Livestock Living Condition

In an effort to produce tenderer, pinker meat in less time and maximum profit, the livestock industry has profoundly altered the natural living conditions of animals.

For example, today most veal is produced by separating calves from their mothers at birth and maintaining them in very small spaces. Chickens are raised in enclosed spaces under artificial light, which keeps them awake and feeding, thus making them ready for market sooner.

How can meat raised under these conditions be as good as that of animals living in a natural environment?

Again, at the beginning of the 20th century the North American author mentioned earlier wrote concerning artificially raised animals: "Shut away from the light and pure air, breathing the atmosphere of filthy stables, perhaps fattening on decaying food, the entire body soon becomes contaminated with foul matter."[42] A century later this remains true.

Time Leading up to Slaughter

Animals that have been well fed, rested, and treated gently in the days or hours before slaughter produce better quality meat. In many countries it is legally mandated that animals rest at least six hours before slaughter. This condition is not always met in modern factory farms and slaughterhouses.

When animals are tired, hungry, or suffering from physical stress just before their death, their muscle glucogen reserves are exhausted (see Vol. 1, p. 269). This prevents the acidification of the meat and makes it more susceptible to bacterial contamination and decay.

Continued on page 302

Drawbacks

Lack of Certain Essential Nutrients

- *The proportion of **carbohydrates** in meat is negligible and is limited to muscle **glycogen**, most of which is converted to lactic acid (see Vol. 1, p. 387).*

- Meat **lacks** cellulose **fiber.**

- The following **vitamins** are present in miniscule amounts or *totally* **absent:**

  – **A** and its provitamin (beta-carotene and other carotenoids).

  – **C, D, E** and **K.** Only variety meats (offal), particularly liver, contain vitamins **A** and **D. Variety meats** contain very high levels of these vitamins, to the point of *risk of* **hypervitaminosis.**

- **Folates** are virtually absent in meat. They are found only in liver and other variety meats.

- *Minerals*

  – **Calcium** and **magnesium** are present in *very small amounts.* One hundred grams of meat provide between 1% and 3% of the RDA for calcium, and between 4% and 7% of the RDA for magnesium. Because of this, **diets rich** in **meat** have a **decalcifying** effect.

  – Iodine, manganese, and selenium are also present in very small amounts.

Waste Products

Meat contains various **nitrogenous** compounds (see Vol. 1, p. 281). Some (urea, uric acid, purines, etc.) are by-products of the animal's metabolism; others (histamine, tyramine) are *produced* by **bacteria** that *proliferate* in the meat.

These by-products cause undesirable effects:

- **Acidification** of the blood and tissues, which predispose to a variety of illnesses such as kidney stones or rheumatism. **Fruit** and **vegetables** produce the *opposite* effect, since they are **alkalizers.**

- They must be eliminated from the body by *overtaxing* the **liver** and, particularly, the **kidneys,** whose function is altered by meat consumption, but *not* by the consumption of **soy** (see Vol. 2, p. 264).[43]

- *Raise* **blood pressure** (especially tyramine) and *foster* **allergies** (above all histamine).

Fat and Cholesterol

Meat, even lean meat, contains a certain amount of saturated fat and cholesterol, both of which are *harmful* to the health of the **heart** and **arteries.**

Chemical Contaminants

Animals *concentrate* chemical contaminants found in the environment such as lead, cadmium, and other heavy metals, as well as pesticides, fungicides, etcetera particularly in their tissues and *especially* their **livers. Humans,** who are at the top of the food chain, **accumulate** *even* **more** of the contaminants, above all with a meat-based diet.

Microbial Contamination

Meat normally contains a **great number of microorganisms** that cause it to *decay* and produce **toxic substances.** Additionally, it can carry pathogens (see Vol. 1, p. 302).

Drug Residue

Particularly **hormones** and **antibiotics,** but *many* **others** used on factory farms (see Vol. 1, p. 303).

Parasites

Parasites are *particularly* **common** in **pork** (see Vol. 1, p. 322), as well as **horsemeat** (see Vol. 1, p. 329).

to Meat

Diseases Produced or Aggravated by Regular Meat Consumption

Heart

The *more* meat one **eats**, the *greater* the *risk* of heart disease, including myocardial **infarction** (see Vol. 1, p. 304).

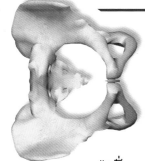

Heart: one of the organs most affected by meat consumption.

Intestinal Disorders

Colon diverticulitis is *more common* among those who eat a great deal of meat.[44] This is also the case with **constipation.**

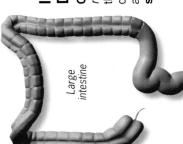

Large intestine

Gout

Meat consumption *produces* or *aggravates* the disease of **gout,** which is characterized by an increase of uric acid in the blood. This is due to two factors:

- The **purine** content of meat which leads to the formation of uric acid (this is particularly true of offal or variety meats), and
- The **acidifying** *action* of meat.

Some plant foods, such as legumes, are also rich in uric acid, even more than meat. However, since **legumes** are *not* as **acidifying** as meat, their uric acid is more easily eliminated through the kidneys, and its negative effect on the body is less (see Vol. 1, p. 85).

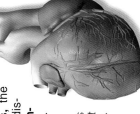

The joints in the foot, particularly the great toe, are affected by gout.

Osteoporosis

The consumption of **animal proteins** such as those in meat, as well as excessive **salt,** increases *calcium loss* through the urine. Thus, both of these dietary factors contribute to the high incidence of osteoporosis seen today in Western countries.[45]

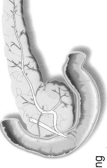

The pelvis, one of the bones affected by osteoporosis.

Rheumatic Disease

There is abundant scientific evidence that rheumatoid arthritis and other chronic rheumatoid diseases *improve substantially* with a **non-meat vegetarian diet.**[46]

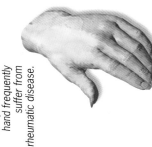

The joints of the hand frequently suffer from rheumatic disease.

Diabetes

It has been proven that *high* meat **consumption** places one at *higher* **risk** for diabetes, and that it is one of the least frequent diseases among vegetarians.[47] Although there is no clear explanation for these epidemiological findings, they do cast doubt on the typical diet prescribed for diabetics, in which roast meat is fundamental.

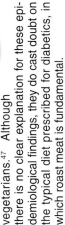

The pancreas: the gland that secretes insulin.

Cancer

Certain types of cancer are closely related to meat consumption (see Vol. 1, p. 306, 325).

Continued from page 299

Specific Problems With Meat

Bacterial Contamination

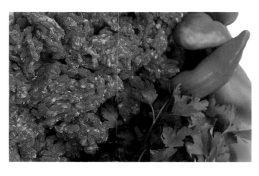

Meat is an *ideal medium* for the *development* of **microorganisms**. Even the highest quality meat always has some bacteria, which can proliferate to dangerous levels if the temperature is favorable.

The bacteria that most frequently contaminate meat are from the genera **Campylobacter, Salmonella,** and **Shigella.** In recent years type O157:H7 Escherichia coli has also been found to cause infections. This microorganism appears with some frequency in ground meat and ham-

burgers, and produces serious cases of **gastroenteritis,** occasionally with bloody feces and kidney impairment (hemolytic-uremic syndrome).[48]

Microorganisms in Meat[4]

Number of microorganisms per gram of meat	quality
100	**Excellent quality** (difficult to find)
10,000	**Good** commercial quality
1,000,000	**Acceptable** limit
100,000,000	The meat **stinks**
1,000,000,000	The meat appears **viscous**

Ground meat and products made from it, such as hamburgers, are very prone to bacterial contamination, particularly the feared Escherichia coli O157:H7. This is due to the huge increase of surface area in contact with the air that results from the grinding process.

Meat and Digestive Infections

Raw meat may contain pathogenic microorganisms that contaminate other foods. At the same time, bacteria present on the hands or utensils used to handle meat can easily contaminate it. To avoid this as much as possible, it is necessary to follow these recommendations:

- **Carefully wash the hands** before and after working with meat.

- **Avoid contact** between raw meat and other foods, particularly with already cooked meat.

- **Carefully wash any utensils** used to prepare meat before touching any other food with them.

- **Avoid pork and poultry cooked "rare,"** since this is the most often contaminated meat. Bear in mind, however, that well-done meat produces carcinogenic substances (see Vol. 1, p. 276).

- **Keep meat in the refrigerator** after it has been cooked, if it is not to be eaten immediately. Refrigeration stops the spread of bacteria, but it does not destroy them. Consequently, refrigerated meat must be **reheated** to at least **70°C** (158°F) for a few minutes **before serving it.**

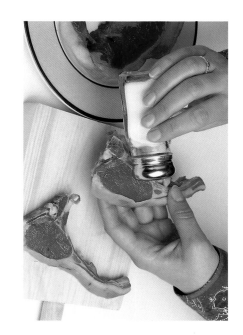

Drug Residue in Meat

Meat producers, driven by the desire for greater income and profit, view themselves as "forced" to use various drugs on their animals. Some of these are authorized; others are not.

Authorities in the European Union, for example, are stricter in the use of hormones and other drugs than their counterparts in the United States, who tend to be more permissive.

Various Health Effects

Drug *residue* in meat can cause the following negative health effects for consumers:

- **Acute poisoning:** Normally no drugs are to be administered to animals some days before slaughter to allow time for any residuals to be eliminated. However, if for any reason this is not done, the resulting meat contains high levels of drugs that may be toxic to the consumer. This has occurred several times in Spain and other European Union countries with the hormonal drug **clembuterol**, which accumulates particularly in the liver. Consumption of meat with high levels of clembuterol causes liver inflammation, skin rash, and headache.

- **Chronic poisoning** takes place when **hormone** levels in the meat are not high enough to cause an acute reaction, but still sufficient to affect consumer health. This is the case of a group of boys that developed gynecomastia (breast enlargement) from eating chicken treated with the female hormone **estrogen.**

- **Sensitization:** Drug residues in meat, even in minute amounts, can sensitize the consumer. If this happens, taking the same drug as a treatment of illness can produce a serious **allergic reaction.** This occurs frequently with **antibiotics.**

- **Bacterial resistance** can occur when **antibiotics** are *systematically* **used** in feed.

The Most Utilized Drugs in Livestock Raising

- **Antibiotics** *are systematically administered to poultry and livestock, resulting in faster growth and fewer deaths of animals due to infections.*

- **Hormones** *are widely used even though they are prohibited in the European Union. However, there are some permitted in the United States. They accelerate the fattening of the animal, increase its muscle mass, and reduce the fat proportion.*

- **Anabolic steroids,** *which are derivatives of hormones, increase protein synthesis and muscle mass in animals. The best known is* **clembuterol,** *which is used in America but prohibited in the European Union.*

- **Beta-adrenergic agonists** *excite the animal causing it to burn more fat.*

- **Antithyroids** *suppress the action of the thyroid gland, which slows the animal's metabolism, causing rapid weight gain.*

- **Sedatives** *cause the animal to tolerate its difficult and unhealthful living conditions better.*

Bacteria simply become *resistant* to these drugs. When these same bacteria infect humans, something quite common with **Salmonella** from poultry, for example, there is a risk that antibiotics will not treat the infection. The germs have developed a resistance to the antibiotics with which they have coexisted in the animal.

- **Unforeseen effects** on the quality of the meat: The use of hormones and other drugs on livestock may produce as yet unknown effects on the meat, which may negatively affect consumers.

The adverse health effects of drug residue in meat are still not well understood, according to the World Health Organization (WHO).[49]

The fact that chemical analysis of meat does not detect drug residue does not mean that they were not used on the animal. It simply means that their use was discontinued some time before slaughter. However, the possible harmful effects of these drugs on the quality of the meat remain.

Meat and the Heart

It is a well-known fact that eating meat high in fat is associated with a greater risk of heart disease, particularly heart attack (myocardial infarction).

However, recent studies prove that meat contains substances *other* than **fat** harmful to the heart. Among the most noteworthy are:

Iron in Meat

- A Finnish study showed that the *greater* amount of **iron taken in**, the *higher the* **risk** of **coronary disease.**

- However, researchers at the Harvard University School of Public Health proved that *only* the *heme* iron **found in** *meat* is heart-harmful (see Vol. 1, p. 401). According to this study, the greater con-

sumption of *heme* iron-rich red meat, the higher the risk of heart attack.

This *heme* iron effect is statistically independent from those of other meat components, such as cholesterol.[50]

Nutritional Balance

Habitual meat consumption alters the proportion of calories coming from each nutrient as compared to the ideal proposed by the WHO (World Health Organization) and most nutrition experts.

A based primarily **diet** on **meat** and its derivatives is *unbalanced* and constitutes an important cardiovascular risk factor according to a study conducted at the Tulane School of Public Health (New Orleans, USA), whose results are shown on the next page.[51]

Continued on page 306

Men who eat beef four or more times a week present a 30% higher risk of heart attack (myocardial infarction) than those who eat it once a month or less, according to studies conducted at the School of Public Health at Harvard University (USA).[50]

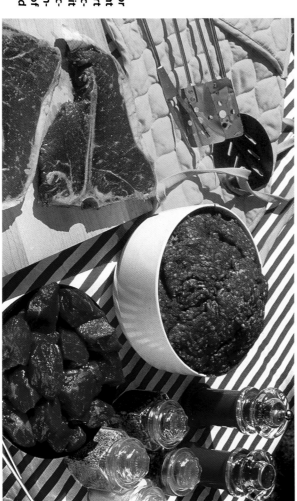

Meat and Balance in the Diet

Results of a study conducted at the Tulane School of Public Health at New Orleans (USA) concerning caloric balance in the diet as it relates to meat consumption.[51]

The dietary characteristics of a large segment of the population were analyzed in relation to meat consumption. The average daily meat intake was 180 grams (about 6.5 ounces). Those that ate more meat displayed a considerable number of significant differences when compared to those who ate less.

High Meat Consumption

Persons whose meat consumption was considerably above the average (>75 percentile) displayed the following characteristics:

- *Unbalanced diet* due to excess calories from proteins and fats (18% and 41%, respectively).
- Intake of **cholesterol**, *heme* **iron**, vitamin B₁₂, niacin, and zinc was *higher.*
- Exhibited *greater* **cardiovascular risk.**

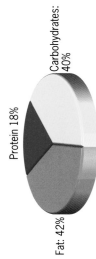

Protein 18%

Carbohydrates: 40%

Fat: 42%

Calorie distribution from each nutrient in a **high** meat diet, according to the study described in this box.

Low Meat Consumption

Persons whose meat consumption was considerably below the average (<25 percentile) displayed the following characteristics:

- *More balanced* diet in terms of **calorie** source, approximating the recommended proportions: *10%* from **protein**, *30%* from **fat**, and *60%* from **carbohydrates** (see Vol. 1, p. 387).
- *Higher* **calcium** intake (a mineral that protects the cardiovascular system and is scarce in meat) and lower amounts of **heme iron and phosphorus.**
- Exhibited *lower* **cardiovascular risk.**

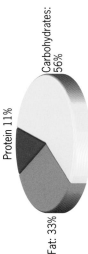

Protein 11%

Carbohydrates: 56%

Fat: 33%

Calorie distribution from each nutrient in a low meat diet, according to the study described in this box.

High meat consumption produces a **dietary imbalance:**

- **It increases** the proportion of **calories** from **protein and fat,** while
- **reducing** the percentage of **calories** from carbohydrates.

This change in calorie ratios **increases** the **risk** of **cardiovascular disease** (arteriosclerosis, myocardial infarction) and metabolic disorders such as **obesity.**

It increases the risk of contracting many other diseases as well (see Vol. 1, pp. 300-301).

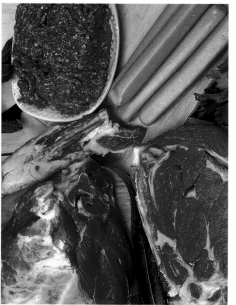

Meat and Cancer

Continued from page 304

First Statistical Confirmation

In 1984 the *American Journal of Epidemiology* published the results of a twenty-one-year-long study entitled Study of Adventist Health. It analyzed the deaths of 27,530 Seventh-day Adventists that followed a basically vegetarian diet. It found that cancer was considerably less frequent than in the general population.[52]

Since then there are an increasing number of experimental and epidemiological studies being conducted that relate meat consumption with cancer (see next page).

Counsel From World Authorities

A variety of public institutions recommend an *increase* in the amount of **plant** foods eaten, particularly grains, legumes, and vegetables, which also implies a *reduction* in the amount of **meat** eaten:

- **The European Union**, with the European Code Against Cancer (Point number three) recommends to increase the daily intake of vegetables, fresh fruit, and cereals with a high fiber content (see Vol. 1, p. 388).

- **The World Health Organization** in all of its publications.[53]

- **The U. S. Department of Agriculture** through its "Dietary Norms for Americans."

Two Changes Are Better Than One

The School of Hygiene and Tropical Medicine in London (UK) performed a large epidemiological study. It proved that persons who do not eat meat have a 39% lower cancer mortality risk than those who do.[54] These researchers attribute the results to greater consumption of plant foods and not as much to the fact that those persons abstained from meat.

However, considerable additional research indicates that the reduction of cancer risk resulting from reduced meat in the diet is due:

- just as much to eating less carcinogen-containing meat;

- as increasing fruit, nut, grain, legume, and vegetable consumption, which have anticarcinogenic properties.

It may be that some scientists give more credence to the former point and others to the latter. But the reality is that the greatest benefit is gained by combining the two dietary changes.

Continued on page 310

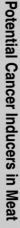

Potential Cancer Inducers in Meat

Meat contains one or more of the following substances capable of inducing cancer:

- **Animal fat**, whose consumption is associated with various types of cancer (see Vol. 1, p. 293).

- **Nitrosamines** formed in **cured meats** and **sausages** (see Vol. 1, p. 271-276).

- **Heterocyclic amines** and **aromatic hydrocarbons**, such as **benzopyrene**, that form when meat is well-done (particularly when grilled or fried, see Vol. 1, p. 276).

- **Hormones** used to fatten livestock, when they are present in meat in elevated amounts.

Meat-related Cancers

Recent studies associate regular meat consumption with these types of cancer:

Cancer of the Mouth and Pharynx

Although the *most important* risk factors for these cancers are **smoking** and **drinking alcoholic beverages,** eating **salted** or **cured meat** also influences its genesis, according to studies conducted in Uruguay.[55]

Colon Cancer

Men who eat red meat (beef, pork, or lamb) as a main dish five or more times a week have four times greater risk of colon cancer than those that eat these meats less than once a month. This is the result of a broad statistical study conducted at the School of Public Health at Harvard University (Massachusetts, USA).[57]

Eating 600 grams (1.32 pounds) of red meat—but not white meat (chicken) or fish—triples the amount of N-nitrous compounds in the feces, which explains the **carcinogenic** *effect* of **red meat** on the colon, according to the Medical Research Council of Cambridge (UK).[58]

A *high* intake of animal **fat** also increases the risk of colon cancer.[33]

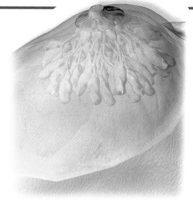

Kidney Cancer

Carcinoma in renal cells is more frequent with greater fat, meat, and meat products, according to the German Institute of Human Nutrition in Bergholz-Rehbrucke.[56]

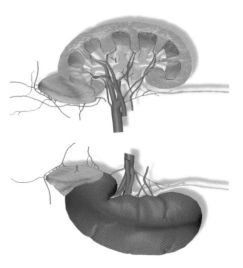

Breast Cancer

Women who eat meat more than five times a week run a two and a half times greater risk of breast cancer than those who eat it two times a week or less, according to the Montebello Institute of Epidemiological Investigation (Oslo, Norway).[59]

Beef

Although beef is the most prevalent of all meats, it has recently suffered a significant drop in popularity due to scandals involving fraudulent use of hormones and mad cow disease.

Beef is meat from the cow, bull, or calves (animals less than one year of age) or steer (castrated bull). These are all bovine, which have these characteristics:

- They are ruminant mammals whose natural food is grass and grain.
- They all belong to the zoological family *Artiodactyla*, ungulates with split hooves and an even number of toes (two or four).

Positive Aspects of Beef

- **Healthy animals:** in an appropriate natural environment with a good diet, bovines are quite healthy animals, which have few diseases or parasites. Unfortunately, few beasts are raised under these optimal conditions.

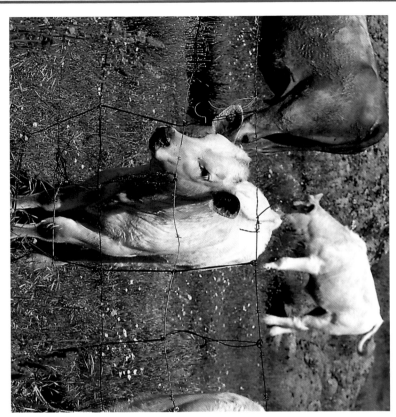

See benefits and drawbacks of meat in general in Vol. 1, pp. 282-300.

VEAL Composition
per 100 g of raw edible portion

Energy	144 kcal = 601 kj
Protein	19.4 g
Carbohydrates	—
Fiber	—
Vitamin A	—
Vitamin B₁	0.080 mg
Vitamin B₂	0.270 mg
Niacin	10.8 mg NE
Vitamin B₆	0.410 mg
Folate	13.0 µg
Vitamin B₁₂	1.34 µg
Vitamin C	—
Vitamin E	0.260 mg α-TE
Calcium	15.0 mg
Phosphorus	203 mg
Magnesium	24.0 mg
Iron	0.830 mg
Potassium	315 mg
Zinc	3.06 mg
Total Fat	6.77 g
Saturated Fat	2.79 g
Cholesterol	82.0 mg
Sodium	82.0 mg

% Daily Value (based on a 2,000 calorie diet) provided by 100 g of this food

1% 2% 4% 10% 20% 40% 100%

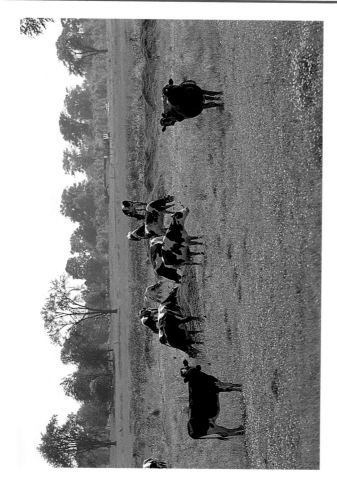

When cattle are raised in a healthy, natural environment, their meat is less harmful than that of animals raised artificially on factory farms.

Negative Aspects of Beef

- **Drug residue:** Cattle are commonly given a variety of drugs to increase meat production. The most common are **hormones** and **antibiotics.** These laboratory products usually leave some residue in the meat.

- **Saturated fat:** Beef fat is among those that *most increase cholesterol* levels. However, some studies show that eating very lean meat does not have an unfavorable effect on cholesterol.[60]

- **Harmful for the heart:** Regular beef consumption increases the risk of arterial hypertension and myocardial infarction.[61]

- **Cooking methods:** Beef is frequently roasted or barbecued. This type of cooking submits it to high temperatures that cause the formation of many proven **carcinogenic** substances (see Vol. 1, p. 276).

- **Cancer:** Much research has been done relating regular consumption of red meat (beef, lamb, and pork) with the incidence of various types of cancer, particularly colon cancer (see Vol. 1, p. 306).

- **Mad cow disease:** To date it has not been shown that bovine muscle tissue transmits this disease to humans or other animals. However, there is growing evidence that other tissues and body parts of these animals are potentially contaminating. Eating any of these may produce, after several years, a variant of Creutzfeldt-Jakob disease in humans (see Vol. 1, p. 311).

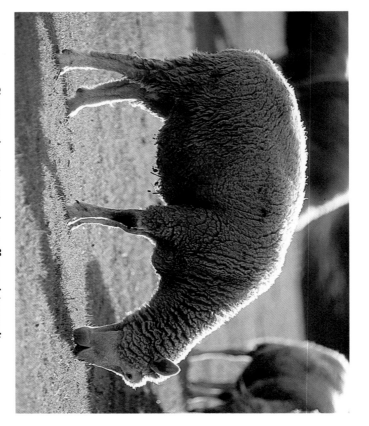

Sheep and goats may also suffer and transmit spongiform encephalitis. **When it affects cattle, this disease is known as "mad cow disease."**

Continued from page 306

Mad Cow Disease

Bovine spongiform encephalopathy or mad cow disease has affected millions of cattle in the United Kingdom and the rest of Europe. However, cattle were not the only animals involved. Sheep and goats can also suffer from this disease. The disease spread because the feed that the cattle ate was prepared using contaminated meat scraps. The practice of feeding cattle with feeds of animal origin was officially prohibited in 1994 in the European Union.

Fortunately, only certain tissues or portions of infected animals can transmit the disease to other animals or persons that eat them. These tissues are referred to as *Specified Risk Materials* (SRM).

As scientific studies have progressed, other tissues or parts have been added to the list of contaminated materials. At first only the brain and lymphatic tissue were listed, but today the list is much broader.

Tissues and Animal Parts That Must Be Discarded

After intense study and broad debate, the European Commission promulgated decision 97/534/EC in 1998, which states the following to be **SRM**:

- The **cranium** (including eyes, brain, and tonsils) and the **spinal chord** of all cattle, sheep, and goats over the age of twelve months;

- The **spleen** of all sheep and goats;

- The **vertebral column** of any animal.

- Recently, the **intestine** of cattle has been added.

Since these tissues or body parts can transmit bovine spongiform encephalopathy, they must be removed from carcasses in slaughterhouses throughout the European Union. They may not be used for human or animal consumption, cosmetics, or medications.

Eliminate Meat With Bone

Since 1998 European health authorities have recommended that beef destined for human consumption not include bone. There are two reasons for this:

- **Nerve ganglions:** Close to the bones and closely united with them are thickenings of the nerve tissue called ganglions. Those beside the vertebral column, called dorsal root ganglions, are particularly notorious. There are two of these for each vertebra. Ganglions in cattle measure approximately a centimeter in diameter.

It has recently been confirmed that the dorsal root ganglions of infected livestock transmit spongiform encephalopathy or mad cow disease to laboratory animals that eat them. Since it is very difficult to separate ganglions from the bones of beef ribs and chops, the safest thing is to avoid those cuts of meat that might include the spinal column or tissues adhered to it.

- There are suspicions that **marrow of all of the bones** of an infected animal can transmit spongiform encephalopathy or mad cow disease. The most prudent course of action is to avoid eating anything related with the bones, like gelatin.

Lean meat from infected cattle does not transmit mad cow disease. However, the bone and nerve ganglions that accompany it have been classified potentially contaminated SRM (Specified Risk Materials).

An Enigmatic Disease

The prestigious British medical journal *The Lancet* published an article suggesting for the first time the possibility that mad cow disease may be transmitted to humans as a *variant* of **Creutzfeldt-Jakob disease,** whit the following characteristics:[62]

- It appears in young people whose common antecedent is beef consumption during the previous ten years.

- The first symptoms are psychiatric: increasing anxiety and depression.

- Some months later, progressive muscular incoordination, gait disturbances, and dementia appear.

- Death results in one to two years, and the victim's brain contains spongiform lesions very similar to those found in mad cows.

Even though there have been few reported cases in humans until now, a surge is foreseen in next years because the long incubating period of this disease. The relationship between this variant of the

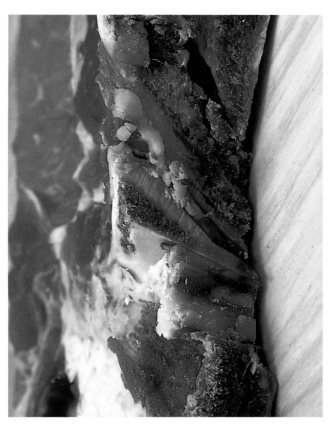

Meat does not transmit mad cow disease, but bone does.

Commercial sale of beef with bone has recently been prohibited in the European Union. This is because the nerve ganglions associated with backbone, as well as the bone marrow of infected animals, can transmit the disease to humans.

Slaughterhouses in the European Union are now forced to dispose of the animal parts that may transmit the disease to humans.

Creutzfeldt-Jakob disease and the consumption of contaminated meat (Specified Risk Materials, SRM) is now clearly established.

The causative agent of this enigmatic disease is no known microorganism, but rather an infectious protein called **prion**[63] by its discoverer, the 1997 winner of the Nobel Prize for Medicine, **Dr. S. B. Prusiner.**

Continued on page 320

Sheep

Very rich in vitamin B₁₂ and iron, but also in saturated fat

Sheep and goats are also ruminants and members of the genus *Artiodactyla* (even split hooves). Just as cattle, they have a stomach divided into four sacs (see Vol. 1, p. 297) where their food experiences profound chemical changes that purify it to some extent before it passes to the intestine and on to the bloodstream.

Unfortunately, the bucolic image of flocks of sheep placidly grazing on green hills is becoming less frequent. Even though sheep are the animals most likely to be raised in a natural, healthful environment, many suffer from infectious diseases such as brucellosis. They also suffer from ill treatment and stress during long trips to city slaughterhouses.

In their greed to increase the financial gain from their flocks, sheep raisers often maintain the animals in unnatural living conditions. This creates a great deal of stress, to which sheep are particularly sensitive; Such **stress** results in higher infection rates and greater need for drugs. The result of all of this is a decline in meat quality from a nutritional and health standpoint.

Sheep and goats are also susceptible to **spongiform encephalitis**, just as are mad cows. In fact, it is believed that the use of sheep by-products in preparing commercial feed has been the cause of its transmission to cattle and other animal species.

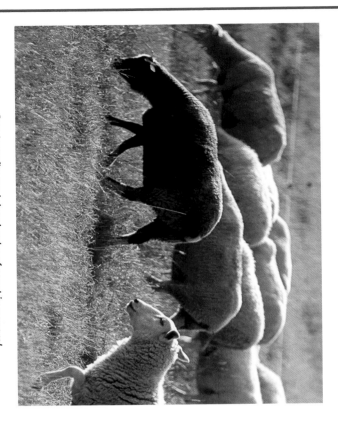

See benefits and drawbacks of meat in general in Vol. 1, pp. 282-300.

LAMB Composition
per 100 g of raw edible portion

Energy	267 kcal = 1117 kJ
Protein	16.9 g
Carbohydrates	—
Fiber	—
Vitamin A	—
Vitamin B₁	0.120 mg
Vitamin B₂	0.220 mg
Niacin	9.38 mg NE
Vitamin B₆	0.130 mg
Folate	18.0 µg
Vitamin B₁₂	2.39 µg
Vitamin C	—
Vitamin E	0.210 mg α-TE
Calcium	12.0 mg
Phosphorus	160 mg
Magnesium	22.0 mg
Iron	1.57 mg
Potassium	230 mg
Zinc	3.33 mg
Total Fat	21.6 g
Saturated Fat	9.47 g
Cholesterol	72.0 mg
Sodium	58.0 mg

% **Daily Value (based on a 2,000 calorie diet)** provided by 100 g of this food

1% 2% 4% 10% 20% 40% 100% 200% 500%

Positive Aspects of Lamb

- ***Better diet:*** sheep and lambs usually live on a *more natural diet* since they live more dynamic lives. It is quite unlikely that they have been fed on commercial feeds made up of by-products and other processed animal proteins, the opposite of that which occurs with cattle and swine.

- *Less chemical contamination:* lamb generally contains less hormone and antibiotic residue.

- **Nutritious:** lamb contains twice as much or more iron and vitamin B₁₂ as beef, pork, or chicken.

Comparison of the Composition of Various Lean Meats
for each 100 grams

	Protein (g)	Vit. B₁₂ (μg)	Iron (mg)
Lamb	20.3	2.62	1.77
Beef	20.2	1.4	0.85
Chicken	21.4	0.37	0.89
Pork	21.1	0.67	0.91

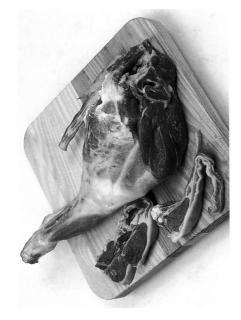

Lamb has one of the highest fat contents of any meat. The portion with the lowest amount is the leg. The highest amount is found on the shoulder and ribs (chops).

Negative Aspects of Lamb

- **Abundant fat:** *After* **pork,** lamb contains the *most* **fat** (21.6%). *Most of* this fat is composed of **saturated fatty acids** (see Vol. 1, p. 292). The fat content of lean meat from animals raised under good conditions, once the visible fat has been removed, drops to 5.25%, which is less harmful.

- **Red meat:** Just as the case of beef, lamb is red meat. Eating it regularly is related with **coronary** artery **disease** and various types of **cancer,** particularly of the colon.

- **Cooking method:** Lamb chops and other fatty parts are usually grilled, which forms a *great* deal of **carcinogenic** substances (see Vol. 1, p. 276).

Chicken

Its fat is less harmful than that of other meats, but it is often contaminated

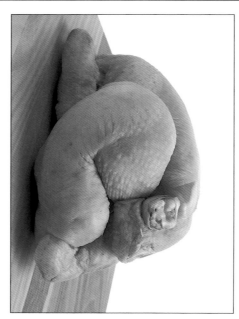

Skinless chicken contains considerably less fat than beef or lamb. However, it has other drawbacks due to the living conditions and forced feeding of these birds in industrial farms. Additionally, poultry contains the highest level of hormone and other drug residues.

Before the advent of intensive poultry raising in the 20th century, chicken and turkey were considered a luxury. Chicken was only served on special days, and turkey was served on Christmas and Thanksgiving in the United States.

Today, poultry is cheap and available year round, but this availability has come at a high cost. When compared to naturally raised chicken, poultry from factory farms generally contains **hormone** and **antibiotic** residues, *more* **saturated fat**, *more* **bacteria**, and less flavor.

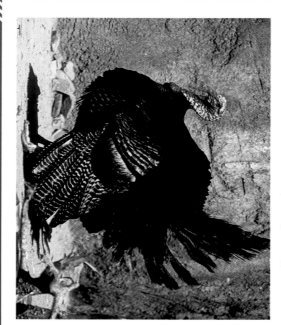

Meat from web-footed birds (ducks and geese) contains more fat and B complex vitamins than that of chickens, turkeys, or partridge.

CHICKEN, MEAT ONLY
Composition
per 100 g of raw edible portion

Energy	119 kcal = 498 kj
Protein	21.4 g
Carbohydrates	—
Fiber	—
Vitamin A	16.0 µg RE
Vitamin B₁	0.073 mg
Vitamin B₂	0.142 mg
Niacin	12.4 mg NE
Vitamin B₆	0.430 mg
Folate	7.00 µg
Vitamin B₁₂	0.370 µg
Vitamin C	2.30 mg
Vitamin E	0.295 mg α-TE
Calcium	12.0 mg
Phosphorus	173 mg
Magnesium	25.0 mg
Iron	0.890 mg
Potassium	229 mg
Zinc	1.54 mg
Total Fat	3.08 g
Saturated Fat	0.790 g
Cholesterol	70.0 mg
Sodium	77.0 mg

% Daily Value (based on a 2,000 calorie diet) provided by 100 g of this food

1%   2%   4%   10%   20%   40%   100%

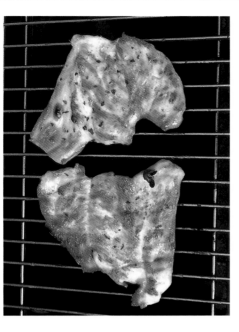

Juicy, lightly grilled chicken breasts can contain pathogens such as salmonella. To avoid this they must be well cooked.

Chicken is one of the most susceptible to bacterial contamination. It is regularly given to children and the elderly, with the thought that it is the most appropriate for them. However, they are precisely the most sensitive to foodborne diseases.

Positive Aspects of Chicken

- Its *fat* is **less harmful:** poultry meat in general and chicken in particular, differs from meat from mammals in that it:
  - contains *less* **fat,** which is easier to eliminate, since it is mostly just below the skin.
  - contains *fewer* **saturated fatty acids,** which increase total cholesterol level, and *more* **polyunsaturated** fatty acids, which partially neutralize the action of the saturated.

Fat Content of Poultry
grams per 100 g

Bird	With skin	Without skin
Chicken	15.1	3.08
Turkey	8	2.86
Goose	33.7	7.13
Duck	39.3	5.95

Negative Aspects of Chicken

- **Cholesterol:** Poultry contains less fat, but its *proportion* of cholesterol is **similar** to that of **red meat.** This is one of the reasons why cholesterol levels are not lowered when chicken or fish replace beef, lamb, or pork in the diet.[64] In reality, there is *no* **food of animal** origin that, when regularly eaten, lowers **cholesterol** level, not even fish or its oil (see Vol. 1, p. 241). It is reasonable to think that eating chicken may be less harmful for the arteries and the heart than red meat. However, there is no evidence that it provides any protection at all for the cardiovascular system.

- **Uric acid:** Chicken, and poultry in general, produce *more* uric acid than any meat (174 mg/100 g), second only to **variety meats** (liver, kidney, 200 mg/100 g).

- **Bacterial contamination:** Massive chicken production fosters the development of numerous microorganisms in these birds. Their transport tends to be unsanitary. The result is that more than 30% of the chickens sold in the United States are contaminated with salmonella. In Spain this same bacterium was found in 23% of chicken breasts sold in a supermarket.[65]
  The bacteria found most frequently in chicken are those of the genera *Salmonella* and *Campylobacter.*[66] Both produce more or less serious **gastroenteritis** and are associated with chicken or turkey that is not well cooked.

  Poultry is **contaminated** by one or more of these ways:
  - by contaminated **feed;**
  - by being **raised, transported,** or **slaughtered** under unsanitary conditions;
  - by **improper handling** of the meat up to the point of sale.

- **Virus:** Chicken and other poultry frequently suffer from various types of **retroviruses** that cause leukemia and lymphoma in fowl. To date, it has not been proven that these viruses in chicken cause any type of disease in humans, particularly leukemia or lymphoma. However, in light of current scientific knowledge it is impossible to assure that they are safe.[67]

Hamburgers

- **Low quality:** hamburgers are usually prepared with low quality meat that may *include* ground **by-products** that would not normally be sold as meat.

- **A great deal of fat:** Its fat proportion is considerably higher than lean meat, and varies between 13% and 16%.

- **Bacterial contamination:** since it is made from ground meat, the risk of bacterial contamination is very high. One of the most pathogenic is the feared *Escherichia coli* O157:H7. The Centers for Disease Control in Atlanta (USA) performed an investigation of a massive food poisoning outbreak in the state of Washington caused by consumption of hamburgers contaminated with this bacteria.[68] Investigators were able to show that, in many cases, the interior temperature of the hamburger was less than 60°C (140°F) during cooking allowing the pathogens to remain alive.

- **Carcinogenic:** a study to analyze *fast food* in California (USA) found that "only" seven of seventeen samples contained detectable levels of carcinogenic **heterocyclic amines.** For this reason, these researchers tend to discount the risk of hamburgers, roast chicken, and hotdogs.[69]

- However, another study conducted by the University of Iowa (USA) School of Medicine found that high consumption of animal proteins (not vegetable), particularly hamburger, increased the risk of lymphoma (cancer of the lymph nodes) by 235% in the population studied (35,156 women over the age of 55).[70]

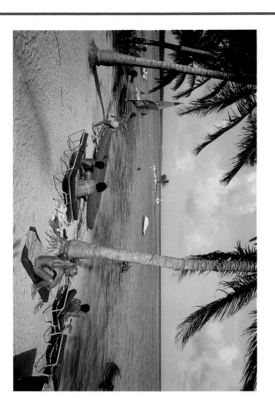

Many cases of traveler's diarrhea are attributed to eating raw vegetables, when the true cause is found in hamburgers and other contaminated meat products, according to the Centers for Disease Control in Atlanta (USA).[71]

Meat Extract Broth

Extracts of meat broths are used to flavor other foods even though they present various drawbacks:

- **They are rich in purines,** which transform into **uric acid** in the body. Meat broths are not advised for those suffering from gout or excess uric acid.

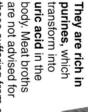

Meat extract cubes

- Meat broths and extracts contain significant amounts of **mutagens,** which are capable of causing genetic mutations that foster cancer development:

  – **Creatine and creatinine** are non-protein nitrogenous compounds (see Vol. 1, p. 281) normally present in meat and concentrated in meat broth. Tests have been conducted showing that they can produce **genetic mutations.**[72]

  – **Heterocyclic amines** are formed in meat by heat. In addition to being **mutagenic,** they are *clearly* **carcinogens.**[73]

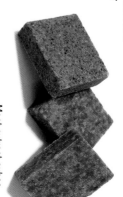

Derivatives

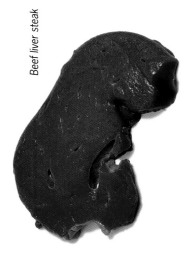

Lamb kidneys

Variety Meats (Offal)

The most utilized of these are brains, sweetbreads, liver, heart, lung, stomach, intestine, kidneys, and testicles.

Variety meats are richer in vitamin B$_{12}$, vitamin A, vitamin D, and iron than meat, but they have several **drawbacks.**

- They contain more than 300 mg/100 g of **cholesterol, *four times more* than meat.**

- The viscera (variety meats) in general, and the **liver** in particular, is where all of the **residue** of hormones, antibiotics, and other drugs **accumulate.**

- **Chemical contaminants** such as lead, cadmium, arsenic, as well as pesticides and other toxins taken in by the animal throughout its life **accumulate** particularly in the **viscera** (variety meats). A study that took place in Denmark shows that the kidneys of livestock more than two years of age contain excess cadmium, a toxic metal with similar effects to those of lead.[74]

- **Excess vitamin A:** 100 grams of beef liver contains almost five times the RDA (Recommended Dietary Allowance) of vitamin A. This vitamin A is in the form of retinol, which accumulates in the body and can produce hypervitaminosis. The **carotenoids** in **plant-based foods** are in reality **provitamin A,** which the body transforms into vitamin A as it is needed. Therefore there is **no risk of overdose** with plant provitamin A (see Vol. 1, p. 389).

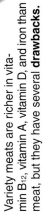

Beef liver steak

Gelatin

Boiling collagen-rich tissues, such as skin, bone, tendons, and ligaments of cattle and swine produces gelatin which, because of its thickening properties and the fact that it is tasteless, is widely used as an **additive** in *many* meat products, as well as in ice cream and jellies. However, it has the following drawbacks:

- **Incomplete *protein*:** as a food, gelatin is one of the poorest protein sources since *it lacks **tryptophan** and is poor* in other **essential amino acids.**

- **Possible relationship with mad cow disease:** There are serious questions whether gelatin from animals with spongiform encephalitis may transmit the disease to the consumer. Consequently, it is much safer to use vegetable gelatin such as agar-agar (see Vol. 1, p. 131).

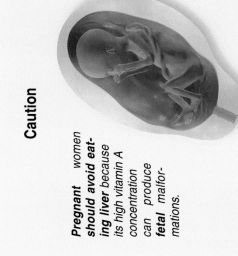

Caution

Pregnant *women* ***should avoid eating liver*** *because its high vitamin A concentration can produce* ***fetal malformations.***

Pork

There are those who think that the taboo concerning swine flesh, based on the practice of Jews, Moslems, and some Christians, is historically attached to sanitary concerns (see Vol. 1, p. 297). They argue that today's hygiene practices, which are far superior to those of antiquity, have made any such prohibitions obsolete, leaving the idea that pork is unhealthful as an ancient myth.

However, in spite of advances in hygiene and veterinary science, there is a growing body of scientific evidence that demonstrates the various negative aspects of pork and its derivatives. Medical literature consistently relates pork consumption with a variety of infections, cancer, liver disease, and parasite infestations.

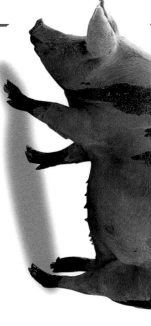

See benefits and drawbacks of meat in general in Vol. 1, pp. 282-300.

Positive Aspects of Pork

- **Rich in *vitamin B₁*:** 100 g of lean pork provides 0.966 mg of vitamin B₁, or thiamin, which represents 64% of the RDA. Pork contains twelve times more vitamin B₁ than beef or chicken, and eight times more than lamb. Even though pork stands out among meat foods as the richest in vitamin B₁, there are various plant-based foods that *compare favorably with it*, such as **soy** and **whole-grain oats**, and others that *easily surpass* it, such as **pine nuts**, **wheat germ**, and **brewer's yeast**.

- **Less *harmful fat*:** pork fat contains a higher proportion of polyunsaturated fatty acids (such as oleic acid) than beef or lamb, but less than chicken. These fatty acids compensate in part for the harmful effects of the saturated fats and cholesterol.

PORK Composition
per 100 g of raw edible portion

Energy	**227 kcal = 948 kj**
Protein	**18.3 g**
Carbohydrates	—
Fiber	—
Vitamin A	2.00 µg RE
Vitamin B₁	0.800 mg
Vitamin B₂	0.242 mg
Niacin	8.13 mg NE
Vitamin B₆	0.415 mg
Folate	6.00 µg
Vitamin B₁₂	0.670 µg
Vitamin C	0.600 mg
Vitamin E	0.290 mg α-TE
Calcium	15.0 mg
Phosphorus	197 mg
Magnesium	20.0 mg
Iron	0.890 mg
Potassium	324 mg
Zinc	2.11 mg
Total Fat	16.5 g
Saturated Fat	5.77 g
Cholesterol	69.0 mg
Sodium	54.0 mg

% **Daily Value** (based on a 2,000 calorie diet) provided by 100 g of this food

1%   2%   4%   10%   20%   40%   100%

Although meat in general is the object of much criticism from a health standpoint today, there is more criticism focused specifically on pork than on any other.

To gain a perspective, simply consult a database on the Internet such as Medline: Most of the articles published about meat, and particularly about pork, point out their negative health effects.

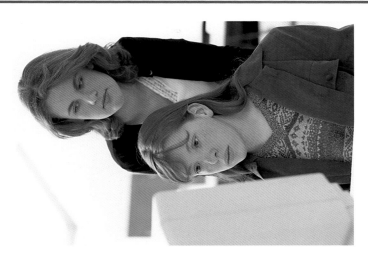

Negative Aspects of Pork

- *High fat content:* although the composition of pork fat is less harmful than that of other red meats, it is present in much higher proportion (see table Vol. 1, p. 290). Consumption of pork fat is related with **cardiovascular disease** and various types of **cancer,** as is animal fat in general (see Vol. 1, p. 325).

- **Harmful substances:** Pork contains *more* histamine (provokes allergies), tyramine (produces hypertension), and hypoxanthine (addictive stimulant, see Vol. 1, p. 283) than any other meat.

- **Bacterial and viral contamination:** Pork can be contaminated with a variety of bacteria that cause gastroenteritis and other diseases, as well as various types of viruses.

- **Parasites:** "The tissues of swine swarm with parasites," wrote Ellen G. White, a well-known North American health reformer at the beginning of the 20th century.[75] Today it is well known that pork is the meat with the *highest incidence* of parasites. **Trichinosis, cysticercosis,** and **toxoplasmosis** are some of the parasitic diseases that may be contracted from pork (see Vol. 1, p. 322).

- **Cancer:** Regular consumption of pork and its derivatives (ham and sausages) is associated with various types of cancer more frequently than with other types of meat, according to epidemiological studies (see Vol. 1, p. 324).

- **Cirrhosis:** Alcohol consumption is not the only risk factor for cirrhosis of the liver, but pork as well.[76] This may be due to its high content of non-protein nitrogenous compounds, which must be metabolized in the liver.

Contraindications to Pork

Pork and its derivatives are specifically contraindicated in cases of:

- *Arterial hypertension,* due to its high salt content and hypertensive effect.

- *Arteriosclerosis* and *coronary heart disease,* due to its high total fat, saturated fat, and cholesterol content.

- Increased level of *uric acid* and *gout.*

- *Kidney failure,* because of its high protein level.

- *Liver disease,* because it overworks that organ and promotes cirrhosis.

- *Skin disease,* due to its histamine content, which fosters eczema and boils.

- *Children* and *the elderly:* since they are more susceptible to infections.

- *Cancer patients,* due to its content of carcinogenic substances.

Pork Consumption and Cervical Cancer[88]

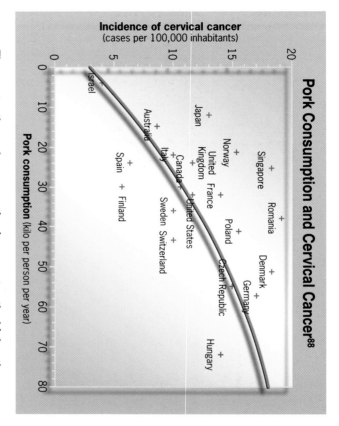

Incidence of cervical cancer
(cases per 100,000 inhabitants)

Pork consumption (kilo per person per year)

Israel · Japan · Singapore · Norway · United Kingdom · France · Romania · Australia · Italy · Canada · United States · Poland · Denmark · Germany · Spain · Sweden · Switzerland · Czech Republic · Finland · Hungary

The greater the pork consumption in a country, the higher the incidence of cervical cancer in women. This is, together with lymphoma, a type of cancer known to be caused by a virus.

Continued from page 311

Principal Drawbacks to Pork

Among the drawbacks to pork described in Vol. 1, p. 319, infections, cancer, and parasites will be examined on this and the following pages.

Pork-produced infections

More than any other type of meat, pork is the best medium for the development of **bacteria, viruses,** and **parasites,** although it is not known exactly why. It may be because of two biochemical peculiarities of this meat:

- It is *rich* in **mucopolysaccharide,** a gelatinous material that infiltrates pork and serves to support bacterial growth.

- Its *high* **free amino acid** content serves as predigested nutrients for germs. **Shell-fish,** *together* with swine, are the animals *richest* in free amino acids (see Vol. 1, p. 254).

Types of Germs

More than twenty species of pathogens have been detected in pork. The most frequent are:

- **Salmonella,** a type of bacterium that frequently causes serious **gastroenteritis,** quite common in pork, as well as in eggs and chicken. A study at the College of Veterinary Medicine of the University of Utrecht (Netherlands) showed that salmonella contaminated from 5% to 30% of the swine carcasses from slaughterhouses throughout the country. The carcasses are contaminated during slaughtering since many swine already have the bacteria in their gut.[77] The situation in other Western countries is quite similar to the Netherlands.

  If salmonella-contaminated pork is not cooked at a high enough temperature, it transmits the disease. These bacteria can even survive the heat of a barbecue, as has been demonstrated by the Center for Disease Control in Atlanta (USA).[78]

- **Gram-positive cocci,** primarily **staphylococcus** and **micrococcus,** are found particularly in Spanish ham (cured ham that has not been cooked). Since these germs produce enterotoxins, they are responsible for **diarrhea** and **gastroenteritis** caused by eating raw cured ham.[79]

- **Enterococci** also cause gastroenteritis. They are found in certain sausages of the bologna type.[80]

- *Staphylococcus aureus* is a germ found in pus. Pork is usually contaminated with it at the slaughterhouse during butchering when abscesses often existing on the animals' feet are inadvertently opened.[81] Pork contaminated with this germ pro-

duces a generalized **toxicity** accompanied by **gastroenteritis**.[82]

- ***Vibrio cholerae:*** Cases of **cholera** are fairly common in Thailand, where eating pork raw with spices is the norm. The sources of contamination tend to be the butchers and cooks, whose hands transmit the microbes. Pork provides the ideal medium for the cholera germ.[83]

- ***Listeria monocytogenes*** bacteria are quite resistant to high temperatures. They are found *primarily* in **cheese** (see Vol. 1, p. 208) and produce serious infections (listeriosis) associated with meningitis. Mortadella sausage can transmit the disease[84] as can cooked ham, as was seen in France where 38 persons were infected.[85]

- ***Yersinia enterocolitica*** bacteria cause numerous cases of **gastroenteritis** in Norway and other Northern European countries. The studies conducted show that those contracting the infection have usually eaten pork or sausage during the two weeks prior to the manifestation of symptoms.[86]

These **bacteria** are *quite resistant*, and in efforts to eliminate them, sausages and hams may be submitted to high doses of radiation (from 3 to 4 kGy).[87]

Viruses in Pork

Swine are the **natural reservoir of** *many* **viruses,** *including* the one that causes **flu** in humans. **Hog cholera or swine fever,** either African or classic, is a *frequent* epidemic in hog farms, killing many animals.

Although it is said that infected pork poses no threat to humans, there are unsettling data to the contrary. For example, swine contain a papilloma (wart)-causing virus similar to the viruses that cause papilloma in humans. Studies at the University of Ulm (Germany) have demonstrated a relationship between the consumption of pork products and the appearance of diseases caused by the papilloma virus in humans.[88]

- **Condylomas** are tumor-like growths of viral origin in the form of huge warts on the anus or external genitalia. There have been cases of condylomas disappearing after simply giving up pork.

- **Cervical cancer in women** is caused by a type of the human papilloma virus. The *more* pork products **consumed,** the *higher* the **risk** of suffering from cervical cancer. According to studies at the University of Ulm, the carcinogenic substances found in pork contribute to the development of cervical cancer, as well.

- **Warts** *are common* on the hands of butchers and slaughterhouse workers that handle pork and other meats. An investigation conducted by the Department of Dermatology of the University of Southampton (UK), demonstrated that these warts are caused by the HPV7 virus, which is found almost exclusively on the hands of those who handle raw meat.[89]

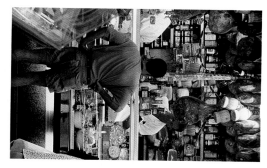

Viral warts are often found on the hands of butchers and slaughterhouse workers that handle meat, in general, and pork in particular.

How Meat Becomes Contaminated

Meat can become contaminated by a variety of microorganisms at any point in its processing:

- *While the **animal** is **alive,** something that occurs frequently due to the **unsanitary living conditions** in which they are raised.*

- *During slaughter and butchering in **slaughterhouses.***

- ***During the processing** of the meat prior to reaching the point of sale, and from there on to the kitchen.*

Trichina Parasites: How To Detect and Destroy Them

*Pork infested with trichina larvae presents a normal appearance. An infestation can **only** be detected by a **microscopic examination** of a meat sample by a veterinarian.*[90]

Curing the hams of swine or wild boar does not affect trichina larvae.[90] *Destroying trichina parasites in pork requires:*

- *Cooking the meat until it is done to the point that it has lost its rosy color. The drawback to this, however, is the formation of carcinogenic substances (see Vol. 1, p. 278).*

- *Freeze the meat for 20 days at -15°C (5°F).*

The foods that most often transmit trichina parasites are:

  ▪ **Wild boar and the products made from it, particularly sausages.**

  ▪ **Pork that has not been properly cooked or roasted, above all when it has been home-slaughtered.**

  ▪ **Uncooked pork sausages.**[91]

Although one might think that trichinosis is a disease of the past, there are continuous outbreaks around the world. In the United States there are some 57 cases annually according to the Centers for Disease Control in Atlanta (USA), even though it is thought that many more cases go undiagnosed.[92] In Spain in the Statutory Community of Navarra alone there were 71 reported cases in the years 1995-1996.[93]

Parasites in Pork

Given its lifestyle and omnivorous diet (eating anything and everything), the pig is the animal whose meat contains the *most* **parasites**. Presented below are the three most important repercussions for human health, but these are by no means unique.

'Trichinella spiralis'

This parasite belongs to the zoological order Nematodes (roundworms), which affect swine and wild boar primarily, but also the horse. One gram of infested pork may contain as many as 3,000 trichina larval cysts.

Consumption of infested pork products leads to the disease of **trichinosis**, which appear typically about 17 days after the intake of contaminated meat. Trichinosis is characterized by the following symptoms:

- **Edema** and swelling of the face or eyelids;

- **Myalgia** (muscular pain), **fever**, and **headache;**

- Blood analysis shows an *increase* in **eosinophilic leukocytes.**

Many cases may be slight and not noticed initially. However, this is a progressive disease and may produce death.

'Toxoplasma gondii'

This is a protozoan (microscopic unicellular animal) that promotes an swelling of the lymph nodes, fever, and asthenia. When pregnant women are infected, it can produce miscarriage or fetal brain damage and blindness.

Toxoplasma **is contracted** in two ways:

- **Contact with** infested **animals,** particularly cats;

- Consumption of infested **raw** or **improperly cooked** meat. Raw pork as is eaten in some Asian countries, is a frequent cause of toxoplasmosis.[94]

An investigation carried out at the Federico II School of Medicine in Naples (Italy) came to the conclusion that the use of **cured pork** (ham, sausage) or *any* type of raw **meat,** *even once a month,* **triples** the risk of **toxoplasmosis.**[95]

'Tenia solium'

Tenia solium or pork tapeworm is a flatworm from two to five meters in length that lives parasitically in the intestine. Its eggs pass to the blood and form cysts in the brain and other organs, causing a disease known as **cysticercosis.**

Contamination is produced by one of these mechanisms:

- Eating pork *not properly cooked* which may contain live larvae. Up to 25% of swine in rural areas of some developing countries are infested.[96]

- Eating **vegetables** containing tenia eggs because of being irrigated with contaminated human **sewage.**

The Trichina Cycle

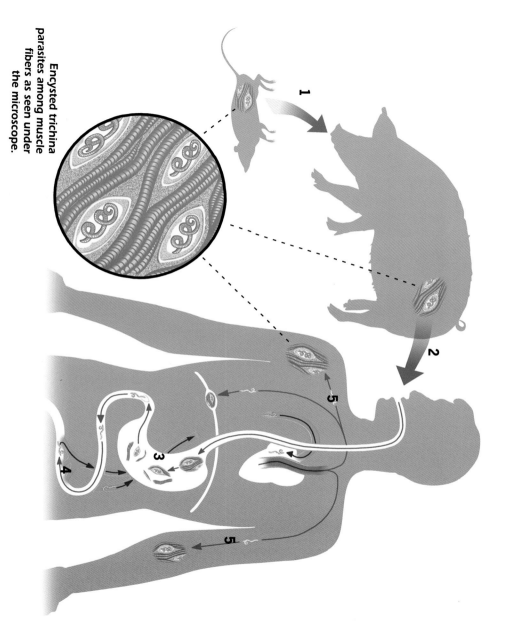

Encysted trichina parasites among muscle fibers as seen under the microscope.

From Rat to Pig to Human

From ancient times it has been known that eating the meat of rats, swine, and even horses can produce a variety of disorders, which, in some cases may prove fatal. 2,700 years ago in ancient Israel, the prophet Isaiah wrote, "…those eat the flesh of pigs and rats and other abominable things—they will meet their end together."[97]

However, it was not until 1835 when the British anatomist and zoologist Sir Richard Owen discovered the parasite that causes trichinosis in humans in the flesh of swine. Today it is well known that the primary vector for the trichina parasite that affects swine and humans is the rat.

1. Swine contract the trichina parasite by eating infested **rats.**

2. **Humans** take in the trichina larvae by eating infested pork or wild boar.

3. **Stomach acid** dissolves the larval cysts, thus releasing the trichina larvae.

4. The larvae mature in the **intestine,** transforming into adults measuring three to four mm in length. Each female lays approximately 1,500 eggs about the size of a red blood cell, which then pass into the bloodstream.

5. The trichina **eggs** are distributed in the bloodstream throughout the body's **muscles,** where they form new larvae-containing **cysts.**

Pork and

There is continually more evidence that one of the greatest drawbacks to meat in general is that its regular consumption increases the risk of certain types of cancers. This risk is particularly high with pork and its derivatives.

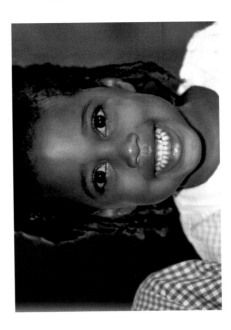

Meat Cooked "Rare"

"Rare" meat produces *less risk* of **cancer**, but a *higher* risk of **infection**.

Uncured and undercooked pork presents the lowest cancer risk, however, it has the drawback of potentially containing pathogens and more live parasites. Nor is it as tasty.

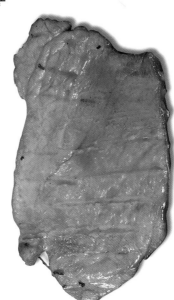

Hot dogs are four times more mutagenic (capable of changing the nuclear material in the cell) than hamburgers according to studies conducted in Canada.[99]

Hot Dogs and Cancer in Children

The school of Public Health at the University of North Carolina (USA) studied 234 cases of cancer in children and found:[98]

- **Children** that eat one or more pork *hot dogs* per week have a 210% **higher risk** of brain **tumors.**
- **Pregnant** women that eat one or more *hot dogs* per week expose their **unborn children** to a 230% **higher risk** of brain **tumors.**

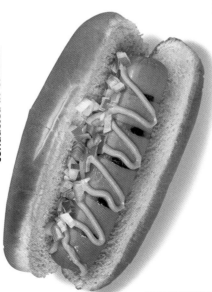

Cancer

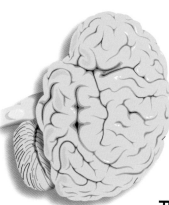

Pork and Brain Cancer

Studies at the Cancer Research Center of Heidelberg (Germany) have concluded that consumption of processed pork increases the risk of cerebral glioma (a type of cancer of the central nervous system).

The risk is highest for those who regularly eat:[100]

- Cooked ham,
- Processed pork, particularly when it is very well done,
- Fried *bacon*.

The **nitrosamine** content of these foods is considered responsible for their carcinogenic effect.

Pork, Wine, and Liver Cancer

Consumption of pork together with wine or other alcoholic beverages significantly increases the risk of hepatocellular carcinoma, a type of liver cancer.[101]

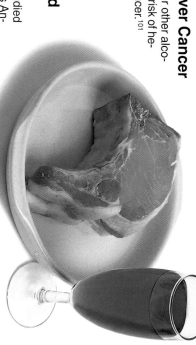

Bacon, Ham, Sausages, and Colon and Pancreatic Cancer

The Massachusetts Institute of Technology (USA) studied the dietary habits of three principal ethnic groups in Los Angeles County (California), and found the following:[102]

- Afro-Americans eat more *bacon*, ham, sausage, and other prepared meats than other groups.

- Those eating more pork derivatives, present three times more carcinogenic heterocyclic amines in the urine than those eating less of these products.

- Within the Afro-American population, pancreatic cancer is 50% more frequent, and colon cancer is 20% more frequent than in the European-American or Hispanic population.

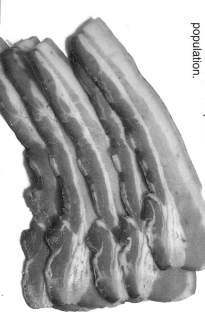

Carcinogenic Substances

Pork, as well as the products derived from it, contains carcinogens such as:

- **Nitrosamines** (see Vol. 1, pp. 271, 276), which come from nitrites and nitrates used to cure the meat. **Ham** and **sausages** are the pork products that **contain** the most nitrosamines.

- **Heterocyclic amines** form with the heat of cooking (see Vol. 1, p. 276).

Pork

*Besides the disadvantages of pork itself,
its derivatives present additional drawbacks resulting from the way they are prepared.*

See benefits and drawbacks of meat in general in Vol. 1, pp. 282-300.

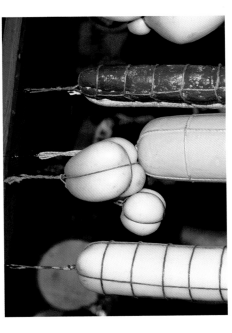

Sausages

- **Ingredients** are basically those listed below, but with many variations, depending on the final product (chorizo, mortadella).

  – Ground **meat** and/or **variety meats.**

  – Pork **fat,** which serves to bind other ingredients as an emulsifier because of its high viscosity.

  – One or **more** of these **ingredients:** blood, blood plasma, rice, soy, bread, onions, etcetera.

  – **Condiments:** paprika, garlic, spices.

  – **Additives:** nitrites and nitrates (to avoid putrefaction and give the sausage a bright color); sulfur dioxide (preservative); polyphosphates (to retain moisture and keep them tender and juicy); glutamate (to enhance flavor).

- **Processing:** After mixing the ingredients and placing the mixture in a recipient (usually pork intestine), the sausages are **cured** or **fermented.**

- **Drawbacks:**

  – *Excessive* **fat:** between 30% and 50% of its weight.

  – **Contamination:** fairly frequently sausages are contaminated with certain pathogenic bacteria, which cause digestive disorders.

  – **Cancer:** sausage consumption is related to various types of cancer (see Vol. 1, p. 324).

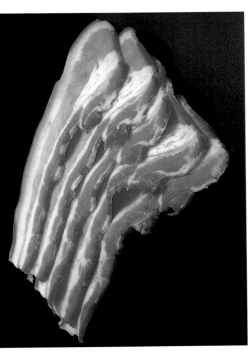

Bacon

Bacon is smoked and cured with salt and nitrites.

- **Drawbacks:** Bacon is possibly the **most unhealthful** of all pork derivatives. Besides being **very salty,** it presents three **carcinogenic** factors:

  – Bacon is **more** than half **fat**—specifically 57.6%. One hundred grams of *bacon* contains 21.3 g of saturated fat. This alone exceeds the acceptable daily limit of 20 grams of saturated fat. The *greater* the *fat consumption,* particularly animal fat, the *higher* the **cancer** *risk* (see Vol. 1, p. 293).

  – Bacon is cured with **nitrites,** which foster the formation of carcinogenic **nitrosamines** (see Vol. 1, pp. 271, 276).

  – Bacon is **smoked,** which adds more carcinogenic substances (see Vol. 1, p. 271).

Products

Ham

Ham is one of the most appreciated pork derivatives, although it cannot be said that it is healthful, as some believe. Its most positive aspect is its *low* **fat** content. Lean ham contains between 8% and 10% fat.

- **Drawbacks:** In *addition* to the drawbacks of meat in general (see Vol. 1, pp. 282, 300), and the negative aspects of pork, ham presents its own:

  – **Nitrosamines:** Cured ham contains **carcinogenic** nitrosamines, which form from the nitrites used in the curing process. Nitrites are **essential** to *avoid* **putrefaction** and the **proliferation** of deadly pathogens such as **botulism.** Whether ham is eaten cured or cooked, it increases the risk of various cancers (see Vol. 1, p. 324).

  – **Negative alterations:** Cured ham is susceptible to a variety of germs and insects. For example:

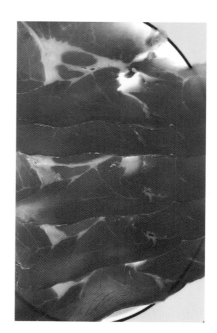

Cooked or York ham is considered milder than cured ham, appropriate even for the infirm. However, it can transmit a variety of germs such as those that cause **listeriosis** (see Vol. 1, p. 321),[85] **and its regular consumption has been related to a type of brain cancer** (see Vol. 1, p. 325).[100]

✓ **Fetid bone** is putrefaction that begins in the vicinity of the bones in the ham and extends throughout the ham producing a nauseating smell.

✓ **Mites** are tiny, seemingly insignificant insects that leave a yellowish dust on the surface of the ham. Mites are an important cause of respiratory **allergies.**

✓ **Insects** may deposit their eggs on the surface of the ham. When the larvae emerge, they penetrate the ham, causing it to decay.

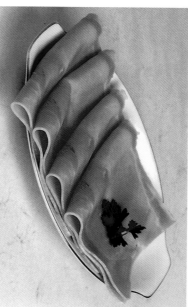

■ ■ ■

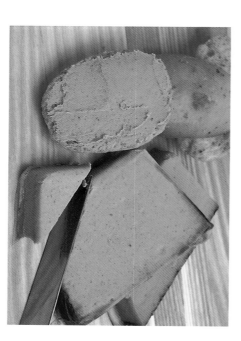

Foie Gras

Foie gras is usually prepared with goose or pork **liver.** As a result, it presents the same benefits and drawbacks as liver, with the aggravating feature of *very high fat content* (between 30% and 40%). In some instances it may contain *Listeria monocytogenes,* the microorganism that causes listeriosis in humans (see Vol. 1, pp. 208, 321).[103]

Paté prepared with animal fat and liver, in many cases, has the same drawbacks as *foie gras.*

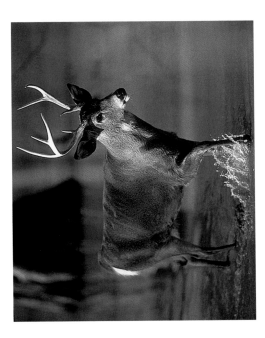

Game

Meat from wild animals such as deer, hare, pheasant, or wild boar, must **not** be eaten *under any circumstances* ***without*** a **veterinary inspection.** Even though wild animals are thought of as "more natural," they suffer from disease that makes consumption of their meat ill advised or dangerous.

- **Benefits:**

  − They contain *no* **hormone, antibiotic or other drug residues,** in contrast to domestic animals.

  − They often contain *less* **fat** since wild animals tend to exercise more and eat a more natural diet.

- **Drawbacks:**

  − Eating game meat presents the possibility of swallowing the **lead shot** used to kill the animal. Given the high toxicity of lead, this presents a health risk.

  − In spite of what one might think, wild animals, wild boar and swine particularly[104], are *more* susceptible to chemical contamination than domestic livestock. This may be due to feeding on domestic crops treated with pesticides and herbicides before the chemicals have disappeared from the plants. It is also possible that they have eaten poisoned bait illegally used to control predators.

  − **Bacterial contamination:** Any projectile used in hunting (shot or bullet) can perforate the animal's intestine, causing spillage of its highly contaminated contents within the carcass. This fosters very rapid contamination of the meat, and can cause decay.

  − They contain *more* **parasites,** as occurs with the wild boar in which **trichina** cysts are frequently found.

See benefits and drawbacks of meat in general in Vol. 1, pp. 282-300.

■ ■ ■

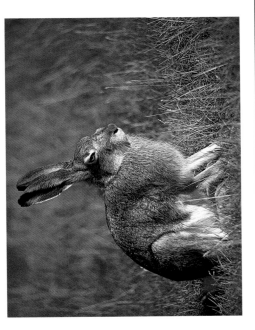

Rabbit and Hare

Neither the rabbit nor the hare are ungulates (they do not have hooves). Like the horse and swine, they are monogastric.

- **Benefits**

  − Their meat contains *little* **fat** (5.6%).

- **Drawbacks**

  − They are **coprophagous** animals, in other words, they feed on their own excrement, and *frequently* suffer from **plagues and epidemics,** such as that caused by the rabbit myxoma virus, which causes a fatal disease in rabbits called myxomatosis.

  − Their meat is rich in waste products and non-protein nitrogenous compounds such as **urea,** which are generally toxic (see Vol. 1, p. 281). This is because the excretory ducts of both the urine and the feces empty into a cavity or cloaca where they are retained for a time. During that time waste products can be reabsorbed into the bloodstream of the animal.

Meats

Horse

The horse is a herbivore, but not a ruminant. Its stomach is monogastric as contrasted with the four-chambered stomach of ruminants such as the cow, sheep and deer.

Horses belong to the order Perissodactyla, so called because their feet are hoofed but have an odd number of toes (one in this case, and not split).

- **Benefits**
  – Horsemeat is relative *low* in *fat* (4.6%).

- **Drawbacks**
  – *Poor* in **vitamins** (except B12) and **minerals.**
  – The anatomy and physiology of the digestive systems of animals influence the quality of their meat. **Monogastric** animals, such as the horse, swine, or the rabbit lack the "purifying filter" that the four gastric chambers of ruminants have. As a result, their meat is more vulnerable to negative effects that their feed may contain in terms of chemical composition, contaminants, pathogens or parasites (see Vol. 1, p. 289).
  – The horse can transmit **trichinosis** as do swine.[105]

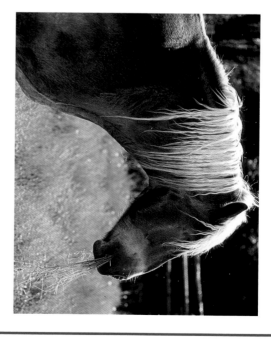

DEER
Composition
per 100 g of raw edible portion

Energy	120 kcal = 502 kj
Protein	23.0 g
Carbohydrates	—
Fiber	—
Vitamin A	—
Vitamin B1	0.220 mg
Vitamin B2	0.480 mg
Niacin	6.37 mg NE
Vitamin B6	0.370 mg
Folate	4.00 µg
Vitamin B12	6.31 µg
Vitamin C	—
Vitamin E	0.200 mg α-TE
Calcium	5.00 mg
Phosphorus	202 mg
Magnesium	23.0 mg
Iron	3.40 mg
Potassium	318 mg
Zinc	2.09 mg
Total Fat	2.42 g
Saturated Fat	0.950 g
Cholesterol	85.0 mg
Sodium	51.0 mg

% Daily Value (based on a 2,000 calorie diet) provided by 100 g of this food
1% 2% 4% 10% 20% 40% 100% 200% 500%

RABBIT MEAT
Composition
per 100 g of raw edible portion

Energy	136 kcal = 568 kj
Protein	20.1 g
Carbohydrates	—
Fiber	—
Vitamin A	—
Vitamin B1	0.100 mg
Vitamin B2	0.150 mg
Niacin	11.7 mg NE
Vitamin B6	0.500 mg
Folate	8.00 µg
Vitamin B12	7.16 µg
Vitamin C	—
Vitamin E	—
Calcium	13.0 mg
Phosphorus	213 mg
Magnesium	19.0 mg
Iron	1.57 mg
Potassium	330 mg
Zinc	1.57 mg
Total Fat	5.55 g
Saturated Fat	1.66 g
Cholesterol	57.0 mg
Sodium	41.0 mg

% Daily Value (based on a 2,000 calorie diet) provided by 100 g of this food
1% 2% 4% 10% 20% 40% 100% 200% 500%

HORSE
Composition
per 100 g of raw edible portion

Energy	133 kcal = 556 kj
Protein	21.4 g
Carbohydrates	—
Fiber	—
Vitamin A	—
Vitamin B1	0.130 mg
Vitamin B2	0.100 mg
Niacin	9.02 mg NE
Vitamin B6	0.380 mg
Folate	—
Vitamin B12	3.00 µg
Vitamin C	1.00 mg
Vitamin E	—
Calcium	6.00 mg
Phosphorus	221 mg
Magnesium	24.0 mg
Iron	3.82 mg
Potassium	360 mg
Zinc	2.90 mg
Total Fat	4.60 g
Saturated Fat	1.44 g
Cholesterol	52.0 mg
Sodium	53.0 mg

% Daily Value (based on a 2,000 calorie diet) provided by 100 g of this food
1% 2% 4% 10% 20% 40% 100% 200% 500%

The Myths

The Myth and the Reality

"Well, it's time to start the baby on meat," the pediatrician told the child's mother.

"Well, I mean, I'm not sure…"

"Is there some problem?"

"Doctor, my husband and I are vegetarians, and we'd like to raise our child without meat," the mother replied.

"I can assure you that animal tissue is a natural food and is necessary for the proper growth of your baby. If you do not feed him meat, you are risking the health of your child," stated the doctor imperiously.

"I don't know what the basis is for your statement, but I will tell you about my own experience. I was raised on an ovolactovegetarian diet, as was my older daughter, and I can assure you that we have never suffered from any nutritional lack."

The doctor was somewhat taken aback, as he recognized his arguments were based more on the myth of meat than on sound scientific fact. Unfortunately, there are many physicians and nutritionists still influenced by the "mythology" surrounding meat.

However, it is notable that more and more pediatricians do not consider meat necessary for child development. In a demonstration of this tendency, a paper in favor of a vegetarian diet for children, was presented in 1995, possibly for the first time in history, to the Spanish Royal Academy of Medicine.[106]

Efforts are being launched by international organizations such as the FAO and the WHO to demolish the myths surrounding meat that persist, with the objective that developing countries not focus their efforts of meat for their population, but rather grain and legume production.[107]

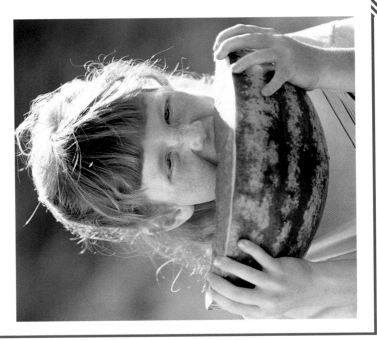

Myth

Meat is necessary for blood formation. In other words, meat ***produces blood.***

Scientific Fact

It is true that the ***iron*** in meat and fish is in a chemical form (called *heme*) easily absorbed by the body. However, the iron in plant foods, eggs, and dairy products is also absorbed, particularly in the presence of ***vitamin C*** (see Vol. 1, p. 401).

Meat is not essential as a source of dietetic iron. In fact, the iron from vegetable sources is just as useful in the formation of red blood cells as that from meat. Blood hemoglobin cannot distinguish whether its iron atoms are from a beefsteak or from a bowl of lentils.

Anemia is as frequent among omnivores as it is among vegetarians.[108] But it is much more prevalent among those whose diet is based on meat. This has been proved with native Alaskans, who frequently suffer from anemia due to lack of iron in addition to other chronic diseases, as a consequence of their typically carnivorous diet.[109]

# of Meat

Myth

*Meat protein is necessary for tissue production during growth periods. In other words, **meat makes meat**. This myth is analogous to that of certain primitive tribes believing that by eating the meat of a strong animal they acquire the same strength.*

Scientific Fact

Protein, whether of animal or vegetable origin, is made up of long chains of **amino acids** that are the same in either case. The **only difference** between animal and plant proteins is the **proportion** of their **amino acids.**

Digestive enzymes break down proteins and free their component amino acids. These amino acids are absorbed into the bloodstream and distributed to the cells where they are used to synthesize the own body proteins.

The body **needs amino acids, not** specific **proteins.** The source of these amino acids, whether from beef, legumes, grain, or other vegetable, is not important.

The **content** of essential amino acids in **meat protein** is quite balanced, but **not ideal**. It is possible to achieve an equal or better amino acid balance than those of meat by combining the proteins of a variety of **plant-based foods** (see Vol. 1, p. 80).

Meat protein does not provide any amino acid that is not available from vegetable sources. In fact, herbivorous animals, whose muscles form what is known as meat, obtain essential amino acids from the plant foods that they eat.

■
■
■

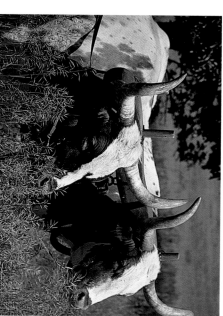

"If you want to be as strong as an ox, eat what the ox eats, but don't eat the ox."

Myth

*Meat provides **essential nutrients** that are unavailable from any other source.*

Scientific Fact

It has been stated that meat protein is of equivalent value to that resulting from the combination of various plant-based foods.

In terms of **essential minerals and trace elements** there are **none** that are present exclusively in **meat** or **fish**; not even iodine or zinc (see Vol. 1, p. 401).

The only **vitamin** that meat contains and plant-based foods do not is vitamin B_{12}. Even so, milk and eggs provide all the vitamin B_{12} the body needs even when they are eaten in moderate amounts. *Tempeh* (a fermented soy product, see Vol. 1, p. 88) contains half as much vitamin B_{12} as meat, and spirulina seaweed contains much more (although some doubt its effectiveness; see Vol. 1, p. 134). Additionally, some vegetable products, such as soy beverage (soymilk) (see Vol. 1, p. 88), are usually enriched with vitamin B_{12}.

It is therefore unnecessary to eat meat to obtain the vitamin B_{12} that the body needs (see Vol. 1, p. 395).

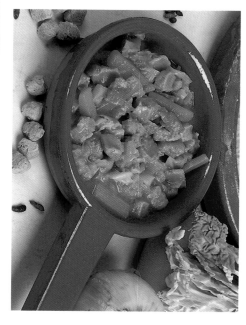

Meat

Meat is not essential in the human diet. By understanding the nutritional value of the available alternatives, eliminating it can be easy and healthful.

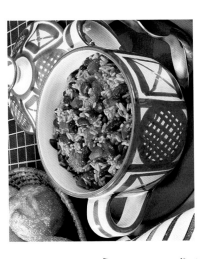

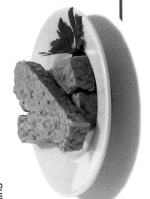

Legumes

A plate of legumes can substitute for a serving of meat in terms of nutrition (see Vol. 1, pp. 80, 287):

- *Protein:* Legumes provide protein that is **equal to or superior** to that of meat in *quality* and *quantity*. However, the digestibility of legume protein is not as good as that of meat. The **biological value** of meat protein as well as that of legumes is *increased* when it is **combined** with that of **grains** (supplementation).

- *Iron:* Legumes generally provide *more* **iron** than meat. This availability compensates for the fact that the iron from legumes is less absorbable.

- **Other differences:** Legumes are a good source of **carbohydrates** and *fiber*, which are missing in meat. Additionally, they do **not** contain **cholesterol**. On the other hand, legumes lack *vitamin B₁₂*, which is abundant in meat.

Legumes, particularly when combined with grains, are comparable or even superior to meat in terms of protein and minerals; although not in vitamin B₁₂.

Vegetable "Meat"

This is a healthy and delicious alternative to meat. It may be prepared at home from a variety of ingredients such as **soy, oatmeal, nuts, or gluten.** Methods of preparation are explained in detail in the accompanying book of recipes.

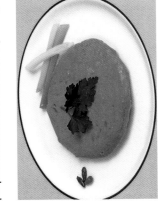

Soy Protein

Texturized soy protein (see Vol. 1, p. 89) has a texture similar to that of meat. It is essentially flavorless, which necessitates its preparation with other vegetables to make "hamburgers," "meat" balls, fillings and other dishes similar to those made with meat.

Their **nutritional value** and **flavor** can be *equal* to or *superior* to those of **meat.**

Oil-bearing Nuts

These constitute an alternative to meat because they are rich in **protein, minerals,** and **vitamins** (see Vol. 1, p. 56).

Gluten

Gluten is **protein** extracted from **wheat** or other **grains** (see Vol. 2, p. 307). It is used in a variety of meatless recipes. Its flavor is neutral so it must be prepared and flavored. Gluten has two important *drawbacks*:

- There are persons who suffer from **celiac disease** (gluten intolerance).
- It is an **incomplete protein** and must be complemented by other vegetable proteins.

Soy Derivatives

Tofu, tempeh (contains vitamin B₁₂) and *miso* present many **advantages** as meat analogs (see Vol. 1, p. 88).

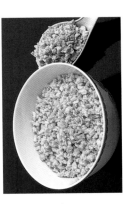

Alternatives

Meat Analogs

Meat analogs are prepared from a soy base. They are useful for those seeking a **transitional diet** from meat to one based on plant foods.

For those whose diet is already formed around vegetables, they can be an occasional complement, but they *should not* constitute *a dietary base.*

Benefits

All of those associated with plant-based foods as opposed to animal-based foods.

- *No cholesterol;*
- They contain *mostly* **unsaturated *fats;***
- They provide **carbohydrates** and in some cases, vegetable **fiber;**
- They do not have the **carcinogenic effect** of meat.

Drawbacks:

- They are **processed foods,** which are generally made from **refined products.** They contain added **salt** and, in *some* cases, **additives** (thickeners, preservatives, and antioxidants). It is important to note, however, that many of these additives are of natural origin.
- *They can be* **difficult to digest,** since they are *concentrated* foods and contain **spices** to compensate for the neutral flavor of the soy protein.

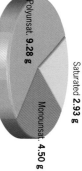

SAUSAGE, MEATLESS
Percentage distribution of **fatty acids**

Polyunsat. 9.28 g | Saturated 2.93 g | Monounsat. 4.50 g

Fiber 2.80%
Minerals 3.07%
Carbohydr. 7.05%
Fat 18.2%
Water 50.4%
Protein 18.5%

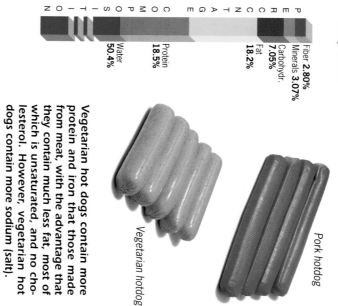

Vegetarian hotdog

Pork hotdog

Vegetarian hot dogs contain more protein and iron that those made from meat, with the advantage that they contain much less fat, most of which is unsaturated, and no cholesterol. However, vegetarian hot dogs contain more sodium (salt).

PORK SAUSAGE
Percentage distribution of **fatty acids**

Polyunsat. 5.24 g | Saturated 14.5 g | Monounsat. 18.5 g

Minerals 2.49%
Carbohydr. 1.02%
Fat 40.3%
Water 44.5%
Protein 11.7%

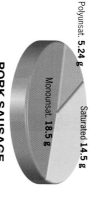

SAUSAGE, MEATLESS Composition
per 100 g of raw edible portion

Energy	256 kcal = 1072 kj
Protein	18.5 g
Carbohydrates	7.05 g
Fiber	2.80 g
Vitamin A	64.0 µg RE
Vitamin B₁	2.34 mg
Vitamin B₂	0.402 mg
Niacin	15.8 mg NE
Vitamin B₆	0.828 mg
Folate	26.0 µg
Vitamin B₁₂	—
Vitamin C	—
Vitamin E	2.10 mg α-TE
Calcium	63.0 mg
Phosphorus	225 mg
Magnesium	36.0 mg
Iron	3.72 mg
Potassium	231 mg
Zinc	1.46 mg
Total Fat	18.2 g
Saturated Fat	2.93 g
Cholesterol	—
Sodium	888 mg

% **Daily Value** (based on a 2,000 calorie diet) provided by 100 g of this food

PORK SAUSAGE Composition
per 100 g of raw edible portion

Energy	417 kcal = 1746 kj
Protein	11.7 g
Carbohydrates	1.02 g
Fiber	—
Vitamin A	—
Vitamin B₁	0.545 mg
Vitamin B₂	0.164 mg
Niacin	4.40 mg NE
Vitamin B₆	0.250 mg
Folate	4.00 µg
Vitamin B₁₂	1.13 µg
Vitamin C	2.00 mg
Vitamin E	—
Calcium	18.0 mg
Phosphorus	118 mg
Magnesium	11.0 mg
Iron	0.910 mg
Potassium	204 mg
Zinc	1.59 mg
Total Fat	40.3 g
Saturated Fat	14.5 g
Cholesterol	68.0 mg
Sodium	667 mg

% **Daily Value** (based on a 2,000 calorie diet) provided by 100 g of this food

15 CONDIMENTS AND SPICES

CHAPTER SUMMARY

*T*HE FLAVORS of condiments are a gift from the Asian continent; on the other hand, most culinary aromatic herbs have their origin around the Mediterranean.

With the exception of vanilla, hot peppers or chilies, and Jamaican pepper, which come from America, most spices come from the Asian region between India and the Moluccas Islands of Indonesia.

In Search of Flavor

From the remotest of times, spices have been the object of international trade. The book of Genesis describes how Joseph was sold to some merchants who were transporting spices from Gilead in Palestine, to Egypt.[1]

In ancient times merchants made long, difficult trips to get spices in Asia and return with them to the West. Nothing deterred the caravans:

Continued on page 336

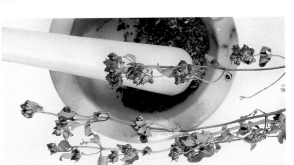

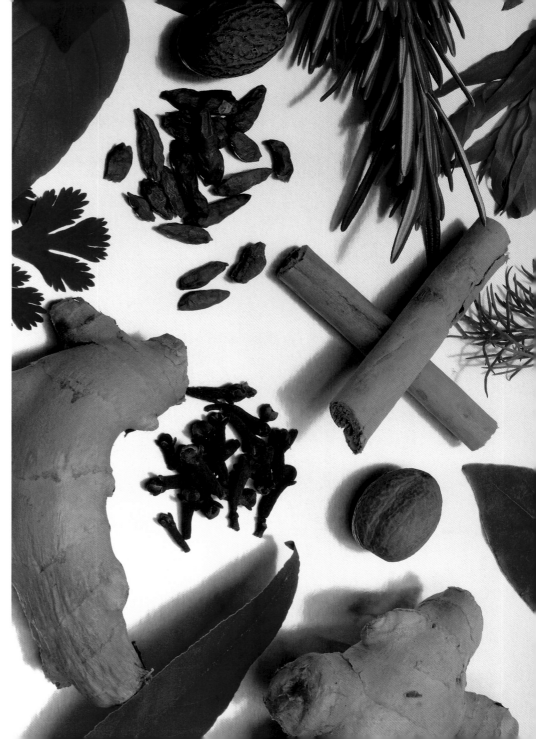

No condiment or spice can be considered essential, or even necessary from a nutritional or dietary standpoint. However, many of them give a touch of flavor that can convert a dull or insipid food or dish into something truly appetizing.

Condiments and Spices

Condiment: Substance with an intense tart, salty, or piquant taste added in small amounts to foods to enhance the food's flavor.

From a **therapeutic dietary** standpoint, there are two distinct types of condiments:

- **Healthful condiments** are those which add dietary or medicinal properties to foods, as well as flavor, thus improving their nutritive value. The most common are:
  - **Lemon, garlic,** and **salt.**
  - **Aromatic herbs:** herbaceous plants with delicate flavors and medicinal properties adding aroma and taste to foods.

- **Spices:** dried portions of generally tropical plants. Their flavors are strong and piquant. Today, the use of many spices is justified more by their **medicinal properties** than by their seasoning ability. Hence their **dosage must be controlled,** keeping **side effects** in mind.

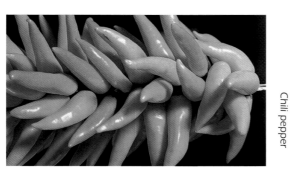

Chili pepper

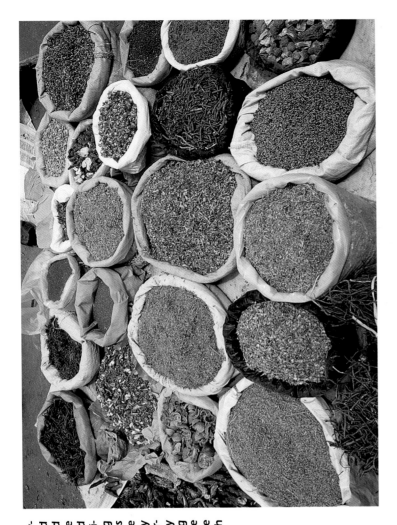

From a gastronomical viewpoint, a properly seasoned dish is always appreciated by all tastes. It is also true that proper digestion, and by extension, proper nutrition, begins with a pleasing meal. Although some spices and condiments may have drawbacks from a dietary standpoint, others are clearly beneficial. It is necessary to learn to select, among the many choices that the market has to offer, the most appropriate from both points of view.

Continued from page 334

not the dangers, the deserts, nor the long distances that had to be traversed to arrive in Egypt, and on to the rest of the known world with their invaluable cargo of spices.

During the Middle Ages, the Arabs continued to bring the precious merchandise from the port of Alexandria in Egypt to Venice and from there to the rest of Europe.

In 1492 Christopher Columbus, convinced that the world was round just as the Bible declares,[2] sailed toward the setting sun searching, among other things, a new, shorter route to the land of spices, India. But instead he reached the unknown lands of America, where spices also abounded.

The Portuguese navigator, Vasco da Gama, sailing around Africa, reached India in 1498. Later, the Dutch and the British established a broad maritime transport network and spice trade.

Pleasure and Fraud

What is it about spices that has prompted so much exploration, travel, and effort to procure them?

Above all, flavor. Europeans were prepared to go to any length, pay any price, and even risk all types of dangers to satisfy the sense of taste.

But *not* **taste** *alone.* Spices were used in Europe for their supposed aphrodisiac effect (clove, for example[3]), as well as to cover the bad taste of decaying foods.

"Pleasure and fraud" are the two words that sum up the history of spices. In our time, spices do not awaken the passions of yesteryear, nor are they typically used fraudulently.

Unfortunately, from a nutritional standpoint, spices offer ***more drawbacks than benefits***. We can imagine that if today it were necessary to go to India for them or pay for

Vinegar: Only Flavor

It has been known from antiquity that wine sours when it is left open to the air. This way "vinum acrus"—"sour wine"—vinegar was obtained, but without knowing why. In 1864 Pasteur discovered that a microorganism called "Mycoderma aceti" ferments wine, transforming its alcohol into acetic acid. Any alcoholic beverage can be used to make vinegar, but the most common are wine and cider.

The Composition of Vinegar

- **Acetic acid** (4% to 12%): This is a toxic substance that if taken in sufficient quantities, produces **serious alterations** in the coagulative properties of the blood known as **disseminated intravascular coagulopathy**,[4] besides **anemia and renal failure**.[5]

- **Minerals** such as potassium, iron, and magnesium are present in small amounts.

- Vinegar **contains no sugars or vitamins**, whereas grape and apple juices are rich in both nutrients.

Use As a Condiment

*Apart from its flavor, which many find disagreeable, vinegar **does not provide** any nutritive or dietary **benefit**. It does not facilitate digestion or improve absorption of other nutrients the way lemons do. To the contrary, **vinegar and pickled foods** prepared with it have several drawbacks:*

- Pickled foods become **tough** due to the protein coagulation caused by the acetic acid, which makes their digestion more difficult.

- **It erodes dental enamel.**[6]

- **It breaks the mucus barrier** that protects the mucous membrane of the stomach and causes **gastritis.**

- As it passes to the bloodstream, it **causes anemia** due to hemolysis (destruction of the red blood cells).

- Although some claim healing properties for **apple cider vinegar**, there is no scientific evidence to confirm it.

---

them at the price of gold as in the distant past, hardly anyone in the West would use them. Additionally, today we are fortunate to have healthful condiments, such as delicate aromatic herbs, making the use of spices even less necessary.

The Art of Seasoning

It is said that the good Hindu cooks combine spices just as artists combine colors. One must find the balance among flavors, not allowing any to dominate and, thus cancel out the flavor of the food. Many piquant spices mask the flavor of the primary ingredient instead of enhancing it.

The **taste buds** only perceive four basic flavors: **sweet, salty, sour, and bitter.** In reality, the wide range of flavors provided by condiments is due to their volatile essential oils. These oils vaporize easily and enter the nasal cavities, stimulating the sense of smell.

Seasoning must be, then, the art of adequately combining tastes and aromas to enhance the flavors of foods without diminishing their nutritional and dietary value.

Sources of spices

Spices are made up of various plant parts, such as:

- **Flower buds:** clove.
- **Bark** of the branches: cinnamon.
- **Fruit:** black and white pepper, and chilies (hot peppers).
- **Rhizomes:** ginger.
- **Seeds:** mustard.

Storage

Both aromatic herbs and spices lose their aroma over time, particularly if they have been exposed to air and light.

Because of this, they should be well dried and stored in opaque, airtight containers.

Vinegar is not a healthful condiment, even though some producers describe it as such. Lemon juice is preferable.

Grape and apple juices lose most of their nutritional and dietary therapeutic properties when they are fermented and converted to wine or cider. When they are transformed to vinegar, the loss is even greater.

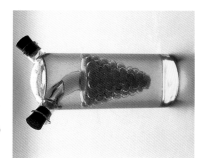

Continued on page 344

The Value of

From a nutritional standpoint, most condiments only provide small amounts of fiber and mineral salts. Their primary value is in their potential medicinal properties.

Benefits of Condiments

- **They stimulate the appetite:** As they improve the flavor of foods, condiments increase the desire to eat them. Healthful condiments are *of particular value for* those with **little or no appetite** or those **recovering** from weakening diseases.

- **They increase digestive secretions:** From saliva to pancreatic and intestinal juices, condiments stimulate an increase of all the secretions normally found in the digestive system (around five liters a day) that are necessary for digestion. *Healthful condiments,* such as **garlic** and **lemon**, *do not irritate or inflame* the mucous membrane of the stomach where digestive juices are produced. On the other hand, **spices** and **alcoholic beverages** achieve greater production of juices, particularly gastric juices, but at the expense of *irritation or inflammation* of the mucous lining of the stomach, producing **gastritis.**

- **They reduce flatulence:** many aromatic herbs have **carminative properties,** and reduce intestinal gas (see *EMP* p. 478). Spices overall have the same effect.

- **They reduce the need for salt:** The use of condiments allows for less salt to be used with foods. This is particularly *beneficial* for those suffering from **hypertension** or some degree of **coronary or renal failure.**

- **They improve food storage:** Many aromatic herbs such as thyme and certain spices such as clove and cinnamon are effective **antimycotics.**[7] It has been proved that lentils were completely free of **aflatoxin**-producing molds (carcinogenic substance, see Vol. 1, p. 140). The **capsaicin** from chili peppers, is also an *antifungal*[8] (destroys fungus and mold),

Healthful Condiments

Lemon (Vol. 2, p. 124)

- Excellent replacement for vinegar.

- It is **antiseptic: limes,** as well as **lemons** *eliminate* the **cholera bacillus** and others that can contaminate the raw vegetables in salads.[9]

- It increases the **secretion of gastric juices** and aids digestion.

- It improves the **absorption of** *non heme iron* (not from meat) found mostly in vegetable foods.

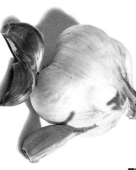

Garlic

- Its piquant flavor makes it an excellent replacement for stronger spices.

- It is a natural **antibiotic** against various microorganisms that may contaminate foods.

- It possesses *many* **medicinal properties:** it reduces cholesterol, combats hypertension, stimulates the immune system, inhibits the formation of malignant tumors, etcetera (see *EMP* p. 231).

Condiments

Aromatic Herbs

- The delicate flavors of aromatic herbs are an excellent **replacement** for many spices.

- They do *not* **mask** the flavor of foods.

- They are **medicinal**: thanks to their essential oils, they are an ideal accompaniment to foods because of their properties:

  – They are *eupeptic, conducive to good* **digestion**, particularly of legumes (see *EMP* p. 419).

  – They are *carminative, avoiding* intestinal **flatulence** (see *EMP* p. 478).

  – They are *antiseptic.* Although all aromatic herbs are antibacterial, **thyme** stands out due to its capacity to inhibit the development of bacteria of the genus *Salmonella*, which cause many cases of food poisoning (see *EMP* p. 770).

Mint

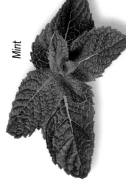

Thyme

Salt (Vol. 1, p. 344)

- When used *in moderation,* it is a universally prized seasoning.

- *Unrefined* **sea salt** or **herb salt** is healthier than common salt since they both contain *potassium*, a mineral that counteracts some of the negative effects of salt's sodium.

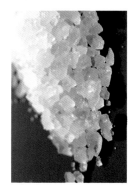

EMP = Encyclopedia of Medicinal Plants, EDUCATION AND HEALTH LIBRARY, Editorial Safeliz.

Drawbacks to Spices

- **They irritate the stomach:** The action of piquant spices such as pepper on the stomach is similar to that of **aspirin**. This has been proven by placing small amounts of pepper (red or black) or aspirin in the stomachs of healthy persons.[10] An endoscope was used to observe the effects of both on the gastric mucosa:

  – reddening and increase of gastric secretions, and

  – tiny hemorrhages or significant bleeding.

  Spices together with certain medications and alcohol *predispose* the body to **gastritis and gastric hemorrhage.**[11]

  A study has been published stating that spices do not produce gastric lesions.[12] But we believe that this finding may be due to the fact that the endoscopies were performed from 12 to 24 hours after eating and not immediately.

- They contribute to **cancer**: a study carried out in Israel[13] shows that spice consumption is related to esophageal cancer in women. Other studies find that hot chili peppers are carcinogenic,[14] while others declare that they protect against cancer.[15]

- They produce **allergies**: There are numerous cases of spice-caused facial[16] (itchy nose, sneezing, coughing), digestive[17] (abdominal pain, anal discomfort), or cutaneous[18] (atopy) allergic reactions.

- They are **habit-forming**: Regular use of spices produces an effect similar to that produced by drugs, called *tolerance*: it is necessary to increase the dose to obtain the same sensation.[19] The sense of taste becomes habituated to spices so that food in its natural state seems insipid.

- **They hide signs of deterioration in foods:** Before modern food preservation methods such as refrigeration, spices were used to mask the unpleasant flavor of contaminated or decaying foods. Spices can help avoid notice of the poor condition of foods, particularly meat and fish.

- **They increase the need for liquids** during a meal, thus *slowing digestion.*

Intense and/or Hot

All of these spices stimulate the digestive process and help avoid flatulence, but they can also cause stomach inflammation (gastritis). Their regular use is no more recommended than the heavy dishes in which they are usually used.

Cinnamon
Cinnamomum zeylanicum
EMP p. 442

Cinnamon is the bark from the young branches of the cinnamon tree, which is similar to the laurel and is grown in Asia and tropical America.

Its flavor is sweet and fragrant. It serves as an **appetizer;** it is **digestive** and **astringent,** but **contraindicated** for persons with gastroduodenal ulcers.

It is used in sticks as is illustrated in the photograph, or ground into powder.

Clove
Eugenia caryophylata
EMP p. 192

These dried buds of an Asian tree are piquant and sweet at the same time..

Clove is a general **stimulant.** It has **aperitif** and **carminative** (antiflatulent) properties.

Clove is **contraindicated** in instances of gastroduodenal ulcers and gastritis. If eaten in large amounts, it **irritates** the digestive tract.

Chili Peppers
Capsicum frutescens
EMP p. 354

This fruit is more or less piquant or hot due to the presence of the alkaloid **capsaicin,** which is eliminated through the urine and feces.

In Mexico there are many popular notions concerning the possible medicinal value of chilies, but these are not scientifically confirmed. It is certain, however, that regular consumption of chili peppers has drawbacks,[20] among them the *possibility* that they may be **carcinogenic.**[16]

There are instances in which chilies are not **recommended** such as cases of gastroduodenal ulcer, gastritis, colitis, hemorrhoids, prostatitis, and cystitis. Some studies suggest that eating chilies may have a positive effect on the stomach, since capsaicin induces greater mucus secretion, which protects the mucous lining of the stomach.[23]

However, *only the* **external** *use* of capsaicin has proven medicinal properties:

• Fungicide[8] (destroys fungi and molds).

• Antirheumatic and analgesic.[21]

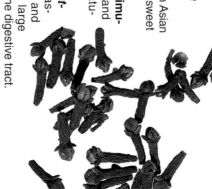

Nutmeg *Myristica fragans*

Nutmeg is the seed of the nutmeg tree, which is native to the Moluccas Islands. It is ovoid in shape, about 4 x 2 cm. It has an intensely sweet, piquant taste.

Mace is a spice prepared from the dried pulp of the nutmeg fruit. It may be purchased whole or powdered. It is hotter than nutmeg and must be used only in **very small amounts.**

The use of nutmeg and mace is not recommended. They contain the **toxic** alkaloid *myristicin,* whose **narcotic effect** depresses the central nervous system. These are possibly the two spices with the most serious health effects.

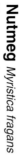

Flavored Spices

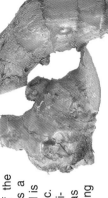

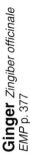

Pepper *Piper nigrum*
EMP p. 370

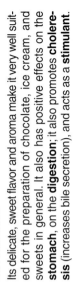

Pepper is the dried fruit with the shell (black pepper) or without the shell (white pepper) from a bush native to India. It is possibly the ***most common*** of all spices.

Its piquant flavor, stronger for black pepper, is due to the alkaloid ***piperidine***, which stimulates the production of gastric juices by **irritating** and **inflaming** the digestive mucosa.

Pepper aids the digestion of rich, heavy foods that contain a great deal of protein and fat. The most healthful is to avoid such foods and, therefore, do without pepper.

The use of pepper ***should be avoided*** in cases of gastritis, gastroduodenal ulcer, pancreatitis, hemorrhoids, and arterial hypertension (pepper raises blood pressure).

Jamaican or English pepper comes from the immature dried berries of a tree native to Jamaica (*Pimenta officinalis*). It is also piquant and its regular use produces **gastritis.**

Vanilla
Vanilla planifolia
EMP p. 376

Vanilla is the pod or shell of the fruit of an orchid native to Mexico and other Central American countries.

Its delicate, sweet flavor and aroma make it very well suited for the preparation of chocolate, ice cream, and sweets in general. It also has positive effects on the **stomach**, on the **digestion**; it also promotes **cholere-sis** (increases bile secretion), and acts as a **stimulant.**

Ginger *Zingiber officinale*
EMP p. 377

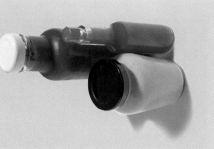

The rhizome of the ginger plant has a sweet flavor and is intensely aromatic. It is used in a variety of dishes as well as in preparing fruit preserves.

If eaten in large amounts, it produces gastritis. It ***should be avoided*** in cases of gastroduodenal ulcer.

Turmeric (see *EMP* p. 450) is another piquant rhizome similar to ginger.

Spice-based Products

Curry

Curry is a piquant sauce typical of India made up of pepper, ginger, clove, nutmeg, turmeric, and up to 14 ingredients. It is used to season protein-rich dishes such as meats and cheeses. It is very strong for sensitive stomachs and is *completely inadvisable* in a healthy diet.

Prepared Mustard

Prepared mustard is made from ground mustard seed (see *EMP* p. 663) mixed with salt, vinegar, and turmeric or saffron, which gives it its yellow color.

It **irritates** the digestive mucosa and is ***contraindicated*** in cases of gastritis or gastroduodenal ulcer.

Ketchup

Ketchup is a mixture of tomato, vinegar, sugar, and a variety of spices. It is not healthful since it is quite **indigestible** and is *inadvisable* from a dietary standpoint.

Tabasco Sauce

Tabasco sauce is made from hot chili peppers, vinegar, and a variety of spices. It is **spicy hot** and **indigestible.**

Worcestershire Sauce

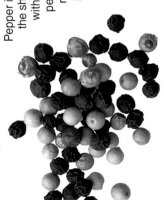

Worcestershire sauce is made from cane sugar molasses and piquant spices. It is used to flavor hamburgers and other meats.

Its regular use causes dyspepsia (indigestion) and gastritis.

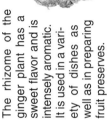

VOLUME 1 / **341**

EMP = *Encyclopedia of Medicinal Plants*, EDUCATION AND HEALTH LIBRARY, Editorial Safeliz.

Aromatic Plants:

The use of these healthful condiments does not mask the true flavor of foods. Additionally, it improves digestion, helps avoid intestinal gas, and disinfects foods. Almost all of them belong to two essence-producing botanical families: *Umbelliferae and Labiatae.*

Caper *Capparis spinosa*

Capers are the buds of a bush native to the Mediterranean region that grows in dry environments. Capers are rich in **fiber, vitamin C,** and **rutin** (an anti-inflammatory and antioxidant glucoside flavonoid).

Fresh, preserved, or pickled, they are used as a condiment in sauces, salads, and pizza, or as an accompaniment to a variety of dishes.

They *stimulate* the **appetite,** *aid digestion,* and are **diuretic.**

Dill

Anethum graveolens
EMP p. 349

Dill stimulates the **appetite** and *eliminates* digestive **gas.** It is similar to fennel (see Vol. 2, p. 161, *EMP* p. 360), in appearance as well as effect.

Coriander

Coriandrum sativum
EMP p. 447

Coriander aids digestion and **invigorates** the nervous system.

Laurel Leaves

Laurus nobilis
EMP p. 457

Bay leaves are used to season legumes because of their **eupeptic** (digestive aid) and **carminative** (antiflatulent) effects.

Sage

Salvia officinalis
EMP p. 638

Sage leaves are di**gestive, carminative** (antiflatulent), and **intestinal antiseptics.** They relieve **menstrual cramps.** They provide good seasoning for legumes, vegetables, soups, and sauces.

Rosemary

Rosmarinus officinalis
EMP p. 674

Rosemary leaves give an exquisite aroma to dishes. It is **digestive, cholagogic** (facilitates the draining of the gall bladder), and **antiflatulent.**

Parsley

Petroselinum sativum
EMP p. 583

Parsley gives a delicate aroma to all kinds of foods. It is di**uretic** and **invigorating,** although it is **not** advised for **pregnant** women, since it may predispose to miscarriage.

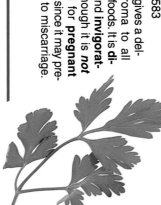

Delicate and Medicinal

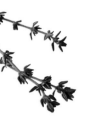

Basil
Ocimum basilicum
EMP p. 368

Basil leaves are used to give a pleasant flavor to salads and soups. Basil relieves nervous **digestive spasms** and **headaches** associated with indigestion.

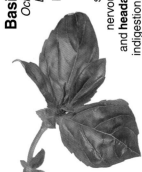

Thyme
Thymus vulgaris
EMP p. 769

Thyme's aroma goes very well with a variety of potato, legume, and vegetable dishes. Besides its **digestive** and **antiflatulent** properties, thyme *combats* intestinal **autointoxication** and is a *good* intestinal **antiseptic.** It is particularly *effective* in cases of **diarrhea caused by salmonella.**

Other Useful Plants

Chervil
Anthriscus cerefolium

Chervil leaves are similar to parsley (CAUTION: they are also similar to poison hemlock!) and are used fresh in salads and vegetable dishes. Its flavor is reminiscent of anise.

Oregano
Origanum vulgare
EMP p. 464

The flowering tips of these plants from the *Labiatae* family are a typical seasoning in the Mediterranean diet. Oregano is ideal for pizza, pasta, and legumes. It is **sedative, antispasmodic** (alleviates digestive organ spasms), and **antiflatulent.**

Lovage
Levisticum officinale
EMP p. 578

Powder made from the lovage root is used as a substitute for pepper in Central Europe. It is very aromatic and **digestive.** It is a very good seasoning for salads, soups, and legumes.

Saffron
Crocus sativus
EMP p. 448

The stigmas of the saffron flower are used as a seasoning because of the pleasant **flavor** and **color** that they give foods. In small amounts (very few threads) saffron is **digestive**, but in larger quantities it may have toxic effects on the nervous system.

Horseradish
Armoracia rusticana
EMP p. 394

The root of this plant is quite pungent due to its high sulfurous essence content. It has an *appetizing* and *invigorating* effect on the digestive system. It has a *mucolytic* and *soothing* effect on the respiratory system. It is recommended for cases of **lack of appetite, sinusitis, bronchitis,** and **asthma.**

Cumin
Cuminum cyminum
EMP p. 449

Invigorates the digestive organs. Its tiny flowers are used for their essence or for infusions.

Savory
Satureja hortensis
EMP p. 374

Savory is a healthy substitute for pepper. Besides being a **digestive** and **carminative**, savory is **invigorating** and an **expectorant**. It is recommended for **gastritis.**

Anise
Pimpinella anisum
EMP p. 465

In general, the fruits of the umbellate plants, such as the anise or the cumin, are used to season breads, rolls, and cookies due to their pleasant aroma and *effective* **carminative** (antiflatulent) **properties.**

Anise is also an **expectorant** and **galactagogue** (increases milk secretion in lactating mothers).

EMP = Encyclopedia of Medicinal Plants, EDUCATION AND HEALTH LIBRARY, Editorial Safeliz.

Sources of Sodium in the Diet

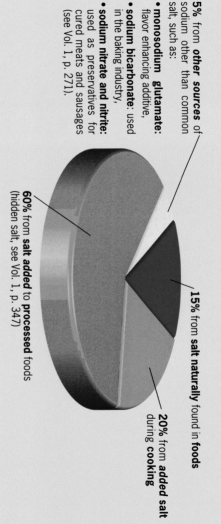

Most of the effects, both beneficial and harmful, of salt, are due to this metal called sodium. Excess salt in the diet is harmful precisely because of its sodium content.

5% from **other sources** of sodium other than common salt, such as:

- **monosodium glutamate:** flavor enhancing additive,
- **sodium bicarbonate:** used in the baking industry,
- **sodium nitrate and nitrite:** used as preservatives for cured meats and sausages (see Vol. 1, p. 271).

15% from **salt naturally** found in **foods**

20% from **added salt** during **cooking**

60% from **salt added** to **processed** foods (hidden salt, see Vol. 1, p. 347)

Benefits of salt

- **Satisfies the body's need for** *sodium*: It provides the sodium necessary to maintain fluid equilibrium and arterial pressure.
- **Flavor:** It helps make foods more flavorful, increases the secretion of juices, and aids digestion.
- **Improves food preservation:** It prevents bacterial proliferation that leads to decay in foods.

Drawbacks of Salt

- **It is habit forming:** Salt diminishes the sensitivity of the taste buds. Over time more salt is required to achieve the same sense of saliness.
- **Arterial hypertension:** *Heavy* salt use fosters an increase in arterial pressure, particularly the diastolic (lower number). It has been demonstrated that this effect is

---

Continued from page 337

Salt

Salt is *much more than* a simple **condiment** that improves the taste of food. It is also *more than* an **additive** that prevents the decay of foods. *Above all* it is the **main** dietary **source** of *sodium* and *chlorine*, two *essential* elements for the function of the body.

Salt and Sodium

Common salt is composed primarily of **sodium chloride**, with 60% chlorine and 40% sodium. Each of these elements performs specific functions within the body.

Chlorine

The body uses chlorine to form the **hydrochloric acid** that the stomach secretes. It forms part of the **blood** and organic **fluids**, as well.

Sodium

Sodium is a very important ingredient in the **blood** and the **extracellular fluid** that bathes all of the cells of the body. It has **water retention** properties.

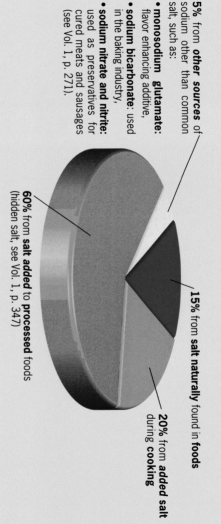

Most of the salt and sodium in the typical Western diet comes from processed foods.

Therefore, eating less processed products and reducing the amount of salt added to foods reduces salt and sodium intake.

When Salt Turns to Poison

The excess sodium taken in with the salt that we customarily add to our foods must be eliminated through the urine.

When the body loses the capacity to do this, this sodium is retained in the tissues. Salt, then, becomes a true poison. This occurs in the following cases in which salt use must be reduced to a necessary minimum:

- *Heart failure,*
- *Renal failure caused by nephritic syndrome or other causes,*
- *Cirrhosis of the liver.*

The minimum daily need for salt (500 mg, which equals 1.25 g of salt) is covered by the salt found in foods in their natural state without need to add any common salt.

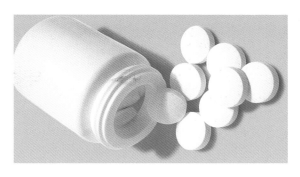

The more salt is consumed, the more calcium is eliminated through the urine. Reducing salt intake is equivalent to taking a calcium tablet a day.

more pronounced in certain sensitive individuals, and increases with age.[24] However, salt use is only one of the diverse factors that play a role in hypertension. For this reason, simply reducing salt use, while necessary, is not the complete solution to hypertension.[25]

- **Cardiovascular disease:** the Intersalt study, an international effort to analyze the effects of salt, found that the *more salt consumed, the higher the probability* of dying from a **stroke**.[26] This may be related to the fact that excess salt makes the arterial walls more rigid.[27]

- **Stomach disorders: Brine-preserved or pickled foods** foster infection of the mucous membrane of the stomach by the *Helicobacter pylori* bacteria. This is a cause of a variety of stomach diseases, such as atrophic gastritis, gastroduodenal ulcers, and cancer. The National Institute for Cancer Research in Tokyo (Japan), arrived at this conclusion after a broad study.[29] The researchers recommended that the Japanese population, which suffers from stomach cancer with considerable frequency, abstain from very salty or pickled foods.

- **Stomach cancer:** A study conducted at Louvain University (Belgium), analyzed data from twenty-four countries, and confirmed that salt consumption is related with stomach cancer in men and women. Additionally, the **nitrates** used as food additives were found to be even *more carcinogenic* the more salt there is in the diet.[30]

- **Asthma:** There is epidemiological and experimental evidence that high salt consumption provokes spasms of the bronchial muscles and asthma.[31] At the University Hospital of Zurich (Switzerland) it has been demonstrated that a low-salt diet improves the condition of asthma patients, and reduces the need for antiasthmatic medication.[32] However, other studies indicate that there is no

clear relationship between salt consumption and asthmatic bronchial hyperactivity.[33]

- **Calcium loss:** *Excessive* salt leads to increased calcium loss through the urine *leading* to **osteoporosis.** A reduction in salt use is beneficial to bone density similarly to increased calcium intake.[28]

- **Kidney stones:** Increased calcium loss through the urine caused by excess salt is detrimental to those suffering from kidney stones, particularly those composed of calcium.[34] A study conducted at Yale University (USA), states the importance of reduction of salt intake as well as calcium rich foods in the prevention of kidney stones.[35]

Salt: Much More

Types of Salt

Sea Salt

In *addition* to **sodium chloride**, sea salt contains *small amounts* of the salts of **calcium**, **potassium**, and **magnesium**. These are very beneficial minerals that partially compensate for the harmful effects of excess sodium. Sea salt also provides a *small* but **important** amount of **iodine**.

The **drawback** to unrefined sea salt is that it *retains* a lot of **moisture**, which makes it harder to handle. But its benefits far outweigh this small inconvenience.

Refined Salt

This is *more common* but *less healthful*. It is prepared by:

- **Removing** the **magnesium** and **calcium** salts that sea salt naturally contains and that cause the salt to clump. This makes the salt easier to use both for the packager and in the kitchen, but at the cost of the mineral content of sea salt.

- Various **additives** are *used* to keep the salt grains free and dry.

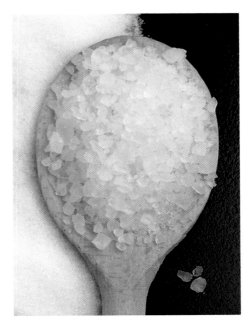

A few grains of rice mixed with salt absorb the moisture it may contain making it easier to pour.

The Need For Salt

The average Western diet provides *eight times* more salt and sodium than the body **needs**.

For some persons, salt can become a **"drug"** almost as dangerous as alcohol or tobacco. Aside from its harmful health effects, salt has the ability to become habit-forming.

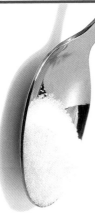

Approximately half a teaspoon of salt a day, 1.25 g, covers the need for **sodium** of an adult with a sedentary **lifestyle. The foods that normally make up the diet provide more than enough sodium without a need to add salt.**

Those involved in intense physical labor or who live in hot climates need more salt: approximately one gram per each hour of sweating.

	Sodium (mg)	Equivalent in common salt (g)*
Minimum daily needs of an adult	500	1.25
Daily Value (acceptable daily intake)	2,400	6
Normal consumption	4,000	10

* *Equivalents:*
1 g of salt contains 0.4 g of sodium (400 mg).
1 g of sodium (1,000 mg) equals 2.5 g of salt.

Than a Seasoning

"Hidden Salt": An Abundant Additive

Grams of salt contained in 100 grams of each of these products:

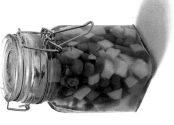

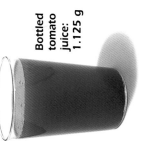

Preserves: 1-2 g

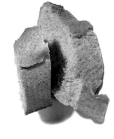

Bread:[36] 1.2 g

Bottled tomato juice: 1.125 g

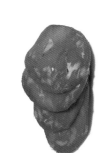

Sausages and cured meats: 3-6 g

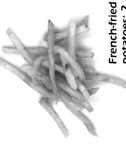

French-fried potatoes: 2.5 g

Fast food and snacks: 2-3 g

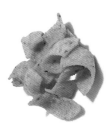

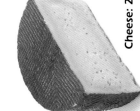

Cheese: 2.5 g

Just as with sugar (see Vol. 1, p. 168) it is possible that the *worst* aspect of salt may not be the sodium chloride itself but the *unhealthful foods* usually *accompanying* it: cured meats, sausages, fried foods, refined products (without fiber), etcetera. These foods *trigger* the *harmful effects* of salt.

There are many specialists, such as Professor Mac-Gregor of the Hypertension Unit of Saint George Hospital in London, who see a clear connection between excess use of common salt (NaCl, sodium chloride) and arterial hypertension, strokes, and osteoporosis. They all question why the food industry is so loath to reduce the amount of salt added to precooked dishes, preserves and other processed foods.[37, 22]

Salt Alternatives

To reduce the use of salt, one must first accustom the palate to a less intense salt taste. The following alternatives may be useful:

- *Other salts such as potassium chloride and potassium iodide. These have a somewhat less salty taste than sodium chloride. They are usually mixed with it to form dietetic salts. Diabetics and those suffering from renal failure must use them with care since an excess of potassium may be harmful in these cases.*

- *Herb salt contains a mixture of common salt, other salts and aromatic herb extracts. It contains ap-*

proximately *half* the *sodium* of the common salt by weight. Its flavor is somewhat less salty than common salt, but it is tastier due to the aromatic herbs.

- *Healthful seasonings provide flavor and health (lemon, aromatic herbs, garlic, onion, etc.; see Vol. 1, pp. 338-339, 342-343).*

- *Sea salt, although it contains practically the same amount of sodium as refined salt, it is somewhat less harmful because it contains other minerals that partially compensate for the undesirable effects of sodium.*

16

NUTRITIONAL SUPPLEMENTS

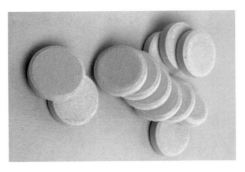

Supplements may improve a healthy diet, but they cannot replace it.

For example, a pharmaceutical vitamin C supplement may complement natural sources of this vitamin such as fresh fruits and vegetables, but it does not eliminate the need to eat them.

M ANY PEOPLE, particularly in industrialized societies, fear that the foods they eat may not provide all of the nutrients that their bodies need.

Others are not aware of or undervalue the preventive and healing properties of simple plant-based foods. Simultaneously, they praise and idealize the virtues of certain sophisticated foods or manufactured products that are very attractively presented and well marketed.

So, they tend to take nutritional supplements of various types. And it is very possible that in many cases these supplements are completely unnecessary.

Simple, natural foods possess healing power, just as is explained in Volume Two of this work, and can be much more effective than many supplements in the maintenance of good health.

Reasons To Take Supplements

This notwithstanding, supporters of supplement usage put forward arguments in their favor. Although many of their claims may be exaggerated, some deserve consideration. Let us assess the most important claims.

Soil Exhaustion

Intensive agriculture makes extensive use of **chemical fertilizers** to increase crop yields and produce multiple crops during the year.

It is possible that these chemical fertilizers do not replace the minerals that the plants use as they develop. These plants, as well as the animals feeding on them, may lack some nutrients that are expected to be present, particularly *trace elements* (minerals that are present in very small amounts: iron, copper, zinc, etc.).

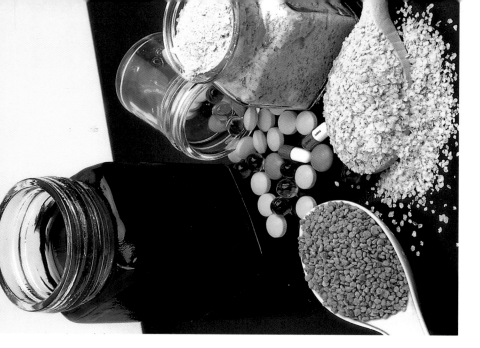

Those Who May Truly Need Supplements

- *Newborns: vitamin K to avoid hemorrhage.*
- *Children who get little sun: vitamin D.*
- *Women with heavy menstruation: iron.*
- *Women before conception and during the first months of pregnancy: folates or folic acid, to avoid malformations of the fetus' neural tube such as spina bifida. Supplemental iron is needed only in few cases.[1]*
- *Women at risk of osteoporosis: calcium.*
- *Strict vegetarians and the elderly: vitamin B$_{12}$, although it is not essential.*
- *Smokers: vitamins C and B.*
- *Men at risk of heart attack: folates[2] and beta-carotene.*
- *Persons under a great deal of stress or nervous tension: wheat germ or B group vitamins.*
- *Patients who are malnourished, have infectious diseases, or are convalescing: multiple vitamins and minerals (see also Vol. 1, p. 353).*

This can be a valid reason to take nutritional supplements unless one eats foods grown naturally using organic fertilizers, which are more nutritious for the plants.

Unripe Crops

The needs of mass commerce and transportation require that many crops be harvested while they are still **immature** or green. In this condition fruits and vegetables in general have not developed their optimal concentration of:

- Sugars, vitamins, and minerals;
- Other non-nutritive substances that have preventive and healing power such as phytochemicals (see Vol. 1, p. 410).

Ripening usually takes place during transport or storage under artificial conditions. These modern techniques make a wider variety of fruits available during more of the year, but of a lower quality than those naturally ripened.

Regular consumption of artificially ripened fruits may be another justification for the use of supplements. However, they are not as necessary if the fruits and vegetables eaten are grown as naturally as pos-

sible. This is the case with organic foods, which are even more flavorful.

Chemical Pollution

For decades most of the inhabitants of Planet Earth, and particularly those living in industrialized countries, have been continually assaulted with thousands of artificial chemical substances that are foreign to humans, for example:

Nutritional Supplements

*Foods or nutrients used specifically to **complement** or **improve** the nutritive value of foods are considered nutritional supplements. They can be of various types:*

- ***Dietary supplements:** Foods or food products particularly rich in specific nutrients.*
- ***Vitamin supplements,** minerals, and other nutrients derived from natural or synthetic sources.*

Pharmaceutical Supplements or Fruit and Vegetable Juices

One of the proven beneficial effects of *vitamin C* is that it **inhibits** the formation of **nitrosamines** in the body. These carcinogenic substances are formed from nitrites and nitrates found in various preserved foods, such as cured meats and sausages (see Vol. 1, pp. 270-271).

An experiment conducted at Cornell University (New York) demonstrated that the **natural juices** of peppers, pineapple, tomatoes, strawberries, and carrots are **much more effective** as **anticarcinogens** than an aqueous solution of the same amount of vitamin C present in those juices.[3]

This investigation illustrates the fact that **natural products** provide much more than isolated chemicals such as vitamin C. Thus, their **healing and preventive power** is **far superior.** Nature's chemistry is far more effective than that of the laboratory.

Pharmaceutical Supplements

Made of isolated and purified vitamins and minerals have the **advantage that dosage can be precisely** known and controlled.

Fruit, vegetables, and their juices

They have the **advantage** of containing vitamins, minerals, and hundreds of accompanying phytochemicals (see Vol. 1, p. 411) that **improve** their assimilation and effects in the body.

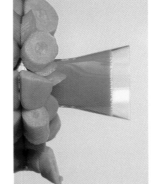

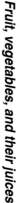

cells, causing alterations called **mutations,** which are a cause of cancer.

Fortunately the human body is capable of:

• Neutralizing and eliminating free radicals, as well as

• Repairing damage to the DNA and other molecules

To accomplish this, the body needs **antioxidant** substances such as **provitamin A** (beta-carotene) and *vitamins C and E,* which are found in plant-based foods.

The growing amount of pollutants acting as free radicals that the body must combat makes eating **vegetable foods *rich* in antioxidants** all the more important (see Vol. 1, p. 354).

Additionally, the use of **antioxidant supplements** *may be necessary* as a complement to a healthy diet, **particularly** if one is exposed to *very high* **pollution** *levels.*

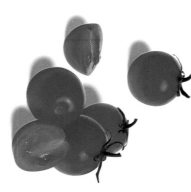

Eating organically grown plant-based foods raised without chemical pesticides can reduce the need for nutritional supplements.

• Carbon monoxide, sulfur dioxide, tobacco smoke, and other atmospheric **fumes and gases;**

• **Heavy metal** residues (lead, mercury, etc.) in the air, the water, and in food;

• **Additives** in processed foods;

• **Pesticide** residues in fresh and processed foods.

All these chemical substances pass to the blood and into the body's cells. While normally present in only small amounts when considered individually, taken together, they represent a serious health threat.

Most of these pollutants act as free radicals, which are *aggressive chemical substances capable of oxidizing and deteriorating* the molecules that form the body's cells. The chemical damage produced by free radicals can even affect the genes in the nuclei of the

Drawbacks to Nutritional Supplements

In addition to some specific issues, nutritional supplements share others with medications. For example:

Objects of Exaggeration and Fraud

There are many healthful and effective nutritional supplements sold with truthful and realistic information.

But there are others marketed with *exaggerated* or *distorted* **claims** regarding their nutritional or medicinal properties, raising *false hopes* for patients.

To *avoid* **deception** and even **fraud** which, unfortunately, are quite common, it is necessary to carefully review any information dispensed with any of the new supplements that continually appear on the market, asking these questions:

- Which **company or laboratory** produces the nutritional supplement? Is it known to be honest and realistic in its dealings?

- **Who is providing the information** regarding the effectiveness of the product? What professional credentials do they have? **What research** forms the base of the claims for the product?

- Does the person responsible for conducting or sponsoring the research have a **commercial interest** in the sale of the product?

- Is the product claimed to cure or prevent multiple deficiencies or diseases?

- Are **exaggerated** claims made about the product such as longer life, eternal youth, unlimited energy, or inexhaustible sexual potency?

- Is the product claimed to **replace** the need to eat fruit, vegetables, or other healthful foods? Is it offered to **compensate** for the negative consequences of unhealthy habits such as smoking?

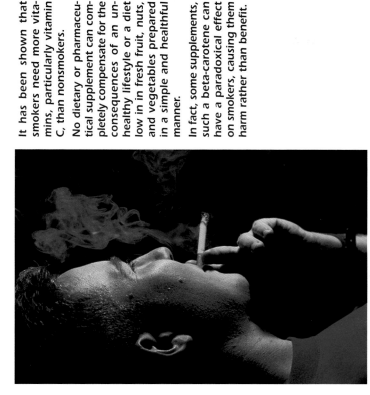

It has been shown that smokers need more vitamins, particularly vitamin C, than nonsmokers.

No dietary or pharmaceutical supplement can completely compensate for the consequences of an unhealthy lifestyle or a diet low in in fresh fruit, nuts, and vegetables prepared in a simple and healthful manner.

In fact, some supplements, such a beta-carotene can have a paradoxical effect on smokers, causing them harm rather than benefit.

Supplements Can Hide Symptoms

Supplements taken to alleviate seemingly minor symptoms such as fatigue, headache, dizziness, rapid weight loss, or sexual impotence can mask the symptoms of serious disease making diagnosis difficult. When one experiences these symptoms, the first step should be a visit to a physician for a medical diagnosis instead of taking supplements.

Toxicity, Interactions and Allergies

Excessive supplements can provide high doses of certain nutrients such as vitamin A (not provitamin A, beta-carotene), vitamin D, selenium, or iron, which can be toxic.[4]

Additionally, high doses of certain nutrients can interfere with the absorption of others. For example, excess fiber interferes with the absorption of iron. An excess of iron interferes with the absorption of zinc.

Besides, certain supplements such as brewer's yeast, pollen, or royal jelly can produce serious allergies.

SUPPLEMENTS

DIETARY SUPPLEMENTS (VARIOUS FOODS)

These are foods with especially high **concentrations** of particular nutrients used to **complement** the nutritional value of regular **foods** in the diet.

Fenugreek

Sesame

Supplement	Vol./Page	Description
WHEAT GERM	2/310	Very rich in **protein** (more complete than that of wheat flour), essential **fatty acids** (including **omega-3**), **vitamins B** and **E**, minerals, and other antioxidant components. It is poor or lacking in calcium, provitamin A and vitamin C. **USE AS A SUPPLEMENT:** From one to four spoonfuls a day. Wheat germ combines very well and complements many foods such as salads, soups, milk, or fruit juices.
MOLASSES	1/167	This natural syrup is normally obtained from sugarcane. It is very rich in minerals, particularly **iron** and **calcium**. **USE AS A SUPPLEMENT:** May be used in place of sugar or jams. It combines well with yogurt and cottage cheese.
SESAME SEED	EMP 611	The seeds from the *Sesamum indicum* are very rich in **unsaturated fatty acids**, high value **proteins** (similar to soy proteins, but without the drawbacks), **lecithin**, **vitamins**, **calcium**, and **trace elements**. It represents a very concentrated food that invigorates the **nervous system** and promotes **sexual vigor**. **USE AS A SUPPLEMENT:** • Toasted whole seeds. • Seeds ground to a paste called **tahini** that makes an excellent substitute for butter and margarine.
BARLEY GREEN		This is the juice of the immature barley plant. It is rich in **chlorophyll** and **trace elements** and is used as an **antioxidant, tonic, and depurant**; it is also useful to slow cellular **aging**.
FENUGREEK	EMP 474	Flour made from fenugreek seeds (*Trigonella foenum-graecum*) is rich in **iron**, easily assimilated **proteins**, **carbohydrates**, and **vitamins**. Calms and reduces inflammation in the digestive tract, and improves the assimilation of other foods. **USE AS A SUPPLEMENT: Anemia, underweight,** malnutrition, and digestive failure due to a variety of illnesses.
PROTEIN POWDER		Dietary protein supplements are generally manufactured from one or more of these ingredients: powdered milk, soy flour or protein, and/or dehydrated egg white. It is typically used by those involved in physical culture, bodybuilding, and weightlifting, with the intention of increasing muscle mass. Since there is no proof that excess dietary protein increases muscle mass, this practice is of doubtful effectiveness.[5] On the other hand, it is known that excess protein produces **undesirable effects** such as an increase of uric acid and cholesterol, calcium loss through the urine,[6] and predisposition to kidney disease.
DESIGNER FOODS OR NUTRICEUTICALS		These are new products that share certain food and supplement characteristics. They are foods developed through **genetic engineering** providing greater proportions of vitamins, minerals, and phytochemicals with preventive and healing properties. Some have great hope for these food-medicines. But it would be very difficult to improve the healing and preventive power of organically grown plant-based foods that have been prepared as simply as possible (washed and cooked, if necessary).

EMP = *Encyclopedia of Medicinal Plants*, Education and Health Library, Editorial Safeliz.

VOLUME 1 / **352**

PRODUCTS OF THE BEEHIVE

These products of bees are noted for their special nutritive and medicinal properties (see Vol. 1, p. 160).

VITAMINS AND MINERALS

These are pharmaceutical preparations, which are generally **artificially** manufactured. Although they may be useful due to ease of use and precise dosages, their nutritional and medicinal value is inferior to those of fresh plant-based foods. Such foods contain, besides vitamins and minerals, a series of complimentary substances known globally as phytochemicals. Even though they are found in minute quantities, these substances possess considerable healing and preventive power.

Supplement	Vol./Page	Description
HONEY	1/160	Honey is much more than sugar. Even though some specialists do not accept its medicinal value, it is used in cases of **asthenia** (debility), **insomnia**, **infectious diarrhea**, **respiratory conditions**, and **liver failure**.
POLLEN	1/359	Nutritious and invigorating. It is used in cases of **anorexia** (lack of appetite) and **asthenia** (fatigue).
ROYAL JELLY	1/360	Used in case of physical or mental **exhaustion**, sexual **impotence, arteriosclerosis,** and **lowered resistance.**
PROPOLIS	1/361	Natural **antibiotic, emollient,** and **antitussive.**
PHARMACEUTICALLY PREPARED VITAMINS		Multivitamin supplements provide no **invigorating effect,** as some believe. Their use is only justified for the elderly or weakened patients who are not properly nourished. The **best multivitamin supplement** for those capable of eating is a diet rich in fresh, raw **fruits** and **vegetables.** Those suffering from debilities may choose freshly squeezed juices. The use of vitamin supplements is only medically justified in specific cases. And even in these cases they are dispensable (see Vol. 1, p. 349). • **Vitamin B12:**for strict **vegetarians.** • **Vitamin C:** for **smokers.** • **Vitamin D:** for children who are **not** exposed to **sunlight** or do not use dairy products. • **Folates** for women who are pregnant or considering becoming **pregnant,** and for men at risk of heart attack. • **Vitamin K** for **newborns.**

PHARMACEUTICALLY PREPARED MINERALS		The same as was said of multivitamin supplements applies to mineral supplements. Mineral supplements are medically indicated in only these cases (see Vol. 1, p. 349):
		
		• **Iron:** may be necessary in cases of hypermenorrhea (excessively prolonged or profuse menses), to avoid anemia. It is usually recommended during pregnancy, but it is not truly necessary if the diet is adequate.[1]
		• **Calcium:** in cases of osteoporosis.
		• Other **dietary supplements** that are rich in minerals that make pharmaceutically prepared supplements unnecessary:
		  – brewer's yeast (Vol. 1, p. 358),
		  – molasses (Vol. 1, p. 352),
		  – bran and wheat germ (Vol. 2, pp. 310, 311),
		  – spirulina (Vol. 1, p. 134).

DOLOMITE		This supplement, prepared by crushing certain rocks, contains inorganic calcium and magnesium. Assimilation of these minerals is more difficult than organic calcium and magnesium found naturally in foods. **Caution:** dolomite powder may contain some amount of heavy metals such as lead, arsenic, or mercury.
KELP TABLETS		These are manufactured by grinding **laminaria seaweed,** also known as kelp (see Vol. 1, p. 134). They are rich in **iodine,** an essential trace element for the proper function of the **thyroid** gland, which may be lacking in the soil and water in regions far from the sea. No more than one a day should be taken to avoid iodine **overdose.**

Supplement	Vol./Page	Description
EVENING PRIMROSE OIL	EMP 237	The primrose (*Oenothera biennis*) is a plant whose seeds are very rich in **essential fatty acids,** particularly **linolenic acid,** which belongs to the **omega-3** series, as do fish oils, and performs various important functions in the body. It is recommended as a compliment in the treatment of **numerous diseases:** thrombosis and cerebral hemorrhage, myocardial infarction, dysmenorreah, nervous system degeneration, rheumatoid arthritis, allergies, eczema, and skin disorders. *USE AS A SUPPLEMENT:* 2 to 4 g in capsules daily.
LECITHIN	1/89	This is a lipid substance obtained *primarily from* **soy.** It is recommended in cases of elevated **cholesterol, liver** disease, and **nervous disorders,** although its effectiveness has not been completely established. *USE AS A SUPPLEMENT:* Granules, 2 to 6 spoonfuls daily.
BRAN	2/311	The cellulose fiber in wheat bran is mostly insoluble (see Vol. 1, p. 388). It is more effective in preventing **constipation** and colon cancer than it is in lowering cholesterol levels. *As A SUPPLEMENT:* Take **no** more than 30 g a day and take care that what is used was grown without pesticides. If whole grains and breads are regularly used there is no need to supplement the diet with bran. Whole grain contains germ and endosperm (the source of flour) in addition to bran.
FLAX	EMP 508	Flaxseeds are rich in **soluble fiber** (mucilage and pectin), which softens the intestinal mucosa and regulate its flora. *As A SUPPLEMENT:* Whole seeds (must be well chewed) or flour may be added to bread and bakery products. Besides fiber, flax provides valuable proteins and fats.
GLUCOMANNAN		This is a type of dietary fiber formed from non-absorbable gum or mucilage extracted from a tuber called konjuc. It lowers **cholesterol** levels and helps *reduce appetite in* **weight loss** diets.
BETA-CAROTENE	1/389	This yellow or orange pigment found in many fruits and vegetables transforms into **vitamin A** in the intestine or the liver. Synthetic beta-carotene (produced in the laboratory) is used as a dietary supplement to reduce the risk of lung cancer and myocardial infarction in smokers. However, this has not been effective. No supplement can reverse the consequences of unhealthy habits such as smoking, or an incorrect diet. There is no need to take supplements of this pro-vitamin if one enjoys a **diet rich in** **fruits** and **vegetables** high in beta-carotene.
VITAMIN C	1/396	Vitamin C is a *potent* **antioxidant** that prevents the oxidation of numerous molecules and their consequent transformation into free radicals. When it is isolated and purified as a supplement, vitamin C is effective, but less so than when it is accompanied by the organic acids and other phytochemicals found in plant foods potentiate the effects of vitamin C. Vitamin C is particularly helpful for smokers and those who are exposed to a high level of chemical pollution.

OILS AND FATS

These can complement the nutritional value of the fats in foods and provide certain medicinal properties.

Primrose

DIETARY FIBER

Fiber is a substance that accompanies all foods, but is not absorbed in the intestine or passed to the bloodstream. It is completely eliminated in the feces. The typical diet in developed countries is poor in fiber because it is removed from many products that would naturally contain it, such as whole grains, through the refining process.

By eating *abundant* **fruits, vegetables and grains** the need for **supplemental fiber** is largely *eliminated.* However, patients who are unable to chew or digest properly do not take in enough whole foods.

ANTIOXIDANTS

These substances have the *capacity to* **prevent** the **oxidation** of various types of molecules within the body. For example:

• **Lipoprotein** molecules are a type of fat that transports cholesterol in the blood. When they oxidize, they deposit on the arterial walls causing arteriosclerosis. This way, antioxidants stop this degenerative disease.

• **Nucleic acid** molecules such as DNA (deoxyribonucleic acid) that form the genes and chromosomes in the nuclei of the cells. The oxidation of a cell's DNA causes mutations that can make the cell become cancerous. Antioxidants are anticarcinogens due to this effect.

• **Free radicals:** these are the most pernicious of oxidizing agents. They are aggressive molecules

EMP = Encyclopedia of Medicinal Plants, EDUCATION AND HEALTH LIBRARY, Editorial Safeliz.

Supplement	Vol./Page	Description
N-ACETYLCYSTEINE		n-Acetylcysteine is also known by its acronym **NAC**. It is a precursor to the nonessential amino acid cysteine that has been used as an oral medication to relieve **excess mucus.** Recently it has begun to be used as a nutritional supplement because its **antioxidant and immune boosting properties.** **Suggestions for use:** There are ongoing studies regarding the use of NAC in AIDS cases. Laboratory investigations have proved that n-acetylcysteine increases glutathione (an antioxidant tripeptide) levels in the lymphocytes and other defensive cells, and improves their function in AIDS patients.[10,11] The clinical effectiveness of this supplement is being studied. ***DOSE:*** from 2 to 4 grams daily by mouth.
COENZYME Q10 (UBIQUINONE)		This is a liposoluble substance that all cells produce, both animal and plant. It is a potent antioxidant that intervenes in the production of energy in the form of ATP in the cells.[12] **Natural sources:** Foods provide an average of 3 to 5 mg daily. It is not considered a vitamin, because the body's own cells can produce it. **Recommendations for use:** Coenzyme Q10 is recommended as a dietary supplement in the following situations: • **Heart:** Improves the heart's activity in case of heart failure, reduces arterial hypertension, and speeds recovery after myocardial infarction. • **Muscles:** Improves performance in athletes without doping. It is used in cases of muscular dystrophy. • **Periodontal disease:** Accelerates the healing of affected gums. ***USE AS A SUPPLEMENT:*** Natural sources of coenzyme Q10 may be insufficient in the above-cited cases. The recommended supplemental dosage is 100 to 200 mg daily for the first weeks. The maintenance dose is 30 mg daily.
GUARANA		The guarana (*Paullinia cupana*) is a vine of the family *Sapindaceae* that grows in the Amazon region of Brazil. Its small red fruit is toasted and ground to a powder, which is mixed with milk or other beverages. **Effects:** • Invigorating, stimulates the nervous system, and relieves headache due toits caffeine, theophylline, and theobromine contains.[13] In this sense, their effect is *similar* to that of **tea** and **coffee.** • Its capacity to improve intellectual activity, memory, and stress resistance has been confirmed in laboratory animals.[14] It appears that this is due to the **essential oils** it contains.[15] • It decreases the tendency of platelets to agglutinate, causing the blood to coagulate within the arteries.[16] **Drawbacks** • Those associated with the **caffeine** that it contains (see *EMP* p. 178). The concentration of caffeine in guarana drinks is generally similar to that of tea, but it depends on the dilution of the powder. • It has been shown that guarana produces **mutations** in the DNA of bacterial cells,[17] which raises the possibility that it could increase cancer risk. This supplement should be used prudently while waiting for further study. ***USE AS A SUPPLEMENT:*** No more than a teaspoon (3 to 5 grams) of powder per day.

Lungs

STIMULANTS

These are products with certain nutritional and medicinal value, but which also stimulate the nervous system. Their regular use as supplements presents mental and physical health drawbacks due to their ability to create addiction or dependency.

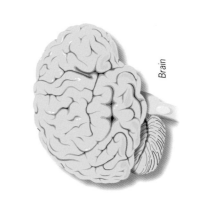

Brain

EMP = Encyclopedia of Medicinal Plants, EDUCATION AND HEALTH LIBRARY, Editorial Safeliz.

VOLUME 1 / **356**

that can cause chemical damage to our own cells. They come primarily from:

– Environmental pollution such as tobacco smoke;
– Metabolic activity of the body, particularly when under stress, either physical (disease, overwork) or psychological (nervous tension).

Antioxidants neutralize the action of free radicals. In this way it has been demonstrated that they are useful in treating various diseases such as:

• Arteriosclerosis,
• Cancer,
• Myocardial infarction,
• Immunodepression (lowering of immunity),
• Poisoning from chemical sources or unhealthful foods.

The levels of pollution and stress in modern life that simply did not exist only a few decades ago increasingly justify the use of antioxidant supplements.

Cabbage

Citrus

Supplement	Vol./Page	Description
VITAMIN E	1/397	Vitamin E acts to inhibit the oxidation of fats, which helps to prevent arteriosclerosis and the deterioration of cell membranes. Beta-carotene, vitamin C, selenium, and other antioxidants potentiate its action. Based on the source, there are two types of vitamin E supplements: • **Synthetic** vitamin E: this supplement contains only **l-alpha-tocopherol**, one of the many types of tocopherol found in foods with vitamin E action. • **Natural** vitamin E: this supplement contains the natural **d-alpha-tocopherol**, which is slightly different from the synthetic, as well as other **tocopherols** such as beta, gamma, and delta tocopherol. It is **more potent** than the synthetic supplement.
SELENIUM		The body needs this mineral in very small amounts (see Vol. 1, p. 409), but it performs very important functions. Minerals such as selenium are called **trace elements**. The entire body contains approximately 1 mg of selenium. Selenium is an **antioxidant** that stimulates the **immune system** and protects against **cancer**, particularly of the **skin**.[7] **USE AS A SUPPLEMENT**: the **amount** of selenium in **foods** is **varied** and **unpredictable**, since it depends on the amount in the soil where the food was grown. For this reason supplemental selenium may be used in addition to foods rich in trace elements (see Vol. 1, p. 409), particularly when there is risk of cancer or cardiovascular disease.
FLAVONOIDS OR BIOFLAVONOIDS		These glucoside-type natural dyes are widespread throughout plant foods and have a significant **antioxidant and anti-inflammatory** effects, as well as protecting the **capillaries**. They potentiate the action of **vitamin C**, with which they are usually found in plant foods. They are non-nutritive components of foods known as **PHYTOCHEMICALS**. The best known are **quercetin, catechin** (primarily in onions and apples), **rutin**, and **hesperidin** (in oranges and other citrus). **Function:** numerous beneficial functions are attributed to flavonoids. Among them are **protection** against **cancer, arteriosclerosis** and cellular **aging**.[8] The beneficial effect of unfermented grape juice, and to a lesser extent, red wine on the arteries and the heart is due to its flavonoid content (see Vol. 1, p. 411).[9] **USE AS A SUPPLEMENT:** A diet rich in fresh **fruits** and **vegetables** provides sufficient flavonoids, but they may be taken as a supplement (30 to 100 mg, two or three times a day).
ANTHOCYANIDINE		This purple or reddish pigment is found in many berries such as black grapes, mulberries, blueberries, and currants. Its action and supplemental dosage are similar to those of **flavonoids**.
CHLOROPHYLL		Plants use chlorophyll to convert light energy into chemical energy to synthesize carbohydrates. It is a **potent antioxidant.** It is found particularly in green leafy vegetables and in tender sprouts of grains and legumes. **Use as a supplement:** Chlorophyll extracts are used as an antioxidant and depurative, and to combat bad breath.

SUPPLEMENTS – continued

Supplement	Vol./Page	Description
CHOCOLATE	EMP 597	Chocolate is considered a supplement due to its energy content and stimulant action.

Composition: Chocolate is made from cocoa, cocoa butter, sugar, vanilla, and, in some cases, milk. It contains the following nutrients and stimulant substances:

- *Carbohydrates* (particularly sugar), 50-55%.
- *Fat*, primarily saturated: 30-35%.
- *Protein:* 3-6%.
- *Vitamins:* particularly B₂ and E. It lacks A and C.
- *Minerals and trace elements:* it is a good source of magnesium, iron, potassium, zinc, and chromium.
- *Stimulant substances:* phenylethylamine (similar to amphetamines), theobromine (similar to caffeine), and variable amounts of caffeine depending on the cocoa used in manufacture (100 g of chocolate may contain as much as 60 mg of caffeine, somewhat less than a cup of coffee).

USE AS A SUPPLEMENT: compared with coffee, tea, and guarana, chocolate provides significant *energy* and *nutrients.* It produces a slight sensation of well-being and euphoria similar to a drug, while at the same time providing nutrients.

Drawbacks: regular chocolate consumption may cause or aggravate the following disorders or diseases:

- **Obesity,** due to its elevated energy content (from 400 to 500 calories [= 400 to 500 kcal] for each 100 g).
- **Dental caries** due to high sugar content.
- **Slow digestion and acne** due to high fat content.
- **Constipation** due to lack of fiber.
- **Insomnia, hyperactivity,** and **tachycardia,** particularly in children, due to its stimulant content, and possibly, because of the sugar it contains.
- **Addiction:** Due to its content of stimulants and psychoactive substances, it can create a certain level of dependence, but much less than coffee or other drugs.

Supplement	Vol./Page	Description
SPIRULINA	EMP 276	These microscopic algae are rich in protein, vitamins, and minerals, particularly **iron.** They provide **vitamin B₁₂,** although some researchers state that its chemical composition cannot be utilized by the body.

USE AS A SUPPLEMENT: Desiccated algae form a powder that is sold in capsules.

Supplement	Vol./Page	Description
LACTOBACILLUS		These germs, produced by the lactic acid fermentation of milk, which converts it to **yogurt,** balance the bacterial flora in the large intestine and improve its function. They also stimulate the immune system.

Foods containing these "friendly" germs are referred to as **"probiotic"** (see Vol. I, p. 203).

USE AS A SUPPLEMENT: These desiccated bacteria may be taken in isolation (without dairy products). They are available as a white powder or as tablets, and should be taken with meals.

Supplement	Vol./Page	Description
TORULA YEAST		This yeast is extracted from a microscopic fungus that ferments wood. Its properties are similar to those of **brewer's yeast.**

Cocoa

Chocolate

MICROORGANISMS

Supplements based on microorganisms are formed by huge numbers of them, generally desiccated and powdered. The most common are microscopic **bacteria, algae, and yeasts.**

Lactobacillus

EMP = Encyclopedia of Medicinal Plants, EDUCATION AND HEALTH LIBRARY, Editorial Safeliz.

SUPPLEMENTS – *continued*

Supplement	Vol./Page	Description

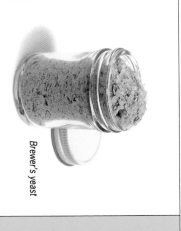

Brewer's yeast

Beer

BREWER'S YEAST

This dry powder is the result of the dehydration of millions of yeast cells (microscopic unicellular fungi) belonging to the genus *Saccharomyces*, similar to those that ferment bread dough. These yeasts proliferate during the brewing process and are used to prepare a dietary supplement referred to as brewer's yeast.

Composition: the most prominent nutrients are:

- **Protein:** 33% of its total weight is protein of **high biological quality.**

- **Vitamins,** *including a small amount of B₁₂. Also contains vitamin D.* all of the **B vitamins,**

- **Minerals and trace elements:** All are present to a greater or lesser degree. Selenium (antioxidant and anticarcinogen[7]) and chromium (whose lack leads to diabetes and arteriosclerosis) stand out.

- **Alpha-lipoic acid** is a potent **antioxidant** whose extracts are used as a complement in the treatment of AIDS because of its antioxidant properties, invigorating effect and as a stimulant of the immune system.

Recommendations for use:

- **Tonic** and **depurant** for the body.

- B group vitamin, mineral, or trace element **deficiency.**

- Liver and skin disorders due to its **antioxidant** and **detoxifying** (promotes the elimination of toxins) properties.

- Radiation therapy for cancer: It has been shown that the use of brewer's yeast reduces undesirable side effects such as loss of appetite and anemia.[18]

Drawbacks:

- It produces **uric acid** and should not be used in cases of gout.

- It can alter the **intestinal flora,** producing flatulence and diarrhea. It is contraindicated in cases of Crohn's disease and ulcerative colitis.[19]

- Contraindicated in cases of yeast infections such as candidiasis caused by *Candida albicans.*

- Unpleasantly bitter taste. Debittered brewer's yeast is commercially available.

USE AS A SUPPLEMENT: 10 to 30 mg a day (1-3 spoonfuls of powder) This is not a supplement for general use due to its drawbacks. It should be used only as recommended.

Pollen: Nutritive Concentrate

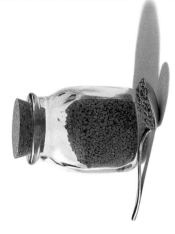

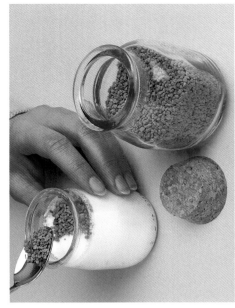

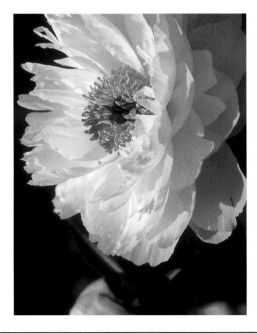

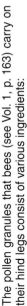

The pollen granules that bees (see Vol. 1, p. 163) carry on their hind legs consist of various ingredients:

- **Pollen** (male germ cells) of flowers (each pollen granule contains between 500,000 and 5,000,000 microscopic pollen grains),
- Flower **nectar,**
- **Secretions** from the bees' hypopharyngeal glands.

By means of a collecting device at the opening to the beehive, bees are forced to drop these granules, which are then bottled and consumed by humans.

Composition

Bee pollen granules are a complex mixture of numerous nutrients:

- *Protein:* 35%, of high biological value and free amino acids;
- *Sugars:* 50%;
- *Fat:* 5% formed of **unsaturated** fatty acids;
- *B vitamins* (including a small amount of B₁₂, C, E, and provitamin A (beta-carotene);
- *Minerals,* among them potassium, calcium, magnesium, and silica;
- *Flavonoids* (see Vol. 1, p. 411) such as *quercetin,* a potent antioxidant.

Properties and Recommendations For Use

Pollen is very nutritious and invigorating. It has a revitalizing effect on the entire body. It is particularly useful in the following cases:

- **Anorexia:** one or two spoonfuls of pollen at breakfast stimulate the appetite by midday.
- **Asthenia** (fatigue), apathy, physical exhaustion.
- **Nervous disorders:** irritability, depression, lowered intellectual performance, scholastic difficulty.
- **Allergies:** taking small quantities of pollen can act as a **desensitizing vaccine** in rhinitis, hay fever, asthma, or migraines caused by allergies. It is important to begin with very low doses (a gram a day, about a pinch), and increase according to tolerance level up to a spoonful (about 15 g) daily.
- **Acne:** from 3 to 5 grams of pollen a day (about one-half dessert spoon) continuously for two to three months contributes to the elimination of acne, possibly due to its effect on hormonal balance. Pollen has a slight estrogenic effect.

Pollen is a highly concentrated food containing a great variety of nutrients. The regular recommended dose is one to two spoonfuls a day (15-30 g), preferably with breakfast. It can be taken with fruit juices, milk, or yogurt.

Royal Jelly: Powerful Tonic

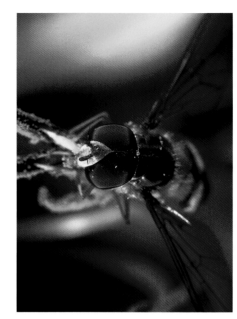

Royal jelly is a creamy whitish fluid that worker bees secrete from their hypopharyngeal glands (see Vol. 1, p. 163). It is designed to feed:

- the larvae of all bees during the first three days of life, and
- the larvae of those bees destined to be queens during their entire life.

Thanks to royal jelly, queens attain greater body development and live 3 to 4 years (workers live only 45 to 50 days).

Composition

The composition of royal jelly is very *similar* to that of **pollen**, but less concentrated (it contains about 68% water).

Its salient feature is its *protein* content (12%) of high biological value, rich in amino acids that are generally missing in other foods, such as lysine and cystine.

From antiquity many have tried to isolate the substance in royal jelly that converts a larva into a queen. This has not yet been accomplished. However, we do know that royal jelly contains protein substances that act in the human body to *stimulate*:

- The function of endocrine glands, particularly the **suprarenal gland**, the **ovaries**, and the **testicles**;
- The **immune system** and the production of **antibodies**;
- The production of **collagen** and the repair of injured **tissue**.

Properties and Recommendations For Use

Although some have idealized and exaggerated its effects, there seems to be evidence confirming that it does possess nutritive and invigorating effects. It also stimulates the hormonal and immune systems and improves blood flow to the body's tissues. It is useful in the following cases:

- As a tonic in case of asthenia, depression, stress, nervousness, physical or mental exhaustion, memory loss.
- **Sexual impotence** in males and lowered libido in both sexes.
- **Arteriosclerosis**, coronary disease, hypertension; lowers cholesterol level, dilates the arteries, improves blood flow.
- **Immunodeficiency** due to lowered resistance; abuse of antibiotics; chronic infectious diseases; flu, and repeated colds.

Use

Since gastric juices can deactivate some of royal jelly's proteins, it should be taken in **capsule** form. The normal dose is 2 to 4 g daily during a month, and may be repeated three or four times a year.

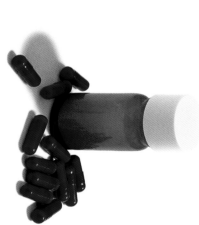

Royal jelly stimulates hormone glands, particularly the suprarenal, the testicles, and the ovaries.

Allergies to Products of the Beehive

Pollen, royal jelly, and propolis can cause allergic reaction in sensitized individuals, particularly children.

Consequently, they must be used *cautiously* with *children, and never with infants under one year of age.*

Propolis: Natural Antibiotic

Propolis is a viscous substance made by bees (see Vol. 1, p. 163) using:

- Their own **secretions,** mixed with
- **Resin** and **sap** from various trees, particularly pines and other conifers, birch, and ash.

A typical beehive produces between 150 and 300 grams of propolis a year. The bees use it as:

- a construction material to repair damage to the hive, and to varnish its interior.
- an antiseptic, due to its ability to destroy fungi, bacteria, and viruses.

Composition

- *Resins:* 55%
- *Waxes:* 25%
- *Essential oils:* 10%
- *Pollen:* 5%
- *Flavonoids, vitamins, organic acids,* and *minerals:* 5%

Properties and Recommendations For Use

Propolis is useful for humans as well as bees.

- **Natural antibiotic:** many of the component substances of propolis arrest the growth of various bacteria such as staphylococcus, streptococcus, salmonella, and a variety of bacteria that cause intestinal infections.

  – It is as effective topically on the skin or mucosa as when taken orally.

  – It does not depress the body's immunity as do other antibiotics, but rather **it stimulates the immune system.**

  – It is particularly recommended for **respiratory** (pharyngitis, bronchitis) or **digestive** (gastroenteritis, colitis) **infections.**

- **Virucide:** Propolis is active against flu and herpes viruses. Its effect on other viruses such as AIDS is under investigation.

- **Fungicide:** It impedes the growth of various microscopic fungi that affect the skin and mucosa such as *Candida albicans.* In these cases it is applied topically as an ointment or other preparations.

- **Emollient and antitussive:** Protects and reduces inflammation of the respiratory system. It is recommended for upper respiratory infections (pharyngitis, laryngitis, sinusitis, etc.), bronchitis and cough from various causes.

- **Anti-inflammatory and antirheumatic.**

- **Local anesthetic:** it is used for dental pain by applying a drop of tincture to the affected area.

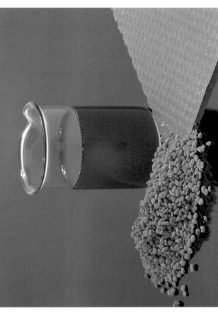

Propolis is a natural antibiotic recommended for respiratory infections.

Dosage and Packaging

Normal dose by mouth is 300 to 500 mg two to three times daily, in any of these forms:

- Syrup or tincture,
- Chewing gum,
- Capsules,
- Ointments or other dermatological preparations.

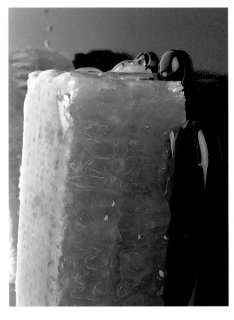

Bees produce propolis from the resins of various trees to protect the beehive from pathogenic microorganisms.

17

BEVERAGES

After the oxygen that we breathe, without which we can survive only a few minutes, there is nothing more essential to our survival than water. When a human is deprived of it, survival is a matter of only a few days.

ALL LIVING creatures need water. Humans take in a certain amount of it as part of their **food**, but this is *not* **sufficient** to satisfy their physiological needs. Even with a diet based on fruits and vegetables that contain up to 95% water, it is essential to drink liquid water.

The *primordial* function of any **beverage** is to supply *water* to the body, with or without other substances dissolved in it. These *accompanying* substances can be of two types:

- **Nutritive,** such as vitamins, minerals, and sugars found in fruit and vegetable juices. Milk is a beverage that, in addition, contains protein and fat (see Vol. 1, p. 180).

- **Non-nutritive,** such as caffeine, alcohol, and various additives. Beverages not containing nutritive substances tend to be **unhealthful,** *even* **dangerous.**

Water

Water is the only **essential beverage,** and the one that most relieves thirst. When the water supply to the body diminishes, health progressively deteriorates. Drinking water is *as* **essential** as **breathing** for good health.

How Much Water Is Needed

The body *continually* **loses** water through numerous physiological processes: breathing, perspiration, and urine and feces production. It is necessary to take in enough water to *compensate* for these **losses** and, if possible, *a little* **more.**

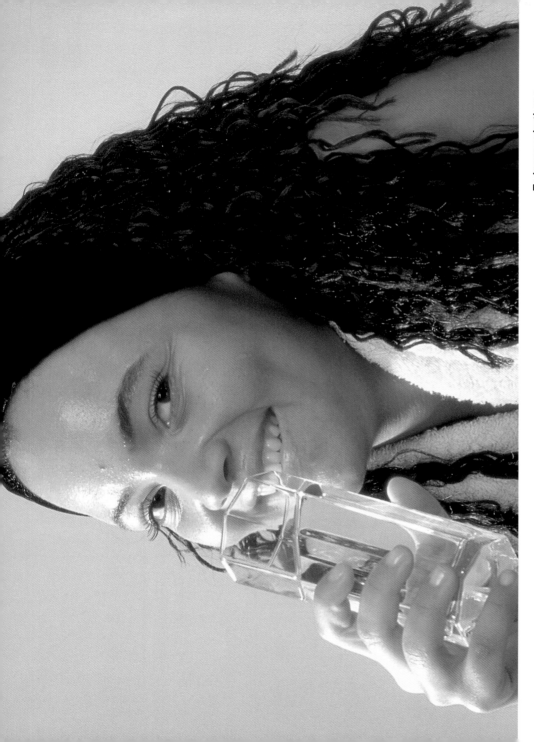

For an adult weighing 70 kilos (154 lbs), these losses are estimated to be about 2,600 ml ($\simeq$ 5.49 pint). Bearing in mind that the water contained in foods plus that obtained through its metabolism sum about 1,100 ml ($\simeq$ 2.32 pint), we should drink another 1,500 ml ($\simeq$ 3.17 pint) to balance the losses (2,600 ml $\simeq$ 5.49 pint). This 1,500 ml (a liter and a half $\simeq$ 3.17 pint) of water can be obtained by drinking a daily average of 6 to 8 glasses. In hot climates double or more water may be necessary.

When To Drink Water

The ideal is to drink water 15 to 30 minutes before meals, and not during or after. By doing so, water increases stomach volume, makes its contractions more difficult, and dilutes gastric juices, all of which slows down digestion.

It is preferable not to drink water two or three hours before bedtime, particularly

To know whether a healthy individual is drinking enough water, it is only necessary to observe the appearance of the urine: a pale yellow color indicates adequate hydration, while a golden or intense yellow signals a lack of water.

Beverages

- **Beverages** *are liquids that **quench the thirst**, and whose basic component is **water** (H_2O), alone or accompanied by other substances.*
- **Nutritive beverages** *are those beverages whose **substances dissolved** in water possess nutritional value. The most common are fruit and vegetable **juices**, and **milk**.*
- **Non-nutritive beverages** *are those providing virtually **no nutrients** other than water and sugar. This is the case with **soft drinks**, **coffee**, and **alcoholic beverages**.*

Daily Balance of the Body's Water

Each day one must **drink** at least **as much** water as is **lost**. This means that an adult must drink 7 or 8 glasses of water of 200 ml each under normal conditions.

Water supply		Water loss	
Foods	850 ml	Perspiration	700 ml
Results of metabolism	250 ml	Breathing	350 ml
Beverages	1,500 ml	Urine	1,400 ml
		Feces	150 ml
Total	2,600 ml	Total	2,600 ml

for men suffering with prostate enlargement. This avoids having to interrupt one's sleep to urinate in the middle of the night.

Benefits of Proper Hydration

The body of a normal **adult** contains approximately 60% water. To maintain this optimum level the daily intake of water must at least equal the loss.

There are persons who, by ignoring their thirst, submit their bodies to a permanent state of dehydration without even being aware of it. This can produce numerous disorders.

However, when one drinks enough water, and the body is properly hydrated, one experiences the following health benefits:

- **Renal function** *improves*, producing *more* and *clearer* **urine**. In this way, the kidneys better purify the blood of waste material and the latter is eliminated more easily.
- There is *less* **risk** of kidney **stones**.
- The **feces** are less dry and are eliminated with less effort.
- The **blood** is less concentrated so there is *less* **risk** of **thrombosis** (clotting within the blood vessels).
- **Fatigue resistance and physical output** *increase*, something of particular importance for athletes.

After physical exercise, drinking one liter of water for each hour of intense activity is recommended. **Isotonic beverages** are particularly useful in replacing mineral salts lost through perspiration.

Isotonic Beverages

Water is a **hypotonic** beverage, *because the concentration of its dissolved substances is less than that of* **perspiration** *and other body* **fluids.** For this reason, when one **perspires** *heavily* or loses liquid due to **diarrhea**, drinking only water is insufficient. It is necessary to drink other beverages or eat foods containing *mineral salts*, as well.

Isotonic beverages are especially formulated to easily replace the mineral salts lost through perspiration, vomiting, or diarrhea. Athletes, who perspire profusely during physical exercise, are the ones who most frequently use them. In addition to water they contain:

- **Salt** (sodium chloride),
- Other **minerals**: potassium and a small amount of magnesium and calcium.
- **Sugar**: 60 to 70 g/l (about 1 ounce per pint), approximately half of that of soft drinks.

Benefits of Isotonic Beverages

- They *rapidly* **replace** minerals lost through perspiration.
- They do *not* contain **stimulants** *or* **carbonation.**

Drawbacks to Isotonic Beverages

- They often contain chemical **sweeteners:** Many isotonic beverages contain **aspartame** (see Vol. 1, p. 179), which, among other drawbacks, increases thirst.
- *They lack* **vitamins,** which are essential for converting carbohydrates into energy. Therefore, although isotonic beverages provide more salt and sodium than fruits, they are *not* as **effective** as **natural fruit juices** in supplying the energy needs of athletes. Fruit juices are rich in vitamins, minerals, and sugars.

Composition of Soft Drinks

Water

Carbon dioxide gas (CO$_2$), which dissolves very well in water (up to 8 g/l).

Chemical Sweeteners do not provide calories, and are used to partially or totally replace sugar. The most common chemical sweetener in soft drinks is **aspartame** (see Vol. 1, p. 179).

Caffeine: Some cola drinks contain **cola nut** *extract*, which is a tropical fruit containing **caffeine** as an ingredient. Caffeine is added directly to other beverages. The proportion of caffeine in soft drinks is usually 0.02%, or 20 mg/100 ml, which is more than 60 mg in a can of soft drink. This is an amount *similar* to that found in a **cup of coffee.**

Common Sugar (saccharose), or other types of sugars such as **glucose** or **fructose.**

Acids: the most common in cola drinks is **phosphoric acid**, an inorganic acid that is **highly acidifying** to the blood. Fruit-flavored soft drinks tend to contain organic acids from fruit such as **citric acid** and **malic acid.**

Other Additives: flavorings, colorings, stabilizers, and preservatives.

Soft Drinks

Soft drinks are beverages, usually carbonated, with *no nutritional value*, except the **sugar** that they may contain. They are made *primarily* from **artificial** ingredients.

Their consumption is very common in many Western countries, to the point that they are normally drunk in place of water or natural juices. This custom is *particularly* **harmful for** *children.*

Soft Drinks and Children

A study conducted at the Hospital of Southampton (UK)[1] has shown that children who drink a great deal of soft drinks experience the following negative health effects:

- They obtain up to *half* of their daily **energy** supply from the **sugar** in soft drinks. This creates a metabolic imbalance that *predisposes* them to **arteriosclerosis** and **diabetes** as adults. It is recommended that sugar make up **no** *more than 10%* of total dietary calories.

- They are **malnourished**, since soft drinks are non-nutritive, but create lack of appetite.

- They exhibit nervous **irritability, lack of appetite,** and **diarrhea.**

All of these symptoms disappear when the amount of soft drinks is reduced.

Water quenches the thirst better than any soft drink. If it is of good quality or bottled mineral water, it is much more healthful.

A good time to drink one or two glasses of room temperature water (not cold) is upon awakening. In this way secretions retained in the stomach overnight are removed and the kidneys are activated.

Continued on page 370

Soft Drinks: Beverages

Fruit-flavored Beverages

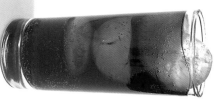

Almost all are carbonated and are referred to as sodas. They *lack nutritional value* except the sugar they contain (90-120 g/l).

Cola Beverages

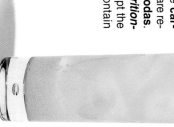

These contain sugar or chemical sweeteners, carbon dioxide, a variety of natural extracts, phosphoric acid, and caffeine. They are simply unhealthful with many *drawbacks.*

Cola beverages are particularly undesirable for children and for those suffering from insomnia or cardiac disease because of their caffeine content.

Tonic Water

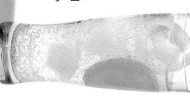

These are sweetened (80-100 grams of sugar per liter, about 1.5 ounces per pint) carbonated beverages, which contain fruit extracts and a small amount of quinine (45-85 mg/l). Quinine is an alkaloid extracted from the quinine tree (see *EMP* p. 752) endowed with fever reducing, antimalarial, and invigorating effects.[2]

Tonic water contains no caffeine or phosphoric acid.

"Bitters"

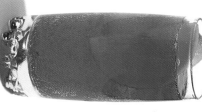

"Bitters" are *similar in* composition to tonic water, but with less quinine and more sugar (up to 135 g/l). Their characteristic ingredient is a bitter natural extract, which increases the appetite and aids digestion. Their primary drawback, however, is that *their high sugar content counteracts any* possible health benefits provided by the plant extracts.

The Calories in a Can of Soft Drink

A *330 ml* (11 ounces) can of soft drink, either cola or *fruit-flavored,* sweetened with sugar contains around *35 g* (1.25 ounces) *of sugar, which provides 140 calories,* approximately the same as:

- *55 g* (2 ounces) *of bread,*
- *400 ml* (about 1 pint) of *nonfat milk,* or
- *240 g* (about half a pound) of *apples* (two medium-sized apples).

However, the calories in soft drinks have a serious drawback: they are *"empty."* This means that vitamins or minerals do not accompany them. Because of this, they *foster obesity and upset metabolism.*

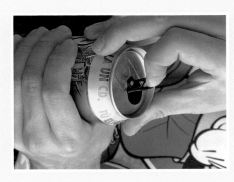

Without Nutritional Value

Benefits of Soft Drinks

- **Water content:** From a health standpoint, the *only positive* aspect of soft drinks is their **water** content. By drinking soft drinks one is drinking water, which improves kidney function.

- **Stimulate digestion:** The carbonation in soft drinks *irritates* the stomach mucosa *to some degree*, resulting in *increased* **gastric juice production**, which speeds digestion.

- **They do *not* contain alcohol.**

The nutritional value of soft drinks is virtually nonexistent, except the sugar they contain. Their many additives present a health risk.

In reality, the only positive aspect to soft drinks is their water content.

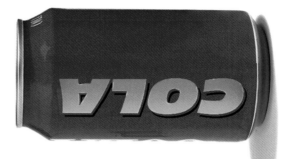

Drawbacks to Soft Drinks

- **They are *not* thirst-quenching:** Because of sugar content and other chemical substances, many soft drinks leave an after-thirst. This leads to even greater thirst than before.

- **"Empty" calories:** Sugar-sweetened soft drinks contain many calories, which are **"empty"** (see box on previous page). In order for the **sugar** in a soft drink to be *transformed* into **energy, *B-group vitamins and minerals*** are *essential*. Since these are absent in soft drinks, they must be obtained from the body's own reserves, thus depleting them. In situations where the individual is not involved in physical exercise, this sugar is *turned to **fat.***

- **Stomach irritation:** Some degree of irritation and inflammation of the mucous lining of the stomach is associated with the digestive process of carbonated beverages. Soft drinks *should be avoided* in cases of **gastritis**, gastroduodenal **ulcer**, and digestive **disorders** in general. [3]

- **Dental caries:** The combination of sugar and acids such as phosphoric acid and others attack dental enamel *very* **aggressively.** Soft drink consumption is a causal factor in dental caries. [3]

- **Decalcification:** Several acids, including phosphoric acid, are added to cola beverages. Phosphoric acid **acidifies** the blood, which the body attempts to neutralize by releasing calcium and other minerals from the bones. That is why cola beverages have a decalcifying action and *should be particularly* ***avoided*** in cases of **rickets** and **osteoporosis.**

- **Allergies:** Many of the additives in soft drinks can cause allergies, which may manifest in many ways:
  - skin eruptions,
  - stomach pain and digestive disorders,
  - nervous irritability and hyperactivity.

- **Urinary stones:** *Regular consumption* of cola **beverages** *increases the **risk*** of urinary stones. This is because they foster elimination of calcium and oxalates through the urine. These substances form most urinary stones. [4]

Nourishing

In addition to quenching the thirst, these beverages provide nutrients and exercise healing and preventive effects on the body.

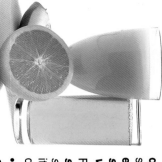

Fruit Juices

Fruit juices are *ideal thirst-quenchers*, while at the same time they supply *energy* in the form of *natural sugars* accompanied with *vitamins and minerals*.

Fresh fruit juice *(fresh-squeezed)* contains the *same nutrients* as the *fruit* itself, *except fiber*, which is discarded with the pulp.

• **Orange juice** is rich in *vitamin C, carotenoids, and flavonoids,* all of which are **antioxidants.** Those suffering from gall bladder disorders may not tolerate orange juice well if drunk on an empty stomach.

• **Apple juice** is digestive, diuretic, depurant, and laxative. It is rich in *potassium* and *iron*. It is suggested for **constipation** and **skin** and **liver** conditions.

• **Peach juice** is rich in provitamin A and vitamins B₁, B₂, B₆, and C. It is *highly recommended* in cases of **heart** and **kidney** disease and arterial **hypertension.**

• **Pineapple juice** is an aperitif and digestive aid. It is very *effective* for **dyspepsia** (indigestion) caused by stomach disorders.

It is important to bear in mind that certain industrially-prepared juices, such as apple juice, can cause digestive disorders and diarrhea (see Vol. 1, p. 35).

Vegetable Juices

Freshly prepared vegetable juices retain all the medicinal properties of the vegetables. They are very rich in vitamins and minerals. Carrot and tomato juices are probably the most used because of their exceptionally *high content* of carotenoids *(provitamin A).*

• **Carrot and tomato juices** are very rich in beta-carotene (provitamin A), which is a *powerful antioxidant.*

• **Celery juice** is a diuretic and depurant.

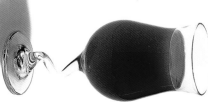

Fruit Nectars

Fruit nectars are fruit juices than have been thickened by *adding* a portion of **fruit pulp.** They also contain added **sugar** (90-120 g/l) and fruit acids. They contain between 400 and 500 calories per liter and less vitamins and minerals than juices.

Drinking a glass of fruit juice, fresh-squeezed if possible, when one gets up in the morning prepares the stomach for breakfast and invigorates the body.

However, the ever-popular orange juice may not go well with those suffering from gallbladder disorders, since it causes abrupt contractions and draining of this organ.

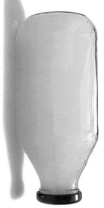

Fruit Drinks

In spite of their commercial name, fruit drinks only contain between **8%** and **12%** fruit juice. The rest is water, sugars, and a variety of additives. Their vitamin and mineral content is ten times less than natural fruit juice. These are the *least nutritious* of those described in this section.

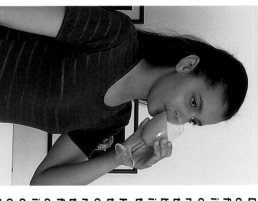

Beverages

Other Nourishing Beverages

- **Cow's milk is the nourishing beverage** *par excellence.* It supplies many nutrients, but it is poor in vitamin C and iron (see chapter 11 Vol. 1, p. 180).

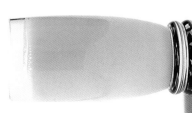

- **Shakes** are prepared with milk and fruit. They are very nutritious, although they may slow digestion somewhat. Shakes containing **artificial** flavors and colors should *be avoided,* particularly by children.

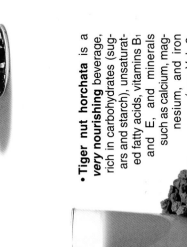

- **Tiger nut horchata** is a *very nourishing* beverage, rich in carbohydrates (sugars and starch), unsaturated fatty acids, vitamins B_1 and E, and minerals such as calcium, magnesium, and iron (see Vol. 2, p. 160).

- **Almond milk** is refreshing, nutritious, and rich in protein and minerals. It can **beneficially** replace **soft drinks** (see Vol. 2, p. 51).

- **Soy milk** may be used to replace milk even though it contains less calcium and lacks vitamin B_{12}. Some commercially available soy beverages are enriched with these nutrients (see Vol. 1, p. 88).

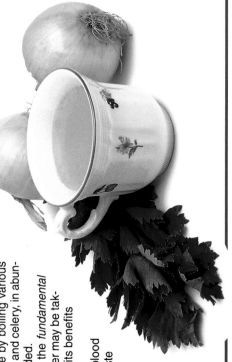

- **Depurant or cleansing vegetable broth** is made by boiling various alkalizing and diuretic vegetables, primarily onions and celery, in abundant water. A small amount of olive oil may be added. This broth is very healthful and constitutes one of the *fundamental* ingredients in a **cleansing diet.** One-half to one liter may be taken a day as a beverage in place of water. Some of its benefits are:

  - **Depurant** or purifying action: It **alkalizes** the blood and urine, which improves the *elimination* of waste products, particularly **uric acid.**
  - **Diuretic:** *Improves* **kidney function** and increases urine output.
  - **Mineralizer:** It supplies a significant amount of *minerals* and *trace elements,* particularly potassium, magnesium, and iron. Potassium prevents arterial hypertension.

Caffeine Content of Various Stimulant Beverages
per 100 ml

Espresso coffee (obtained by pressure)	212 mg
Regular brewed coffee (obtained by brewing and filtration)	58 mg
Brewed black or green tea (obtained by brewing)	30-40 mg
Maté	25-50 mg
Cola beverages (see Vol. 1, p. 366)	20 mg
Iced tea	8-15 mg
Decaffeinated coffee	1-2 mg

Continued from page 365

Stimulant Beverages

The common element in stimulant beverages is their greater or lesser caffeine content. This type of beverage is used more for its stimulant effect than to quench the thirst.

Caffeine

Caffeine is a *toxic* **alkaloid** belonging to the purine chemical group. It is produced in the leaves, seeds, and fruit of some 60 plants throughout the world.

Caffeine *easily* **penetrates** *every* **cell** in the body, *particularly* those of the **nervous system.** Its most important effect is that of stimulating the transmission of nervous impulses between the neurons. It affects the function of the brain, the heart, the stomach, and the kidneys. It is eliminated

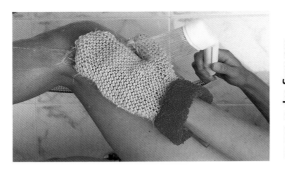

Cold-water friction and other hydrotherapeutic techniques produce natural, healthy stimulation.

When done in the morning and followed by a nutritious breakfast rich in grains and fruits, they are an excellent replacement for a morning cup of coffee.

through the urine between 3 and 6 hours after it is ingested. It is *not* **accumulated** in the body.

Beneficial Effects of Caffeine

When used *as* a **medicine**, caffeine in stimulant beverages may be useful in the following cases:

- **Fainting,** arterial **hypotension,** or **fatigue:** caffeine provides *emergency* stimulation but it does **not resolve** the cause of these disorders.

- **Headache:** caffeine reduces the blood supply to the brain, thus relieving pressure.

Undesirable Effects of Caffeine

- *Reduces* **performance** capacity: stimulant beverages tend to **"fool" the brain,** *masking* **fatigue,** but not truly relieving it. The real performance capacity of the nervous system diminishes after intake of a moderate amount of caffeine, according to a study at Yale University (USA).[5]

- **Cerebral hypoglycemia:** Caffeine creates a transient stimulation, but finishes with a greater sense of fatigue, similar to that of hypoglycemia or fainting. This is due to a reduction in glucose arriving at the brain, which results in *lowered* **mental performance.**[5]

- **Addiction:** In spite of their apparent innocence, stimulant beverages constitute a *true* **drug,** with **great** *capacity* to create physical as well as psychological **dependence.**

- **Abstinence syndrome:** those addicted to coffee or other stimulant beverages often suffer various symptoms when they miss their regular dose of caffeine: tiredness, nervous irritability, inability to concentrate, anxiety, headache, or even tremors or other physical symptoms.

- **Functional changes:** Stimulant beverages foster insomnia, gastritis, and arrhythmia (alterations in cardiac rhythm). Their use is particularly **discouraged** in cases of nervous, digestive, and cardiac disorders. The drawbacks to coffee are described in Vol. 1, p. 374.

Healthy Alternatives to Coffee and Other Stimulant Beverages

There are a variety of beverages suitable to replace coffee, tea, and other stimulants; some of these have additional health benefits.

Malt and Chicory

Malt (see Vol. 2, p. 164) is nutritious and easily digested, and has a flavor similar to that of coffee.

Chicory root (see Vol. 2, p. 176; *EMP* p. 440) is used to brew a slightly bitter beverage suitable to replace coffee. It is highly digestible and improves liver function.

Various Plant Infusions

Those products whose flavor allows them to replace coffee and tea are described in detail in the *Encyclopedia of Medicinal Plants* (*EMP*).

Decaffeinated Coffee

The composition of decaffeinated coffee is identical to that of regular coffee, with the difference that it does not contain caffeine, which is tasteless. As a result decaffeinated coffee retains the same aroma and flavor as regular.

It *cannot* be said, however, that it is **a healthful** beverage. It provides no nutrients other than the water with which it is brewed. However, it is *preferable* to regular coffee, because it has been proved that by replacing regular with decaffeinated coffee:

- Arterial pressure *is reduced,*[6,7]
- Gastroesophageal **reflux** and **heartburn** are *reduced,*[8]

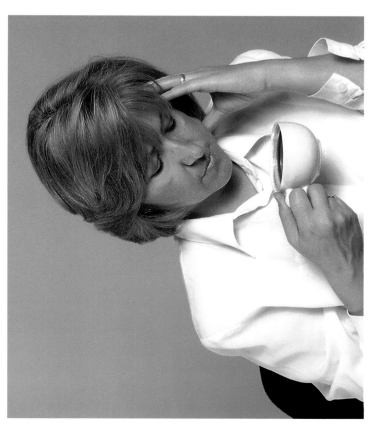

Coffee, tea, maté, and cola beverages excite the nervous system, but provide no nutrients essential to its proper function. Due to this, exhaustion results from habitual use of these products.

- The **harmful effects** of caffeine on the nervous system, the heart, and the digestive system *are avoided* (see Vol. 1, p. 375).

However, certain negative effects of coffee are not due to caffeine, but rather other substances in the coffee also present in the decaffeinated, as well.

Therefore, replacing regular coffee with decaffeinated coffee, has *no lowering effect* on **cholesterol** level.[9] On the other hand, the use of malt, chicory, or other plants in place of coffee does have this effect.

Continued on page 376

Stimulant

All of these have the alkaloid caffeine in common, to which they owe most of their effects and drawbacks.

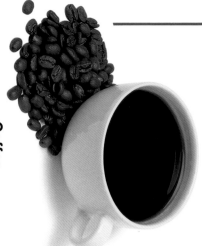

Coffee

See *EMP* p. 178

Coffee is the most consumed of all stimulant beverages, and the one with the highest caffeine content (see Vol. 1, p. 370).

Maté

See *EMP* p. 182

Maté is a uniquely South American beverage prepared by steeping in hot water the leaves of a small tree or bush, whose scientific name is *Ilex paraguayensis.*

Its caffeine concentration and effects are *similar* to **tea.** Maté has some degree of antioxidant effect, just as tea does. However, it has the drawbacks associated with the caffeine it contains. *Heavy use of maté* can lead to **esophageal or pharyngeal cancer,** *particularly if* combined with **alcohol** use.[16]

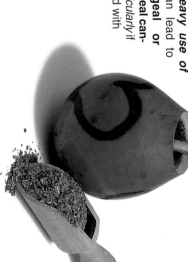

Cola Soft Drinks

These contain a certain amount of **caffeine** in addition to *numerous* **additives** (see Vol. 2, p. 398-399). They are *particularly* **damaging** for *children.*

When a school-aged *child* drinks a cola soft drink (330 ml = 11 ounces), he or she is taking in an amount of caffeine equivalent to an adult drinking *four cups* of **coffee.**[5]

The effects of caffeine on children are more intense than on adults: nervous excitation, hyperactivity, behavioral problems, and sleep disorders.

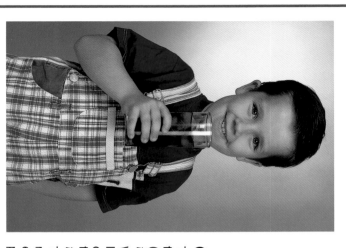

Volume 1 / **372**

EMP = Encyclopedia of Medicinal Plants, Education and Health Library, Editorial Safeliz.

Beverages

Tea

See *EMP* p. 185

Tea is prepared by steeping the leaves of the *Thea sinensis* bush in hot water. There are two types of tea: **green** (*unfermented*) and **black** (the leaves have been *fermented*). Both contain a similar percentage of caffeine.

Tea is *less* **harmful** than coffee since it contains *less* **caffeine** and *does contain* two types of medically active **phytochemicals:**

- **Astringent *phenolic tannins*.** It has been seen that these substances, present in many other plants as well, *partially* **neutralize** the **carcinogenic** effect of the **nitrosamines** that form in cured meats and sausages (see Vol. 1, p. 271). When these nitrosamine-containing foods are eaten with tea, their carcinogenic action is reduced.[10]

- **Antioxidant *flavonoids*.** Tea drinkers are presumably at lower risk of arteriosclerosis[11] and cardiovascular conditions[12] due to the presence of these substances. Fortunately, there are many other plant foods rich in flavonoids (see Vol. 1, p. 411) and free from the drawbacks of caffeine.

However, the beneficial effect of tea on cancer and cardiovascular disease is not clear. A broad study conducted in Great Britain shows that those drinking more than 8 cups of tea a day are 2.4 times more likely to die of a heart attack or a stroke than those who drink less than two cups a day.[13]

Investigators have attributed this negative effect of tea to the British custom of taking tea with milk. This cancels the antioxidant properties of the flavonoids in tea.

Tea contains a substance that **destroys *vitamin B₁***. Because of this, those who drink a great deal of tea may experience a deficiency in this important vitamin to the nervous system.[14]

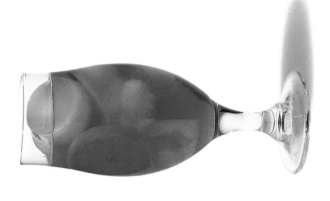

Iced Tea

Commercial iced tea is a cold beverage prepared from water, tea extract, lemon juice (sometimes replaced by citric acid), sugar, and various additives. Its caffeine content should not exceed 15 mg/100 ml. Even though it is refreshing, it is an unhealthful drink since it has *all* of the ***drawbacks*** of **caffeine** and **additives.**

A study in the Netherlands involving more than 120,000 persons has shown that tea drinking does not protect against cancer as was once thought, but neither does it foster it.[15]

The phenolic tannins and flavonoids in tea do give it certain medicinal properties. But there are many medicinal plants, fruits, and vegetables containing these same substances, while being completely free from the negative effects of caffeine.

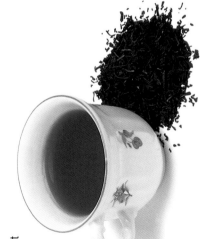

Coffee: a Stimulating

Coffee is a highly aromatic stimulant beverage prepared from roasted and ground coffee beans. Coffee beans are the seeds of the *Coffea arabica* or the *Coffea robusta* plants.

Coffee is a *true* **drug** due to its caffeine content. It meets the criteria set by the World Health Organization (WHO) for drug addiction:

- It creates **addiction** or dependency;
- Produces **tolerance** (the dose must be increased to achieve the same effect);
- Its elimination results in **abstinence syndrome**;
- Its *regular use* is **harmful** to health.

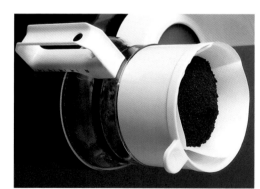

Coffee-drinking raises cholesterol levels. However, this effect is eliminated when it is brewed using a paper filter. The substance that raises cholesterol is not caffeine, but rather an aromatic substance in the coffee that remains in the paper filter.[17, 18]

Contents of a Cup of Coffee

Water makes up between 97.8% and 99.3% by weight, depending on the brewing method.

Carbohydrates make up an irrelevant 0.4% to 1.5%. These are composed of sugars and a miniscule amount of starch.

Coffee contains from 58 to 212 mg/100 l of **caffeine**, which represents 0.058% to 0.212%. Coffee is the **richest** in **caffeine** of any **beverage**. This is particularly so for espresso, which is prepared by forcing steam and hot water through coffee grounds. Espresso is more highly concentrated than that prepared with a regular coffee maker by brewing and filtration.

Vitamins and minerals: There are only *very small* amounts of niacin (0.22 mg/100 g), magnesium (5 mg/100 g), and potassium (54 mg/100 g).

Caffeic and chlorogenic acids, which act as diuretics and irritate the digestive tract.

Essential oil: this is what gives coffee its unique flavor and aroma, but it irritates the mucosa of the stomach and intestine.

The only nutrient that may be found in any significant amount in a cup of coffee is the sugar that may have been added.

and Aromatic Drug

Harmful Effects of Coffee

The harmfulness of coffee is the subject of broad debate among researchers. While some feel that moderate amounts (2 to 3 cups a day) is safe, others are equally certain that it produces numerous disorders.

This page illustrates its proven harmful effects (see Vol. 1, p. 370), which it has in common with other stimulant beverages.

Changes in intellectual performance: An experiment conducted in the psychology department at Nene College in Northampton (UK) shows that more errors are produced in identifying pairs of equal (for example A/a) or different (for example P/a) letters.[19] Although other studies demonstrate that coffee stimulates mental activity, more errors are produced after drinking it as well. This is possibly due to the fact that caffeine reduces the brain's glucose supply[5] (see Vol. 1, p. 370).

Arterial hypertension: when one stops drinking coffee blood pressure drops.[20] This also results from changing to decaffeinated coffee, but not to the same degree.[7]

Acid stomach: coffee increases the production of acid juices in the stomach. It also promotes acid reflux, causing **heartburn** and **esophagitis**. This has been well demonstrated at the Bogenhausen Hospital in Munich (Germany).[23]

Urinary bladder cancer: coffee consumption, *particularly* if *combined* with **alcohol** use, significantly raises the risk of this type of cancer.[24, 25]

Myocardial infarction risk is slightly higher in coffee drinkers, according to a meta-analysis (a compendium of a large body of previous statistics) carried out at Harvard University (USA).[21]

Arrhythmia: Coffee may lead to changes in cardiac rhythm.

Mammary nodules: No statistical relationship has been found between coffee consumption and breast cancer.[26] However, when it is removed from the diet, there is a reduction in the number of mammary nodules in women with fibrocystic dysplasia.[27]

Osteoporosis: Coffee *fosters calcium loss* through the urine.[28] Even though moderate coffee consumption (2 to 3 cups a day) increases calcium loss very little, it does contribute to osteoporosis.

Cholesterol: A study at the University of South Carolina (USA) demonstrated that increasing unfiltered coffee consumption by one cup a day on a regular basis raises blood cholesterol by 20 mg/100 ml.[22]

Compared to the tremendous number of diseases and accidents caused by wine and other alcoholic beverages, the possibly beneficial effects on the heart are insignificant from a public health standpoint.

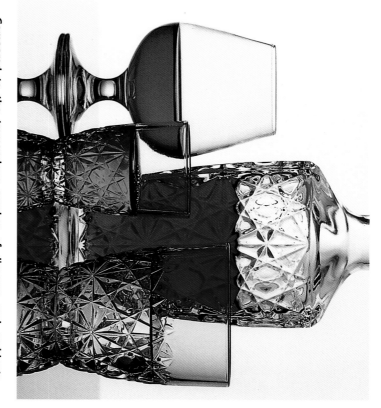

icinal property of alcoholic beverages has been known for thousands of years.

An example is the Good Samaritan of the biblical parable, who treated the wounds of the victim he found by the road with wine and oil.[29]

The Most Pernicious Drug

Alcoholic beverages cause much *more* **physical disease** and moral **suffering** throughout the world, than any other drug, whether legal or illegal. Taken together, they are a true scourge and a curse on humanity. Only certain beverages such as red wine, drunk in very limited amounts by certain individuals (adult males), may have some statistically beneficial effect.

This *possible* **beneficial action** of red wine on cardiovascular health has been *intentionally* **exaggerated** *for commercial reasons*, as has been recognized by the World Health Organization (WHO).[30] At the same time the numerous negative effects of their consumption are silenced, even when the consumption is moderate.

Continued from page 371

Alcoholic Beverages

All alcoholic beverages contain a certain proportion of **ethyl alcohol**. This substance is produced by a variety of yeasts or microscopic fungi as they decompose fruit glucose in a process known as **alcoholic fermentation**.

Medicinal, Yes, But For External Application Only

Many medicinal properties have been attributed to alcoholic beverages throughout history. However, the only one completely proven and lacking undesirable side effects is its **antiseptic action** when applied externally.

Because of their **ethyl alcohol** content, *all* alcoholic beverages act as **disinfectants** and **antiseptics** when they are applied to wounds and lesions of the skin. This med-

From a health point of view, nothing positive can be said for spirits, in spite of the folklore surrounding whisky. They are all extremely detrimental, and are classified within the group of hard, dangerous drugs.

Contraindications to Alcoholic Beverages

• They give a *sense* of **power and ability** but *in reality* they **diminish** physical and mental **capacity**. A half-gram of alcohol per liter of blood, (0.5 g/l, the amount reached after drinking a glass of wine), is enough to dangerously reduce one's ability to drive an automobile.

• They *increase sexual desire*, but *diminish* the **capacity** to perform.

• They give a *sense* of **energy**, but *in reality* they **reduce** it, since the calories released from alcohol as it metabolizes in the body cannot be used to produce muscular work.

• They give a **warm sensation**, but *in reality* they **cool** the body by increasing the blood flow near the skin, causing the loss of body heat.

• They give a *sense* of **health**, but *in reality* they **ruin it**. Alcoholic beverages **do not nourish**, and alcohol is not a nutrient, but rather a poison.

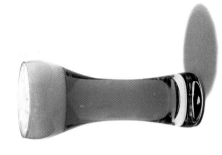

Non-alcoholic beer is a good alternative to regular beer. It provides a small amount of vitamin B$_{12}$ as well as other B vitamins and trace elements, such as chromium.

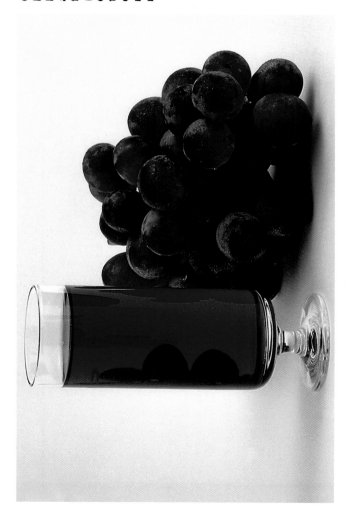

Grape juice has true healing properties. It contains the same antioxidant flavonoids as wine (resveratrol and quercetin), but with the added benefits of vitamins and minerals and no alcohol.

"Alcoholic" Beverages Without Alcohol

Alcohol is the primary drawback of alcoholic beverages from a health standpoint. Because of this, efforts have been made to eliminate it from such popular beverages as beer, liqueurs, and even wine.

Non-alcoholic Beer

So-called non-alcoholic beer usually contains a small amount of ethyl alcohol, equal to or less than 1% (regular beer contains from 5% to 7%). This amount of alcohol has no perceptible effects on the mind or the nervous system in most individuals, and does not create addiction.

Its consumption is increasing since its flavor and refreshing effect are very similar to regular beer, but without the drawbacks. It also supplies a variety of vitamins such as B$_{12}$ and trace elements such as chromium, which is highly recommended for diabetics.

Reliable scientific data is not yet available regarding the carcinogenic **nitrosamine** content of non-alcoholic beer, but it is sus-

pected that it is less than that of regular beer.

Although non-alcoholic beer has certain negative aspects such as its carbonation and subsequent irritating effect on the stomach, it is a good alternative for those wishing to avoid alcoholic beverages.

Non-alcoholic Wine

Recently wines with most of the alcohol removed have appeared on the market. These non-alcoholic wines contain the same antioxidant flavonoids from the grape that are in regular wine. Non-alcoholic wine is recommended for those wishing to reduce the risk of heart attack, as a healthy alternative to regular wine.

In contrast to unfermented grape juice, which is sweet, non-alcoholic wine has almost no natural sugars (glucose and fructose). Due to this, its flavor is quite similar to regular wine.

Non-alcoholic wine is preferable to regular wine. However, **unfermented grape juice** is *superior* to it in medicinal properties and healing power.

Scientific investigation has uncovered more negative aspects than positive to wine and other alcoholic beverages, even in low to moderate doses. However, these are seldom spoken of.

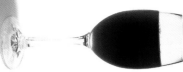

Various statistical studies have shown that drinking one or two small glasses of wine a day may reduce myocardial infarction risk in men fifty years old and older.

However, many other studies demonstrate that moderate consumption of wine or other alcoholic beverages increases risk of arterial hypertension, esophageal reflux, gastritis, liver disease, and various types of cancer, among other diseases.[35]

So the benefit-risk ratio for wine is much lower than reported. Compared to unfermented grape juice, wine offers very little benefit at a very high risk.

Positive Aspects of Wine

- **Stimulates digestion:** Alcohol *irritates* the mucosa of the digestive tract much in the same way it irritates the tissue of a wound on the skin. The cells of the stomach's mucosa secrete more juices to counteract this irritation. This, in turn, promotes digestion. In other words, the digestive stimulation produced by alcohol is at the expense of *irritation and inflammation* of the stomach mucosa, which can result in **gastritis**, gastroduodenal **ulcer,** or **cancer** of the esophagus or stomach. These diseases are more common among drinkers, even moderate drinkers.

- **Beneficial action on the heart:** Various statistical studies show that drinking between *100 and 200 ml* (1/2-1 cup) of red wine a day (not white wine) lowers the risk of death from heart attack.[31,32,33] This effect *only* seems to involve *men* over the *age of 50.*

  These same statistics report that when more than this amount of wine (*200 ml* or about 1 cup of wine or 20 g of pure alcohol) is *exceeded,* the *mortality rate* due to *cardiovascular* disease *increases,* and *many other disorders* are fostered.[34]

  The possible beneficial effect of red wine has been attributed to two of its ingredients:

  - **Ethyl alcohol:** Some statistical studies have shown that any alcoholic beverage, even in small amounts, has a protective effect on the heart.[35] However, experiments conducted with laboratory animals show that only high blood alcohol levels, at least 2 grams per liter (2 g/l) of blood, is enough to reduce the platelets' tendency to clot within the arteries.[36] In other words, in order for alcohol to affect blood clotting positively, one would need to be intoxicated, with all of the health concerns that entails.

    Smaller amounts of alcohol, such as one or two glasses of wine a day, have been proved insufficient to protect the cardiovascular system.

  - *Phenolic* *flavonoids:* these substances come from the grape and its skin, which give red wine its color.[32] They act to inhibit the oxidation of lipoproteins, and by so doing, prevent cholesterol deposits within the arteries known as **arteriosclerosis.**[37] **Fruit** in general, and **grapes** in particular, are the best sources of *flavonoids.*

    In other words, whatever small benefit may come from wine is from the grape. Eating **grapes** themselves or drinking **grape juice** is *much more healthful* for the heart and the entire body.

About Wine

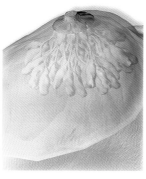

Women who drink alcoholic beverages, including wine, even in small amounts, are at higher risk for breast cancer and other disorders.

Drawbacks to Wine and Other Alcoholic Beverages

Virtually *everyone recognizes* that consuming *large amounts* of alcohol is **harmful**. However, numerous studies confirm undesirable effects of even reduced amounts of alcohol, such as the wine recommended to reduce heart attack risk:

- **Cerebral hemorrhage** is more frequent among drinkers.[38]

- **Arterial hypertension:** It has been shown that three or more glasses of wine a day can increase arterial pressure, which represents a risk factor to the cardiovascular system.[39]

- **Cancer in general** is more frequent among moderate drinkers than nondrinkers.[40]

- **Colon cancer** is also more frequent among those who drink moderately than those who do not drink at all.[41]

- **Breast cancer:** Women who consume moderate amounts of alcohol are at higher risk of breast cancer, as is confirmed by studies throughout the world. For example:
  - The University of Milan (Italy) has verified that women who drink 24.3 g of alcohol (one-fourth liter or 1 cup of wine, approximately) or more a day, are at twice the risk of breast cancer than nondrinkers.[42]
  - A study in the United States involving 89,539 women showed that those who consumed 15 g of alcohol a day (about 150 ml of wine) are at 2.5 times higher risk of breast cancer than those who do not drink.[43]

- **Stomach cancer:** The relationship between alcohol use and cancers of the esophagus and the stomach has been well known for many years. The General Direction of Health in Portugal conducted a study to quantify this relationship. It was observed that the greater the wine consumption, the higher the risk of stomach cancer.[44]
  - Drinkers that consume less than one glass of wine with a meal are at a 36% higher risk than nondrinkers.

  - Those who consume a bottle or more a day are at almost four times greater risk than nondrinkers.

- **Esophageal reflux:** The Clinic Hospital of Barcelona (Spain) has confirmed that men who drink 360 ml of wine during meals (somewhat less than two glasses) experience 70% more esophageal reflux than those who drink the same amount of water. Reflux is the ascension of the acid content of the stomach into the esophagus, causing heartburn (a burning sensation and inflammation of the esophagus, called esophagitis).[45]

- **Bone fracture:** women who drink 25 grams of alcohol (one large glass of wine) or more a day are at 2.33 times greater risk of hip fracture than those who do not drink.[46] Moderate amounts of alcohol, as well as coffee (see Vol. 1, p. 375), promote osteoporosis and possible bone fractures.

- **Fetal alterations:** Pregnant women who drink 400 ml (two glasses) or more of wine a day, or its equivalent in other alcoholic beverages, have a higher incidence than nondrinkers of:[47]
  - Premature births,
  - Low birthweight babies, and
  - Immature placentas.

  Greater amounts of alcohol during pregnancy affect the fetus even more seriously and may lead to birth defects (fetal alcohol syndrome).

- **Other diseases:** Alcohol consumption is associated with *higher* risk of cirrhosis of the liver, **cerebral atrophy, arrhythmia, cardiomyopathy** (degeneration of the heart muscle itself), and **gout**.
  Any **possible benefit** that *small amounts* of wine or other alcoholic beverage may have on the heart is far *outweighed* by its **drawbacks**. As a result, the World Health Organization and other specialists state categorically that alcohol intake as a prophylaxis for heart disease should not be promoted as a public health measure. In other words, *no health benefits* are obtained by **recommending** that *nondrinkers* should *drink* a little wine.[31, 36]

Beer,

Positive Characteristics of Beer

- **Lower alcohol content:** beer contains from 5% to 7% alcohol, approximately half that of wine and eight times less than whisky and other liquors. Because alcohol is the most injurious component in alcoholic beverages, when **equal volumes** are compared beer is **less harmful** than wine or other liquors.

- **Nutrients:** Beer contains small amounts of **vitamins** and **minerals**, which come in large part from the brewer's yeast used in its manufacture. Brewer's yeast (see Vol. 1, p. 358) is very rich in B group vitamins, minerals, and trace elements. However, brewer's yeast is very diluted in beer. Therefore, the vitamins and minerals are only found in small quantities, although greater than other alcoholic beverages. In 100 g of beer there is:

  — **Vitamins B₂, B₆, niacin,** and **folates:** from 2% to 3% of RDA (recommended dietary allowance). Vitamins C and E are not found in beer.

  — **Vitamin B₁₂:** 1% of RDA. This is an interesting fact for strict vegetarians, who can obtain small amounts of this vitamin from **non-alcoholic** beer, since alcohol is destructive to B group vitamins, and possibly B₁₂, as well.

  — Very small amounts of **minerals:** from 1% to 2% of RDA of calcium, phosphorous, magnesium, and potassium.

  — **Chromium:** beer is one of the **best sources** of this **trace element**, whose lack is involved in the onset of diabetes. **Diabetics** may benefit from beer consumption, preferably without alcohol.

- **Protection against myocardial infarction:** a study carried out at the University of Munster (Germany) shows that Southern Germans who drink moderate amounts of beer suffer fewer heart attacks than non-drinkers.[49]

  However, similar studies conducted at Kiruna Hospital (Sweden) demonstrate the complete opposite: the consumption of beer and other alcoholic beverages provides no heart attack protection for the Swedish population.[50]

  It has been suggested that only dark beer, rich in antioxidant flavonoids similar to those in red wine, provides any protection to the heart.[32] However, the results of research are inconclusive in terms of beer's potential benefits to the cardiovascular system. On the other hand, its negative effect on the cardiac muscle (heart failure) and on other organs is quite clear.

The Ingredients in Beer

Beer is an alcoholic beverage with a fairly low alcohol content, obtained by fermenting malt. These are the primary ingredients involved in its manufacture:

- **Malt** is the aqueous extract of sprouted and toasted grains of barley (see Vol. 1, p. 371). It contains carbohydrates that convert to alcohol when fermented by the action of brewer's yeast.

- **Brewer's yeast** is added to malt to cause fermentation. It is composed of a mold (a special type of microscopic fungus) called Saccharonices cerevisae.

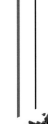

- **Hops extract** is added to beer to give it its typical flavor. Hops (Humulus lupulus) is a bitter-tasting plant with sedative medicinal properties.[48]

- **Carbon dioxide (CO₂):** from 3 to 5 grams of gas per liter.

a Harmless Beverage?

Negative Characteristics of Beer With Alcohol

In addition to the general drawbacks of alcoholic beverages, described in Vol. 1, p. 376, beer has the following:

- **Gastritis:** the carbonation in beer, together with the irritating effect of alcohol, produces a permanent inflammation of the stomach mucosa. Indigestion, slow digestion, gastritis, and gastroduodenal ulcer are the most common among beer drinkers.

- **Cardiac failure:** Beer contains less alcohol by volume. To compensate for this, and reach the alcohol level necessary for the desired state of inebriation, beer drinkers must take great quantities of this beverage. As a consequence of excess liquid, and the harmful action of alcohol on the cardiac muscle, heart failure (incapacity of the heart to pump blood correctly) is common among beer drinkers.

- **Carcinogenic substances:** Beer contains carcinogenic **nitrosamines** (see Vol. 1, p. 271), which explains its relationship with certain types of cancer. These substances are possibly formed during the fermentation process. A study conducted in the German Institute of Cancer Research in Heidelberg

(Germany) demonstrates that beer is the primary source of carcinogenic nitrosamines and supplies 31% of those taken in daily by German men.[51]

- **Rectal cancer:** There are numerous studies that relate consumption of various alcoholic beverages with cancer (see Vol. 1, p. 379), including small to moderate amounts. It has been proven that beer drinkers are at an especially high risk of rectal cancer: 73% higher than that of nondrinkers. The International Cancer Research Agency in Lyon (France) attributes this effect to beer's elevated carcinogenic nitrosamine content.[52]

- **Gout:** *All* alcoholic beverages increase uric acid levels in the blood, but *beer has the greatest impact.*[53] Because of this, beer is contraindicated for those suffering from gout or a tendency toward excess uric acid levels.

- **Migraines:** It is well known that cheese, chocolate, red wine, and beer are the food products that are most frequently responsible for initiating migraine headaches. A study performed at Charing Cross Hospital in London (UK) confirms that beer, specifically, is the product responsible for most migraines.[54]

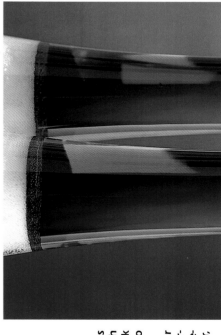

Even though there are studies relating beer consumption with the reduction of heart attack risk,[49] others state that it has no such effect.[50]

One thing clear is that regular beer consumption causes cardiac failure and fosters the development of rectal cancer, gout, and migraines.

18

THE COMPONENTS OF FOODS

The history of the discovery of the components of foods is a lesson in humility for human science. There is more in the plant-based foods provided by nature than can be analyzed in today's laboratory.

WHAT IS an apple made of? What is the composition of an onion? What substances form part of a piece of cheese? Throughout history many have asked similar questions. But it has only been within the last 150 years that science has begun to identify the components of foods; and the search continues.

The Discovery of the Components of Foods

At the beginning of the 20th century, only four food components were known: water, carbohydrates, fats, and proteins. Scientists thought that a diet that supplied these four nutrients was complete.

Vitamins and Minerals

However, even those who ate sufficient amounts of these four nutrients continued to contract diet-related diseases. Some of these, such as beriberi and scurvy, were attributed to unidentified toxic substances, when in reality they were caused by the lack of certain nutritional components, as yet undiscovered, such as vitamin B₁ and vitamin C.

Little by little during the first half of the 20th century, vitamins and minerals present in small amounts in foods began to be identified. The first vitamin to be discovered was A in 1913; the last, B₁₂, in 1955.

Mission Accomplished?

Since the 1960s the list of food components necessary for humans, that is, the list of nutrients, was considered finished. It totaled some fifty different substances, including the 22 types of amino acids that form proteins.

However, it is not possible to nourish a human being indefinitely using only these nutrients or chemical substances in a pure state.

Surprise: New Components in Plant Foods

Therefore there must be other substances in foods required for the body in order to remain healthy and avoid disease; other substances than those already known.

Beyond doubt: During the 1980's, advances in methods of chemical analysis permitted the discovery of hundreds of new components, specifically in plant-based foods, which are called ***phytochemicals*** (see Vol. 1, p. 410).

And the research continues to surprise with new components that, although present in minute amounts in fruits, vegetables, grains, and legumes, exercise significant preventive and healing activity.

One might well ask:

- *How many more components are left to be discovered in oranges, oats, or lentils?*
- *Of those vegetable components known, how many more health benefits do they hide?*

It is only logical to infer that a superior Intelligence placed all of these healing substances precisely there, in plant-based foods (see Vol. 1, p. 22). And for good reason this same creative Being placed these vegetable foods before humans as their ideal food.

Components of a Food

The proportion of weight of each component found in the edible portion of the food shown in the example is presented in parentheses.

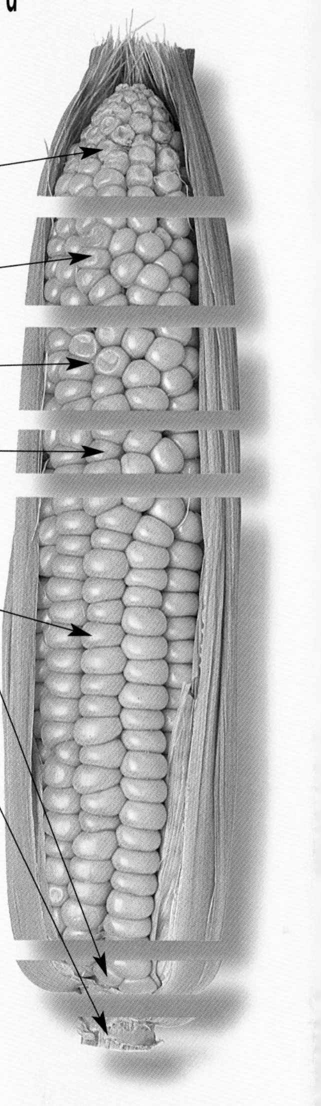

Fiber (2.7%)

Carbohydrates (16.3%)

Proteins (3.22%)

Fats (1.18%)

Water (76%)

Minerals (0.82%)

Other Natural Components

The total weight of these is negligible; therefore, they are not included in the graph of percentage distribution (see Vol. 1, p. 160). Although there may be others, these are the most important:

Vitamins (a few milligrams for each 100 grams of food); ***phytochemicals*** (see Vol. 1, p. 410); ***aromatic compounds; phytosterols*** (in foods of animal origin, cholesterol); **antinutritive factors** (as found in raw legumes, see Vol. 1, p. 84).

Accidental contamination

These may be **chemical** or **biological** (bacteria, viruses, and parasites). Generally, the most common and dangerous are those found in animal-based foods (see Vol. 1, pp. 300, 302, 303).

Added Components (additives)

Definitions

- ***Component:*** *chemical substances present in whatever form in foods:*
  - ***natural,*** *as is the case with nutrients;*
  - ***accidental,*** *as is the case with biological or chemical contaminants;*
  - ***intentional,*** *as additives.*
- ***Nutrient:*** *a food component that the body needs in order to carry out vital functions. Its chemical composition must be known. A food component is classified as a nutrient when its lack in the diet provokes a pathologic condition which disappears when this food component is again available in the body.*

Daily Requirements For A Nutrient

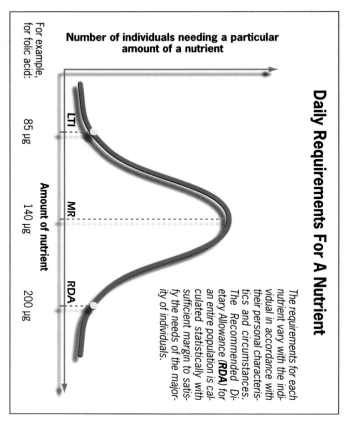

Number of individuals needing a particular amount of a nutrient

Amount of nutrient

For example, for folic acid: 85 µg   140 µg   200 µg
                              LTI   MR   RDA

The requirements for each nutrient vary with the individual in accordance with their personal characteristics and circumstances. The Recommended Dietary Allowance (**RDA**) for an entire population is calculated statistically with sufficient margin to satisfy the needs of the majority of individuals.

Plant-based foods provide all the nutrients necessary, with the exception (doubtful for some) of vitamin B₁₂.

Endogenous Production

The body can synthesize some nutrients: vitamin D is synthesized in the skin; choline, in the liver; biotin and vitamins B₁₂ and K, in the intestinal bacteria. However, endogenous production may be insufficient to cover all nutritional needs, particularly during infancy.

RDA / MR
LTI / ADI

RDA (recommended dietary allowance). In some countries RDA is also referred to as the **Daily Value** or **reference intake for the population.**

RDA for a nutrient is the recommended amount which meets the needs of 97.5% of the population. Ingesting this amount, the needs of the majority of the population will be met, although some may need considerably less. Only 2.5% of individuals may need more.

MR (mean requisite). It is the amount of a nutrient that meets the needs of the average individual in the population. It is always lower than the RDA.

LTI (less tolerable ingestion). It is the amount of nutrients that meets the needs of 2.5% of the population with lowest needs. Most need higher amounts.

For example, in the case of folic acid the RDA is 200 µg, the MR is 140 µg, and the LTI is 85 µg. The acronym **ADI (acceptable daily intake)** is used for harmful or toxic components or products.

Nutrients

When human physiology is studied, two things stand out: the variety and the high number of substances, possibly thousands, that the body's cells are capable of synthesizing. For example, all types of proteins, such as enzymes, hormones, neurotransmitters, sedating endorphins, and even hydrochloric acid in the stomach!

However, there are a few substances that the body needs and cannot synthesize, at least in sufficient amounts. For this reason, they must be taken in from outside the body in the form of food nutrients.

Sources of Nutrients

Foods

Foods are the primary source of nutrients, even though no single food provides everything that is needed (except milk during lactation). Therefore, it is important to combine various types of foods appropriately.

Types of Nutrients

Classically, water, carbohydrates, proteins, fats, minerals, and vitamins are considered nutrients.

There is still no unanimity concerning fiber and phytochemicals. Even though these food components are necessary for good health, they are not considered nutrients in the strict sense.

Types of Nutrients Based on Function

- **Energy generators:** Carbohydrates (4 calories per gram), fats (9 calories per gram), and proteins (4 calories per gram).

- **Plastics:** These contribute substantially to growth and tissue repair. They are proteins, fats, and some minerals such as calcium and phosphorus.

- **Regulators:** These intervene in the various processes and functions of the body. They are vitamins, minerals, and, in the broadest sense, fiber and phytochemicals.

The Most Important Components of Foods

These are described on the following pages. All, except cholesterol (Vol. 1, p. 406) and saturated fat (Vol. 1, p. 405), may be considered nutrients.

Energy

Energy is defined in physics as *"the capacity to perform work."* It is not a component of foods, but rather the *result of the combustion of the so-called energy-producing nutrients: carbohydrates, fats, and proteins.*

- **Units of measure:** the calorie, or more specifically *the kilocalorie (kcal),* which is equivalent to *4.184 kilojoules (kJ).*

- **Sources:** *All* of the energy supplied by food comes, ultimately, from the **sun.** Plants transform solar energy into chemical energy by synthesizing carbohydrates, fats, and proteins.

  Humans can obtain the energy they need from two sources:

  – **Plant-based foods:** In this manner they *directly* utilize the nutrients produced by the sun's energy, which is more healthful.

  – **Animal-based products:** Animals assimilate and process nutrients from plants and other animals. By eating meat, eggs, or milk and its derivatives, one is eating *second-hand* nutrients, which have been transformed by animals and, therefore, are less healthful (see following pages).

- **Proportional distribution among energy-producing nutrients:** *Ideally,* from a health standpoint there should be a **balance** among those nutrients producing energy: *60%* of calories should come from *carbohydrates, 30%* from *fats,* and *10%* from *proteins* (see Chapter 37, *The Proper use of Foods*). The more plant-based foods are eaten, the easier it is to meet these recommendations.

- **Function:** The body produces work for all bodily functions in the broadest sense whether physical, mental, or physiological, from the energy in foods,

- **Symptoms of deficiency:** Growth retardation in children, weight loss, physical weakness.

- **Consequences of excess:** Obesity.

- **Increased need:** Intense physical exercise, trauma, and severe burns.

- **Loss during processing of foods:** None or very little, since energy-producing nutrients are affected very little by cooking or other processes.

ENERGY
per each 100 g of raw edible portion

Vol./ Page	Food	Quantity
2/275	**Tomato**	21.0 kcal
2/251	**Watermelon**	32.0 kcal
1/132	**Kelp**	43.0 kcal
2/360	**Orange**	47.0 kcal
2/233	**Plum**	55.0 kcal
2/229	**Apple**	59.0 kcal
2/201	**Potato**	79.0 kcal
2/70	**Banana**	92.0 kcal
2/127	**Lentils, cooked without salt**	116 kcal
2/108	**Avocado**	161 kcal
2/322	**Chestnut**	213 kcal
1/72	**White bread**	267 kcal
2/205	**Potatoes fried in vegetable oil**	309 kcal
1/170	**White sugar**	387 kcal
2/336	**Peanut**	567 kcal
2/64	**Walnut**	642 kcal
1/126	**Olive oil**	884 kcal
1/182	**Whole cow's milk**	61.4 kcal
2/202	**Nonfat fruit-flavored yogurt**	102 kcal
2/314	**Skinless chicken**	119 kcal
2/239	**Sardine**	178 kcal
1/239	**Tuna, canned in oil**	198 kcal
1/308	**Beefsteak**	283 kcal
2/204	**Whipping cream**	345 kcal
1/318	**Pork**	376 kcal
2/210	**Gruyere cheese**	413 kcal
1/326	**Beef or pork sausage**	455 kcal
1/326	**Bacon**	556 kcal
1/204	**Unsalted butter**	717 kcal
1/318	**Lard**	902 kcal

1% 2% 4% 10% 20% 40% 100% 200% 500%

% Daily Value (based on a 2,000 calorie diet) provided by 100 g of this food

Plant-based foods provide as much or more energy as animal-based products, with the advantage that vegetables are more healthful and are endowed with healing power.

Daily Energy Needs

Average for an adult: *2,000 calories.*

This is the amount used for graphs of the composition of foods. The needs of the individual vary based on the physical makeup and physical activity.

Proteins

- **Chemical composition:** Proteins are formed by the union of various **amino acids** (usually from 50 to 1,000). Proteins differ from one another by the amino acids forming them and by the *order* in which they are joined.
  The body requires amino acids to synthesize its own proteins. These may be:

  - *Essential amino acids:* Those that the *body cannot produce*, and therefore *must be supplied by foods*. These are *isoleucine, leucine, lysine, methionine, phenylalanine, threonine, tryptophan, valine*, and in children, *histidine*.

  - *Nonessential amino acids:* These are those that the *body can produce from other substances*.

- **Sources:** Both plant and animal-based foods contain proteins. All of these contain the eight essential amino acids (nine for children). The difference is in the **proportion** in which these amino acids are found:

  - *Animal proteins:* The proportions of the various amino acids that form animal protein **approximate** the **ideal** for humans, particularly with the egg (see Vol. 1, p. 287). Because of this, they are referred to as **complete**.

  - *Vegetable proteins:* The proportion of amino acids of each type of vegetable protein is **not ideal**, except with **legumes,** which *approximate* it. However, by adequately **combining** two or more vegetable proteins in the same meal, or within an interval of a few hours, these deficiencies are overcome. Hence, vegetable proteins behave as a complete protein. (**Supplementation** phenomenon, see Chapter 37).

- **Function:** The formation and maintenance of tissues, synthesis of antibodies (defense against infection), formation of blood hemoglobin, production of enzymes, and energy production.

- **Deficiency symptoms:** weakness, apathy, immunodepression (low disease resistance), edema, and liver failure.

- **Consequences of excess:** renal and rheumatic disease, gout, and acidification of the blood.

- **Increased need:** infancy and adolescence, trauma, and serious burns.

Daily Value (Recommended Dietary Allowance) of proteins

Average for adult: 50 g.

There are two ways to calculate protein need precisely:

- Based on **body weight:** For an adult, *0.75 g per kilo* of weight (the **ideal**, not true weight; 52.5 g for a 70 kg person); from *1 to 2 g* per kilo of weight for **children.**

- Based on **caloric intake: 10%** (15% maximum) should come from proteins. For a 2,000 calorie diet, this amounts to 50 grams of proteins.

PROTEINS
per each 100 g of raw edible portion

% Daily Value (based on a 2,000 calorie diet) provided by 100 g of this food

Vol./Page	Food	Quantity
2/112	Pear	0.390 g
2/275	Red tomato	0.850 g
2/159	Zucchini	1.16 g
2/147	Date	1.97 g
2/294	Mushroom	2.09 g
2/250	Canned asparagus	2.14 g
2/28	Spinach	2.86 g
2/145	Dried fig	3.05 g
2/201	Baked potato	4.29 g
1/74	Cooked macaroni	4.77 g
2/225	White rice	6.61 g
2/227	Whole-grain rice	7.50 g
1/88	Tofu	8.08 g
1/72	White bread	8.20 g
1/72	Whole-grain bread	9.70 g
1/77	Amaranth	14.5 g
2/266	Mung bean	23.9 g
2/127	Lentil	28.1 g
2/264	Soybean	36.5 g
1/183	Nonfat milk	3.41 g
1/202	Natural yogurt	5.25 g
1/212	Cottage cheese, 1% fat	12.4 g
1/218	Fresh egg	12.5 g
1/239	Flatfish	18.8 g
1/308	Lean beef	20.2 g
1/312	Lean lamb	20.3 g
1/318	Lean pork	21.1 g
1/314	Baked chicken	27.3 g
1/239	Tuna, canned in oil	29.1 g
1/210	Gruyere cheese	29.8 g

% Daily Value: 1% 2% 4% 10% 20% 40% 100% 200% 500%

What the body needs is not a specific type of protein, but rather amino acids, and these are found in meat, milk, and eggs, as well as in vegetables.

The **biological value** of proteins is described in Vol. 1, p. 286.

Carbohydrates

- **Chemical composition and sources:** Carbohydrates constitute a broad group of substances that are mostly present in plant-based foods.

  – Absorbable *carbohydrates* are those that *the body can assimilate* and transform into energy.

  ✓ **Simple:** The most abundant simple carbohydrates in foods are **monosaccharides** (*glucose* and *fructose*) and **disaccharides** (*saccharose* or common sugar, *maltose*, and *lactose*, or milk sugar). These are the so-called *sugars*. They are found primarily in *fruits* and *honey*.

  ✓ **Complex:** These are **polysaccharides**, whose molecule is formed by the union of thousands of monosaccharide molecules. They are *starch* (abundant in grains, legumes, and tubers) and *glycogen* (this is found in small, nutritionally insignificant amounts in the liver and meat of animals).

  The *starch* in grains (particularly whole grains) and legumes is *slowly* transformed into *glucose* in the intestine, without provoking an abrupt increase in the glycemia (the level of sugar in the blood). Starch is *preferable* to sugars. It is the *most healthful* of carbohydrates and the *best tolerated* by diabetics.

  – *Non-absorbable carbohydrates:* This is dietary *fiber* (see Vol. 1, p. 388).

- **Function:** Carbohydrates constitute the *primary source of energy* for the body. Consequently, it is important to include abundant **plant-based foods** in the diet, since they are the almost the *only* source of *carbohydrates.*

- **Deficiency symptoms:** Ketosis (acidification of the blood), internal consumption of proteins, mineral loss, dehydration. This occurs in diets rich in animal-based proteins and fats, but lacking plant-based foods.

- **Consequences of excess:** Malnutrition with farinaceous dystrophy in children (see Vol. 1, p. 65).

- **Increased need:** physical exercise, growth periods.

- **Loss during processing of foods:** virtually none.

CARBOHYDRATES
per each 100 g of raw edible portion

Vol./Page	Food	Quantity
2/45	Lettuce	0.670 g
2/130	Alfalfa sprouts	1.28 g
2/97	Squash	6.00 g
1/132	Kelp	8.27 g
2/75	Peach	9.10 g
2/229	Apple	12.6 g
1/371	Malt beverage	13.4 g
2/135	Pistachio	14.0 g
2/304	Cherry	14.3 g
2/145	Fig	15.9 g
2/201	Potato	16.4 g
2/70	Banana	21.0 g
2/322	Chestnut	37.4 g
1/72	Whole-grain bread	39.2 g
2/241	Corn tortilla	41.4 g
1/72	White bread	47.2 g
2/145	Dried fig	56.1 g
2/306	Whole-wheat flour	60.4 g
1/69	Light rye flour	65.6 g
2/78	Raisin	71.7 g
1/69	Raw cuscus	72.4 g
2/306	White wheat flour	73.6 g
2/225	White rice	79.3 g
1/230	Fish	0.000 g
1/262	Meat	0.000 g
1/210	Camembert cheese	0.460 g
1/218	Fresh egg	1.22 g
1/317	Beef liver	4.59 g
1/183	Nonfat milk	4.85 g
1/202	Natural yogurt	7.04 g

% Daily Value (based on a 2,000 calorie diet) provided by 100 g of this food

1% 2% 4% 10% 20% 40% 100% 200% 500%

Carbohydrates, which are found almost exclusively in plant-based foods, are the nutrient most needed by the body. Grains, legumes, and tubers are the best sources of carbohydrates (the most healthful); fruits and honey are the best source of simple carbohydrates (sugars).

Daily Value (Recommended Daily Intake) of Carbohydrate

Average for an adult: *300 grams* a day, for a 2,000 calorie diet (375 g for a 2,500 calorie diet). This supposes that *60%* of daily *caloric* intake must come from carbohydrates.

Most of these carbohydrates must be complex (polysaccharides). **Refined sugars** must not make up *more* than *10%* of total calories (50 g of sugar a day maximum).

Fiber

- **Chemical composition and description:** Dietetic fiber if formed by various substances such as *cellulose, hemicellulose, pectin, gums, mucilage,* and other **polysaccharides** sharing the following characteristics:

  – They are of **plant** origin.

  – They are generally found in the **walls of plant cells**, although some types of fiber, such as gums and mucilage, are found in the cellular **cytoplasm,** as well.

  – They are **indigestible** in the small intestine. Some are partially digested by bacteria in the colon, causing flatulence.

- **Sources:** Fiber is found **exclusively** in **plant-based** foods. Milk, eggs, fish, meat and their derivatives contain *no* fiber.

  – Water-**insoluble** fiber is found primarily in grain bran. It is formed by *cellulose, hemicellulose,* and occasionally *lignin,* which give it a woody consistency.

  – Water-**soluble** fiber is found in oat bran (beta-glucan, see Vol. 2, p. 43), flax, and fruit seeds. They are formed by viscous substances such as *pectin, gums,* and *mucilage.*

- **Function:**

  – It reduces the risk of **constipation** and accompanying disorders, such as colon **diverticulosis,** colon **cancer,** and **hemorrhoids.** This protective effect is *mainly performed by insoluble fiber.*

  – It contributes to the avoidance of excess **cholesterol,** particularly *soluble fiber.*

  – It serves as an *emollient* and *protects* the **intestinal mucosa,** particularly *soluble fiber.*

  – It improves **diabetes.**

- **Deficiency symptoms:** constipation, diverticulosis, arteriosclerosis, greater cancer risk.

- **Consequences of excess:** May reduce the absorption of iron, zinc, and other minerals. Excessive insoluble fiber can irritate the intestine producing colitis.

- **Loss during processing of foods:** Refined grains lose as much as 95% of their fiber.

see Vol. 2, p. 43

Daily Value (Recommended Daily Intake) of Fiber

Average for an adult: 25 grams daily (between 20 and 35 g according to the American Dietetic Association).[25] To achieve this amount is not a problem with a plant-based diet. However this is not the case in diets primarily based on animal products.

Children older than three years: The minimum amount of daily grams may be determined by adding five to the child's age in years (years + 5). For example, for a ten-year-old child the amount would be 15 grams.[26]

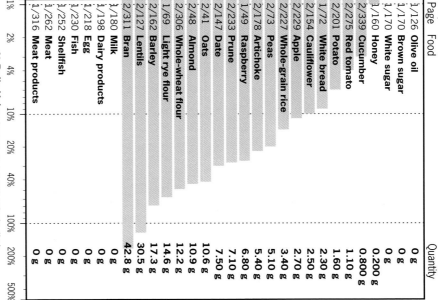

FIBER
per each 100 g of raw edible portion

Vol./Page	Food	% Daily Value (based on a 2,000 calorie diet) provided by 100 g of this food	Quantity
1/126	Olive oil		0 g
1/170	Brown sugar		0 g
1/170	White sugar		0 g
1/160	Honey		0.200 g
2/339	Cucumber		0.800 g
2/275	Red tomato		1.10 g
2/201	Potato		1.60 g
1/72	White bread		2.30 g
2/154	Cauliflower		2.50 g
2/229	Apple		2.70 g
2/227	Whole-grain rice		3.40 g
2/73	Peas		5.10 g
1/49	Artichoke		5.40 g
2/178	Raspberry		6.80 g
2/233	Prune		7.10 g
2/147	Date		7.50 g
2/41	Oats		10.6 g
2/48	Almond		10.9 g
2/306	Whole-wheat flour		12.2 g
1/69	Light rye flour		14.6 g
2/162	Barley		17.3 g
2/127	Lentils		30.5 g
2/311	Bran		42.8 g
1/180	Milk		0 g
1/198	Dairy products		0 g
1/218	Egg		0 g
1/230	Fish		0 g
1/252	Shellfish		0 g
1/262	Meat		0 g
1/316	Meat products		0 g

Dietary fiber is found exclusively in plant-based foods. In their natural state plant-based foods all contain some fiber, particularly whole grains (unrefined) and legumes.

Vitamin A

- **Chemical composition:** two substances are included under the name vitamin A:

  – *Vitamin A* itself: *retinol* and *dehydroretinol*. They are found in **animal**-based foods. In large **amounts** they are **toxic.**

  – *Provitamin A: carotenes* and similar substances called *carotenoids*. There are about ten different carotenes, the *most active* of which is *beta-carotene*. They transform to vitamin A in the intestine answering to the body's needs, and present *no risk of* **toxicity.**

- **Sources:**

  – *Vitamin A* (*retinol*): animal liver and milk fat are the richest sources.

  – *Provitamin A* (*carotenes* and *carotenoids*): all red and orange vegetables, particularly carrots and peppers, and some dark green as spinach.

- **Units of measurement:** the amount of active vitamin A in foods is measured in micrograms of retinol equivalent (µg RE).

  1 µg RE = 1 µg of retinol = 6 µg of beta-carotene = 12 µg of other carotenoids = 3.33 IU of vitamin A = 10 IU of carotenes

  1IU of vitamin A = 0.3 µg RE

- **Function:** vitamin A is involved in numerous bodily processes: vision, growth, bone and tooth development, maintenance of the health of the skin and mucosa, and protection against cancer. Additionally, carotenes and carotenoids are **antioxidants**, so they *protect* the **heart** and the **arteries.**

- **Deficiency symptoms:** vision disorders, dry skin, and fetal developmental disorders.

- **Increased need:** growth periods (children and adolescents), pregnancy, and nursing.

- **Loss during processing of foods:** 15% to 35% of the vitamin A is lost through cooking. Dehydration and exposure to light, particularly ultraviolet, destroy provitamin and vitamin A. Freezing has little effect on vitamin A.

Vitamin A
per each 100 g of raw edible portion

Vol./ Page	Food	Quantity
2/238	**Sweet corn**	28.0 µg RE
2/275	**Red tomato**	62.0 µg RE
2/298	**Loquat**	153 µg RE
2/63	**Broccoli**	154 µg RE
2/97	**Squash**	160 µg RE
2/45	**Lettuce**	260 µg RE
2/255	**Cantaloupe melon**	322 µg RE
2/341	**Mango**	389 µg RE
2/132	**Watercress**	470 µg RE
2/198	**Sweet red pepper**	570 µg RE
2/297	**Chard**	610 µg RE
2/28	**Spinach**	672 µg RE
2/136	**Lamb's lettuce**	709 µg RE
2/26	**Dried apricot**	724 µg RE
1/121	**Corn oil margarine**	799 µg RE
2/25	**Carrot**	2,813 µg RE
1/308	**Beef**	0.000 µg RE
1/318	**Pork**	2.00 µg RE
1/314	**Chicken**	16.0 µg RE
1/239	**Tuna, canned in oil**	23.0 µg RE
1/239	**Herring**	28.0 µg RE
1/182	**Whole cow's milk**	31.0 µg RE
1/239	**Grouper**	43.0 µg RE
1/314	**Baked chicken**	47.0 µg RE
1/183	**Nonfat milk**	61.0 µg RE
1/239	**Sardine**	70.0 µg RE
1/218	**Fresh egg**	191 µg RE
1/204	**Whipping cream**	421 µg RE
1/204	**Butter**	754 µg RE
1/317	**Beef liver**	4,427 µg RE

% Daily Value (based on a 2,000 calorie diet) provided by 100 g of this food

1%   2%   4%   10%   20%   40%   100%   200%   500%

Plant-based foods provide more vitamin A than animal products, and without the risk of over-accumulation and toxic effects.

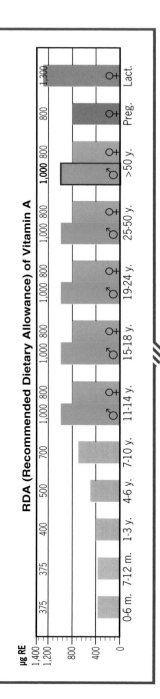

RDA (Recommended Dietary Allowance) of Vitamin A

µg RE													
375	375	400	500	700	1,000	1,000	1,000	1,000	1,000	800	1,000	800	1,300
0-6 m.	7-12 m.	1-3 y.	4-6 y.	7-10 y.	♂ 11-14 y.	♂ 15-18 y.	♂♀ 19-24 y.	♂♀ 25-50 y.	♂ >50 y. ♀	Preg.	Lact.		

Vitamin B₁

- **Chemical composition:** vitamin B₁ or *thiamin* is a substance formed by carbon, hydrogen, oxygen, nitrogen, and sulfur.

- **Sources:** Thiamin is found in a wide variety of foods, although in small amounts. Sunflower seeds, wheat germ, whole grains, and brewer's yeast are the best sources. All of these are better than pork, which is erroneously considered the best source of this vitamin. Refined products such as flour, sugar, and white rice contain very little.

- **Antivitamin B₁ factors:** There are substances in tea that are antagonistic to vitamin B₁. There is an enzyme in raw or poorly cooked fish and shellfish called **thiaminase** that destroys this vitamin.

- **Function:**
  - The production of **energy:** Thiamin is *essential* for the **metabolism** of *carbohydrates* in the energy-producing process in the body. Hence the importance of eating *unrefined* carbohydrates (whole grains, brown sugar, or molasses), which contain the vitamin B₁ necessary for these processes.
  - Stability of the **nervous system:** Vitamin B₁, thanks to its ability to maintain the nervous system in optimal condition, promotes mental and psychological health and balance.

- **Deficiency symptoms:** nervous disorders (apathy, fatigue, irritability, depression), digestive disorders (lack of appetite, slow digestion, constipation), circulatory disorders (cardiac failure). In serious cases, polyneuritis (inflammation of the peripheral nerves) and beriberi.

- **Increased need:** nervous disorders, nicotine addiction, drug addiction, and alcoholism.

- **Loss during processing of foods:** Bread baking causes a 15% to 20% loss of vitamin B₁; cooking vegetables or grains, 25%; cooking meat or fish, from 30% to 50%.

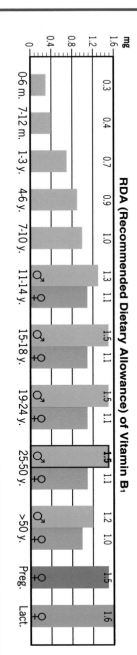

Sunflower

B complex or B group vitamins are formed by **B₁, B₂, B₆, B₁₂, niacin,** and **folates** (which are described on these pages), and **biotin, choline,** and **pantothenic acid** (Vol. 1, p. 408-409).

VITAMIN B₁
per each 100 g of raw edible portion

Vol./Page	Food	% Daily Value	Quantity
1/170	**Brown sugar**		0.008 mg
1/74	**Cooked macaroni**		0.020 mg
2/225	**White rice**		0.070 mg
2/108	**Avocado**		0.108 mg
2/306	**White wheat flour**		0.120 mg
2/322	**Chestnut**		0.238 mg
2/73	**Peas**		0.266 mg
2/227	**Whole-grain rice**		0.413 mg
2/306	**Whole-wheat flour**		0.447 mg
2/91	**Chickpea**		0.477 mg
2/41	**Oats**		0.763 mg
1/352	**Sesame**		0.791 mg
1/58	**Pecan**		0.848 mg
2/264	**Soybean**		0.874 mg
2/44	**Brazil nut**		1.00 mg
2/47	**Pine nut**		1.24 mg
2/310	**Wheat germ**		1.88 mg
2/105	**Sunflower seeds**		2.29 mg
1/212	**Cream cheese**		0.017 mg
1/202	**Natural yogurt**		0.048 mg
1/218	**Fresh egg**		0.062 mg
1/308	**Beef**		0.080 mg
1/239	**Flatfish**		0.089 mg
1/253	**Oyster**		0.105 mg
1/312	**Lamb**		0.120 mg
1/239	**Trout**		0.203 mg
1/314	**Duck**		0.360 mg
1/316	**Hamburger**		0.370 mg
1/327	**Ham**		0.863 mg
1/318	**Pork loin**		0.901 mg

% Daily Value (based on a 2,000 calorie diet) provided by 100 g of this food

RDA (Recommended Dietary Allowance) of Vitamin B₁

mg

Age	mg
0-6 m.	
7-12 m.	
1-3 y.	
4-6 y.	
7-10 y.	
11-14 y. ♂	1.3
11-14 y. ♀	1.1
15-18 y. ♂	1.5
15-18 y. ♀	1.1
19-24 y. ♂	1.5
19-24 y. ♀	1.1
25-50 y. ♂	1.5
25-50 y. ♀	1.1
>50 y. ♂	1.2
>50 y. ♀	1.0
Preg.	1.5
Lact.	1.6

Vitamin B₂

- **Chemical composition:** *riboflavin.*

- **Sources:** widely distributed in all natural foods of both plant and animal origin.

- **Function:**

  - **Energy** production: Riboflavin is necessary in all chemical reactions in which energy is produced in the body from carbohydrates, fats, and when the former are lacking, from proteins.

  - Formation of **pigments in the retina** involved with vision.

  - *Necessary* for the **synthesis** of **corticoid** hormones in the cortex of the suprarenal glands. These hormones prepare the body to confront stress, among many other functions.

- **Deficiency symptoms:** fatigue, weakness, apathy, vision disorders, seborrheic dermatitis, skin eruptions, anemia.

- **Increased need:** stress, fatigue, dermatitis and eczema, vision disorders.

- **Loss during processing of foods:** Even though riboflavin is quite heat resistant, 10% to 20% is lost during cooking. Dehydration and freezing have little effect.

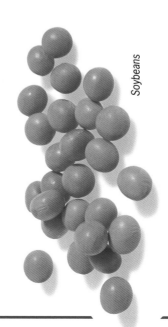

Soybeans

VITAMIN B₂
per each 100 g of raw edible portion

Vol./Page	Food	Quantity
1/108	Cassava	0.101 mg
2/108	Avocado	0.122 mg
2/130	Alfalfa sprouts	0.126 mg
2/336	Peanut	0.135 mg
2/239	Popcorn with oil	0.136 mg
2/41	Oats	0.139 mg
2/64	English walnut	0.148 mg
2/358	Borage	0.150 mg
2/91	Chickpea	0.212 mg
2/297	Chard	0.220 mg
2/116	Rye	0.251 mg
1/72	White bread	0.341 mg
2/102	Buckwheat	0.425 mg
2/294	Mushroom	0.449 mg
2/310	Wheat germ	0.499 mg
2/311	Bran	0.577 mg
2/264	Soybean	0.870 mg
1/239	Flatfish	0.076 mg
1/204	Cream	0.149 mg
1/182	Whole cow's milk	0.162 mg
1/314	Baked chicken	0.168 mg
1/202	Natural yogurt	0.214 mg
1/327	Ham	0.252 mg
1/308	Beef	0.280 mg
1/316	Hamburger	0.300 mg
1/239	Salmon	0.380 mg
1/314	Duck	0.450 mg
1/218	Fresh egg	0.508 mg
1/210	Roquefort cheese	0.586 mg
1/218	Fresh egg yolk	0.639 mg

% Daily Value (based on a 2,000 calorie diet)
provided by 100 g of this food

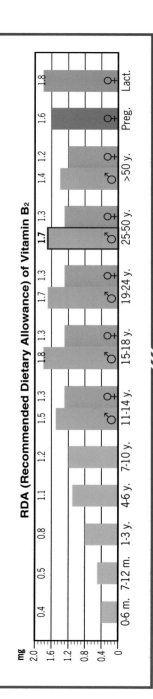

RDA (Recommended Dietary Allowance) of Vitamin B₂

	0-6 m.	7-12 m.	1-3 y.	4-6 y.	7-10 y.	11-14 y.	15-18 y.	19-24 y.	25-50 y.	>50 y.	Preg.	Lact.
mg	0.4	0.5	0.8	1.1	1.2	♂ 1.5 / ♀ 1.3	♂ 1.8 / ♀ 1.3	♂ 1.7 / ♀ 1.3	♂ 1.7 / ♀ 1.3	♂ 1.4 / ♀ 1.2	♀ 1.6	1.8

Niacin

- **Chemical composition:** Under the names *niacin*, *PP factor*, or *vitamin B$_3$*, two equally active natural substances are included: *nicotinic acid* (this has nothing to do with the nicotine in tobacco), which is present in plant-based foods, and *nicotinamide*, which is found in milk, eggs, fish, and meat.

- **Sources:** Foods provide niacin in either of these forms or both:

  – **Preformed *niacin*,** which is found in foods in the form of nicotinic acid or nicotinamide.

  – **Transformed *niacin*** by the modification of *tryptophan* (essential amino acid) contained in food proteins. Tryp-

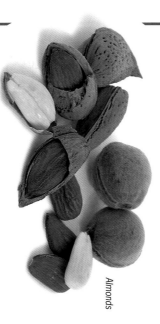

Almonds

tophan transforms in the body in such a way that 60 mg of this amino acid becomes 1 mg of niacin.

- **Units of measure:** The niacin content of foods is measured in mg of niacin equivalents (mg NE). This measure includes both the preformed niacin present in a food and that formed from tryptophan.

- **Function:** Intervenes as a coenzyme in energy production in the cells. It is necessary for body growth. *Niacin from plant sources* (nicotinic acid) *reduces cholesterol levels.* Niacin from animal sources (nicotinamide) does *not* have the same effect.

- **Deficiency symptoms:** skin disorders (dermatitis, pellagra in advanced cases) and nervous system disorders (depression, anxiety).

- **Increased need:** Periods of growth, pregnancy, skin and nervous system disorders.

- **Loss during processing of foods:** Niacin is the *most stable* of all vitamins and deteriorates very little with heat, freezing, or long-term food storage.

NIACIN
per each 100 g of raw edible portion

Vol./Page	Food	% Daily Value (based on a 2,000 calorie diet) provided by 100 g of this food	Quantity
2/75	Peach		1.02 mg NE
2/178	Artichoke		1.05 mg NE
2/59	Cherimoya		1.30 mg NE
2/250	Asparagus		1.54 mg NE
2/201	Potato		2.02 mg NE
2/238	Sweet corn		2.08 mg NE
2/108	Avocado		2.27 mg NE
1/88	Tofu		2.30 mg NE
2/225	White rice		2.88 mg NE
2/147	Date		3.03 mg NE
2/64	English walnut		4.19 mg NE
2/227	Whole-grain rice		5.91 mg NE
1/72	Whole-grain bread		6.17 mg NE
2/48	Almond		9.33 mg NE
2/102	Buckwheat		10.2 mg NE
1/352	Sesame		11.0 mg NE
2/310	Wheat germ		12.1 mg NE
1/55	Peanut butter		17.6 mg NE
2/311	Bran		18.3 mg NE
1/202	Natural yogurt		0.657 mg NE
1/183	Nonfat milk		0.888 mg NE
1/218	Fresh egg		2.61 mg NE
1/239	Cod		5.38 mg NE
1/210	Gruyere cheese		7.12 mg NE
1/318	Pork loin		8.65 mg NE
1/239	Salmon		11.6 mg NE
1/308	Beefsteak		11.7 mg NE
1/314	Baked chicken		13.6 mg NE
1/317	Beef liver		14.9 mg NE
1/239	Tuna, canned in oil		17.8 mg NE

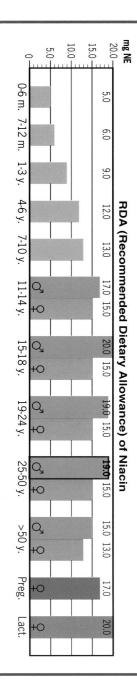

RDA (Recommended Dietary Allowance) of Niacin

mg NE

Age	♂	♀
0-6 m.	5.0	
7-12 m.	6.0	
1-3 y.	9.0	
4-6 y.	12.0	
7-10 y.	13.0	
11-14 y.	17.0	15.0
15-18 y.	20.0	15.0
19-24 y.	19.0	15.0
25-50 y.	19.0	15.0
>50 y.	15.0	13.0
Preg.	17.0	
Lact.	20.0	

Vitamin B₆

- **Chemical composition:** Vitamin B₆ is found in foods in three chemical forms, which are interchangeable within the body: *pyridoxine, pyridoxal,* and *pyridoxamine.*

- **Sources:** Whole grains, legumes, and some fruits such as the banana are equal or superior to animal-based foods in vitamin B₆. Vegetables are also a good source.

- **Function:**

  – *Metabolism of proteins:* It facilitates the absorption of amino acids and their assimilation to form body proteins.

  – *Metabolism of carbohydrates and fats:* Allows these nutrients to be transformed into energy.

  – **Energy** production within the cells of the **nervous system.**

  – **Blood formation:** it is involved in the synthesis of hemoglobin that forms the red blood cells.

- **Deficiency symptoms:** fatigue, nervousness, anemia, skin disorders.

- **Increased need:**

  – Women taking oral contraceptives, pregnant, or who are nursing.

  – Tuberculosis patients being treated with isoniazid.

  – Neuropsychological patients.

- **Loss during processing of foods:**

  – Refining grains: up to 75%; because of this, white bread and pasta are poor in this vitamin.

  – Refined sugar: loss of all vitamin B₆.

  – Cooking: 25% to 50% loss.

    – Freezing: 37% to 56% loss.

    – Canning: 40% to 50% loss.

Wheat germ

VITAMIN B₆
per each 100 g of raw edible portion

Vol./Page	Food	Quantity
2/250	Canned asparagus	0.110 mg
2/251	Watermelon	0.144 mg
2/78	Raisin	0.188 mg
2/147	Date	0.192 mg
2/154	Cauliflower	0.222 mg
2/319	Leek	0.233 mg
2/198	Sweet red pepper	0.248 mg
2/201	Potato	0.260 mg
2/306	Wheat	0.272 mg
2/108	Avocado	0.500 mg
2/227	Whole-grain rice	0.509 mg
2/91	Chickpea	0.535 mg
2/70	Banana	0.578 mg
1/175	Blackstrap molasses	0.700 mg
1/352	Sesame	0.790 mg
1/109	Garlic	1.24 mg
2/310	Wheat germ	1.30 mg
2/311	Bran	1.30 mg
1/204	Unsalted butter	0.003 mg
1/183	Nonfat milk	0.040 mg
1/202	Natural yogurt	0.053 mg
1/316	Hamburger	0.070 mg
1/218	Fresh egg	0.139 mg
1/210	Camembert cheese	0.227 mg
1/239	Cod	0.245 mg
1/239	Herring	0.302 mg
1/329	Rabbit	0.500 mg
1/318	Lean pork loin	0.500 mg
1/308	Beefsteak	0.527 mg
1/239	Salmon	0.530 mg
		0.818 mg

% Daily Value (based on a 2,000 calorie diet) provided by 100 g of this food

1% 2% 4% 10% 20% 40% 100% 200% 500%

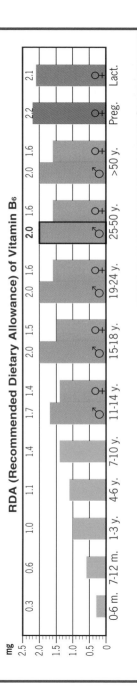

RDA (Recommended Dietary Allowance) of Vitamin B₆

	0-6 m.	7-12 m.	1-3 y.	4-6 y.	7-10 y.	11-14 y.	15-18 y.	19-24 y.	25-50 y.	>50 y.	Preg.	Lact.
	0.3	0.6	1.0	1.1	1.4	♂ 1.7	♂♀ 2.0 1.5	♂♀ 2.0 1.6	♂ 2.0	♂ 2.0 ♀ 1.6	♀ 2.2	♀ 2.1

mg: 0 0.5 1.0 1.5 2.0 2.5

Folates

- **Chemical composition:** the name folate describes *folic acid* as well as *its salts* (folates). Some researchers include all these substances, which possess the same physiological properties, under the term *folacin.*

- **Sources:** Legumes are the major source, followed by green leafy vegetables (spinach, lettuce) and nuts. Milk, fish, and meat are poor in folates.

- **Units of measurement:** micrograms (millionths of gram), represented by the symbol µg (1 mg = 1,000 µg).

- **Function:** Folates are *essential for the* **synthesis of DNA** (deoxyribonucleic acid) and **RNA** (ribonucleic acid), which make up the biochemical base of life. Folates are also involved in the production of hemoglobin and many other physiological processes.

- **Deficiency symptoms:** A particular type of anemia, called megaloblastic or macrocytic anemia (few, very large red blood cells); glossitis (inflammation of the tongue); mental deterioration; congenital malformations of the fetal nervous system.

- **Increased need:** In these cases it is recommended that folates intake be double the RDA, or to about 400 µg:
  - Growth periods: infancy and adolescence.
  - When taking oral contraceptives (these may interfere with the absorption of folates).
  - Pregnancy (to avoid fetal malformations).
  - Persons at high risk of cardiac disease (to lower the heart attack risk, see Vol. 2, p. 57).
  - Anemia in general, and macrocytic anemia in particular.
  - Intestinal parasitosis.
  - Regular alcohol consumption, which blocks the absorption and assimilation of folates; intake of certain medications, such as anti-epileptics and chemotherapeutic drugs used to combat cancer, which counteract folates.

- **Loss during processing of foods:** Folates are *quite unstable,* and are easily destroyed by heat and light.
  - Cooking and canning: 50% to 95% of folates are lost.
  - Storage: Vegetables lose 50% to 70% of their folates at room temperature. When refrigerated, however, folates are little affected.

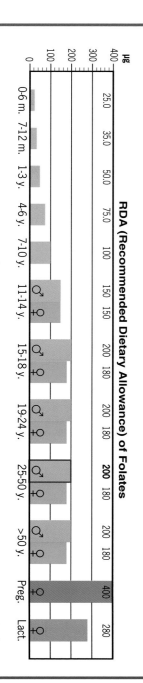

RDA (Recommended Dietary Allowance) of Folates

FOLATES
per each 100 g of raw edible portion

Vol./ Page	Food	% Daily Value (based on a 2,000 calorie diet) provided by 100 g of this food	Quantity
2/103	Strawberry		17.7 µg
2/360	Orange		30.3 µg
2/263	Feijoa		38.0 µg
1/72	Whole-grain bread		50.0 µg
2/73	Peas		65.0 µg
2/64	Walnut		66.0 µg
2/178	Artichoke		68.0 µg
2/200	Okra		87.8 µg
2/122	Red beet		109 µg
2/250	Asparagus		128 µg
2/45	Lettuce		136 µg
2/176	Endive		142 µg
1/132	Kelp		180 µg
2/28	Spinach		194 µg
2/310	Wheat germ		281 µg
2/127	Lentil		433 µg
2/91	Chickpea		557 µg
2/266	Adzuki		622 µg
2/266	Mung bean		625 µg
1/324	Pork sausage		4.00 µg
1/314	Baked chicken		5.00 µg
1/183	Nonfat milk		5.20 µg
1/239	Grouper		8.80 µg
1/202	Natural yogurt		11.2 µg
1/308	Lean beef		13.0 µg
1/210	Cottage cheese, 2% fat		13.1 µg
1/312	Lean lamb		23.0 µg
1/316	Hamburger		28.0 µg
1/218	Fresh egg		47.0 µg
1/210	Camembert cheese		62.2 µg

Vitamin B₁₂

- **Chemical composition:** *cyanocobalamin* and other similar substances.

- **Sources:** The *only* living things capable of synthesizing this vitamin are **bacteria** and other microorganisms such as **yeasts.** The bacteria usually found in the mouth or the intestine also produce vitamin B₁₂, although it is not assured that the body can assimilate it.

  – Higher animals (fish, mammals) do not produce this vitamin, but they store it in their tissues, particularly in the liver. Milk and eggs also contain vitamin B₁₂, as do meat and fish.

  – Plants and higher algae do not produce or store vitamin B₁₂. However, they may provide it in small amounts:

    ✓ through contamination by certain bacteria that produce vitamin B₁₂ as is the case with certain seaweed;[1]

    ✓ by containing yeasts that produce vitamin B₁₂. This is the case with certain fermented products such as beer (with or without alcohol), *tempeh* (fermented soybean), and even bread (in very small amounts).

  – Unicellular or blue-green algae such as spirulina (see Vol. 1, p. 134), which produce significant amounts.

- **Function:** Cell division, formation of red blood cells, formation of myelin (substance that protects the nerve fibers).

- **Deficiency symptoms:** Pernicious anemia, nervous disorders. Most cases involving lack of this vitamin are due to difficulty of absorption, and not lack of availability.

- **Deficiency risk:** In theory it could be said that strict vegetarians are at risk. However, in reality, there are very few cases. An ovolactovegetarian diet generally supplies sufficient vitamin B₁₂.

  The possibility exists that the vitamin B₁₂ found in spirulina and plant-based foods such as tempeh is not well assimilated by the body. Due to this, it is suggested that *strict vegetarians* take B₁₂ supplements.

- **Loss during processing of foods:** cooking destroys 30% of vitamin B₁₂; the pasteurization of milk, about 10%.

VITAMIN B₁₂
per each 100 g of raw edible portion

Vol./Page	Food	Quantity
1/380	Beer	0.020 µg
1/371	Malt beverage	0.020 µg
1/72	White bread	0.020 µg
1/88	Tempeh	1.00 µg
1/204	Salted butter	0.125 µg
1/314	Baked chicken	0.300 µg
1/182	Whole cow's milk	0.357 µg
1/183	Nonfat milk	0.378 µg
1/202	Natural yogurt	0.562 µg
1/212	Cottage cheese, 1% fat	0.633 µg
1/327	Ham	0.830 µg
1/218	Fresh egg	1.00 µg
1/210	Camembert cheese	1.30 µg
1/308	Lean beef	1.40 µg
1/239	Tuna, canned in oil	2.20 µg
1/312	Lamb	2.39 µg
1/218	Fresh egg yolk	3.11 µg
1/239	Trout	3.77 µg
1/239	Sardine	9.00 µg
1/239	Herring	13.7 µg
1/253	Oyster	16.2 µg
1/239	Caviar	20.0 µg
1/317	Beef liver	46.8 µg

% Daily Value (based on a 2,000 calorie diet) provided by 100 g of this food

1% — 2% — 4% — 10% — 20% — 40% — 100% — 200% — 500%

Liver, caviar, and oysters are the *richest* sources of vitamin B₁₂. However, due to the drawbacks they present, they are not recommended.

There is no need to take vitamin B₁₂ every day since the livers of healthy persons contain enough reserves for at least five years.

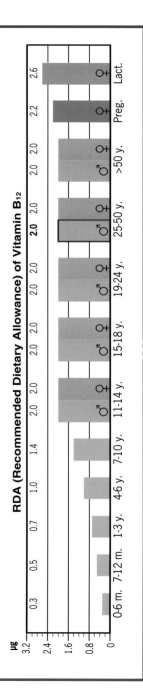

RDA (Recommended Dietary Allowance) of Vitamin B₁₂

µg										
	0.3	0.5	0.7	1.0	1.4	2.0	2.0	2.0	2.0	2.0	2.0	2.0	2.0	2.0	2.0	2.6
	0-6 m.	7-12 m.	1-3 y.	4-6 y.	7-10 y.	♂♀ 11-14 y.	♂♀ 15-18 y.	♂♀ 19-24 y.	♂ 25-50 y.	♂♀ >50 y.	♀ Preg.	♀ Lact.

Vitamin C

- **Chemical composition:** *ascorbic acid.* Plants and most **animals** produce it from *glucose.* **Humans** *cannot* **synthesize** this vitamin, *nor* can they **store it** in significant amounts, therefore it must be **taken in** *daily.*

- **Sources:** fruits and vegetables, particularly if they are fresh.

- **Function:**

  - **Antioxidant:** It neutralizes free radicals, which are substances causing cellular aging, DNA deterioration, and cancer.

  - **Antitoxin:** Neutralizes the action of a variety of toxic substances, such as nitrosamines found in cured meats (see Vol. 1, p. 270).

  - *Strengthens* the **immune system** against infections.

  - *Contributes to the formation of* **collagen,** fibrous tissue necessary for wound healing.

  - *Improves* the **consistency** of **bones** and **teeth.**

  - *Strengthens* **capillary** and **arterial** walls.

  - *Facilitates* the **absorption** of *nonheme iron* (that contained in plant-based foods, dairy products, and eggs).

- **Deficiency symptoms:** fatigue, poor wound healing, tiny subcutaneous hemorrhages, scurvy.

- **Increased need:** nicotine addiction, stress, infections, wounds, and burns.

- **Loss during processing of foods:** Vitamin C is the *most* **unstable** of all. Heat, light, dehydration, and all food-processing methods destroy up to 75% of this vitamin.

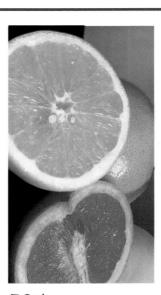

To take full advantage of the vitamin C in fruits and vegetables, they **must** be eaten fresh and raw.

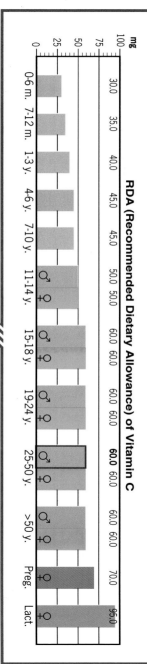

RDA (Recommended Dietary Allowance) of Vitamin C

mg

0-6 m.	30.0
7-12 m.	35.0
1-3 y.	40.0
4-6 y.	45.0
7-10 y.	45.0
11-14 y. ♂ ♀	50.0 50.0
15-18 y. ♂ ♀	60.0 60.0
19-24 y. ♂ ♀	60.0 60.0
25-50 y. ♂ ♀	60.0 60.0
>50 y. ♂ ♀	60.0 60.0
Preg. ♀	70.0
Lact. ♀	95.0

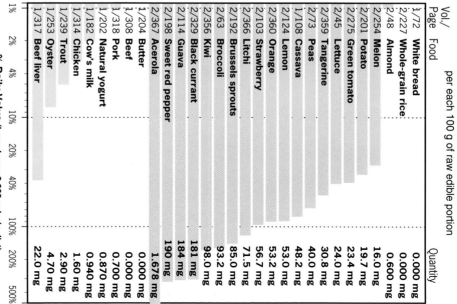

VITAMIN C
per each 100 g of raw edible portion

% **Daily Value** (based on a 2,000 calorie diet) provided by 100 g of this food

Vol./Page	Food	Quantity
1/72	White bread	0.000 mg
2/227	Whole-grain rice	0.000 mg
2/48	Almond	0.600 mg
2/254	Melon	16.0 mg
2/201	Potato	19.7 mg
2/275	Green tomato	23.4 mg
2/45	Lettuce	24.0 mg
2/359	Tangerine	30.8 mg
2/73	Peas	40.0 mg
1/108	Cassava	48.2 mg
2/124	Lemon	53.0 mg
2/360	Orange	53.2 mg
2/103	Strawberry	56.7 mg
2/366	Litchi	71.5 mg
2/192	Brussels sprouts	85.0 mg
2/63	Broccoli	93.2 mg
2/356	Kiwi	98.0 mg
2/329	Black currant	181 mg
2/114	Guava	184 mg
2/198	Sweet red pepper	190 mg
2/367	Acerola	1,678 mg
1/204	Butter	0.000 mg
1/308	Beef	0.000 mg
1/318	Pork	0.700 mg
1/202	Natural yogurt	0.870 mg
1/182	Cow's milk	0.940 mg
1/314	Chicken	1.60 mg
1/239	Trout	2.90 mg
1/253	Oyster	4.70 mg
1/317	Beef liver	22.0 mg

Vitamin E

- **Chemical composition:** There are eight different substances of the *tocopherol* and *tocotrienol* groups under the name vitamin E. The *most active* of these is *alpha-tocopherol.*

- **Sources:** Grain germ, particularly that of wheat, sunflower seeds, oil-bearing nuts, and some fleshy fruits such as the olive and avocado. Milk and meat are very poor in this vitamin.

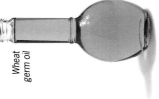

Wheat germ oil

- **Unit of measurement:** alpha-tocopherol is used as a reference to evaluate the activity of vitamin E in a food. This is expressed in milligrams of of alpha-tocopherol equivalents (mg α-TE).

  1 mg α-TE = 1.5 IU
  (International Units) of vitamin E

  1 IU of vitamin E = 0.66 mg α-TE

- **Functions:**
  - It protects the integrity of the **cells** and *prolongs* their life span.
  - **Antioxidant:** Prevents the oxidation of vegetable oils. It *neutralizes* the harmful effect of *free radicals* from chemical contamination and body activity within the cells.
    - *Facilitates* the activity of other **antioxidants** such as vitamins A and C.
  - Exercises a *protective* action against **cancer** and **arteriosclerosis.**
  - Is involved in the formation of germinal cells (**spermatozoids** and **ova**).

- **Deficiency symptoms:** These are not well known, due to the broad range of activities with which it is involved.

- **Increased need:** Consumption of vegetable oils rich in polyunsaturated fatty acids increases the need for this vitamin. Fortunately, nature has provided that many of the foods rich in these types of fatty acids are also rich in vitamin E.

- **Loss during processing of foods:** Refined grains lose up to 80%; roasted nuts, 80%; frying the oil, from 32% to 75%; in preserves, from 41% to 65%.

VITAMIN E
per each 100 g of raw edible portion

Vol./ Page	Food	Quantity
2/250	Canned asparagus	0.430 mg α-TE
2/78	Grape	0.700 mg α-TE
1/36	Tamarind	0.700 mg α-TE
2/145	Fig	0.890 mg α-TE
2/114	Guava	1.12 mg α-TE
2/341	Mango	1.12 mg α-TE
2/63	Broccoli	1.66 mg α-TE
2/116	Rye	1.87 mg α-TE
2/28	Spinach	1.89 mg α-TE
1/352	Sesame	2.27 mg α-TE
2/108	Avocado	2.30 mg α-TE
2/165	Olive	3.00 mg α-TE
2/44	Brazil nut	7.60 mg α-TE
2/336	Peanut	9.13 mg α-TE
1/121	Margarine, various oils, salted	12.0 mg α-TE
1/126	Olive oil	12.4 mg α-TE
2/310	Wheat germ	13.5 mg α-TE
2/252	Hazelnut	23.9 mg α-TE
2/48	Almond	24.0 mg α-TE
2/105	Sunflower seeds	50.3 mg α-TE
1/125	Sunflower oil	50.6 mg α-TE
1/127	Wheat germ oil	192 mg α-TE
1/202	Natural yogurt	0.042 mg α-TE
1/182	Whole cow's milk	0.100 mg α-TE
1/314	Baked chicken	0.265 mg α-TE
1/316	Hamburger	0.550 mg α-TE
1/218	Fresh egg	1.05 mg α-TE
1/204	Butter	1.58 mg α-TE
1/239	Flatfish	1.89 mg α-TE
1/239	Caviar	7.00 mg α-TE

% Daily Value (based on a **2,000 calorie diet**) provided by 100 g of this food

1% 2% 4% 10% 20% 40% 100% 200% 500%

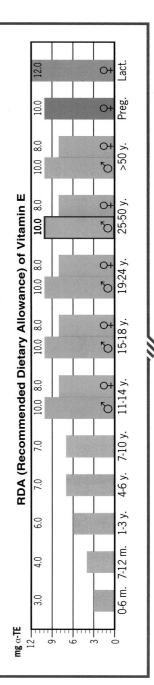

RDA (Recommended Dietary Allowance) of Vitamin E

mg α-TE

0-6 m.	7-12 m.	1-3 y.	4-6 y.	7-10 y.	11-14 y.	15-18 y.	19-24 y.	25-50 y.	>50 y.	Preg.	Lact.

0-6 m. 3.0 — 7-12 m. 4.0 — 1-3 y. 6.0 — 4-6 y. 7.0 — 7-10 y. 7.0 — 11-14 y. ♂♀ 10.0 — 15-18 y. ♂♀ 10.0 — 19-24 y. ♂♀ 10.0 — 25-50 y. ♂♀ 10.0 / 8.0 — >50 y. ♂♀ 10.0 / 8.0 — Preg. ♀ 10.0 — Lact. ♀ 12.0

Calcium

- **Chemical composition:** *mineral* element.

- **Sources:** Milk and dairy products are well known as the best sources of calcium. However, there are a variety of plant-based foods providing as much or more calcium as milk: sesame, blackstrap molasses, almonds, beans, and corn. Cabbage, broccoli and, oranges are also good sources of calcium.

- **Absorption:** Only 20% to 30% of the calcium present in foods is absorbed in the intestine, even though at times of rapid growth, pregnancy, or nursing it may rise to 40%. The rest is lost through the feces.

  - **Facilitators of absorption:** vitamin D, proteins in the diet, the lactose in milk, and acidity in the intestinal bolus.

  - *Inhibitors of absorption:* excess phosphorus, as occurs in diets rich in fish and meat; the phytates found in bran (see Vol. 2, p. 311), even though the leavening in whole bread causes phytates to partially disappear; oxalates present in rhubarb, spinach, and other green leafy vegetables; excess fat in the diet.

    Although phytates and oxalates reduce calcium absorption from grains and vegetables, respectively, both types of foods remain good sources of calcium.

    Meat and fish, with the exception of sardines, are poor in calcium.

- **Function:** Calcium is involved in bone and tooth formation, muscular contraction, nerve impulse transmission, and in blood coagulation.

- **Deficiency symptoms:** rickets; osteoporosis.

- **Increased need:** adolescence, pregnancy, and nursing.

- **Loss during processing of foods:** Lost only as calcium salts are dissolved in cooking water.

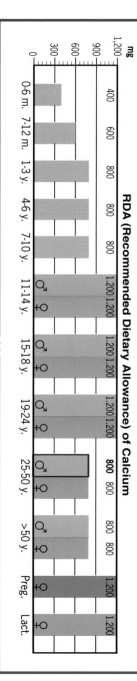

RDA (Recommended Dietary Allowance) of Calcium

mg axis: 0, 300, 600, 900, 1,200

Age group	mg
0-6 m.	400
7-12 m.	600
1-3 y.	800
4-6 y.	800
7-10 y.	800
11-14 y. ♂♀	1,200 1,200
15-18 y. ♂♀	1,200 1,200
19-24 y. ♂♀	1,200 1,200
25-50 y. ♂♀	800 800
>50 y. ♂♀	800 800
Preg.	1,200
Lact.	1,200

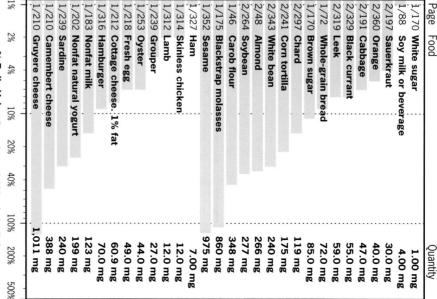

CALCIUM per each 100 g of raw edible portion

Vol./ Page	Food	Quantity
1/170	White sugar	1.00 mg
1/88	Soy milk or beverage	4.00 mg
2/197	Sauerkraut	30.0 mg
2/360	Orange	40.0 mg
2/191	Cabbage	47.0 mg
2/329	Black currant	55.0 mg
2/319	Leek	59.0 mg
1/72	Whole-grain bread	72.0 mg
1/170	Brown sugar	85.0 mg
2/297	Chard	119 mg
2/241	Corn tortilla	175 mg
2/343	White bean	240 mg
2/48	Almond	266 mg
2/264	Soybean	277 mg
1/46	Carob flour	348 mg
1/175	Blackstrap molasses	860 mg
1/352	Sesame	975 mg
1/327	Ham	7.00 mg
1/314	Skinless chicken	12.0 mg
1/312	Lamb	12.0 mg
1/183	Hamburger	12.0 mg
1/316	Nonfat milk	70.0 mg
1/212	Cottage cheese .1% fat	60.9 mg
1/218	Fresh egg	49.0 mg
1/253	Oyster	44.0 mg
1/239	Grouper	27.0 mg
1/202	Nonfat natural yogurt	123 mg
1/239	Sardine	199 mg
1/210	Camembert cheese	240 mg
1/210	Gruyere cheese	388 mg
		1,011 mg

% Daily Value (based on a 2,000 calorie diet) provided by 100 g of this food

% axis: 1%, 2%, 4%, 10%, 20%, 40%, 100%, 200%, 500%

Milk and dairy products are not by any means the only source of calcium.
Sesame, for example, is the richest plant source of calcium,
much richer than most cheeses.
The orange is one of the fresh fruits richest in calcium.

Phosphorus

- **Chemical composition:** *mineral* element.

- **Sources:** Phosphorus is widely distributed in both plant and animal-based foods, although it is found primarily in the latter. Meat-based diets present the *risk* of **excess** phosphorus rather than a lack.

- **Absorption:** Phosphorus is much more easily absorbed than calcium. About 70% of the phosphorus present in foods is absorbed.

- **Function:**
  - It is involved along with calcium in the formation of bones and teeth.
  - It is involved in the chemical reactions that release energy.
  - It forms part of the nucleic acids DNA and RNA.

- **Deficiency symptoms:** muscle weakness, loss of appetite, bone pain.

- **Increased need:** As important as or more than the absolute amount of phosphorus taken in with foods, is the need for a 1:1 balance with calcium. Adolescence, pregnancy, and nursing increase the need for both minerals.

- **Loss during processing of foods:** very slight.

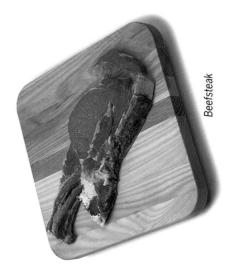

Beefsteak

PHOSPHORUS
per each 100 g of raw edible portion

Vol./Page	Food	Quantity
2/93	Grapefruit	8.00 mg
2/78	Grape	13.0 mg
2/304	Cherry	19.0 mg
2/275	Green tomato	28.0 mg
2/25	Carrot	44.0 mg
2/45	Lettuce	45.0 mg
2/201	Potato	46.0 mg
2/28	Spinach	49.0 mg
2/178	Artichoke	90.0 mg
1/72	White bread	94.0 mg
2/225	White rice	108 mg
2/343	White bean	301 mg
2/64	English walnut	317 mg
2/41	Oats	523 mg
1/352	Sesame	629 mg
2/264	Soybean	704 mg
2/105	Sunflower seeds	705 mg
2/310	Wheat germ	842 mg
2/311	Bran	1.013 mg
1/253	Oyster	93.0 mg
1/212	Cottage cheese, 1% fat	134 mg
1/202	Natural yogurt	144 mg
1/218	Fresh egg	178 mg
1/318	Pork loin	197 mg
1/314	Skinless duck	203 mg
1/239	Cod	203 mg
1/308	Lean beef	211 mg
1/239	Herring	236 mg
1/239	Tuna, canned in oil	311 mg
1/210	Gruyere cheese	605 mg

% Daily Value (based on a 2,000 calorie diet) provided by 100 g of this food

1% 2% 4% 10% 20% 40% 100% 200% 500%

Meat and fish contain a great deal of phosphorus but little calcium. This deficiency fosters osteoporosis because excess phosphorus reduces calcium absorption.

On the other hand, grains, legumes, fruits, and vegetables maintain close to the ideal 1:1 balance between these two minerals.

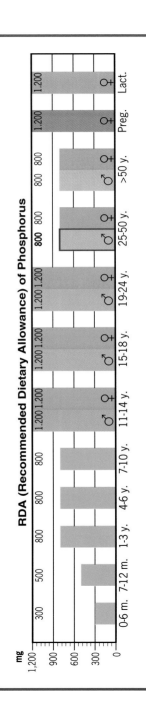

RDA (Recommended Dietary Allowance) of Phosphorus

mg
1,200
900
600
300
0

0-6 m.	7-12 m.	1-3 y.	4-6 y.	7-10 y.	11-14 y.	15-18 y.	19-24 y.	25-50 y.	>50 y.	Preg.	Lact.
300	500	800	800	800	1.200 1.200	1.200 1.200	1.200 1.200	800	800	1.200	1.200

Magnesium

- **Chemical composition:** *mineral* element.

- **Sources:** wheat bran is the richest product in magnesium: it contains 20 times more than meat or milk. However, because of the presence of phytates, only a portion is absorbed. Seeds are very good sources of magnesium, including wheat germ, sesame, oil-bearing nuts, and legumes.

- **Absorption:** From 30% to 50% of that which is taken in is absorbed into the blood.

  - *Facilitators of absorption:* food proteins, lactose from milk, and vitamin D, among other factors.

  - *Inhibitors of absorption:* excess calcium or phosphorus. The same as with calcium, the phytates from whole grains and the oxalic acid from certain green leafy vegetables partly decrease the absorption of magnesium. In spite of this, these foods remain a good source of magnesium since they contain a great deal of this mineral.

- **Function:** Magnesium is involved in the formation of bones and teeth; serves as a catalyst in energy-producing reactions within the cells; facilitates the transmission of nerve impulses; is involved in muscle relaxation, as opposed to calcium, which activates contraction.

- **Deficiency symptoms:** muscle spasms that may become generalized, known as tetania.

- **Increased need:** Cases of alcoholism, serious diarrhea, and kidney disorder can produce a lack of magnesium due to lack of absorption or increased loss through the urine or feces.

  - **Loss during processing of foods:** Magnesium is not affected by heat. Any loss is due to the dissolution of its salts in cooking water.

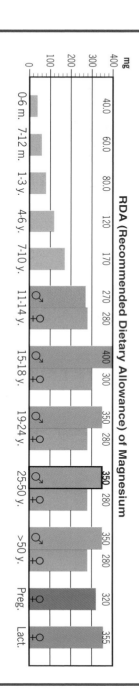

Squash seeds

RDA (Recommended Dietary Allowance) of Magnesium

mg

Age	mg
0-6 m.	40.0
7-12 m.	60.0
1-3 y.	80.0
4-6 y.	120
7-10 y.	170
11-14 y. ♂	270
11-14 y. ♀	280
15-18 y. ♂	400
15-18 y. ♀	300
19-24 y. ♂	350
19-24 y. ♀	280
25-50 y. ♂	350
25-50 y. ♀	280
>50 y. ♂	350
>50 y. ♀	280
Preg.	320
Lact.	355

MAGNESIUM

per each 100 g of raw edible portion

% Daily Value (based on a 2,000 calorie diet) provided by 100 g of this food

Vol./Page	Food	Quantity
2/360	Orange	10.0 mg
2/201	Potato	21.0 mg
2/356	Kiwi	30.0 mg
2/147	Date	35.0 mg
2/178	Artichoke	60.0 mg
1/357	Chocolate syrup	65.0 mg
2/28	Spinach	79.0 mg
1/88	Tofu	103 mg
1/132	Kelp	121 mg
2/306	White bean	138 mg
2/343	Whole-wheat flour	190 mg
2/102	Buckwheat	231 mg
2/310	Wheat germ	239 mg
1/175	Molasses	242 mg
2/40	Cashew	260 mg
2/252	Hazelnut	285 mg
2/48	Almond	296 mg
1/352	Sesame	351 mg
2/99	Dried squash seeds	535 mg
2/311	Bran	611 mg
1/218	Fresh egg	10.0 mg
1/183	Nonfat milk	11.4 mg
1/202	Nonfat natural yogurt	19.1 mg
1/308	Beefsteak	23.0 mg
1/314	Skinless chicken	25.0 mg
1/253	Oyster	33.0 mg
1/239	Sardine	34.0 mg
1/210	Gruyere cheese	35.9 mg
1/253	Shrimp	37.0 mg
1/239	Turbot	51.0 mg

Iron

- **Chemical composition and sources:** Iron is a *mineral* element present in foods in two chemical forms:

  – *Nonheme iron,* also referred to as non-hemic or inorganic iron. Plant-based foods, milk, and eggs contain only this type of iron. In meat and fish nonheme iron constitutes 66% of the total.

  – *Heme iron,* hemic or organic: This is only present in meat and fish, and constitutes 33.3% of the total iron they contain (see Vol. 1, p. 304).

- **Absorption:** *Heme* iron from meat and fish, as well as nonheme iron from other foods *is absorbed with difficulty.* Percentages of absorption are as follows:[2]

  – Iron in **vegetables:** *10%*

  – Iron in **fish:** *15%*

  – Iron in **soybean** and its derivatives: *20%*

  – Iron in **meat:** *30%*

  Once absorbed, the body does not distinguish between iron from meat and from plant sources. Both are equally used by the body, which puts to rest the myth that "the iron from meat is better." In reality, the opposite is true since heme iron is harmful to the heart (see Vol. 1, p. 304).

  – *Facilitators* of absorption: *Vitamin C* and *calcium* present in plant-based foods, but very rare in meat, increase the absorption of *nonheme* iron.

  – *Inhibitors* of absorption: the phytates present in grain bran, the oxalates in some vegetables, and the polyphenols or tannins in tea and certain plant-based foods may interfere with the absorption of iron, if they are present in excessive amounts (this does not occur at normal levels).

- **Function:** the formation of hemoglobin of the red blood cells, cellular respiration.

- **Deficiency symptoms:** anemia, cracked lips, brittle hair.

- **Increased need:** adolescence, excessive menstruation, pregnancy, visible or occult hemorrhages.

- **Loss during processing of foods:** very slight.

IRON
per each 100 g of raw edible portion

Vol./Page	Food	Quantity
2/130	Alfalfa sprouts	0.960 mg
2/45	Lettuce	1.10 mg
2/73	Peas	1.47 mg
2/64	English walnut	2.44 mg
2/28	Spinach	2.71 mg
2/165	Olive	3.30 mg
2/227	Parboiled rice	3.56 mg
2/41	Oats	4.72 mg
1/88	Tofu	5.36 mg
2/310	Wheat germ	6.26 mg
2/127	Lentils	9.02 mg
2/311	Bran	10.6 mg
1/352	Sesame	14.6 mg
2/264	Soybean	15.7 mg
1/175	Blackstrap molasses	17.5 mg
1/134	Dried spirulina	28.5 mg
1/352	Fenugreek	33.5 mg
1/182	Cow's milk	0.050 mg
1/202	Natural yogurt	0.080 mg
1/239	Salmon	0.800 mg
1/308	Lean beef	0.850 mg
1/314	Baked chicken	0.890 mg
1/239	Tuna canned in oil	1.39 mg
1/218	Fresh egg	1.44 mg
1/312	Lamb	1.57 mg
1/239	Sardine	2.30 mg
1/316	Hamburger	2.67 mg
1/317	Beef liver	4.79 mg
1/253	Oyster	5.78 mg
1/239	Caviar	11.9 mg

% Daily Value (based on a 2,000 calorie diet) provided by 100 g of this food

1% — 2% — 4% — 10% — 20% — 40% — 100% — 200% — 500%

The nonheme iron found in plant-based foods is absorbed in lower proportion than the heme iron of meat.

However, this is compensated for by the fact that nuts, whole grains, and legumes contain up to 5 or 6 times the iron as meat by weight.

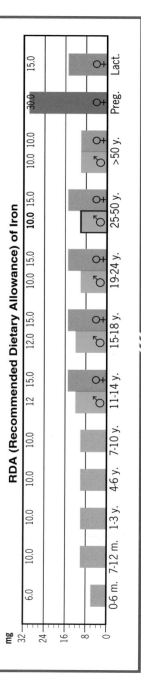

RDA (Recommended Dietary Allowance) of Iron

Potassium

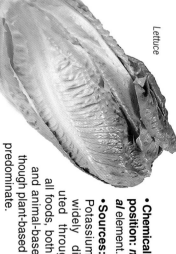

Lettuce

- **Chemical composition:** *mineral* element.

- **Sources:** Potassium is widely distributed throughout all foods, both plant and animal-based, although plant-based foods predominate.

- **Absorption:** Potassium is absorbed easily in the small intestine. Normally 90% of potassium in foods is absorbed.

- **Function:** Potassium is the third most abundant mineral in the body after calcium and phosphorus, and is the ion present in the highest concentration within the cells. It is involved particularly in the following processes:
  – Acid-base balance,
  – Muscular relaxation,
  – Secretion of insulin in the pancreas.

- **Deficiency symptoms:** muscle weakness and cardiac rhythm disorders. When there is a sodium-potassium imbalance with predominant sodium arterial hypertension is the result.

- **Increased need:**
  – **Excess sodium:** when a great deal of sodium is taken in due to a diet rich in meat derivatives, preserves, and salt-preserved foods, the need for potassium increases. This is because there must be a sodium-potassium balance in the blood and in all body fluids, and by extension, foods.
  – **Loss through body fluids** rich in potassium: intense vomiting or diarrhea, polyuria (excess urine production).

- **Loss during processing of foods:** Only that dissolved in cooking water.

Natural fruits and vegetables are a good source of potassium, as are all plant-based foods.

They also have the advantage of being low in sodium, an advantage that protects against arterial hypertension, as opposed to meat derivatives, preserves and salt-preserved foods.

POTASSIUM
per each 100 g of raw edible portion

% Daily Value (based on a 2,000 calorie diet) provided by 100 g of this food

Vol./Page	Food	Quantity
2/339	Cucumber	144 mg
2/78	Grape	185 mg
2/254	Melon	210 mg
2/275	Red tomato	222 mg
1/72	Coconut milk	250 mg
2/325	Whole-grain bread	252 mg
2/250	Asparagus	273 mg
2/248	Celery	287 mg
2/176	Endive	314 mg
2/25	Carrot	323 mg
2/63	Broccoli	325 mg
2/161	Fennel	414 mg
2/201	Potato	543 mg
2/28	Spinach	558 mg
2/108	Avocado	599 mg
2/147	Date	652 mg
2/48	Almond	732 mg
2/310	Wheat germ	892 mg
2/264	Soybean	1,797 mg
1/175	Blackstrap molasses	2,492 mg
1/212	Cottage cheese, 1% fat	85.5 mg
1/218	Fresh egg	121 mg
1/182	Cow's milk	152 mg
1/316	Hamburger	161 mg
1/210	Camembert cheese	187 mg
1/239	Tuna canned in oil	207 mg
1/314	Turkey, meat	296 mg
1/308	Beefsteak	304 mg
1/239	Cod	413 mg
1/239	Salmon	490 mg

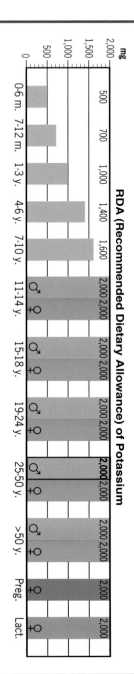

RDA (Recommended Dietary Allowance) of Potassium

Zinc

- **Chemical composition:** *mineral* considered a trace element because it is necessary only in very small amounts, as are other minerals such as iron.

- **Sources:** Among animal-based foods only the oyster is noted as a rich source of zinc. Wheat germ, sesame, maple sugar, oil-bearing nuts, and legumes, equal or exceed the amount of zinc in meat and cured cheeses.

- **Absorption:** Although there are many plant-based foods rich in zinc, some of their components inhibit its absorption and that of other minerals:

  — phytates (see Vol. 2, p. 311) in whole grains,

  — oxalates in some green leafy vegetables such as spinach,

  — vegetable fiber.

  This interference with absorption of minerals is only of concern if one regularly consumes large amounts of bran, whole-grain cereals or other fiber-rich foods. In spite of this, it is perfectly possible to obtain sufficient zinc with a healthful plant-food-based diet.

- **Function:** Most of the zinc in the body (some 2.2 g) is found in the skin, the hair, the nails, and the prostate. It is involved in numerous chemical reactions within the body, since it forms part of various enzymes. Its two most evident functions are:

  — Maintaining the skin, hair, and nails in good condition;

  — Development and functioning of the reproductive organs.

- **Deficiency symptoms:** retardation of physical growth, poor wound healing, lack of development of the gonads (testicles or ovaries).

- **Increased need:** excess fiber consumption, pregnancy, nursing.

- **Loss during processing of foods:** very slight.

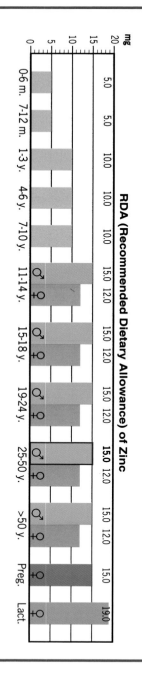

RDA (Recommended Dietary Allowance) of Zinc

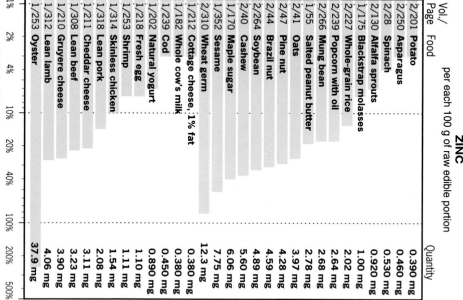

ZINC
per each 100 g of raw edible portion

Vol./Page	Food	Quantity
2/201	Potato	0.390 mg
2/250	Asparagus	0.460 mg
2/28	Spinach	0.530 mg
2/130	Alfalfa sprouts	0.920 mg
1/175	Blackstrap molasses	1.00 mg
2/227	Whole-grain rice	2.02 mg
2/239	Popcorn with oil	2.64 mg
2/266	Mung bean	2.68 mg
1/55	Salted peanut butter	2.78 mg
2/41	Oats	3.97 mg
2/47	Pine nut	4.28 mg
2/44	Brazil nut	4.59 mg
2/264	Soybean	4.89 mg
2/40	Cashew	5.60 mg
1/170	Maple sugar	6.06 mg
1/352	Sesame	7.75 mg
2/310	Wheat germ	12.3 mg
1/212	Cottage cheese, 1% fat	0.380 mg
1/182	Whole cow's milk	0.380 mg
1/239	Cod	0.450 mg
1/202	Natural yogurt	0.890 mg
1/218	Fresh egg	1.10 mg
1/253	Shrimp	1.11 mg
1/314	Skinless chicken	1.54 mg
1/318	Lean pork	2.08 mg
1/211	Cheddar cheese	3.11 mg
1/308	Lean beef	3.23 mg
1/210	Gruyere cheese	3.90 mg
1/312	Lean lamb	4.06 mg
1/253	Oyster	37.9 mg

% Daily Value (based on a 2,000 calorie diet) provided by 100 g of this food

There are plant-based foods such as wheat germ, sesame, and some nuts and legumes that exceed all animal-based foods, with the exception of the oyster, in zinc. With a healthy diet based on plant-based foods, there is no risk of suffering a lack of zinc, particularly if one eats wheat germ and sesame.

Total Fat

TOTAL FAT
per each 100 g of raw edible portion

Vol./Page	Food	% Daily Value (based on a 2,000 calorie diet) provided by 100 g of this food	Quantity
2/225	**White rice**		0.580 g
2/343	**White bean**		0.850 g
2/304	**Cherry**		0.960 g
1/74	**Dry macaroni**		1.58 g
1/88	**Soy milk or beverage**		1.91 g
1/72	**White bread**		3.60 g
1/88	**Tofu**		4.78 g
2/41	**Oats**		6.90 g
2/108	**Avocado**		15.3 g
2/205	**Potatoes fried in vegetable oil**		16.1 g
2/325	**Coconut**		33.5 g
2/64	**English walnut**		61.9 g
1/126	**Olive oil**		100 g
1/183	**Nonfat milk**		0.180 g
1/239	**Flatfish**		1.19 g
1/308	**Lean beef**		2.87 g
1/314	**Skinless chicken**		3.08 g
1/182	**Whole cow's milk**		3.34 g
1/239	**Tuna canned in oil**		8.21 g
1/218	**Fresh egg**		10.0 g
1/327	**Ham**		10.6 g
1/239	**Sardine**		12.0 g
1/314	**Baked chicken**		13.6 g
1/318	**Pork (various cuts)**		16.5 g
1/312	**Lamb**		21.6 g
1/210	**Camembert cheese**		24.3 g
1/210	**Gruyere cheese**		32.3 g
1/324	**Pork sausage**		40.3 g
1/326	**Bacon**		57.5 g
1/204	**Butter**		81.1 g

Scale: 1% — 2% — 4% — 10% — 20% — 40% — 100% — 200% — 500%

- **Chemical composition:** the fats present in all foods are composed primarily (96% to 98%) of *triglycerides*, which are a type of simple lipid composed of glycerin and fatty acids. The quality and properties of fats depend on the type of fatty acids they contain (see chapter 22, Vol. 2, p. 82).

- **Sources:**

  – **Plant-based** foods in their natural state generally contain little fat, with the exception of oil-bearing nuts. **Vegetable fats** have several *advantages* over animal fats:

    ✓ They are predominantly *unsaturated fatty acids,* which reduce blood cholesterol level.

    ✓ They contain substances beneficial to the health, such as *lecithin, phytosterols,* and *vitamin E* (see Vol. 1, p. 116).

  – **Animal-based** foods and products are *all high* in *fats,* except nonfat milk and dairy products, lean fish, and very lean meat. There are various *drawbacks:*

    ✓ Elevated proportion of **saturated fatty acids,** which *increase cholesterol* production within the body.

    ✓ They *contain cholesterol,* which also contributes to increased blood cholesterol levels.

    ✓ They contain *no vitamin E.*

- **Function:** Fats act as a reserve energy source. They transport and facilitate the absorption of liposoluble vitamins, such as A, D, E, and K in the intestine.

- **Deficiency symptoms:** The body can produce its own fats from carbohydrates and proteins; therefore, **lack of dietary fats** is generally of *little concern.* The *only* fatty acids that *cannot be synthesized* within the body and must be **supplied** through the diet are *linoleic, linolenic* and *arachidonic acids,* all of them abundant in nuts.

- **Consequences of excess:** obesity, raised cholesterol levels. Excess fat in the diet is harmful, particularly when it is of animal origin.

- **Loss during processing of foods:** degraded during frying (see Vol. 1, p. 122).

The problem with dietary fats is not their lack, but rather their excess, which is harmful even where vegetable fats are concerned.

Daily Value (Acceptable Daily Intake) of Total Fat

For an adult: An amount of fat that supplies *less* than *30%* of **total calorie** intake. Excess fats of any kind, including vegetable fats, is harmful to health.

For a 2,000 calorie diet, this represents about *65 g* of fats daily.

A typical omnivorous diet usually provides about 40% of calories from fats (from 85 g to 100 g daily), which represents a serious health risk.

Saturated Fat

- **Chemical composition:** Saturated fats are formed by *triglycerides* whose **fatty acids** are of the **saturated** type. These are so named because *all of their carbon atoms have their full complement of hydrogen atoms.*

- **Sources:**

  - **Plant-based** foods: These are all **low** in **saturated** fats, with some exceptions, such as coconut and palm oils. These contain a special type of **medium-chain fatty acids** (8 to 12 carbon atoms) that do not increase blood cholesterol levels.

  - **Animal-based** foods and products: All of these contain a great deal of **saturated fat,** particularly cured cheeses, sausages, and bacon.

- **Function:** Reserve energy source. **Saturated fat is solid** at *room temperature* and tends to be deposited within body tissues, particularly:

  - beneath the skin, causing obesity,

  - on artery walls, causing arteriosclerosis.

- **Deficiency symptoms:** *None.* The body has no need for saturated fat. *The less taken in, the better.*

- **Consequences of excess:** obesity, raised cholesterol levels, arteriosclerosis, and a variety of cancers (see Vol. 1, p. 291). Saturated fats, particularly those of animal origin, are harmful to health.

- **Loss during processing of foods:** degraded during frying (see Vol. 1, p. 122).

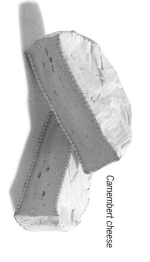

Camembert cheese

Daily Value (Acceptable Daily Intake) of Saturated Fat

Ideal: *0 mg*

For an adult it should not represent more than **10%** of **total calorie** intake.

For a 2,000 calorie diet, this represents about **20 g** of saturated fat daily.

A typical omnivorous diet usually provides about 30 g to 60 g of saturated fat daily. A much more healthful diet formed of plant-based foods, between 5 g and 10 g.

Saturated fats predominate in animal-based foods, while unsaturated fats come mainly from vegetables. Saturated fats increase the production of cholesterol in the body, while unsaturated fats, lower it.

SATURATED FAT
per each 100 g of raw edible portion

Vol./Page	Food	% Daily Value (based on a 2,000 calorie diet) provided by 100 g of this food	Quantity
2/225	White rice		0.158 g
1/88	Soy milk or beverage		0.214 g
2/304	Cherry		0.216 g
2/343	White bean		0.219 g
1/74	Dry macaroni		0.225 g
1/88	Tofu		0.691 g
1/72	White bread		0.811 g
2/41	Oats		1.22 g
2/108	Avocado		2.44 g
2/205	Potatoes fried in vegetable oil		4.99 g
2/64	English walnut		5.59 g
1/126	Olive oil		13.5 g
2/325	Coconut		29.7 g
1/183	Nonfat milk		0.117 g
1/239	Flatfish		0.283 g
1/314	Skinless chicken		0.790 g
1/308	Lean beef		0.860 g
1/239	Tuna canned in oil		1.53 g
1/182	Whole cow's milk		2.08 g
1/239	Sardine		3.09 g
1/218	Fresh egg		3.10 g
1/327	Ham		3.39 g
1/314	Baked chicken		3.79 g
1/318	Pork (various cuts)		5.77 g
1/312	Lamb		9.47 g
1/324	Pork sausage		14.5 g
1/210	Camembert cheese		15.3 g
1/210	Gruyere cheese		18.9 g
1/326	Bacon		21.3 g
1/204	Butter		50.5 g

% Daily Value scale: 1% 2% 4% 10% 20% 40% 100% 200% 500%

Cholesterol

- **Chemical composition:** Cholesterol is a *lipoid* (a substance similar to fats) whose chemical structure is similar to steroid hormones.

- **Sources:**

  - **Animal-based** foods and products: All of these contain cholesterol: milk and its derivatives, eggs, fish, shellfish, and all types of meat. **Variety meats** of animals and **eggs** have the *highest* cholesterol content.

  - **Plant-based foods:** In broad lines, it may be broadly stated that *none* contains cholesterol. However, there are minute amounts in some vegetable oils, such as olive oil, and may be considered incidental (see Vol. 1, p. 116). This small amount of cholesterol is considered of external origin.

  - **Mushrooms:** These are not true vegetables (see Vol. 1, p. 136), and share some characteristics with animals. Certain species may contain minimal amounts of cholesterol (1-3 mg/100 g).

- **Absorption:** An omnivorous diet provides an average of between 500 and 800 mg of cholesterol a day. Of this amount only between 20% and 80% is absorbed; the rest is eliminated through the feces.

  - *Facilitates absorption:* The amount of total fat in the diet (the more fat consumed, the more cholesterol absorbed and produced by the liver).

  - *Reduces absorption:* The amount of fiber present in the diet (the more fiber is present, the less cholesterol is absorbed); *phytosterols* found in unrefined oils (see Vol. 1, p. 116).

- **Function:** Cholesterol forms part of the membranes that protect the cells of animals. It is the raw material for the production of sex and suprarenal (corticoid) hormones, as well as bile, which is necessary for the digestion of fats.

- **Consequences of excess:** arteriosclerosis (narrowing and hardening of the arteries due to deposits of cholesterol) and increased risk of heart attack (myocardial infarction) and stroke (thrombosis). The primary problem with cholesterol is its excess: it is *not only taken in* as part of the diet; the body *also produces it*.

CHOLESTEROL
per each 100 g of raw edible portion

Vol./Page	Food	Quantity
1/183	Nonfat milk	1.80 mg
1/202	Nonfat natural yogurt	1.80 mg
1/202	Natural yogurt	6.10 mg
1/182	Whole cow's milk	13.6 mg
1/239	Tuna canned in oil	18.0 mg
1/239	Salmon	55.0 mg
1/318	Lean pork	61.0 mg
1/318	Pork (various cuts)	69.0 mg
1/314	Skinless chicken	70.0 mg
1/327	Lean cured ham	70.0 mg
1/308	Beefsteak	79.0 mg
1/308	Lean beef	83.0 mg
1/326	Beef or pork sausage	88.0 mg
1/210	Gruyere cheese	110 mg
1/204	Whipping cream	137 mg
1/253	Shrimp	152 mg
1/204	Butter	219 mg
1/327	Paté	255 mg
1/317	Beef liver	309 mg
1/218	Fresh egg	425 mg
1/241	Salmon oil	485 mg
1/239	Caviar	588 mg
1/218	Fresh egg yolk	1,281 mg
1/317	Beef brains	1,590 mg

% Daily Value (based on a 2,000 calorie diet) provided by 100 g of this food

1% — 2% — 4% — 10% — 20% — 40% — 100% — 200% — 500%

Cholesterol is an *undesirable component* of animal-based foods.

It is not necessary to consume cholesterol, and avoiding it is more healthful. This is achieved with a diet of plant-based foods. The liver is more than capable of synthesizing all the cholesterol needed by the body.

Daily Value (Acceptable Daily Intake) of Cholesterol

Ideal: *0 mg* daily
Acceptable Daily Intake for an adult: *300 mg*.

Sodium

- **Chemical composition:** *mineral* element. Combined with another element, chlorine, it forms *common salt* (see Vol. 1, p. 344). Sodium also forms part of many other mineral salts such as **sodium iodide** or **sodium nitrate.**

- **Sources:** Sodium is present in almost all foods, forming different salts. Its origin may be triple:

  - *Naturally* present sodium in foods:

    ✓ **Plant-based foods:** All of these are low in sodium. It is practically nonexistent in fruits, and there are only slight amounts in legumes and grains. Vegetables such as celery, spinach, and particularly seaweed are the plant-based foods richest in sodium.

    ✓ **Animal-based foods:** Sodium is present in rather *high* levels in all of these: milk, meat, eggs, and fish (listed in increasing order).

  - **Added sodium in the form of common salt:** Salt is added to most processed foods, particularly cured meats such as sausages and ham (see Vol. 1, p. 347 *"Hidden salt": an abundant additive*).

  - Sodium added specifically as an **additive:** Many additives used in food processing are sodium salts such as sodium alginate, sodium benzoate, and others.

- **Absorption:** Almost all sodium taken in is absorbed into the bloodstream. The kidneys must eliminate the excess, which tends to be up to 90% of that taken in with foods.

- **Function:** sodium retains water and contributes to the maintenance of the acid-base and water balances in the body. It is the *most important extracellular ion.*

- **Consequences of excess:** arterial hypertension, edema (fluid retention), calcium loss through the urine.

- **Increased need:** Heavy perspiration, intense vomiting or diarrhea.

- **Sodium/potassium balance:** Animal-based and processed foods, bread, preserves, sausages, etc. contain more sodium than potassium. Their regular consumption alters the essential balance between sodium and potassium and is a factor in hypertension and other diseases.

SODIUM
per each 100 g of raw edible portion

Vol./Page	Food	Quantity
2/41	Oats	2.00 mg
2/142	Onion	3.00 mg
2/73	Peas	5.00 mg
2/201	Potato	6.00 mg
2/73	Red tomato	9.00 mg
2/108	Avocado	10.0 mg
2/343	White bean	16.0 mg
2/191	Cabbage	18.0 mg
2/319	Leek	20.0 mg
2/28	Spinach	79.0 mg
2/248	Celery	87.0 mg
1/132	Kelp	233 mg
1/55	Salted peanut butter	486 mg
1/72	White bread	538 mg
2/197	Sauerkraut	661 mg
1/332	Vegetarian hotdog	888 mg
1/183	Nonfat milk	51.5 mg
1/202	Natural yogurt	70.2 mg
1/314	Skinless chicken	77.0 mg
1/308	Lean beef	86.0 mg
1/218	Fresh egg	126 mg
1/239	Hake	135 mg
1/239	Tuna canned in oil	354 mg
1/316	Hamburger	430 mg
1/211	Cheddar cheese	621 mg
1/326	Bacon	730 mg
1/204	Salted butter	826 mg
1/210	Camembert cheese	842 mg
1/326	Pork or beef sausage	1.235 mg
1/327	Lean cured ham	2.695 mg

% Daily Value (based on a 2,000 calorie diet) provided by 100 g of this food

1% — 2% — 4% — 10% — 20% — 40% — 100% — 200% — 500%

The western diet provides an average of **4,000 mg of sodium (10 g of salt), which is excessive and overburdens the body.**

To reduce sodium intake:

- **Reduce the consumption of processed foods.**
- **Do not use salt at the table.**

Daily Value (Acceptable Daily Intake) of Sodium

Minimum: *500 mg* a day, equivalent to *1.25 g* of common table salt.

Acceptable Daily Intake: *2,400 mg* a day, equivalent to *6 g* of common table salt.

Other Nutrients

Nutrient	Function	Sources	Daily Need
VITAMIN D **Cholecalciferol** or **vitamin D₃** of natural origin; **ergocalciferol** or **vitamin D₂** of synthetic origin.	Facilitates intestinal **absorption** of **calcium** and **phosphorus.** Involved in growth and hardening or mineralization of the **bones** and **teeth.**	Only animal-based foods provide significant amounts. In reverse order: fatty fish, particularly liver; mammal liver; egg yolk; butter; whole milk. Nonfat milk does not contain vitamin D unless it has been fortified. Meat contains very little.	• **Children, adolescents and young adults:** 10 µg (400 IU) • **Adults** in general: 5 µg (200 IU) • **Pregnant and nursing women:** 10 µg (400 IU) A fair-skinned individual exposing the face, hands and arms to the **sun** for 5 to 10 minutes gets the equivalent to the 5 µg adult daily requirement of vitamin D.[3] Since the body can produce its own vitamin D through solar action, it is not normally necessary to take it with foods or in the form of supplements. **Excess** vitamin D is **toxic** (renal and cardiac calcification).
VITAMIN K **Phylloquinone** or **vitamin K₁**— plant origin; **menaquinone** or **vitamin K₂** produced by intestinal bacteria.	Necessary for **protein** synthesis in the liver that facilitates blood coagulation. Its action is **anti hemorrhagic.**	• **Dietary sources:** the best sources are vegetables, particularly greens such as spinach, broccoli, and green peas. Animal-based foods such as cheese and meat also contain it. • **Endogenous sources** (from within the body): produced by intestinal bacteria.	• **Infants:** 5-10 µg • **Children:** 15-30 µg • **Adolescents:** 45-70 µg • **Adults:** 60-80 µg Under normal conditions the intestinal bacteria supply sufficient vitamin K to meet daily need, except in the following cases, in which pharmaceutical **supplements** may be necessary: • Newborns. • Individuals undergoing antibiotic or sulfonamide treatment, which destroys the intestinal flora. • Intestinal disorders such as celiac disease. • Obstructive jaundice patients.
BIOTIN	Hydrosoluble B complex vitamin that acts as a **coenzyme** in numerous metabolic reactions.	• **Dietary sources:** this is found in most foods, particularly in brewer's yeast, cheese, soybean, eggs, and spinach. • **Endogenous sources** (from within the body): produced by intestinal bacteria.	Estimated at between 10 and 30 µg for **children** and 30 and 100 µg for **adults.** Normally the **intestinal bacteria** produce the biotin necessary.
CHOLINE	Hydrosoluble **B complex** vitamin that is one of the constituents of **lecithin** (see Vol. 1, p. 89). • Inhibits the accumulation of fats in the liver. • Involved in transmission of nerve impulses.	• **Dietary sources:** this is widely distributed in foods, particularly plant-based (soybean, wheat germ, cabbage, oil-bearing nuts) and in eggs and mammal liver. • **Endogenous sources:** the body can synthesize choline, but not in sufficient quantities, particularly during infancy.	Has not been established, but varies between 300 and 500 mg a day for **adults** and about 100 mg for **children.** It is estimated that an average Western diet provides from 400 to 900 mg daily, particularly if it includes sufficient legumes, eggs, grains, and oil-bearing seeds.

Nutrient	Function	Sources	Daily Need
PANTOTHENIC ACID **vitamin B₃**	Hydrosoluble **B complex** vitamin that forms part of the **A coenzyme**, one of the most active substances in the metabolic processes. Pantothenic acid is necessary to: • Synthesize fatty acids, burn them, and convert them into energy. • Produce energy in the cells through the Krebs cycle. • Produce antibodies.	This is found in virtually all foods (in Greek "pantothen" means "in all"), but particularly in the following: • Of **plant** origin: bran and whole grains, mushrooms, oil-bearing nuts, soybean, avocado. • Of **animal** origin: variety meats, salmon, and other fatty fish.	Has not been determined, but is estimated between 4 and 7 mg daily. Eating enough natural or minimally processed foods amply satisfies the need. There is a risk, however of deficiency if the diet is predominantly processed foods, since it is easily **destroyed** by various processes: • Refining of grains: up to 60% loss • Canning, cooking and freezing: up to 50% loss.
IODINE	Mineral element *(trace element)* whose only known function is to form part of the secretions of the **thyroid** gland. These regulate the rate at which energy-producing nutrients are oxidized or burned in the cells.	• Of **plant** origin: seaweed and vegetables grown in iodine-rich soil. • Of **animal** origin: fish and shellfish. The iodine content of vegetables varies a great deal since it depends on the richness of the soil in this mineral. That found in animal products depends on their diet.	• **Infants:** from 40 to 50 µg • **Children:** from 70 to 120 µg • **Adults:** 150 µg • **Pregnant and nursing women:** 200 µg Since the iodine content of foods is practically unpredictable, **iodized** salt is recommended, particularly in areas away from the sea.
SELENIUM (see Vol. 1, p. 355)	Mineral element *(trace element)* that performs the following functions: • **Antioxidant:** Acts together with **vitamin E. Protects** the cells from damage by **free radicals,** and protects against cancer, arteriosclerosis, and degenerative diseases. • **Stimulates the immune system:** contributes to the formation of antibodies against infectious agents. • **Anticarcinogen:** protects against various types of cancer such as that of the breast[4] and the skin.[5]	The selenium content of foods varies a great deal according to the natural richness of this mineral in the soil. It is scant in processed foods. • **Plant-based:** Brazil nuts, brewer's yeast, wheat germ, and molasses are the best sources. It is also abundant in legumes and other oil bearing nuts.[6] • **Animal-based:** it is present in fish, shellfish, and meat, although in unpredictable amounts.	The following are estimates: • **Infants:** 10-15 µg • **Children:** 20-30 µg • **Adolescents:** 30-50 µg • **Men:** 70 µg • **Women:** 55 µg • **Pregnant women:** 65 µg • **Nursing mothers:** 75 µg Overall, the average intake throughout the population is less than RDA. For example, studies carried out in Germany demonstrate that it is 38 µg for women and 47 µg for men,[7] which confirms the **need to *increase*** selenium intake or take **supplements** (see Vol. 1, p. 355).
CHROMIUM	Mineral element *(trace element)* that increases glucose tolerance and protects against diabetes.	Molasses, eggs, fresh fruits and vegetables, wheat germ, brewer's yeast. It is insignificant in refined and processed foods, or in foods from factory agriculture.	• **Infants:** 10-60 µg • **Children and adults:** 50-200 µg
COPPER	Mineral element *(trace element)* that facilitates the **absorption** of **iron** and is involved in the formation of hemoglobin.[8]	Molasses, oil-bearing nuts, wheat germ, brewer's yeast, oysters.	• **Infants:** 0.4-0.6 mg • **Children:** 0.7-2 mg • **Adolescents and adults:** 1.5-3 mg
MANGANESE	Mineral element *(trace element)* involved in the formation of **bone** and the production of **insulin.**	Whole grains, oil-bearing nuts, fresh vegetables, molasses, brewer's yeast. Present only in minute amounts in vegetables grown in alkaline or impoverished soils.	• **Infants:** 0.3-1 mg • **Children:** 1-3 mg • **Adolescents and adults:** 3-5 mg

Phytochemicals

Phytochemicals are the latest discovery in the components of foods.
They are attributed with a large portion of the healing properties of plant-based foods.

Vegetable Pharmacy

The composition of plant-based foods is very complex. In addition to water, proteins, carbohydrates, fats, minerals, and fiber, in recent years *hundreds* of other substances, now known as *phytochemicals*, have been discovered.

At one time it was thought that these were inert materials, and were therefore called "accompanying substances." Some, such as *phytates*, were considered harmful.

But as research progressed there were surprising discoveries concerning the healing and preventive properties in the phytochemicals found in plant-based foods.

Some phytochemicals have been chemically isolated and are sold as pharmaceutical preparations the same as vitamin supplements. However, *none* of these products *substitutes* the need to follow a *healthy diet* of fruits, grains, legumes, and vegetables. These natural products constitute a true **vegetable pharmacy.**

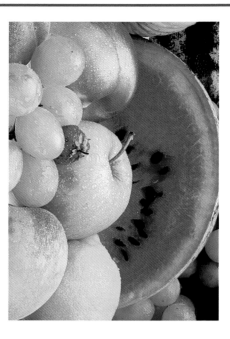

Phytochemical elements are authentic natural medicines present in plant-based foods.

Characteristics of Phytochemicals

- **Synonyms:** they may also be referred to as *phytochemical elements* (Greek *phyto* = "vegetable"); *accompanying or non-nutritive substances; nutraceuticals* (contraction of nutrient and pharmaceutical); *metanutrients* ("beyond" classical nutrients).

- **Chemical composition:** in spite of their name, they are *not elements* in the chemical sense, rather they are complex substances of a diverse nature.

- **Only in plant-based foods:** they are chemical substances found only in **plant-based** foods, above all fruits, vegetables, legumes, and grains.

- **Very small amounts:** they are present in amounts of milligrams (mg) and even micrograms (μg) per 100 grams (g), only detectable using modern methods of chemical analysis.

- **Numerous:** it is known that hundreds, possibly thousands, of different phytochemicals exist, although the health properties of only a few dozen have been investigated.

- **They are not nutrients:** they are not considered "nutrients" in the classical sense since it has not been shown that their lack produces any pathological symptoms and it has not been possible to determine the RDA (Recommended Dietary Allowance) for them.
  Although they are not nutrients, many facilitate the action of some vitamins, such as the case of flavonoids and vitamin C.

- **They do not supply calories:** As happens with vitamins and minerals, phytochemicals have no caloric value.

- **Antioxidants:** Most phytochemicals act as antioxidants, which explains in part the preventive and healing action of fruits, legumes, grains, and vegetables.

- **Preventive and healing:** in spite of being present in minute quantities and not being considered nutrients, phytochemicals perform numerous preventive and healing functions within the body.

A Sampling of Phytochemicals

Phytochemical	Function	Sources
FLAVONOIDS OR BIOFLAVONOIDS	Natural coloring in plant-based foods with **antioxidant, anti-inflammatory, diuretic effects**. They also protect the **capillaries** and **arteries**. A large part of the healing power of plant-based foods is due to flavonoids. They facilitate the action of vitamin C. • **They protect** the **arteries** and the **heart:** flavonoids stop the degenerative process of arteriosclerosis and provide moderate protection against **heart attack** (myocardial infarction).[9, 10] The cardio-protective effect of grapes and grape juice, and, to a lesser degree, wine, is due to the phenolic flavonoids they contain (see Vol. 1, p. 378).[11, 12] • **They prevent stroke** (thrombosis and other vascular accidents).[13] • **They protect** against **cancer.**[14, 15]	They are found in all fruits and many vegetables, but particularly in the following: • Citrus:[16] orange (rutin), grapefruit (naringin), lemon (hesperidin and diosmin), and others. • Cherries (ellagic acid). • Apples and onions: contain quercetin, one of the most studied flavonoids, which has been shown to be very effective in preventing platelet stickiness and clotting (thrombosis). Flavonoids avoid the oxidation of lipoproteins,[17, 18] which improves cardiovascular health. • Grapes (phenolic flavonoids or polyphenols). • Other vegetables: tea, currant (rutin), acerola, squash flower, pepper.
ANTHOCYANIDINES	Vegetable pigments similar to flavonoids that give certain fruits their red or purple color.[19] They are also known as **protoanthocyanidines.** • They are **antioxidants;** they decrease cholesterol synthesis in the liver.[20] • They **protect the heart.** • They **tone** venous circulation. • They regenerate the pigments in the **retina** and improve **vision.** • They are a **urinary antiseptic.**	Black grape,[21] strawberry, pomegranate, blueberry.
ISOFLAVONES	These are a type of **phytoestrogen** (female hormone of plant origin), which facilitates the mineralization of bone and protects against arteriosclerosis and cancer (see Vol. 2, p. 268).	Soybean and all of its derivatives, particularly *tofu.* Other legumes also contain some amount of isoflavones.
LIGNANS	Substances related to phytoestrogens with great preventive capabilities:[22] • They *protect* against **cancer** (particularly of the breast and prostate). • They are **antioxidants** that *eliminate* destructive **free radicals,** *stop* **arteriosclerosis,** and *prevent* **heart attack.**	Actually, what plants provide are lignan precursors, with which bacteria in the colon produce true lignans. The foods richest in these precursors are flax seed, fruits and vegetables,[23] whole grains,[22] and legumes.[24]
SULFUROUS COMPOUNDS	These are diverse substances that contain sulfur and the typical aroma and flavor to cruciferous vegetables (botanical family *Cruciferae*). The best known are **indoles** and **glucosinolates.** These phytochemicals are very effective **anticarcinogenic** agents.	All cruciferous vegetables (the greener the better): cabbage, broccoli, turnip, watercress, etcetera (see Vol. 1, p. 106).
TERPENES OR MONOTERPENES	These interfere with cancer-promoting substances, impeding their action.	Citrus, cabbage, aromatic herbs such as caraway, parsley, and mint.
CAROTENOIDS	A variety of substances that give a yellowish or reddish color to fruits and vegetables. In addition to transforming to vitamin A in the body, they act as potent **antioxidants** and **anticarcinogens.**	Carrot (**beta-carotene,** see Vol. 1, p. 389), red tomato (**lycopene,** see Vol. 2, p. 276), oranges and spinach (**lutein** and **zeaxanthin**).
PHYTATES	When these were discovered, they were considered an antinutritive factor because they reduce the absorption of iron, zinc, and other minerals. However, this is not a serious drawback since plants containing phytates also contain abundant iron and other minerals. Additionally, it has been recently discovered that phytates are effective **antioxidants and anticarcinogens** (see Vol. 2, p. 311).	Whole grains (particularly the bran) and legumes.

Table of the Composition of Foods per 100 g of raw edible portion

NDB_No*	FRUITS	Vol./page	Energy kcal	Pro-teins g	CHO g	Fiber g	Vit. A µg RE	Vit. B1 mg	Vit. B2 mg	Niacin mg NE	Vit. B6 mg	Fola-tes µg	Vit. B12 µg	Vit. C mg	Vit. E mg α-TE	Ca mg	P mg	Mg mg	Fe mg	K mg	Zn mg	Total fat g	Satur. fat g	Cho-lesterol mg	Na mg
09001	Acerola	2/367	32	0.4	6.59	1.1	77	0.02	0.06	0.4	0.009	14	—	1,678	0.13	12	11	18	0.2	146	0.1	0.3	0.068	—	7
09003	Apple	2/229	59	0.19	12.6	2.7	5	0.017	0.014	0.11	0.048	2.8	—	5.7	0.32	7	7	5	0.18	115	0.04	0.36	0.058	—	1.5
09016	Apple juice	2/229	47	0.06	11.6	0.1	—	0.021	0.017	0.1	0.03	0.1	—	0.9	0.01	7	7	3	0.37	119	0.03	0.11	0.019	—	3
09021	Apricot	2/26	48	1.4	8.72	2.4	261	0.03	0.04	0.85	0.054	8.6	—	10	0.89	14	19	8	0.54	296	0.26	0.39	0.027	—	1
09032	Apricot, dried	2/26	238	3.65	52.8	9	724	0.008	0.151	4.08	0.156	10.3	—	2.4	1.5	45	117	47	4.7	1,378	0.74	0.46	0.032	—	10
09040	Banana	2/70	92	1.03	21	2.4	8	0.045	0.1	0.74	0.578	19.1	—	9.1	0.27	6	20	29	0.31	396	0.16	0.48	0.185	—	1
09042	Blackberry	1/49	52	0.72	7.46	5.3	16	0.03	0.04	0.4	0.058	34	—	21	0.71	32	21	20	0.57	196	0.27	0.39	0.014	—	—
09050	Blueberry	2/257	56	0.67	11.4	2.7	10	0.048	0.05	0.409	0.036	6.4	—	13	1	6	10	5	0.17	89	0.11	0.38	0.032	—	6
09059	Breadfruit	2/295	103	1.07	22.2	4.9	4	0.11	0.03	0.9	0.1	14	—	29	1.12	17	30	25	0.54	490	0.12	0.23	0.048	—	2
09138	Cape gooseberry	1/51	53	1.9	11.2	—	72	0.11	0.04	2.8	—	—	—	11	—	9	40	—	1	—	—	0.7	—	—	—
09060	Carambola	2/219	33	0.54	5.13	2.7	49	0.028	0.027	0.478	0.1	14	—	21.2	0.37	4	16	9	0.26	163	0.11	0.35	0.023	—	2
09062	Cherimoya	2/59	94	1.3	21.6	2.4	1	0.1	0.11	1.3	0.2	14	—	9	—	23	40	—	0.5	264	—	0.4	—	—	5
09070	Cherry	2/304	72	1.2	14.3	2.3	21	0.05	0.06	0.4	0.036	4.2	—	7	0.13	15	19	11	0.39	224	0.06	0.96	0.216	—	2
12097	Chestnut	2/322	213	2.42	37.4	8.1	3	0.238	0.168	1.63	0.376	62	—	43	—	27	93	32	1.01	518	0.52	2.26	0.425	—	3
09146	Chinese date (jujube)	2/149	79	1.2	20.2	—	4	0.02	0.04	0.9	0.081	—	—	69	—	21	23	10	0.48	250	0.05	0.2	—	—	3
09078	Cranberry	2/259	49	0.39	8.48	4.2	5	0.03	0.02	0.1	0.065	1.7	—	13.5	0.1	7	9	5	0.2	71	0.13	0.2	0.017	—	1
09083	Currant, black	2/329	63	1.4	13.4	2	23	0.05	0.05	0.3	0.066	—	—	181	0.1	55	59	24	1.54	322	0.27	0.41	0.034	—	2
09084	Currant, red and white	1/51	56	1.4	9.5	4.3	12	0.04	0.05	0.1	0.07	8	—	41	0.1	33	44	13	1	275	0.23	0.2	0.017	—	1
09086	Custard apple	2/62	101	1.7	25.2	—	3	0.08	0.1	0.617	0.221	—	—	19.2	—	30	21	18	0.71	382	—	0.6	—	—	4
09087	Date	2/147	275	1.97	66	7.5	5	0.09	0.1	3.03	0.192	12.6	—	3	0.1	32	40	35	1.15	652	0.29	0.45	0.191	—	3
09088	Elderberry	1/44	73	0.66	11.4	7	60	0.07	0.06	0.717	0.23	6	—	36	1	38	39	5	1.6	280	0.11	0.5	0.023	—	6
09334	Feijoa	2/263	49	1.24	6.13	4.5	—	0.008	0.032	0.289	0.05	38	—	20.3	—	17	20	9	0.08	155	0.04	0.78	—	—	3
09089	Fig	2/145	74	0.75	15.9	3.3	14	0.06	0.05	0.5	0.113	6	—	2	0.89	35	14	17	0.37	232	0.15	0.3	0.06	—	1
09094	Fig, dried	2/145	255	3.05	56.1	9.3	13	0.071	0.088	1.13	0.224	7.5	—	0.8	—	144	68	59	2.23	712	0.51	1.17	0.234	—	11
09111	Grapefruit	2/93	32	0.63	6.98	1.1	12	0.036	0.02	0.283	0.042	10.2	—	34.4	0.25	12	8	8	0.09	139	0.07	0.1	0.014	—	—
09112	Grapefruit, pink and red	2/93	30	0.55	7.68	—	26	0.034	0.02	0.224	0.042	12.2	—	38.1	—	11	9	8	0.12	129	0.07	0.1	0.014	—	—
09132	Grapes	2/78	71	0.66	16.8	1	7	0.092	0.057	0.35	0.11	3.9	—	10.8	0.7	11	13	6	0.26	185	0.05	0.58	0.189	—	2
09139	Guava	2/114	51	0.82	6.48	5.4	79	0.05	0.05	1.32	0.143	14	—	184	1.12	20	25	10	0.31	284	0.23	0.6	0.172	—	3
11620	Horseradish-tree, pods	1/110	37	2.1	5.33	3.2	7	0.053	0.074	0.62	0.12	44.3	—	141	0.095	30	50	45	0.36	461	0.45	0.2	0.033	—	42
09144	Jackfruit	1/46	94	1.47	22.4	1.6	30	0.03	0.11	0.4	0.108	14	—	6.7	0.15	34	36	37	0.6	303	0.42	0.3	0.063	—	3
09148	Kiwi	2/356	61	0.99	11.5	3.4	18	0.02	0.05	0.5	0.09	38	—	98	1.12	26	40	30	0.41	332	0.17	0.44	0.029	—	5
09149	Kumquat	2/364	63	0.9	9.83	6.6	30	0.08	0.1	0.5	0.06	16	—	37.4	0.24	44	19	13	0.39	195	0.08	0.1	0.014	—	6
09150	Lemon	2/124	29	1.1	6.52	2.8	3	0.04	0.02	0.1	0.08	10.6	—	53	0.24	26	16	8	0.6	138	0.06	0.3	0.039	—	2
09159	Lime	2/364	30	0.7	7.74	2.8	1	0.03	0.02	0.25	0.043	8.2	—	29.1	0.24	33	18	6	0.6	102	0.11	0.2	0.022	—	2
09164	Litchi	2/366	66	0.83	15.2	1.3	—	0.011	0.065	0.72	0.1	14	—	71.5	0.7	5	31	10	0.31	171	0.07	0.44	0.099	—	1
09172	Longan	1/50	60	1.31	14	1.1	—	0.031	0.14	0.3	—	—	—	84	—	1	21	10	0.13	266	0.05	0.1	—	—	—

* NDB_No column shows the unique 5-digit code identifying each food in the USDA Nutrient Database, http://www.nal.usda.gov/fnic/foodcomp

		Vol./ page	Energy	Proteins	CHO	Fiber	Vit. A	Vit. B₁	Vit. B₂	Niacin	Vit. B₆	Folates	Vit. B₁₂	Vit. C	Vit. E	Ca	P	Mg	Fe	K	Zn	Total fat	Satur. fat	Cholesterol	Na
			kcal	g	g	g	µg RE	mg	mg	mg NE	mg	µg	µg	mg	mg α-TE	mg	mg	mg	mg	mg	mg	g	g	mg	mg
09174	Loquat	2/298	47	0.43	10.4	1.7	153	0.019	0.024	0.263	0.1	14	—	1	0.89	16	27	13	0.28	266	0.05	0.2	0.04	—	1
09175	Mamey	1/45	51	0.5	9.5	3	23	0.02	0.04	0.483	0.1	14	—	14	0.59	11	11	16	0.7	47	0.1	0.5	0.136	—	15
09176	Mango	2/341	65	0.51	15.2	1.8	389	0.058	0.057	0.717	0.134	14	—	27.7	1.12	10	11	9	0.13	156	0.04	0.27	0.066	—	2
09183	Melon	2/254	26	0.9	5.4	0.8	3	0.06	0.02	0.4	0.12	17	—	16	0.15	5	7	8	0.4	210	0.16	0.1	0.025	—	12
09181	Melon, cantaloupe	2/255	35	0.88	7.56	0.8	322	0.036	0.021	0.574	0.115	17	—	42.2	0.15	11	17	11	0.21	309	0.16	0.28	0.071	—	9
09190	Mulberry	1/46	43	1.44	8.1	1.7	3	0.029	0.101	0.62	0.05	6	—	36.4	0.45	39	38	18	1.85	194	0.12	0.39	0.027	—	10
09191	Nectarine	2/77	49	0.94	10.2	1.6	74	0.017	0.041	0.99	0.025	3.7	—	5.4	0.89	5	16	8	0.15	212	0.09	0.46	0.051	—	—
09200	Orange	2/360	47	0.94	9.35	2.4	21	0.087	0.04	0.432	0.06	30.3	—	53.2	0.24	40	14	10	0.1	181	0.07	0.12	0.015	—	—
09226	Papaya	2/157	39	0.61	8.01	1.8	175 RE	0.027	0.032	0.471	0.019	38	—	61.8	1.12	24	5	10	0.1	257	0.07	0.14	0.043	—	3
09231	Passion fruit (granadilla)	2/133	97	2.2	13	10.4	70	—	0.13	1.5	0.1	14	—	30	1.12	12	68	29	1.6	348	0.1	0.7	0.059	—	28
09236	Peach	2/75	43	0.7	9.1	2	54	0.017	0.041	1.02	0.018	3.4	—	6.6	0.7	5	12	7	0.11	197	0.14	0.09	0.01	—	1
09240	Peach, canned	2/75	54	0.45	13.3	1.3	35	0.009	0.025	0.61	0.019	3.3	—	2.4	0.89	3	11	5	0.36	97	0.09	0.03	0.003	—	5
09252	Pear	2/112	59	0.39	12.7	2.4	2	0.02	0.04	0.1	0.018	7.3	—	4	0.5	11	11	6	0.25	125	0.12	0.4	0.022	—	—
09263	Persimmon	2/222	70	0.58	15	3.6	217	0.03	0.02	0.267	0.1	7.5	—	16	0.5	8	17	9	0.37	161	0.11	0.19	0.02	—	1
09265	Persimmon, American	2/224	127	0.8	33.5	—	—	—	—	0.233	—	—	—	66	—	27	26	—	2.5	310	—	0.4	—	—	1
09266	Pineapple	2/189	49	0.39	11.2	1.2	2	0.092	0.036	0.503	0.087	10.6	—	15.4	0.1	7	7	14	0.37	113	0.08	0.43	0.032	—	1
09276	Pitanga	1/47	33	0.8	7.49	—	150	0.03	0.04	0.3	—	—	—	26.3	—	9	11	12	0.2	103	—	0.4	—	—	3
09277	Plantain	2/72	122	1.3	29.6	2.3	113	0.052	0.054	0.936	0.299	22	—	18.4	0.27	3	34	37	0.6	499	0.14	0.37	0.143	—	4
09279	Plum	2/233	55	0.79	11.5	1.5	32	0.043	0.096	0.5	0.081	2.2	—	9.5	0.6	4	10	7	0.1	172	0.1	0.62	0.049	—	—
09286	Pomegranate	2/236	68	0.95	16.6	0.6	—	0.03	0.03	0.3	0.105	6	—	6.1	0.55	3	8	3	0.3	259	0.12	0.3	0.038	—	3
09287	Prickly pear	1/43	41	0.73	5.97	3.6	5	0.014	0.06	0.46	0.06	6	—	14	0.01	56	24	85	0.3	220	0.12	0.51	0.067	—	5
09291	Prune, dried	2/233	239	2.61	55.6	7.1	199	0.081	0.162	1.96	0.264	3.7	—	3.3	1.45	51	79	45	2.48	745	0.53	0.52	0.041	—	4
09296	Quince	2/221	57	0.4	13.4	1.9	4	0.02	0.03	0.2	0.04	3	—	15	0.55	11	17	8	0.7	197	0.04	0.1	0.01	—	4
09299	Raisin, seeded	2/78	296	2.52	71.7	6.8	—	0.112	0.182	1.11	0.188	3.3	—	5.4	0.7	28	75	30	2.59	825	0.18	0.54	0.178	—	28
09302	Raspberry	1/49	49	0.91	4.77	6.8	13	0.03	0.09	0.9	0.057	26	—	25	0.45	22	12	18	0.57	152	0.46	0.55	0.019	—	—
09312	Rose apple	1/47	25	0.6	5.7	—	34	0.02	0.03	0.8	—	—	—	22.3	—	29	8	5	0.07	123	0.06	0.3	—	—	—
09313	Sapodilla	1/51	83	0.44	14.7	5.3	6	—	0.02	0.283	0.037	14	—	14.7	0.25	21	12	12	0.8	193	0.1	1.1	0.194	—	12
09314	Sapote	2/220	134	2.12	31.2	2.6	41	0.01	0.02	2.18	—	—	—	20	—	39	28	30	1	344	—	0.6	—	—	10
09315	Soursop	2/62	66	1	13.5	3.3	—	0.07	0.05	1.08	0.059	14	—	20.6	0.4	14	27	21	0.6	278	0.1	0.3	0.051	—	14
09316	Strawberry	2/103	30	0.61	4.72	2.3	3	0.02	0.066	0.347	0.059	17.7	—	56.7	0.14	14	19	10	0.38	166	0.13	0.37	0.02	—	1
09321	Sugar apple	2/62	94	2.06	19.2	4.4	1	0.11	0.113	1.05	0.2	14	—	36.3	0.59	24	32	21	0.6	247	0.1	0.29	0.048	—	9
09322	Tamarind	1/36	239	2.8	57.4	5.1	3	0.428	0.152	2.24	0.066	14	—	3.5	0.7	74	113	92	2.8	628	0.1	0.6	0.272	—	28
09218	Tangerine	2/359	44	0.63	8.89	2.3	92	0.105	0.022	0.26	0.067	20.4	—	30.8	0.24	14	10	12	0.1	157	0.24	0.19	0.022	—	1
09326	Watermelon	2/251	32	0.62	6.68	0.5	37	0.08	0.02	0.317	0.144	2.2	—	9.6	0.15	8	9	11	0.17	116	0.07	0.43	0.048	—	2

NUTS

		Vol./ page	Energy	Proteins	CHO	Fiber	Vit. A	Vit. B₁	Vit. B₂	Niacin	Vit. B₆	Folates	Vit. B₁₂	Vit. C	Vit. E	Ca	P	Mg	Fe	K	Zn	Total fat	Satur. fat	Cholesterol	Na
12058	Acorn	1/58	387	6.15	40.8	—	4	0.112	0.118	3.06	0.528	87	—	—	12	41	79	62	0.79	539	0.51	23.9	3.1	—	—
12060	Acorn flour	1/58	501	7.49	54.7	—	5	0.146	0.154	3.88	0.688	114	—	—	12	43	103	110	1.21	712	0.64	30.2	3.92	—	—
12061	Almond	2/48	589	20	9.5	10.9	—	0.211	0.779	9.33	0.113	58.7	—	0.6	24	266	520	296	3.66	732	2.92	52.2	4.95	—	11
12195	Almond butter	2/48	633	15.1	17.5	3.7	—	0.133	0.611	7.39	0.076	65.2	—	0.7	20.3	270	523	303	3.7	758	3.05	59.1	5.6	—	11
12078	Brazilnut	2/44	656	14.3	7.4	5.4	1	0.122		5.96	0.251	4	—	0.7	7.6	176	600	225	3.4	600	4.59	66.2	16.2	—	2

		Vol./page	Energy	Proteins	CHO	Fiber	Vit. A	Vit. B1	Vit. B2	Niacin	Vit. B6	Folates	Vit. B12	Vit. C	Vit. E	Ca	P	Mg	Fe	K	Zn	Total fat	Satur. fat	Cholesterol	Na
			kcal	g	g	g	µg RE	mg	mg	mg NE	mg	µg	µg	mg	mg α-TE	mg	mg	mg	mg	mg	mg	g	g	mg	mg
12085	Cashew, roasted	2/40	574	15.3	29.7	3	—	0.2	0.2	5.35	0.256	69.2	—	—	0.57	45	490	260	6	565	5.6	46.4	9.16	—	16
12104	Coconut	2/325	354	3.33	6.23	9	—	0.066	0.02	1.19	0.054	26.4	—	3.3	0.73	14	113	32	2.43	356	1.1	33.5	29.7	—	20
12119	Coconut water	2/325	19	0.72	2.61	1.1	—	0.03	0.057	0.213	0.032	2.5	—	2.4	—	24	20	25	0.29	250	0.1	0.2	0.176	—	105
12120	Hazelnut (filbert)	2/252	632	13	9.2	6.1	7	0.5	0.11	4.74	0.612	71.8	—	1	23.9	188	312	285	3.27	445	2.4	62.6	4.6	—	3
12131	Macadamia	2/69	702	8.3	4.43	9.3	—	0.35	0.11	5.69	0.196	15.7	—	—	0.41	70	136	116	2.41	368	1.71	73.7	11	—	5
16087	Peanut	2/336	567	25.8	7.64	8.5	—	0.64	0.135	16.2	0.348	240	—	—	9.13	92	376	168	4.58	705	3.27	49.2	6.83	—	18
16099	Peanut flour, defatted	2/336	327	52.2	18.9	15.8	—	0.7	0.48	35.5	0.504	248	—	—	0.05	140	760	370	2.1	1,290	5.1	0.55	0.063	—	180
12142	Pecan	1/58	667	7.75	10.6	7.6	13	0.848	0.128	4.2	0.188	39.2	—	2	3.1	36	291	128	2.13	392	5.47	67.6	5.42	—	1
12149	Pine nut	2/47	629	11.6	8.6	10.7	3	1.24	0.223	6.8	0.111	57.8	—	2	—	8	35	234	3.06	628	4.28	61	9.38	—	72
12151	Pistachio	2/135	577	20.6	14	10.8	23	0.82	0.174	5.8	0.25	58	—	7.2	5.21	135	503	158	6.78	1,093	1.34	48.4	6.13	—	6
12014	Squash blossoms	2/99	541	24.5	13.9	3.9	38	0.21	0.32	8.93	0.224	57.5	—	1.9	1	43	1174	535	15	807	7.46	45.9	8.67	—	18
12036	Sunflower seed	2/105	570	22.8	8.26	10.5	5	2.29	0.25	10.3	0.77	227	—	1.4	50.3	116	705	354	6.77	689	5.06	49.6	5.2	—	3
12155	English walnut	2/64	642	14.3	13.5	4.8	12	0.382	0.148	4.19	0.558	66	—	3.2	2.62	94	317	169	2.44	502	2.73	61.9	5.59	—	10

CEREALS AND GRAINS

		Vol./page	Energy	Proteins	CHO	Fiber	Vit. A	Vit. B1	Vit. B2	Niacin	Vit. B6	Folates	Vit. B12	Vit. C	Vit. E	Ca	P	Mg	Fe	K	Zn	Total fat	Satur. fat	Cholesterol	Na
20001	Amaranth	1/77	374	14.5	51	15.2	—	0.08	0.208	4.3	0.223	49	—	4.20	1.03	153	455	266	7.59	366	3.18	6.51	1.66	—	21
20004	Barley	2/162	354	12.5	56.2	17.3	2	0.646	0.285	8.07	0.318	19	—	—	0.6	33	264	133	3.6	452	2.77	2.3	0.482	—	12
18044	Bread, pumpernickel	2/117	250	8.7	41	6.5	—	0.327	0.305	4.71	0.126	34	—	—	0.507	68	178	54	2.87	208	1.48	3.1	0.437	—	671
18066	Bread, wheat bran	1/72	248	8.8	43.8	4	—	0.397	0.287	6.25	0.176	25	—	—	0.674	74	185	81	3.07	227	1.35	3.4	0.779	—	486
18069	Bread, white	1/72	267	8.2	47.2	2.3	—	0.472	0.341	5.57	0.064	34	0.02	—	0.286	108	94	24	3.03	119	0.62	3.6	0.811	1	538
18070	Bread, white, toasted	1/73	293	9	51.9	2.5	—	0.415	0.337	5.69	0.063	26	0.02	—	0.315	119	103	26	3.33	131	0.68	4	0.892	1	592
18075	Bread, whole-wheat	1/72	246	9.7	39.2	6.9	—	0.351	0.205	6.17	0.179	50	0.01	—	1.04	72	229	86	3.3	252	1.94	4.2	0.917	—	527
20008	Buckwheat	2/102	343	13.3	61.5	10	—	0.101	0.425	10.2	0.21	30	—	—	1.03	18	347	231	2.2	460	2.4	3.4	0.741	—	1
20016	Corn flour, whole-grain	1/69	361	6.93	63.5	13.4	47	0.246	0.08	2.72	0.37	25	—	—	0.25	7	272	93	2.38	315	1.73	3.86	0.543	—	5
11167	Corn, sweet	2/238	86	3.22	16.3	2.7	28	0.2	0.06	2.08	0.055	45.8	—	6.8	0.09	2	89	37	0.52	270	0.45	1.18	0.182	—	15
20028	Couscous, dry	1/69	376	12.8	72.4	5	—	0.163	0.078	6.21	0.11	20	—	—	—	24	170	44	1.08	166	0.83	0.64	0.117	—	10
18239	Croissants, butter		406	8.2	43.2	2.6	137	0.388	0.241	3.84	0.058	28	0.3	0.2	0.43	37	105	16	2.03	118	0.75	21	11.7	75	744
20400	Macaroni, cooked	1/74	141	4.77	27	1.3	—	0.02	0.02	1.42	0.035	7	—	—	0.03	7	54	18	0.5	31	0.53	0.67	0.095	—	1
20499	Macaroni, dry	1/74	371	12.8	72.3	2.4	—	0.09	0.06	4.43	0.106	18	—	—	0.13	18	150	48	1.3	162	1.21	1.58	0.225	—	7
20031	Millet	1/76	378	11	64.4	8.5	—	0.421	0.29	6.7	0.384	85	—	—	0.18	8	285	114	3.01	195	1.68	4.22	0.723	—	5
20038	Oats	2/41	389	16.9	55.7	10.6	—	0.763	0.139	4.86	0.119	56	—	—	0.7	54	523	177	4.72	429	3.97	6.9	1.22	—	2
20097	Pasta, with egg, cooked	1/74	130	5.28	23.5	—	17	0.173	0.174	2.37	0.037	19	0.1	—	—	10	52	14	1.16	21	0.44	1.74	0.408	41	83
19035	Popcorn	2/239	500	9	47.2	10	15	0.134	0.136	2.6	0.209	17	—	0.3	0.12	10	250	108	2.78	225	2.64	28.1	4.89	—	884
20035	Quinoa	1/77	374	13.1	63	5.9	—	0.198	0.396	2.93	0.223	49	—	—	—	60	41	210	9.25	740	3.3	5.8	0.59	—	21
20040	Rice, brown	2/227	362	7.5	72.8	3.4	—	0.413	0.043	5.91	0.509	20	—	—	0.661	33	264	143	1.8	268	2.02	2.68	0.536	—	4
20041	Rice, brown, cooked	2/227	112	2.32	21.7	1.8	—	0.102	0.012	1.83	0.149	4	—	—	—	10	77	44	0.53	79	0.62	0.83	0.165	—	1
20046	Rice, brown, parboiled	2/227	371	6.79	80	1.7	—	0.596	0.07	4.95	0.35	17	—	—	0.13	60	136	31	3.56	120	0.96	0.56	0.151	—	5
20450	Rice, white	2/225	360	6.61	79.3	—	—	0.07	0.048	2.88	0.145	9	—	—	—	9	108	35	0.8	86	1.16	0.58	0.158	—	1
20062	Rye	2/116	335	14.8	55.2	14.6	—	0.316	0.251	6.84	0.294	60	—	—	1.87	33	374	121	2.67	264	3.73	2.5	0.287	—	6
20063	Rye flour, dark	1/69	324	14	46.1	22.6	—	0.316	0.251	6.92	0.443	60	—	—	2.58	56	632	248	6.45	730	5.62	2.69	0.309	—	1
20065	Rye flour, light	1/69	367	8.39	65.6	14.6	—	0.331	0.09	2.38	0.234	22	—	—	0.56	21	194	70	1.8	233	1.75	1.36	0.145	—	2
20067	Sorghum	1/76	339	11.3	74.6	—	—	0.237	0.142	4.99	—	—	—	—	—	28	287	—	4.4	350	—	3.3	0.457	—	6

		Vol./page	Energy	Pro-teins	CHO	Fiber	Vit. A	Vit. B1	Vit. B2	Niacin	Vit. B6	Fola-tes	Vit. B12	Vit. C	Vit. E	Ca	P	Mg	Fe	K	Zn	Total fat	Satur. fat	Cho-lesterol	Na
			kcal	g	g	g	µg RE	mg	mg	mg NE	mg	µg	µg	mg	mg α-TE	mg	mg	mg	mg	mg	mg	g	g	mg	mg
20121	Spaghetti, cooked	1/74	141	4.77	26.6	1.7	—	0.204	0.098	2.69	0.035	7	—	—	0.06	7	54	18	1.4	31	0.53	0.67	0.095	—	1
20120	Spaghetti, dry	1/74	371	12.8	72.3	2.4	—	1.03	0.444	10.2	0.106	18	—	—	0.16	18	150	48	3.86	162	1.21	1.58	0.225	—	7
18449	Tortilla	2/241	222	5.7	41.4	5.2	24	0.112	0.073	2.2	0.219	15	—	—	—	175	314	65	1.4	154	0.94	2.5	0.334	—	11
20073	Wheat	2/306	331	10.4	61.7	12.5	—	0.394	0.096	4.8	0.272	41	—	—	1.44	27	493	126	3.21	397	2.63	1.56	0.289	—	2
20077	Bran	2/311	216	15.6	21.7	42.8	—	0.523	0.577	18.3	1.3	79	—	—	2.32	73	1,013	611	10.6	1,182	7.27	4.25	0.63	—	2
20481	Wheat flour, white	2/306	364	10.3	73.6	2.7	—	0.12	0.04	3.37	0.044	26	—	—	0.06	15	108	22	1.17	107	0.7	0.98	0.155	—	2
20080	Wheat flour, whole-grain	2/306	339	13.7	60.4	12.2	—	0.447	0.215	9.9	0.341	44	—	—	1.23	34	346	138	3.88	405	2.93	1.87	0.322	—	5
20078	Wheat germ	2/310	360	23.2	38.6	13.2	—	1.88	0.499	12.1	1.3	281	—	—	13.5	39	842	239	6.26	892	12.3	9.72	1.67	—	12
20087	Wheat, sprouted	1/86	198	7.49	41.4	1.1	—	0.225	0.155	5	0.265	38	—	2.6	0.05	28	200	82	2.14	169	1.65	1.27	0.206	—	16
20088	Wild rice	1/77	357	14.7	68.7	6.2	2	0.115	0.262	9.72	0.391	95	—	—	0.72	21	433	177	1.96	427	5.96	1.08	0.156	—	7
03217	Zwieback	1/73	426	10.1	71.7	2.5	6	0.208	0.239	1.32	0.082	20	—	5.3	0.4	20	55	14	0.6	305	0.54	9.7	3.95	20.8	232

LEGUMES

		Vol./page	Energy	Pro-teins	CHO	Fiber	Vit. A	Vit. B1	Vit. B2	Niacin	Vit. B6	Fola-tes	Vit. B12	Vit. C	Vit. E	Ca	P	Mg	Fe	K	Zn	Total fat	Satur. fat	Cho-lesterol	Na
16001	Adzuki	2/266	329	19.9	50.2	12.7	2	0.455	0.22	5.81	0.351	622	—	—	—	66	381	127	4.98	1,254	5.04	0.53	0.191	—	5
11001	Alfalfa seeds, sprouted	2/130	29	3.99	1.28	2.5	16	0.076	0.126	0.481	0.034	36	—	8.2	0.02	32	70	27	0.96	79	0.92	0.69	0.069	—	6
16006	Bean, baked	2/343	93	4.79	15.5	5	17	0.153	0.06	1.38	0.134	23.9	—	3.1	0.53	50	104	32	0.29	296	1.4	0.45	0.116	—	397
16014	Bean, black	2/347	341	21.6	47.2	15.2	2	0.9	0.193	6.22	0.286	444	—	—	0.21	123	352	171	5.02	1,483	3.65	1.42	0.366	—	5
11029	Bean, kidney, sprouted	2/343	29	4.2	4.1	—	—	0.37	0.25	3.65	0.085	58.9	—	38.7	—	17	37	21	0.81	187	0.4	0.5	0.072	—	6
16049	Bean, white	2/343	333	23.4	45.1	15.2	—	0.437	0.146	5.1	0.318	388	—	—	0.53	240	301	190	10.4	1,795	3.67	0.85	0.219	—	16
16056	Chickpea	2/91	364	19.3	43.3	17.4	7	0.477	0.212	4.62	0.535	557	—	4	0.82	105	366	115	6.24	875	3.43	6.04	0.626	—	24
16069	Lentil	2/127	338	28.1	26.6	30.5	4	0.475	0.245	6.8	0.535	433	—	6.2	0.33	51	454	107	9.02	905	3.61	0.96	0.135	—	10
16070	Lentil, cooked	2/127	116	9.02	12.2	7.9	1	0.169	0.073	2.41	0.178	181	—	1.5	0.11	19	180	36	3.33	369	1.27	0.38	0.053	—	2
11248	Lentil, sprouted	2/127	106	8.96	22.1	—	5	0.228	0.128	1.13	0.19	99.9	—	16.5	—	25	173	37	3.21	322	1.51	0.55	0.057	—	11
11031	Lima bean	2/347	113	6.84	15.3	4.9	30	0.217	0.103	2.97	0.204	34	—	23.4	0.72	34	136	58	3.14	467	0.78	0.86	0.198	—	8
16076	Lupin	2/303	371	36.2	40.4	—	2	0.64	0.22	7.01	0.357	355	—	4.8	—	176	440	198	4.36	1,013	4.75	9.74	1.16	—	15
16080	Mung bean	2/266	347	23.9	46.3	16.3	11	0.621	0.233	6.58	0.382	625	—	4.8	0.51	132	367	189	6.74	1,246	2.68	1.15	0.348	—	15
11043	Mung bean, sprouted	1/87	30	3.04	4.13	1.8	2	0.084	0.124	1.37	0.088	60.8	—	13.2	0.01	13	54	21	0.91	149	0.41	0.18	0.046	—	6
16097	Peanut butter	1/55	589	24.1	15	6.6	—	0.125	0.112	17.6	0.45	92	—	—	—	41	317	159	1.9	747	2.78	49.9	9.58	—	486
16101	Pigeon peas	1/90	343	21.7	47.8	15	3	0.643	0.187	6.5	0.283	456	—	—	—	130	367	183	5.23	1,392	2.76	1.49	0.33	—	17
16117	Soy flour, defatted	1/89	329	47	20.9	17.5	4	0.698	0.253	14	0.574	305	—	—	0.195	241	674	290	9.24	2,384	2.46	1.22	0.136	—	20
16115	Soy flour, full-fat	1/89	436	34.5	25.6	9.6	12	0.581	1.16	12.7	0.461	345	—	—	1.95	206	494	429	6.37	2,515	3.92	20.7	2.99	—	13
16122	Soy protein isolate	1/89	338	80.7	1.76	5.6	—	0.176	0.1	20	0.1	176	—	—	—	178	776	39	14.5	81	4.03	3.39	0.422	—	1,005
16108	Soybean	2/264	416	36.5	20.9	9.3	2	0.874	0.87	10.5	0.377	375	—	6	1.95	277	704	280	15.7	1,797	4.89	19.9	2.88	—	2
16114	Tempeh	1/88	199	19	17	—	69	0.131	0.111	9.33	0.299	52	1	—	—	93	206	70	2.26	367	1.81	7.68	1.11	—	6
16127	Tofu	1/88	76	8.08	0.68	1.2	9	0.081	0.052	2.3	0.047	15	—	0.1	0.01	105	97	103	5.36	121	0.8	4.78	0.691	—	7

VEGETABLES

		Vol./page	Energy	Pro-teins	CHO	Fiber	Vit. A	Vit. B1	Vit. B2	Niacin	Vit. B6	Fola-tes	Vit. B12	Vit. C	Vit. E	Ca	P	Mg	Fe	K	Zn	Total fat	Satur. fat	Cho-lesterol	Na
11003	Amaranth leaves	1/104	26	2.46	4.03	—	292	0.027	0.158	1.18	0.192	85.3	—	43.3	—	215	50	55	2.32	611	0.9	0.33	0.091	—	20
20003	Arrowroot flour	1/109	357	0.3	84.8	3.4	—	0.001	—	0.067	0.005	7	—	—	—	40	5	3	0.33	11	0.07	0.1	0.019	—	2
11007	Artichoke	2/178	47	3.27	5.11	5.4	18	0.072	0.066	1.05	0.116	68	—	11.7	0.19	44	90	60	1.28	37	0.49	0.15	0.035	—	94
11011	Asparagus	2/250	23	2.28	2.44	2.1	58	0.14	0.128	1.54	0.131	128	—	13.2	2	21	56	18	0.87	273	0.46	0.2	0.046	—	2

		Vol./page	Energy	Proteins	CHO	Fiber	Vit. A	Vit. B1	Vit. B2	Niacin	Vit. B6	Folates	Vit. B12	Vit. C	Vit. E	Ca	P	Mg	Fe	K	Zn	Total fat	Satur. fat	Cholesterol	Na
			kcal	g	g	g	µg RE	mg	mg	mg NE	mg	µg	µg	mg	mg α-TE	mg	mg	mg	mg	mg	mg	g	g	mg	mg
11015	Asparagus, canned	2/250	19	2.14	0.88	1.6	53	0.061	0.1	1.3	0.11	95.6	—	18.4	0.43	16	43	10	1.83	172	0.4	0.65	0.147	—	287
09037	Avocado	2/108	161	1.98	2.39	5	61	0.108	0.122	2.27	0.5	61.9	—	7.9	2.3	11	41	39	1.02	599	0.42	15.3	2.44	—	10
11026	Bamboo shoots	1/108	27	2.6	3	2.2	2	0.15	0.07	1.05	0.24	7.1	—	4	1	13	59	3	0.5	533	1.1	0.3	0.069	—	4
11086	Beet greens	2/297	19	1.82	0.27	3.7	610	0.1	0.22	0.883	0.106	14.8	—	30	1.5	119	40	72	3.3	547	0.38	0.06	0.009	—	201
11151	Belgian endive (witloof)	2/175	17	0.9	0.9	3.1	3	0.062	0.027	0.427	0.042	37	—	2.8	—	19	26	10	0.24	211	0.16	0.1	0.024	—	2
11024	Bitter melon (balsam pear), pods	1/107	17	1	0.9	2.8	38	0.04	0.04	0.4	0.043	72	—	84	—	19	31	17	0.43	296	0.8	0.17	—	—	5
11022	Bitter melon (balsam pear), tips	1/107	30	5.3	3.29	—	173	0.181	0.362	1.11	0.803	128	—	88	—	84	99	85	2.04	608	0.3	0.69	—	—	11
11613	Borage	2/358	21	1.8	1.8	3.7	420	0.06	0.15	0.9	0.084	13.2	—	35	—	93	53	52	3.3	470	0.2	0.7	0.17	—	80
11218	Bottle gourd	1/107	14	0.62	3.39	—	2	0.029	0.022	0.37	0.04	5.9	—	10.1	—	26	13	11	0.2	150	0.7	0.02	0.002	—	2
11088	Broadbean	2/137	72	5.6	7.5	4.2	35	0.17	0.11	2.43	0.038	96.3	—	33	—	22	95	38	1.9	250	0.58	0.6	0.138	—	50
11090	Broccoli	2/63	28	2.98	2.24	3	154	0.065	0.119	1.12	0.159	71	—	93.2	1.66	48	66	25	0.88	325	0.4	0.35	0.054	—	27
11098	Brussels sprouts	2/192	43	3.38	5.16	3.8	88	0.139	0.09	1.36	0.219	61.1	—	85	0.88	42	69	23	1.4	389	0.42	0.3	0.062	—	25
11109	Cabbage	2/191	25	1.44	3.13	2.3	13	0.05	0.04	0.55	0.096	43	—	32.2	0.105	47	23	15	0.59	246	0.18	0.27	0.033	—	18
11119	Cabbage, chinese	2/193	16	1.2	0.13	3.1	120	0.04	0.05	0.6	0.232	78.7	—	27	0.12	77	29	13	0.31	238	0.23	0.2	0.043	—	9
11112	Cabbage, red	2/193	27	1.39	4.12	2	4	0.05	0.03	0.533	0.21	20.7	—	57	0.105	51	42	15	0.49	206	0.21	0.26	0.034	—	11
11122	Cardoon	2/177	20	0.7	3.29	1.6	12	0.02	0.03	0.3	0.043	28.3	—	2	—	70	23	42	0.7	400	0.17	0.1	0.011	—	81
11124	Carrot	2/25	43	1.03	7.14	3	2,813	0.097	0.059	1.11	0.147	14	—	9.3	0.46	27	44	15	0.5	323	0.2	0.19	0.03	—	35
11655	Carrot juice, canned	2/25	40	0.95	8.49	0.8	2,575	0.092	0.055	0.386	0.217	3.8	—	8.5	0.01	24	42	14	0.46	292	0.18	0.15	0.027	—	29
11134	Cassava	1/108	120	3.1	25.3	1.6	1	0.225	0.101	2.12	0.304	22.1	—	48.2	0.19	91	70	66	3.6	764	0.25	0.39	0.103	—	8
11135	Cauliflower	2/154	25	1.98	2.7	2.5	2	0.057	0.063	0.959	0.222	57	—	46.4	0.04	22	44	15	0.44	303	0.28	0.21	0.032	—	30
11143	Celery	2/248	16	0.75	1.95	1.7	13	0.046	0.045	0.49	0.087	28	—	7	0.36	40	25	11	0.4	287	0.13	0.14	0.037	—	87
11149	Chayote	1/107	24	0.9	2.4	3	6	0.03	0.04	0.7	0.132	27.6	—	11	0.12	19	26	14	0.4	150	0.35	0.3	0.063	—	4
11588	Chinese water-chestnut	2/323	106	1.4	20.9	3	—	0.14	0.2	1	0.328	16.1	—	4	1.2	11	63	22	0.06	584	0.5	0.1	0.026	—	14
11156	Chives	1/109	30	3.27	1.85	2.5	435	0.078	0.115	1.26	0.138	105	—	58.1	0.21	92	58	42	1.6	296	0.56	0.73	0.146	—	3
11190	Lamb's lettuce	2/136	21	2	2.4	1.2	709	0.071	0.087	0.848	0.273	13.6	—	38.2	—	38	53	13	2.18	459	0.59	0.4	—	—	4
11205	Cucumber	2/339	13	0.69	1.96	0.8	21	0.024	0.022	0.304	0.042	13	—	5.3	0.079	14	20	11	0.26	144	0.2	0.13	0.034	—	2
11616	Sorrel	1/110	22	2	0.3	2.9	400	0.04	0.1	0.5	0.122	13.2	—	48	—	44	63	103	2.4	390	0.2	0.7	—	—	4
11209	Eggplant	2/256	26	1.02	3.57	2.5	8	0.052	0.034	0.748	0.084	19	—	1.7	0.03	7	22	14	0.27	217	0.14	0.18	0.034	—	3
11213	Endive	2/176	17	1.25	0.25	3.1	205	0.08	0.075	0.483	0.02	142	—	6.5	0.44	52	28	15	0.83	314	0.79	0.2	0.048	—	22
16052	Fava bean	2/137	341	26.1	33.3	25	5	0.555	0.333	6.95	0.366	423	—	1.4	0.09	103	421	192	6.7	1,062	3.14	1.53	0.254	—	13
11957	Fennel, bulb	2/161	31	1.24	4.19	3.1	13	0.01	0.032	0.64	0.047	27	—	12	—	49	50	17	0.73	414	0.2	0.2	—	—	52
11052	Green bean	1/109	31	1.82	3.74	3.4	67	0.084	0.105	1.07	0.074	36.5	—	16.3	0.41	37	38	25	1.04	209	0.24	0.12	0.026	—	6
11961	Hearts of palm, canned	1/110	28	2.52	2.22	2.4	—	0.011	0.057	0.82	0.022	39	—	7.9	—	58	65	38	3.13	177	1.15	0.62	0.13	—	426
11222	Horseradish-tree leafy tips	1/110	64	9.4	6.28	2	756	0.257	0.66	4.62	1.2	40.2	—	51.7	—	185	112	147	4	337	0.6	1.4	—	—	9
11226	Jerusalem artichoke	2/300	76	2	15.8	1.6	2	0.2	0.06	1.3	0.077	13.4	—	4	0.19	14	78	17	3.4	429	0.12	0.01	—	—	4
11241	Kohlrabi	2/193	27	1.7	2.6	3.6	4	0.05	0.02	0.567	0.15	16.1	—	62	0.48	24	46	19	0.4	350	0.03	0.1	0.013	—	20
11246	Leek	2/319	61	1.5	12.4	1.8	10	0.06	0.03	0.6	0.233	64.1	—	12	0.92	59	35	28	2.1	180	0.12	0.3	0.04	—	20
11251	Lettuce	2/45	16	1.62	0.67	1.7	260	0.1	0.1	0.7	0.047	136	—	24	0.44	36	45	6	1.1	290	0.25	0.2	0.026	—	8
11220	Luffa	1/107	20	1.2	4.36	—	41	0.05	0.06	0.4	0.043	6.7	—	12	—	20	32	14	0.36	139	0.07	0.2	0.016	—	3
11278	Okra	2/200	38	2	4.43	3.2	66	0.2	0.06	1.28	0.215	87.8	—	21.1	0.69	81	63	57	0.80	303	0.6	0.1	0.026	—	8

		Vol./page	Energy	Proteins	CHO	Fiber	Vit. A	Vit. B1	Vit. B2	Niacin	Vit. B6	Folates	Vit. B12	Vit. C	Vit. E	Ca	P	Mg	Fe	K	Zn	Total fat	Satur. fat	Cholesterol	Na
			kcal	g	g	g	µg RE	mg	mg	mg NE	mg	µg	µg	mg	mg α-TE	mg	mg	mg	mg	mg	mg	g	g	mg	mg
11282	Onion	2/142	38	1.16	6.83	1.8	—	0.042	0.02	0.431	0.116	19	—	6.4	0.13	20	33	10	0.22	157	0.19	0.16	0.026	—	3
11298	Parsnip	1/111	75	1.2	13.1	4.9	—	0.09	0.05	0.7	0.09	66.8	—	17	—	36	71	29	0.59	375	0.59	0.3	0.05	—	10
11304	Peas	2/73	81	5.42	9.36	5.1	64	0.266	0.132	2.71	0.169	65	—	40	0.39	25	108	33	1.47	244	1.24	0.4	0.071	—	5
11316	Peas, sprouted	2/73	128	8.8	28.3	—	17	0.225	0.155	3.09	0.265	144	—	10.4	—	36	165	56	2.26	381	1.05	0.68	0.124	—	20
11821	Pepper, sweet	2/198	27	0.89	4.43	2	570	0.066	0.03	0.692	0.248	22	—	190	0.69	9	19	10	0.46	177	0.12	0.19	0.028	—	2
11333	Pepper, sweet, green	2/198	27	0.89	4.63	1.8	63	0.066	0.03	0.692	0.248	22	—	89.3	0.69	9	19	10	0.46	177	0.12	0.19	0.028	—	2
11352	Potato	2/201	79	2.07	16.4	1.6	—	0.088	0.035	2.02	0.26	12.8	—	19.7	0.06	7	46	21	0.76	543	0.39	0.1	0.026	—	6
11364	Potato, baked	2/201	198	4.29	38.2	7.9		0.122	0.106	3.07	0.614	21.6	—	13.5	0.04	34	101	43	7.04	573	0.49	0.1	0.026	—	21
21138	Potato, french fried	2/205	309	3.99	35.4	3.2	3	0.14	0.04	3.16	0.26	33	0.12	5.3	0.19	16	133	33	1.35	712	0.52	16.1	4.99	—	163
11422	Squash	2/97	26	1	6	0.5	160	0.05	0.11	0.8	0.061	16.2	—	9	1.06	21	44	12	0.8	340	0.32	0.1	0.052	—	1
11416	Squash blossoms	1/107	15	1.03	3.28	—	195	0.042	0.075	0.69	—	58.9	—	28	—	39	49	24	0.7	173	—	0.07	0.036	—	5
11427	Purslane	1/111	16	1.3	3.43	—	132	0.047	0.112	0.713	0.073	11.5	—	21	—	65	44	68	1.99	494	0.17	0.1	—	—	45
11952	Radicchio	1/105	23	1.43	3.58	0.9	3	0.016	0.028	0.688	0.057	60	—	8	2.26	19	40	13	0.57	302	0.62	0.25	0.06	—	22
11429	Radish	2/181	17	0.6	1.99	1.6	1	0.005	0.045	0.367	0.071	27	—	22.8	0.001	21	18	9	0.29	232	0.3	0.54	0.03	—	24
11430	Radish, oriental	2/181	18	0.6	2.51	1.6	—	0.02	0.02	0.25	0.046	28.2	—	22	0.001	27	23	16	0.4	227	0.15	0.1	0.03	—	21
11080	Red beet	2/122	43	1.61	6.76	2.8	4	0.031	0.04	0.651	0.067	109	—	4.9	0.3	16	40	23	0.8	325	0.35	0.17	0.027	—	78
09307	Rhubarb	1/110	21	0.9	2.74	1.8	10	0.02	0.03	0.3	0.024	7.1	—	8	0.2	86	14	12	0.22	288	0.1	0.2	0.053	—	4
11437	Salsify	1/105	82	3.3	15.3	3.3	—	0.08	0.22	0.5	0.277	26.3	—	8	—	60	75	23	0.7	380	0.38	0.2	—	—	20
11439	Sauerkraut	2/197	19	0.91	1.78	2.5	2	0.021	0.022	0.143	0.13	23.7	—	14.7	0.1	30	20	13	1.47	170	0.19	0.14	0.035	—	661
11114	Savoy cabbage	2/192	27	2	3	3.1	100	0.07	0.03	0.633	0.19	80.2	—	31	0.105	35	42	28	0.4	230	0.27	0.1	0.013	—	28
11677	Shallot	1/109	72	2.5	16.8	—	1,248	0.06	0.02	0.667	0.345	34.2	—	8	—	37	60	21	1.2	334	0.4	0.1	0.017	—	12
11300	Snow pea	2/74	42	2.8	4.96	2.6	14	0.15	0.08	1.05	0.16	41.7	—	60	0.39	43	53	24	2.08	200	0.27	0.2	0.039	—	4
11457	Spinach	2/28	22	2.86	0.8	2.7	672	0.078	0.189	1.37	0.195	194	—	28.1	1.89	99	49	79	2.71	558	0.53	0.35	0.056	—	79
11507	Sweet potato	2/301	105	1.65	21.3	3	2,006	0.066	0.147	1.01	0.257	13.8	—	22.7	0.28	22	28	10	0.59	204	0.28	0.3	0.064	—	13
11505	Sweet potato leaves	2/301	35	4	4.38	2	103	0.156	0.345	1.71	0.19	80	—	11	—	37	94	61	1.01	518	0.29	0.3	0.065	—	9
11518	Taro	1/104	107	1.5	22.4	4.1	—	0.095	0.025	0.983	0.283	22.2	—	4.5	2.38	43	84	33	0.55	591	0.23	0.2	0.041	—	11
11520	Taro leaves	1/104	42	4.98	3.01	3.7	483	0.209	0.456	2.31	0.146	126	—	52	2.02	107	60	45	2.25	648	0.41	0.74	0.151	—	3
11529	Tomato	2/275	21	0.85	3.54	1.1	62	0.059	0.048	0.728	0.08	15	—	19.1	0.38	5	24	11	0.45	222	0.09	0.33	0.045	—	9
11527	Tomato, green	2/275	24	1.2	4	1.1	64	0.06	0.04	0.65	0.081	8.8	—	23.4	0.38	13	28	10	0.51	204	0.07	0.2	0.028	—	13
11564	Turnip	2/320	27	0.9	4.43	1.8	—	0.04	0.03	0.55	0.09	14.5	—	21	0.03	30	27	11	0.3	191	0.27	0.1	0.011	—	67
11568	Turnip greens	2/320	27	1.5	2.53	3.2	760	0.07	0.1	1.03	0.263	194	—	60	2.9	190	42	31	1.1	296	0.19	0.3	0.07	—	40
11591	Watercress	2/132	19	2.2	3	0.7	470	0.09	0.12	0.7	0.129	9.2	—	43	1	120	60	21	0.2	33	0.11	0.1	0.027	—	41
11293	Welsh onion	2/144	34	1.9	6.5	—	116	0.05	0.09	0.75	0.072	16.1	—	27	—	18	49	23	1.22	212	0.52	0.4	0.067	—	17
11601	Yam	2/101	118	1.53	23.8	4.1	—	0.112	0.032	0.752	0.293	23	—	17.1	0.16	17	55	21	0.54	816	0.24	0.17	0.037	—	9
11603	Yambean (jicama)	1/105	38	0.72	3.92	4.9	2	0.02	0.029	0.2	0.042	12	—	20.2	0.457	12	18	12	0.6	15	0.16	0.09	0.021	—	4
11477	Zucchini	2/159	14	1.16	1.7	1.2	34	0.07	0.03	0.567	0.089	22.1	—	9	0.12	15	32	22	0.42	248	0.2	0.14	0.029	—	3

OILS AND MARGARINE

		Vol./page	Energy	Proteins	CHO	Fiber	Vit. A	Vit. B1	Vit. B2	Niacin	Vit. B6	Folates	Vit. B12	Vit. C	Vit. E	Ca	P	Mg	Fe	K	Zn	Total fat	Satur. fat	Cholesterol	Na
04529	Almond oil	2/48	884	—	—	—	—	—	—	—	—	—	—	—	39.3	—	—	—	—	—	—	100	8.2	—	—
04582	Canola oil	1/124	884	—	—	—	—	—	—	—	—	—	—	—	21	—	—	—	—	—	—	100	7.1	—	—
04501	Cocoa butter oil	2/325	884	—	—	—	—	—	—	—	—	—	—	—	—	—	—	—	—	—	—	100	59.7	—	—

		Vol./page	Energy	Proteins	CHO	Fiber	Vit. A	Vit. B1	Vit. B2	Niacin	Vit. B6	Folates	Vit. B12	Vit. C	Vit. E	Ca	P	Mg	Fe	K	Zn	Total fat	Satur. fat	Cholesterol	Na
			kcal	g	g	g	µg RE	mg	mg	mg NE	mg	µg	µg	mg	mg α-TE	mg	mg	mg	mg	mg	mg	g	g	mg	mg
04047	**Coconut oil**	1/124	862	—	—	—	—	—	—	—	—	—	—	—	0.28	—	—	—	0.04	—	—	100	86.5	—	—
04589	**Cod liver oil**	1/239	902	—	—	—	30,003	—	—	—	—	—	—	—	—	—	—	—	—	—	—	100	22.6	570	—
04518	**Corn oil**	1/127	884	—	—	—	—	—	—	—	—	—	—	—	21.1	—	—	—	—	—	—	100	12.7	—	—
04502	**Cottonseed oil**	1/125	884	—	—	—	—	—	—	—	—	—	—	—	38.3	—	—	—	—	—	—	100	25.9	—	—
04517	**Grapeseed oil**	1/127	884	—	—	—	—	—	—	—	—	—	—	—	—	—	—	—	—	—	—	100	9.6	—	—
04532	**Hazelnut oil**	2/252	884	—	—	—	—	—	—	—	—	—	—	—	—	—	—	—	—	—	—	100	7.4	—	—
04092	**Margarine, corn**	1/121	716	0.8	0.5	—	799	0.009	0.032	0.203	0.008	1.05	0.084	0.14	—	26.5	20.3	2.31	—	37.7	—	80.4	14.1	—	1,079
04130	**Margarine, unspec. oils**	1/121	716	0.8	0.5	—	799	0.009	0.032	0.203	0.008	1.05	0.084	0.14	12	26.5	20.3	2.31	—	37.7	—	80.4	13.8	—	1,079
04053	**Olive oil**	1/126	884	—	—	—	—	—	—	—	—	—	—	—	12.4	0.18	1.22	0.01	0.38	—	0.06	100	13.5	—	0.04
09193	**Olives, ripe**	2/165	115	0.84	3.06	3.2	40	0.003	—	0.037	0.009	—	—	0.9	3	88	3	4	3.3	8	0.22	10.7	1.42	—	872
04055	**Palm oil**	1/125	884	—	—	—	—	—	—	—	—	—	—	—	21.8	—	0.15	—	0.01	—	—	100	49.3	—	—
04042	**Peanut oil**	1/124	884	—	—	—	—	—	—	—	—	—	—	—	12.9	0.09	—	0.04	0.03	0.0	0.01	100	16.9	—	0.11
04514	**Poppy seed oil**	1/126	884	—	—	—	—	—	—	—	—	—	—	—	—	—	—	—	—	—	—	100	13.5	—	—
04037	**Rice bran oil**	2/228	884	—	—	—	—	—	—	—	—	—	—	—	—	—	—	—	0.07	—	—	100	19.7	—	—
04510	**Safflower oil**	1/124	884	—	—	—	—	—	—	—	—	—	—	—	43.1	—	—	—	—	—	—	100	9.1	—	—
04114	**Salad dressing, italian**		467	0.7	10.2	—	24	0.01	0.019	0.17	0.013	4.89	0.162	—	10.4	10	5	0.64	0.2	15	0.11	48.3	7	—	787
04593	**Salmon oil**	1/241	902	—	—	—	—	—	—	—	—	—	—	—	—	—	—	—	—	—	—	100	19.9	485	—
04058	**Sesame oil**	1/126	884	—	—	—	—	—	—	—	—	—	—	—	4.09	—	—	—	—	—	—	100	14.2	—	—
04044	**Soybean oil**	1/125	884	—	—	—	—	—	—	—	—	—	—	—	18.2	0.04	0.25	0.03	0.02	—	—	100	14.4	—	—
04506	**Sunflower oil**	1/125	884	—	—	—	—	—	—	—	—	—	—	—	50.6	—	—	—	—	—	—	100	10.3	—	—
04528	**Walnut oil**	1/126	884	—	—	—	—	—	—	—	—	—	—	—	3.22	—	—	—	—	—	—	100	9.1	—	—
04038	**Wheat germ oil**	1/127	884	—	—	—	—	—	—	—	—	—	—	—	192	—	—	—	—	—	—	100	18.8	—	—

SEAWEED

		Vol./page	Energy	Proteins	CHO	Fiber	Vit. A	Vit. B1	Vit. B2	Niacin	Vit. B6	Folates	Vit. B12	Vit. C	Vit. E	Ca	P	Mg	Fe	K	Zn	Total fat	Satur. fat	Cholesterol	Na
11663	**Agar, dried**	1/130	306	6.21	73.2	7.7	—	0.01	0.222	0.202	0.303	580	—	—	5	625	52	770	21.4	1125	5.8	0.3	0.061	—	102
11442	**Agar, raw**	1/130	26	0.54	6.25	0.5	—	0.005	0.022	0.055	0.032	84.8	—	—	0.87	54	5	67	1.86	226	0.58	0.03	0.006	—	9
11445	**Kelp**	1/132	43	1.68	8.27	1.3	12	0.05	0.15	1.27	0.002	180	—	3	0.87	168	42	121	2.85	89	1.23	0.56	0.247	—	233

MUSHROOMS

		Vol./page	Energy	Proteins	CHO	Fiber	Vit. A	Vit. B1	Vit. B2	Niacin	Vit. B6	Folates	Vit. B12	Vit. C	Vit. E	Ca	P	Mg	Fe	K	Zn	Total fat	Satur. fat	Cholesterol	Na
11260	**Mushroom**	2/294	25	2.09	3.45	1.2	—	0.102	0.449	4.9	0.097	21.1	—	3.5	0.12	5	104	10	1.24	370	0.73	0.42	0.056	—	4
11269	**Shiitake, cooked**	1/151	55	1.56	12.2	2.1	—	0.037	0.17	1.57	0.159	20.9	—	0.3	0.12	3	29	14	0.44	117	1.33	0.22	0.055	—	4

HONEY AND SUGARS

		Vol./page	Energy	Proteins	CHO	Fiber	Vit. A	Vit. B1	Vit. B2	Niacin	Vit. B6	Folates	Vit. B12	Vit. C	Vit. E	Ca	P	Mg	Fe	K	Zn	Total fat	Satur. fat	Cholesterol	Na
19349	**Corn syrup, dark**	1/174	282	—	76.6	—	—	0.011	0.009	0.02	0.009	—	—	—	—	18	11	8	0.37	44	0.04	—	—	—	155
19296	**Honey**	1/160	304	0.3	82.2	0.2	—	—	0.038	0.188	0.024	2	—	0.5	—	6	4	2	0.42	52	0.22	—	—	—	4
19304	**Molasses**	1/175	266	—	68.8	—	—	0.041	0.002	0.93	0.67	—	—	—	—	205	31	242	4.72	1,464	0.29	0.1	0.018	—	37
19305	**Molasses, blackstrap**	1/175	235	—	60.8	—	—	0.033	0.052	1.08	0.7	1	—	—	—	860	40	215	17.5	2,492	1.	—	—	—	55
19303	**Orange marmalade**	2/360	246	0.3	66.1	0.2	5	0.005	0.006	0.102	0.014	36	—	4.8	—	38	6	2	0.15	37	0.04	—	—	—	56
19334	**Sugar, brown**	1/170	376	—	97.3	—	—	0.008	0.007	0.082	0.026	1	—	—	—	85	22	29	1.91	346	0.18	—	—	—	39
19335	**Sugar, granulated**	1/170	387	—	99.9	—	—	—	0.019	—	—	—	—	—	—	1	2	—	0.06	2	0.03	—	—	—	1
19340	**Sugar, maple**	1/170	354	0.1	90.9	—	2	0.009	0.013	0.04	0.003	—	—	—	—	90	3	19	1.61	274	6.06	0.2	0.036	—	11
19353	**Syrup, maple**	1/174	262	—	67.2	—	—	0.006	0.01	0.03	0.002	—	—	—	—	67	2	14	1.2	204	4.16	0.2	0.036	—	9

		Vol./page	Energy	Proteins	CHO	Fiber	Vit. A	Vit. B₁	Vit. B₂	Niacin	Vit. B₆	Folates	Vit. B₁₂	Vit. C	Vit. E	Ca	P	Mg	Fe	K	Zn	Total fat	Satur. fat	Cholesterol	Na
			kcal	g	g	g	µg RE	mg	mg	mg NE	mg	µg	µg	mg	mg α-TE	mg	mg	mg	mg	mg	mg	g	g	mg	mg
DAIRY																									
01001	**Butter, with salt**	1/204	717	0.85	0.06	—	754	0.005	0.034	0.242	0.003	3	0.125	—	1.58	24	23	2	0.16	26	0.05	81.1	50.5	219	826
01145	**Butter, without salt**	1/204	717	0.85	0.06	—	754	0.005	0.034	0.242	0.003	2.8	0.13	—	1.58	23.5	22.8	2	0.16	26	0.05	81.1	50.5	219	11
01004	**Cheese, blue**		353	21.4	2.34	—	228	0.029	0.382	6.22	0.166	36.4	1.22	—	0.64	528	387	22.9	0.31	256	2.66	28.7	18.7	75.2	1,395
01006	**Cheese, brie**		334	20.8	0.45	—	182	0.07	0.52	5.75	0.235	65	1.65	—	0.655	184	188	20	0.5	152	2.38	27.7	17.4	100	629
01007	**Cheese, camembert**	1/210	300	19.8	0.46	—	252	0.028	0.488	5.75	0.227	62.2	1.3	—	0.655	388	347	20	0.33	187	2.38	24.3	15.3	72	842
01009	**Cheese, cheddar**	1/211	403	24.9	1.28	—	303	0.027	0.375	5.41	0.074	18.2	0.827	—	0.36	721	512	27.8	0.68	98.4	3.11	33.1	21.1	105	621
01016	**Cheese, cottage, 1% fat**	1/212	72.4	12.4	2.72	—	11	0.021	0.165	2.43	0.068	12.4	0.633	—	0.11	60.9	134	5.34	0.14	85.5	0.38	1.02	0.645	4.4	406
01015	**Cheese, cottage, 2% fat**	1/210	89.7	13.7	3.63	—	20	0.024	0.185	2.69	0.076	13.1	0.712	—	0.056	68.5	151	6	0.16	96.2	0.42	1.93	1.22	8.4	406
01017	**Cheese, cream**	1/212	349	7.55	2.66	—	437	0.017	0.197	1.22	0.047	13.2	0.424	—	0.941	79.9	104	6.44	1.2	119	0.54	34.9	22	110	296
01186	**Cheese, cream, fat free**	1/212	96	14.4	5.8	—	279	0.05	0.172	0.16	0.05	37	0.55	—	0.03	185	434	14	0.18	163	0.88	1.36	0.899	8	545
01019	**Cheese, feta**		264	14.2	4.09	—	128	0.154	0.844	4.32	0.424	32	1.69	—	0.03	493	337	19.2	0.65	61.8	2.88	21.3	14.9	89	1,116
01159	**Cheese, goat, soft type**		268	18.5	0.89	—	283	0.07	0.38	3.68	0.25	12	0.19	—	0.457	140	256	16	1.9	26	0.92	21.1	14.6	46	368
01023	**Cheese, gruyere**	1/210	413	29.8	0.36	—	301	0.06	0.279	7.12	0.081	10.4	1.6	—	0.35	1,011	605	35.9	0.17	81	3.9	32.3	18.9	110	336
01028	**Cheese, mozzarella**		254	24.3	2.77	—	177	0.018	0.303	5.76	0.07	8.8	0.817	—	0.43	646	463	23.2	0.22	83.7	2.76	15.9	10.1	57.8	466
01039	**Cheese, roquefort**	1/210	369	21.5	2	—	299	0.04	0.586	5.78	0.124	49	0.643	—	—	662	392	29.5	0.56	90.7	2.08	30.6	19.3	90	1809
01049	**Cream, half and half**	1/204	130	2.96	4.3	—	107	0.035	0.149	0.778	0.039	2.5	0.329	0.86	0.11	105	95.2	10.2	0.07	130	0.51	11.5	7.16	36.9	40.7
01053	**Cream, heavy whipping**	1/204	345	2.05	2.79	—	421	0.022	0.11	0.522	0.026	3.7	0.18	0.58	0.63	64.6	62.4	7.03	0.03	75.4	0.23	37	23	137	37.6
01056	**Cream, sour, cultured**	1/200	214	3.16	4.27	—	195	0.035	0.149	0.8	0.016	10.8	0.3	0.86	0.566	116	84.9	11.2	0.06	144	0.27	21	13	44.4	53.3
01108	**Milk, buffalo**	1/187	96.6	3.75	5.18	—	53	0.052	0.135	0.974	0.023	5.6	0.363	2.25	—	169	117	31.1	0.12	178	0.22	6.89	4.6	19	52.2
01091	**Milk, dry, skim**	1/183	362	36.2	52	—	8	0.415	1.55	9.45	0.361	50.1	4.03	6.76	0.021	1,257	968	110	0.32	1794	4.08	0.77	0.499	19.6	535
01106	**Milk, goat**	1/186	68.8	3.56	4.45	—	56	0.048	0.138	1.01	0.046	0.6	0.065	1.29	0.09	134	111	14	0.05	204	0.3	4.14	2.67	11.4	49.8
01107	**Milk, human**	1/186	69.6	1.03	6.89	—	64	0.014	0.036	0.46	0.011	5.2	0.045	5	0.9	32.2	13.7	3.4	0.03	51.2	0.17	4.38	2.01	13.9	16.9
01082	**Milk, low fat, 1% fat**	1/183	41.9	3.29	4.78	—	59	0.039	0.167	0.854	0.043	5.1	0.368	0.97	0.04	123	96.2	13.8	0.05	156	0.39	1.06	0.66	4	50.5
01079	**Milk, low fat, 2% fat**	1/183	49.7	3.33	4.8	—	57	0.039	0.165	0.869	0.043	5.1	0.364	0.95	0.07	122	95.1	13.7	0.05	154	0.39	1.92	1.2	7.5	49.9
01109	**Milk, sheep**	1/187	108	5.98	5.36	—	42	0.065	0.355	1.82	0.06	7	0.711	4.16	—	193	158	18.4	0.1	137	0.54	7	4.6	27	44.1
01085	**Milk, skim**	1/183	34.9	3.41	4.85	—	61	0.036	0.14	0.888	0.04	5.2	0.378	0.98	0.04	123	101	11.4	0.04	166	0.4	0.18	0.117	1.8	51.5
01077	**Milk, whole**	1/182	61.4	3.29	4.66	—	31	0.038	0.162	0.851	0.042	5	0.357	0.94	0.1	119	93.4	13.4	0.05	152	0.38	3.34	2.08	13.6	49
01088	**Muttermilk, cultured, skim**	1/204	40.4	3.31	4.79	—	8	0.034	0.154	0.658	0.034	5	0.219	0.98	0.06	116	89.2	11	0.05	151	0.42	0.88	0.548	3.5	105
01114	**Whey, sweet**	1/199	26.7	0.85	5.14	—	4	0.036	0.158	0.291	0.031	0.8	0.277	0.1	0.01	46.8	45.6	8.26	0.06	161	0.13	0.36	0.23	2	53.5
01121	**Yogurt, fruit, low fat**	1/202	102	4.37	19.1	—	11	0.037	0.178	0.512	0.04	9.3	0.467	0.66	0.029	152	119	14.6	0.07	195	0.74	1.08	0.697	4.2	58.4
01117	**Yogurt, plain, low fat**	1/202	63.3	5.25	7.04	—	16	0.044	0.214	0.614	0.049	11.2	0.562	0.8	0.042	183	144	17.5	0.08	234	0.89	1.55	1	6.1	70.2
01118	**Yogurt, plain, skim milk**	1/202	55.8	5.73	7.68	—	2	0.048	0.234	0.657	0.053	12.2	0.613	0.87	0.005	199	157	19.1	0.09	255	0.97	0.18	0.116	1.8	76.5
EGGS																									
01124	**Egg, white**	1/218	50	10.5	1.03	—	—	0.006	0.452	2.26	0.004	3	0.2	—	—	6	13	11	0.03	143	0.01	—	—	—	164
01123	**Egg, whole**	1/218	149	12.5	1.22	—	191	0.062	0.508	2.61	0.139	47	1	—	1.05	49	178	10	1.44	121	1.1	10	3.1	425	126
01125	**Egg, yolk**	1/218	358	16.8	1.78	—	584	0.17	0.639	3.28	0.392	146	3.11	—	3.16	137	488	9	3.53	94	3.11	30.9	9.55	1,281	43
01057	**Eggnog**		135	3.81	13.5	—	80	0.034	0.19	1.01	0.05	0.9	0.45	1.5	0.227	130	109	18.5	0.2	165	0.46	7.48	4.44	58.7	54.4

		Vol./page	Energy	Proteins	CHO	Fiber	Vit. A	Vit. B1	Vit. B2	Niacin	Vit. B6	Folates	Vit. B12	Vit. C	Vit. E	Ca	P	Mg	Fe	K	Zn	Total fat	Satur. fat	Cholesterol	Na
			kcal	g	g	g	µg RE	mg	mg	mg NE	mg	µg	µg	mg	mg α-TE	mg	mg	mg	mg	mg	mg	g	g	mg	mg
FISH AND SEAFOOD																									
15001	Anchovy	1/239	131	20.4	—	—	15	0.055	0.256	17.8	0.143	8.8	0.62	—	—	147	174	41	3.25	383	1.72	4.84	1.28	60	104
15004	Bass	1/239	97	17.7	—	—	27	0.1	0.03	5.42	0.3	9	3.82	—	0.5	15	198	40	0.84	256	0.4	2.33	0.507	80	69
15008	Carp	1/239	127	17.8	—	—	9	0.115	0.055	4.97	0.19	15	1.53	1.6	0.63	41	415	29	1.24	333	1.48	5.6	1.08	66	49
15010	Catfish	1/244	95	16.4	—	—	15	0.21	0.072	4.96	0.116	10	2.23	0.7	0.6	14	209	23	0.3	358	0.51	2.82	0.722	58	43
15012	Caviar, black and red	1/238	252	24.6	4	—	560	0.19	0.62	5.5	0.32	50	20	—	7	275	356	300	11.9	181	0.95	17.9	4.06	588	1,500
15015	Cod	1/239	82	17.8	—	—	12	0.076	0.065	5.38	0.245	7	0.908	1	0.23	16	203	32	0.38	413	0.45	0.67	0.131	43	54
15025	Eel	1/244	184	18.4	—	—	1,043	0.15	0.04	6.95	0.067	15	3	1.8	4	20	216	20	0.5	272	1.62	11.7	2.36	126	51
15028	Flatfish (flounder and sole)	1/239	91	18.8	—	—	10	0.089	0.076	6.42	0.208	8	1.52	1.7	1.89	18	184	31	0.36	361	0.45	1.19	0.283	48	81
15031	Grouper	1/239	92	19.4	—	—	43	0.07	0.005	3.93	0.3	8.8	0.6	—	0.5	27	162	31	0.89	483	0.48	1.02	0.233	37	53
15039	Herring	1/239	158	18.0	—	—	28	0.092	0.233	6.57	0.302	10	13.7	0.7	1.07	57	236	32	1.1	327	0.99	9.04	2.04	60	90
15044	Ling	1/239	87	19	—	—	30	0.11	0.19	5.85	0.304	7	0.56	—	—	34	198	63	0.65	379	0.78	0.64	0.12	40	135
15051	Mackerel, Spanish	1/239	139	19.3	—	—	30	0.13	0.17	5.9	0.4	1	2.4	1.6	0.689	11	205	33	0.44	446	0.49	6.3	1.83	76	59
15054	Monkfish	1/239	76	14.5	—	—	12	0.025	0.06	4.8	0.24	7	0.9	1	—	8	200	21	0.32	400	0.41	1.52	0.34	25	18
15245	Oyster	1/254	59	5.22	5.53	—	8	0.105	0.065	2.25	0.06	18	16.2	4.7	—	44	93	33	5.78	124	37.9	1.55	0.443	25	178
15062	Pike, northern	1/239	88	19.3	—	—	21	0.058	0.063	5.9	0.117	15	2	3.8	0.2	57	220	31	0.55	259	0.67	0.69	0.118	39	39
15065	Pollock, Atlantic	1/239	92	19.4	—	—	11	0.047	0.185	6.9	0.287	3	3.19	—	0.23	60	221	67	0.46	356	0.47	0.98	0.135	71	86
15076	Salmon	1/239	142	19.8	—	—	12	0.226	0.38	11.6	0.818	25	3.18	—	—	12	200	29	0.8	490	0.64	6.34	0.981	55	44
15089	Sardine, canned	1/239	178	16.4	—	—	70	0.044	0.233	6.82	0.123	24.3	9	1	3.7	240	366	34	2.3	341	1.4	12	3.09	61	414
15095	Shark	1/244	130	21	—	—	70	0.042	0.062	6.86	0.4	3.2	1.49	—	1	34	210	49	0.84	160	0.43	4.51	0.925	51	79
15149	Shrimp	1/254	106	20.3	0.91	—	54	0.028	0.034	7.27	0.104	3	1.16	2	0.82	52	205	37	2.41	185	1.11	1.73	0.328	152	148
15110	Swordfish	1/245	121	19.8	—	—	36	0.037	0.095	13.4	0.33	2	1.75	1.1	1	4	263	27	0.81	288	1.15	4.01	1.1	39	90
15240	Trout, rainbow	1/239	138	20.9	—	—	84	0.203	0.073	12.1	0.619	11	3.77	2.9	0.03	67	282	32	0.27	451	0.41	5.4	1.55	59	35
15119	Tuna, canned in oil	1/239	198	29.1	—	—	23	0.038	0.12	17.8	0.11	5.3	2.2	—	1.2	13	311	31	1.39	207	0.9	8.21	1.53	18	354
15117	Tuna, fresh	1/239	144	23.3	—	—	655	0.241	0.251	13	0.455	1.9	9.43	—	1	8	254	50	1.02	252	0.6	4.9	1.26	38	39
15129	Turbot	1/239	95	16.1	—	—	11	0.066	0.08	5.2	0.21	8	2.2	1.7	—	18	129	51	0.36	238	0.22	2.95	0.75	48	150
MEAT AND MEAT PRODUCTS																									
10123	Bacon	1/326	556	8.66	0.09	—	—	0.368	0.104	4.16	0.14	2	0.93	—	0.49	7	142	9	0.6	153	1.15	57.5	21.3	67	730
13001	Beef, carcass	1/308	291	17.3	—	—	—	0.08	0.16	6.89	0.33	7	2.67	—	0.19	8	154	17	1.83	267	3.57	24.1	9.75	74	59
13237	Beef, tenderloin	1/308	283	17.8	—	—	—	0.11	0.2	6.25	0.37	6	2.55	—	—	7	177	19	2.29	295	2.97	23	9.31	71	48
05006	Chicken, meat and skin	1/314	215	18.6	—	—	41	0.06	0.12	10.3	0.35	6	0.31	1.6	0.295	11	147	20	0.9	189	1.31	15.1	4.31	75	70
05009	Chicken, meat & skin, roasted	1/314	239	27.3	—	—	47	0.063	0.168	13.6	0.4	5	0.3	—	0.265	15	182	23	1.26	223	1.94	13.6	3.79	88	82
05011	Chicken, meat only	1/314	119	21.4	—	—	16	0.073	0.142	12.4	0.43	7	0.37	2.3	0.295	12	173	25	0.89	229	1.54	3.08	0.79	70	77
07019	Chorizo, pork and beef	1/326	455	24.1	1.86	—	—	0.63	0.3	9.76	0.53	2	2	—	0.22	8	150	18	1.59	398	3.41	38.3	14.4	88	1,235
17164	Deer	1/328	120	23	—	—	—	0.22	0.48	6.37	0.37	4	6.31	—	0.2	5	202	23	3.4	318	2.09	2.42	0.95	85	51
05139	Duck, meat and skin	1/314	404	11.5	—	—	51	0.197	0.21	6.33	0.19	13	0.25	2.8	0.7	11	139	15	2.4	209	1.36	39.3	13.2	76	63
05141	Duck, meat only	1/314	132	18.3	—	—	24	0.36	0.45	9.53	0.34	25	0.4	5.8	0.7	11	203	19	2.4	271	1.9	5.95	2.32	77	74
07022	Frankfurter, beef	1/308	315	12	1.8	—	—	0.051	0.102	4.22	0.12	4	1.54	—	0.19	20	87	3	1.43	166	2.17	28.5	12.1	61	1,026
07023	Frankfurter, beef and pork	1/326	320	11.3	2.55	—	—	0.199	0.12	4	0.13	4	1.3	—	0.25	11	86	10	1.15	167	1.84	29.2	10.8	50	1,120
05146	Goose, meat and skin	1/315	371	15.9	—	—	17	0.085	0.245	7.06	0.39	4	0.34	4.2	1.74	12	234	18	2.5	308	1.72	33.6	9.78	80	73

		Vol./page	Energy	Pro-teins	CHO	Fiber	Vit. A	Vit. B₁	Vit. B₂	Niacin	Vit. B₆	Fola-tes	Vit. B₁₂	Vit. C	Vit. E	Ca	P	Mg	Fe	K	Zn	Total fat	Satur. fat	Cho-lesterol	Na
			kcal	g	g	g	µg RE	mg	mg	mg NE	mg	µg	µg	mg	mg α-TE	mg	mg	mg	mg	mg	mg	g	g	mg	mg
05148	Goose, meat only	1/315	161	22.8	—	—	12	0.129	0.377	9.56	0.64	31	0.49	7.2	—	13	312	24	2.57	420	2.34	7.13	2.79	84	87
07026	Ham, chopped, canned	1/327	239	16.1	0.28	—	—	0.535	0.165	6.23	0.32	1	0.7	2	0.25	7	139	13	0.95	284	1.83	18.8	6.28	49	1,365
10141	Ham, cured	1/327	195	27.8	0.3	—	—	0.567	0.242	9.45	0.42	5	0.88	—	0.26	10	318	25	1.11	510	2.81	8.32	2.78	70	2,695
07029	Ham, sliced, regular	1/327	182	17.6	3.11	—	—	0.863	0.252	8.77	0.34	3	0.83	—	0.29	7	247	19	0.99	332	2.14	10.6	3.39	57	1,317
21107	Hamburger	1/316	305	13.7	33.9	—	—	0.37	0.3	6.93	0.07	28	0.99	—	0.55	70	114	21	2.67	161	2.22	13.1	4.6	39	430
17170	Horse	1/329	133	21.4	—	—	—	0.13	0.1	9.02	0.38	—	3	1	—	6	221	24	3.82	360	2.9	4.6	1.44	52	53
19300	Jellies	1/317	271	0.4	69.8	1	2	0.001	0.026	0.036	0.02	1	—	0.9	—	8	5	6	0.2	64	0.04	0.1	0.018	—	36
17001	Lamb	1/312	267	16.9	—	—	—	0.12	0.22	9.38	0.13	18	2.39	—	0.21	12	160	22	1.57	230	3.33	21.6	9.47	72	58
17003	Lamb, lean	1/312	134	20.3	—	—	—	0.13	0.23	9.95	0.16	23	2.62	—	0.21	10	189	26	1.77	280	4.06	5.25	1.88	65	66
17011	Lamb, leg	1/312	230	17.9	—	—	—	0.13	0.23	9.74	0.15	19	2.5	—	0.21	9	170	23	1.66	249	3.32	17.1	7.43	69	56
04002	Lard	1/318	902	—	—	—	—	—	—	—	—	—	—	—	1.2	0.07	—	0.02	—	0.1	0.11	100	39.2	95	0.01
07055	Pate, liver	1/327	319	14.2	1.5	—	999	0.03	0.6	5.92	0.06	60	3.2	2	—	70	200	13	5.5	138	2.85	28	9.57	255	697
10003	Pork	1/318	227	18.3	—	—	2	0.8	0.242	8.13	0.415	6	0.67	0.6	0.29	15	197	20	0.89	324	2.11	16.5	5.77	69	54
07063	Pork sausage	1/333	417	11.7	1.02	—	—	0.545	0.164	4.4	0.25	4	1.13	2	—	18	118	11	0.91	204	1.59	40.3	14.5	68	667
10001	Pork, carcass	1/318	376	13.9	—	—	3	0.595	0.207	6.51	0.284	4	0.61	0.4	0.29	19	155	13	0.69	253	1.59	35.1	12.4	74	42
10002	Pork, lean	1/318	143	21.1	—	—	2	0.966	0.273	9.3	0.508	5	0.67	0.7	0.29	16	211	23	0.91	380	2.08	5.88	2.03	61	57
10020	Pork, loin	1/318	198	19.7	—	—	2	0.901	0.248	8.65	0.472	5	0.53	0.6	0.29	18	197	21	0.79	356	1.74	12.6	4.36	63	50
10024	Pork, loin, lean	1/318	143	21.4	—	—	2	0.989	0.267	9.45	0.527	5	0.63	0.6	0.29	17	211	23	0.84	389	1.84	5.66	1.95	59	52
05157	Quail, meat and skin		192	19.6	—	—	73	0.244	0.26	12.3	0.6	8	0.43	6.1	0.701	13	275	23	3.97	216	2.42	12.1	3.38	76	53
05158	Quail, meat only		134	21.8	—	—	17	0.283	0.285	13.9	0.53	7	0.47	7.2	—	13	307	25	4.51	237	2.7	4.53	1.32	70	51
17177	Rabbit meat	1/329	136	20.1	—	—	—	0.1	0.15	11.7	0.5	8	7.16	—	—	13	213	19	1.57	330	1.57	5.55	1.66	57	41
07071	Salami, dry or hard, pork	1/326	407	22.6	1.6	—	—	0.93	0.33	9.82	0.55	2	2.8	—	0.28	13	229	22	1.3	378	4.2	33.7	11.9	79	2,260
16107	Sausage, meatless	1/333	256	18.5	7.05	2.8	64	2.34	0.402	15.8	0.828	26	—	—	2.1	63	225	36	3.72	231	1.46	18.2	2.93	—	888
05160	Squab (pigeon), meat and skin		294	18.5	—	—	73	0.212	0.224	10.5	0.41	6	0.4	5.2	—	12	248	22	3.54	199	2.2	23.8	8.43	95	54
05161	Squab (pigeon), meat only		142	17.5	—	—	28	0.283	0.285	11.4	0.53	7	0.47	7.2	—	13	307	25	4.51	237	2.7	7.5	1.96	90	51
05165	Turkey, meat and skin	1/314	160	20.4	—	—	2	0.064	0.155	7.85	0.41	8	0.4	—	0.353	15	178	22	1.43	266	2.2	8.02	2.26	68	65
05167	Turkey, meat only	1/314	119	21.8	—	—	—	0.072	0.168	8.66	0.47	9	0.43	—	0.345	14	195	25	1.45	296	2.37	2.86	0.95	65	70
17088	Veal	1/308	144	19.4	—	—	—	0.08	0.27	10.8	0.41	13	1.34	—	0.26	15	203	24	0.83	315	3.06	6.77	2.79	82	82
17188	Veal, brain	1/317	118	10.3	—	—	—	0.13	0.26	6.02	0.28	3	12.2	14	—	10	274	14	2.13	315	1.11	8.21	1.91	1,590	127
17193	Veal, heart	1/317	110	17.2	0.08	—	—	0.52	1	9.45	0.43	2	13.8	8	—	5	211	18	4.24	261	1.47	3.98	1.07	104	77
17197	Veal, kidneys	1/317	99	15.8	0.85	—	92	0.32	1.9	10.4	0.37	21	28.2	5	0.18	11	241	16	3.36	272	1.97	3.12	0.96	364	178
17090	Veal, lean	1/308	112	20.2	—	—	—	0.08	0.28	11.2	0.43	13	1.4	—	0.26	15	211	25	0.85	328	3.23	2.87	0.86	83	86
17094	Veal, leg (top round)	1/308	117	21	—	—	—	0.08	0.27	13	0.46	14	1.04	—	0.15	5	220	26	0.79	367	2.3	3.08	1.18	78	63
17202	Veal, liver	1/317	134	17.9	4.59	—	4,427	0.19	1.76	14.9	0.74	642	46.8	22	0.34	9	268	18	4.79	292	4.03	4.38	1.63	309	62
17104	Veal, loin	1/308	163	18.9	—	—	—	0.07	0.24	11.7	0.53	13	1.11	—	0.26	16	199	23	0.73	304	2.32	9.14	3.88	79	85
17116	Veal, shoulder	1/308	130	19.3	—	—	—	0.09	0.29	9.44	0.39	12	1.67	—	0.27	22	203	23	0.91	302	3.93	5.28	2.05	87	91
17134	Veal, sirloin	1/308	152	19.1	—	—	—	0.08	0.3	11.7	0.49	13	1.27	—	0.25	11	209	24	0.78	329	2.55	7.81	3.35	78	76

CONDIMENTS AND SPICES

		Vol./page	Energy	Pro-teins	CHO	Fiber	Vit. A	Vit. B₁	Vit. B₂	Niacin	Vit. B₆	Fola-tes	Vit. B₁₂	Vit. C	Vit. E	Ca	P	Mg	Fe	K	Zn	Total fat	Satur. fat	Cho-lesterol	Na
11935	Catsup	1/341	104	1.52	26	1.3	102	0.089	0.073	1.53	0.175	15	—	15.1	1.47	19	39	22	0.7	481	0.23	0.36	0.049	—	1,186
11215	Garlic	1/109	149	6.36	31	2.1	—	0.2	0.11	1.8	1.24	3.1	—	31.2	0.01	181	153	25	1.7	401	1.16	0.5	0.089	—	17

		Vol./page	Energy	Pro-teins	CHO	Fiber	Vit. A	Vit. B₁	Vit. B₂	Niacin	Vit. B₆	Fola-tes	Vit. B₁₂	Vit. C	Vit. E	Ca	P	Mg	Fe	K	Zn	Total fat	Satur. fat	Cho-lesterol	Na
			kcal	g	g	g	µg RE	mg	mg	mg NE	mg	µg	µg	mg	mg α-TE	mg	mg	mg	mg	mg	mg	g	g	mg	mg
11216	**Ginger root**	1/341	69	1.74	13.1	2	—	0.023	0.029	0.9	0.16	11.2	—	5	0.26	18	27	43	0.5	415	0.34	0.73	0.203	—	13
11297	**Parsley**	1/342	36	2.97	3.03	3.3	520	0.086	0.098	2.06	0.09	152	—	133	1.79	138	58	50	6.2	554	1.07	0.79	0.132	—	56
11670	**Peppers, hot chili**	1/340	40	2	7.96	1.5	77	0.09	0.09	1.38	0.278	23.4	—	243	0.69	18	46	25	1.2	340	0.3	0.2	0.021	—	7

NUTRITIONAL SUPPLEMENTS

		Vol./page	Energy	Pro-teins	CHO	Fiber	Vit. A	Vit. B₁	Vit. B₂	Niacin	Vit. B₆	Fola-tes	Vit. B₁₂	Vit. C	Vit. E	Ca	P	Mg	Fe	K	Zn	Total fat	Satur. fat	Cho-lesterol	Na
16055	**Carob flour**	1/46	180	4.62	49.1	39.8	1	0.053	0.461	2.7	0.366	29	—	0.2	0.63	348	79	54	2.94	827	0.92	0.65	0.09	—	35
14181	**Chocolate syrup**	1/358	218	1.9	57.1	1.8	3	0.009	0.050	0.755	0.006	4	—	0.2	0.027	14	129	65	2.11	224	0.73	0.9	0.519	—	96
14182	**Chocolate syrup, with milk**	1/358	82	3.1	11.7	0.2	27	0.034	0.147	0.833	0.037	4.9	0.310	0.8	—	105	98	20	0.32	161	0.43	3	1.87	12	55
02019	**Fenugreek seed**	1/352	323	23	33.7	24.6	6	0.322	0.366	8.16	—	57	—	3	—	176	296	191	33.5	770	2.5	6.41	1.46	—	67.3
19120	**Milk chocolate**	1/358	513	6.9	55.8	3.4	55	0.079	0.301	1.71	0.042	8	0.390	0.4	1.24	191	216	60	1.39	385	1.38	30.7	18.5	22	82
12023	**Sesame seeds**	1/352	573	17.7	11.7	11.8	1	0.791	0.247	11	0.79	96.7	—	—	2.27	975	629	351	14.6	468	7.75	49.7	6.96	—	11
11666	**Spirulina**	1/134	26	5.92	2.42	—	6	0.222	0.342	2.8	0.034	9.2	—	0.9	—	12	11	19	2.79	127	0.2	0.39	0.135	—	98
11667	**Spirulina, dried**	1/134	290	57.5	20.3	3.6	57	2.38	3.67	28.3	0.364	94	—	10.1	5	120	118	195	28.5	1,363	2	7.72	2.65	—	1,048
19081	**Sweet chocolate**	1/358	505	3.9	54.1	5.5	2	0.02	0.24	1.64	0.043	3	—	—	1.19	24	147	113	2.76	290	1.5	34.2	20.1	—	16
02048	**Vinegar, cider**	1/337	14	—	5.9	—	—	—	—	—	—	—	—	—	—	6	9	22	0.6	100	—	—	—	—	1

BEVERAGES

		Vol./page	Energy	Pro-teins	CHO	Fiber	Vit. A	Vit. B₁	Vit. B₂	Niacin	Vit. B₆	Fola-tes	Vit. B₁₂	Vit. C	Vit. E	Ca	P	Mg	Fe	K	Zn	Total fat	Satur. fat	Cho-lesterol	Na
09036	**Apricot nectar**	2/26	56	0.37	13.8	0.6	132	0.009	0.014	0.26	0.022	1.3	—	0.6	0.08	7	9	5	0.38	114	0.09	0.09	0.006	—	3
14003	**Beer**	1/380	41	0.3	3.5	0.2	—	0.006	0.026	0.503	0.05	6	0.02	—	—	5	12	6	0.03	25	0.02	—	—	—	5
14209	**Coffee, brewed**	1/374	2	0.1	0.4	—	—	—	—	0.222	—	0.1	—	—	—	2	1	5	0.05	54	0.02	—	0.002	—	2
14210	**Coffee, brewed, espresso**	1/374	9	0.01	1.53	—	—	0.001	0.177	5.21	0.002	1	—	0.2	—	2	7	80	0.13	115	0.05	0.18	0.092	—	14
14400	**Cola soft drink**	1/366	41	—	10.4	—	—	—	—	—	—	—	—	—	—	3	12	1	0.03	1	0.01	—	—	—	4
09135	**Grape juice**	2/78	61	0.56	14.9	0.1	1	0.026	0.037	0.262	0.065	2.6	—	0.1	—	9	11	10	0.24	132	0.05	0.08	0.025	—	3
09123	**Grapefruit juice**	2/93	38	0.52	8.86	0.1	1	0.042	0.02	0.231	0.02	10.4	—	29.2	0.05	7	11	10	0.2	153	0.09	0.1	0.013	—	1
09404	**Grapefruit juice, pink**	2/93	39	0.5	9.2	—	44	0.04	0.02	0.2	0.044	10.2	—	38	—	9	15	12	0.2	162	0.05	0.1	0.014	—	1
09152	**Lemon juice**	2/124	25	0.38	8.23	0.4	2	0.03	0.01	0.1	0.051	12.9	—	46	0.09	7	6	6	0.03	124	0.05	—	—	—	1
09160	**Lime juice**	2/364	27	0.44	8.61	0.4	1	0.02	0.01	0.1	0.043	8.2	—	29.3	0.09	9	7	6	0.03	109	0.06	0.1	0.011	—	1
14305	**Malt beverage**	2/164	60	0.29	13.4	—	—	0.016	0.048	1.11	0.027	14	0.02	0.5	—	5	22	7	0.04	8	0.02	0.12	0.024	—	13
09206	**Orange juice**	2/360	45	0.7	10.2	0.2	20	0.09	0.03	0.433	0.04	30.3	—	50	0.09	11	17	11	0.2	200	0.05	0.2	0.024	—	1
14150	**Orange soft drink**	1/366	48	—	12.3	—	—	—	—	—	—	—	—	—	—	5	1	1	0.06	2	0.1	—	—	—	12
09229	**Papaya nectar**	2/157	57	0.17	13.9	0.6	11	0.006	0.004	0.15	0.009	2.1	—	3	0.02	10	—	3	0.34	31	0.15	0.15	0.047	—	5
09251	**Peach nectar**	2/75	54	0.27	13.3	0.6	26	0.003	0.014	0.288	0.007	1.4	—	5.3	0.01	5	6	4	0.19	40	0.08	0.02	0.002	—	7
09262	**Pear nectar**	2/112	60	0.11	15.2	0.6	—	0.002	0.013	0.128	0.014	1.2	—	1.1	0.101	5	3	3	0.26	13	0.07	0.01	0.001	—	4
09273	**Pineapple juice**	2/189	56	0.32	13.6	0.2	—	0.055	0.022	0.257	0.096	23.1	—	10.7	0.02	17	8	13	0.26	134	0.11	0.08	0.005	—	1
16120	**Soy milk**	1/88	33	2.75	0.51	1.3	3	0.161	0.07	0.864	0.041	1.5	—	—	0.01	4	49	19	0.58	141	0.23	1.91	0.214	—	12
09221	**Tangerine juice**	2/359	43	0.5	9.9	0.2	42	0.06	0.02	0.117	0.042	4.6	—	31	0.09	18	14	8	0.2	178	0.03	0.2	0.024	—	1
14355	**Tea, brewed**	1/372	1	—	0.3	—	—	—	0.014	—	—	5.2	—	—	—	—	1	3	0.02	37	0.02	—	0.002	—	3
11540	**Tomato juice**	2/275	17	0.76	3.83	0.4	56	0.047	0.031	0.756	0.111	19.9	—	18.3	0.91	9	19	11	0.58	220	0.14	0.06	0.008	—	361
14084	**Wine**	1/378	70	0.2	1.4	—	—	0.004	0.016	0.074	0.024	1.1	0.01	—	—	8	14	10	0.41	89	0.07	—	—	—	8

BIBLIOGRAPHY

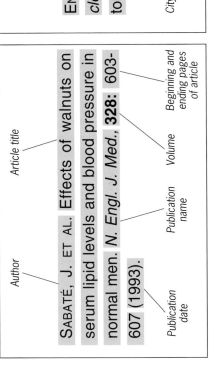

Author — *Article title*

SABATÉ, J., ET AL. Effects of walnuts on serum lipid levels and blood pressure in normal men. *N. Engl. J. Med.,* **328:** 603-607 (1993).

Publication date — *Publication name* — *Volume* — *Beginning and ending pages of article*

Journal references

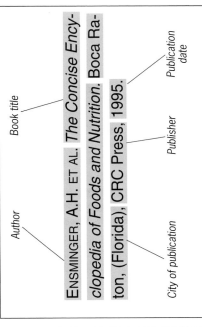

Author — *Book title*

ENSMINGER, A.H. ET AL. *The Concise Encyclopedia of Foods and Nutrition.* Boca Raton, (Florida), CRC Press, 1995.

Publication date — *City of publication* — *Publisher* — *Publication date*

Book references

CHAP. 1: FOODS FOR HUMANS

1. Genesis 1: 29.
2. Genesis 3: 18.
3. NOBMANN, E.D.; BYERS, T.; LANIER, A.P. ET AL. The diet of Alaska Native adults: 1987-1988 [see comments]. *Am. J. Clin. Nutr.,* **55:** 1024-1032 (1992).
4. HEBER, D. The stinking rose: organosulfur compounds and cancer. *Am. J. Clin. Nutr.,* **66:** 425-426 (1997).
5. BERGMAN, J. Diet, Health and Evolution. *Creation Research Society Quarterly,* **34:** 209-217 (1998).
6. MARTINS, Y.; PELCHAT, M.L.; PLINER, P. "Try it; it's good and it's good for you" effects of taste and nutrition information on willingness to try novel foods. *Appetite,* **28:** 89-102 (1997).

CHAP. 2: FRUITS

1. Genesis 2: 9.
2. ENSMINGER, A. H.ET AL. *The Concise Encyclopedia of Foods and Nutrition.* Boca Raton (Florida), CRC Press, 1995, p. 481.
3. HOEKSTRA, J.H. ET AL. Fluid intake and industrial processing in apple juice induced chronic non-specific diarrhoea. *Archives of Disease in Childhood,* **73:** 126-130 (1995).
4. RANKEN, M.D. *Food Industries Manual,* Glasgow, Blackie & Son Ltd., 22nd ed. 1988.
5. DENNISON, B.A.; ROCKWELL, H.L.; BAKER, S.L. Excess fruit juice consumption by preschool-aged children is associated with short stature and obesity. *Pediatrics,* **99:** 15-22 (1997).
6. DENNISON, B.A. Fruit juice consumption by infants and children: a review. *J. Am. Coll. Nutr.,* **15:** 4S-11S (1996).
7. TOUYZ, LZ. The acidity (pH) and buffering capacity of Canadian fruit juice and dental implications. *J. Can. Dent. Assoc.,* **60:** 454-458 (1994).
8. GROBLER, S.R. The effect of a high consumption of citrus fruit and a mixture of other fruits on dental caries in man. *Clin. Prev. Dent.,* **13:** 13-17 (1991).

9. NESS, A.R.; POWLES, J.W. Fruit and vegetables, and cardiovascular disease: a review. *Int. J. Epidemiol.,* **26:** 1-13 (1997).
10. GILLMAN, M.W. ET AL. Protective effect of fruits and vegetables on development of stroke in men. *JAMA,* **273:** 1113-1117 (1995).
11. NEGRI, E. ET AL. Vegetable and fruit consumption and cancer risk. *Int. J. Cancer,* **48:** 350-354 (1991).
12. HEIMENDINGER, J.; VAN DUYN, M.A. Dietary behavior change: the challenge of recasting the role of fruit and vegetables in the American diet. *Am. J. Clin. Nutr.,* **61:** 1397S-1401S (1995).
13. FAO. *Production Yearbook 1990,* vol. 44. FAO/UN, Roma.
14. OBIZOBA, I.C.; ANYIKA, J.U. Nutritive value of baobab milk (gubdi) and mixtures of baobab (Adansonia digitata) and hungry rice, acha (Digitaria exilis) flours. *Plant. Foods. Hum. Nutr.,* **46:** 157-165 (1994).
15. AALBERSBERG, W.G.L. ET AL. Carotenoids in the leaves of Morinda citrifolia. *Journal of Herbs, Spices and Medicinal Plants,* **2:** 51-54 (1993).
16. FRATI, A.C.; GORDILLO, B.E.; ALTAMIRANO, P. ET AL. Influence of nopal intake upon fasting glycemia in type II diabetics and healthy subjects. *Arch. Invest. Med. Mex.,* **22:** 51-56 (1991).

CHAP. 3: NUTS

1. ABBEY, M. ET AL. Partial replacement of saturated fatty acids with almonds or walnuts lowers total plasma cholesterol and low-density-lipoprotein cholesterol. *Am. J. Clin. Nutr.,* **59:** 995-999 (1994).
2. SABATE, J. ET AL. Effects of walnuts on serum lipid levels and blood pressure in normal men. *N. Engl. J. Med.,* **328:** 603-607 (1993).
3. SPILLER, G.A. ET AL. Effect of a diet high in monounsaturated fat from almonds on plasma cholesterol and lipoproteins. *J. Am. Coll. Nutr.,* **11:** 126-130 (1992).
4. DREHER, M.L.; MAHER, C.V.; KEARNEY, P. The traditional and emerging role of nuts in healthful diets. *Nutrition Reviews,* **54:** 241-245 (1996).

5. REDDY, N.S.; HOTWANI, M.S. In vitro availability of iron from selected nuts and oilseeds. *Plant Foods Hum. Nutr.,* **43:** 247-250 (1993).
6. GARG, A. ET AL. Effects of varying carbohydrate content of diet in patients with non-insulin-dependent diabetes mellitus. *JAMA,* **271:** 1421-1428 (1994).

CHAP. 4: CEREALS AND GRAINS

1. Deuteronomy 24: 6.
2. FAO. *Production Yearbook 1990,* vol. 44. FAO/UN, Rome.
3. SLAVIN, J.L. Epidemiological evidence for the impact of whole grains on health. *Crit. Rev. Food Sci. Nutr.,* **34:** 427-434 (1994).
4. KASHTAN, H. ET AL. Wheat-bran and oat-bran supplements' effects on blood lipids and lipoproteins. *Am. J. Clin. Nutr.,* **55:** 976-980 (1992).
5. LAMPE, J.W. ET AL. Effects of cereal and vegetable fiber feeding on potential risk factors for colon cancer. *Cancer Epidemiol. Biomarkers Prev.,* **1:** 207-211 (1992).
6. JACOBS, D.R. JR; SLAVIN, J.; MARQUART, L. Whole grain intake and cancer: a review of the literature. *Nutr. Cancer,* **24:** 221-229 (1995).
7. SLAVIN, J.L. Whole grains and health: separating the wheat from the chaff. *Nutr. Today,* **29:** 6-11 (1994).
8. THOMPSON, L.U. Antioxidants and hormone-mediated health benefits of whole grains. *Crit. Rev. Food Sci. Nutr.,* **34:** 473-497 (1994).
9. SALMERON, J. ET AL. Dietary fiber, glycemic load, and risk of NIDDM in men. *Diabetes Care,* **20:** 545-550 (1997).
10. RASANEN, L. Allergy to ingested cereals in atopic children. *Allergy,* **49:** 871-876 (1994).
11. SANDBERG, A.S. The effect of food processing on phytate hydrolysis and availability of iron and zinc. *Adv. Exp. Med. Biol.,* **289:** 499-508 (1991).
12. TORRE, M.; RODRIGUEZ, A.R.; SAURA-CALIXTO, F. Effects of dietary fiber and phytic acid on mineral availability. *Crit. Rev. Food Sci. Nutr.,* **30:** 1-22 (1991).

13. LECHKY, O. If children are developing poorly, ask what they had for breakfast. *CMAJ*, **143**: 210-213 (1990).

14. SUÁREZ FRAGA ET AL. Valor nutritivo del gofio [Nutritional value of gofio]. *Nutrición Clínica*, **10**: 126-136 (1990).

15. 1 Corinthians 11: 23-26.

16. BUDIN, J.T.; BREENE, W.M.; PUTNAM, D.H. Some compositional properties of seeds and oils of eight Amaranthus species. *Journal of the American Oil Chemists' Society*, **73**: 475-481 (1996).

17. BRESSANI, R.; DE MARTELL, E.C.; DE GODINEZ, C.M. Protein quality evaluation of amaranth in adult humans. *Plant Foods Hum. Nutr.*, **43**: 123-143 (1993).

18. PRAKASH, D.; JOSH, B.D.; PAL, M. Vitamin C in leaves and seed oil composition of the Amaranthus species. *Int. J. Food Sci. Nutr.*, **46**: 47-51 (1995).

19. CHATURVEDI, A.; SAROJINI, G.; DEVI, N.L. Hypocholesterolemic effect of amaranth seeds (Amaranthus esculentus). *Plant Foods Hum. Nutr.*, **44**: 63-70 (1993).

20. RUALES, J.; NAIR, B.M. Nutritional quality of the protein in quinoa (Chenopodium quinoa Willd) seeds. *Plant Foods Hum. Nutr.*, **42**: 1-11 (1992).

21. GONZALEZ, J.A.; ROLDAN, A.; GALLARDO, M. ET AL. Quantitative determinations of chemical compounds with nutritional value from Inca crops: Chenopodium quinoa ("quinoa"). *Plant Foods Hum. Nutr.*, **39**: 331-337 (1989).

22. RUALES, J.; NAIR, B.M. Properties of starch and dietary fibre in raw and processed quinoa (Chenopodium quinoa, Willd) seeds. *Plant Foods Hum. Nutr.*, **45**: 223-246 (1994).

23. LORENZ, K.; COULTER, L. Quinoa flour in baked products. *Plant Foods Hum. Nutr.*, **41**: 213-223 (1991).

CHAP. 5: LEGUMES

1. ESTEVEZ, A.M. ET AL. Effect of processing on some chemical and nutritional characteristics of pre-cooked and dehydrated legumes. *Plant Foods Hum. Nutr.*, **41**: 193-201 (1991).

2. BARAMPAMA, Z.; SIMARD, R.E. Effects of soaking, cooking and fermentation on composition, in-vitro starch digestibility and nutritive value of common beans. *Plant Foods Hum. Nutr.*, **48**: 349-365 (1995).

3. FAO Production Yearbook 1990, vol. 44. FAO/UN, Rome.

4. GANIATS, T.G. Does bano prevent gas? A double-blind crossover study of oral alpha-galactosidase to treat dietary oligosaccharide intolerance. *The Journal of Family Practice*, **39**: 441-445 (1994).

5. VIDAL-VALVERDE, C.; FRÍAS, J.; VALVERDE, S. Changes in the carbohydrate composition of legumes after soaking and cooking. *J. Am. Diet. Assoc.*, **93**: 547-550 (1993).

6. ENSMINGER, A.H. ET AL. *The Concise Encyclopedia of Foods and Nutrition*. Boca Raton (Florida), CRC Press, 1995, p. 609.

7. BONILLA, A.R.; CALZADA, C.; COOKE, R. [Effects of traditional cooking on antinutritional factors of the black beans (Phaseolus vulgaris) of Costa Rica] *Arch. Latinoam Nutr.*, **41**: 609-619 (1991).

8. ANDERSON J.W. ET AL. Serum lipid response of hypercholesterolemic men to single and divided doses of canned beans. *Am. J. Clin. Nutr.*, **51(6)**: 1013-1019 (1990).

9. STEPHEN, A.M. ET AL. Effect of green lentils on colonic function, nitrogen balance, and serum lipids in healthy human subjects. *American*

Journal of Clinical Nutrition, **62**: 1261-1267 (1995).

10. DABAI, F.D. ET AL. Comparative effects on blood lipids and faecal steroids of five legume species incorporated into a semi-purified, hypercholesterolaemic rat diet. *Br. J. Nutr.*, **75**: 557-571 (1996).

11. PANLASIGUI, L.N.; PANLILIO, L.M.; MADRID, J.C. Glycaemic response in normal subjects to five different legumes commonly used in the Philippines. *Int. J. Food Sci. Nutr.*, **46**: 155-160 (1995).

12. FESKENS, E.J. ET AL. Dietary factors determining diabetes and impaired glucose tolerance. A 20-year follow-up of the Finnish and Dutch cohorts of the Seven Countries Study. *Diabetes Care*, **18**: 1104-1112 (1995).

13. THIJS, C.; KNIPSCHILD, P. Legume intake and gallstone risk: results from a case-control study. *Int. J. Epidemiol.*, **19**: 660-663 (1990).

14. NIELSEN, S.S.; LIENER, I.E. Effect of germination on trypsin inhibitor and hemoagglutinating activities in Phaseolus vulgaris. *J. Food Sci.*, **53**: 298-301 (1988).

15. KHADER, V. Nutritional studies on fermented, germinated and baked soybean preparations. *J. Plant Foods* **5**: 31-37 (1983).

16. BATRA, V. Effects of cooking and germination on hemagglutinin activity in lentil. *Ind. J. Nutr. Diet.*, **24**: 15-19 (1987).

17. SANDBERG, A.S. The effect of food processing on phytate hydrolysis and availability of iron and zinc. *Adv. Exp. Med. Biol.*, **289**: 499-508 (1991).

18. STORY, J.A. ET AL. Interactions of alfalfa plant and sprout saponins with cholesterol in vitro and in cholesterol-fed rats. *Am. J. Clin. Nutr.*, **39**: 917-929 (1984).

19. SIDHU, G.S.; OAKENFULL, D.G. A mechanism for the hypocholesterolaemic activity of saponins. *Br. J. Nutr.*, **55**: 643-649 (1986).

20. RAO, A.V.; SUNG, M.K. Saponins as anticarcinogens. *J. Nutr.*, **125** (3 Suppl): 717S-724S (1995).

21. MAHON, B.E. ET AL. An international outbreak of Salmonella infections caused by alfalfa sprouts grown from contaminated seeds. *J. Infect. Dis.*, **175**: 876-882 (1997).

22. BEUCHAT, L.R. Comparison of chemical treatments to kill Salmonella on alfalfa seeds destined for sprout production. *Int. J. Food Microbiol*, **34**: 329-333 (1997).

23. JAQUETTE, C.B.; BEUCHAT, L.R.; MAHON, B.E. Efficacy of chlorine and heat treatment in killing Salmonella stanley inoculated onto alfalfa seeds and growth and survival of the pathogen during sprouting and storage. *Appl. Environ. Microbiol.*, **62**: 2212-2215 (1996).

24. WU, A.H. ET AL. Tofu and risk of breast cancer in Asian-Americans. *Cancer Epidemiol. Biomarkers Prev.*, **5**: 901-906 (1996).

CHAP. 6: VEGETABLES

1. Numbers 11:5.

2. THIEL, C.; HEINEMANN, L. Nutritional behaviour differences in Germany. *Rev. Environ. Health*, **11**: 35-40 (1996).

3. HEIMENDINGER, J.; VAN-DUYN, M.A. Dietary behavior change: the challenge of recasting the role of fruit and vegetables in the American diet. *Am. J. Clin. Nutr.*, **616 Suppl**): 1397S-1401S (1995).

4. KREBS-SMITH, S.M. ET AL. Fruit and vegetable intakes of children and adolescents in United States. *Arch. Pediatr. Adolesc. Med.*, **150**: 81-86 (1996).

CHAP. 7: OILS AND MARGARINE

1. PEREZ-JIMENEZ, F. ET AL. Lipoprotein concentrations in normolipidemic males consuming oleic acid-rich diets from two different sources: olive oil and oleic acid-rich sunflower oil. *Am. J. Clin. Nutr.*, **62**: 769-775 (1995).

2. HEYDEN, S. Polyunsaturated and monounsaturated fatty acids in the diet to prevent coronary heart disease via cholesterol reduction. *Ann. Nutr. Metab.*, **38**: 117-122 (1994).

3. WHO. Technical Report Series, 797. Diet, Nutrition, and the Prevention of Chronic Diseases. Report of a WHO Study Group. Geneva, 1990, pp. 111-113.

4. OOSTHUIZEN, W. ET AL. Both fish oil and olive oil lowered plasma fibrinogen in women with high baseline fibrinogen levels. *Thromb. Haemost.*, **72**: 557-562 (1994).

5. LICHTENSTEIN, A.H. Effects of canola, corn, and olive oils on fasting and postprandial plasma lipoproteins in humans as part of a National Cholesterol Education Program Step 2 diet. *Arterioscler. Thromb.*, **13**: 1533-1542 (1993).

5. BRUG, J.; LECHNER, L.; DE-VRIES, H. Psychosocial determinants of fruit and vegetable consumption. *Appetite*, **25**: 285-296 (1995).

6. MARTINS, Y.; PELCHAT, M.L.; PLINER, P. "Try it, it's good and it's good for you": effects of taste and nutrition information on willingness to try novel foods. *Appetite*, **28**: 89-102 (1997).

7. SERDULA, M.K. ET AL. The association between fruit and vegetable intake and chronic disease risk factors. *Epidemiology*, **7**: 161-165 (1996).

8. KEY, T.; THOROGOOD, M.; APPLEBY, P.N. ET AL. Dietary habits and mortality in 11,000 vegetarians and health conscious people: results of the 17-year follow up. *British Medical Journal*, **313**: 775-779 (1996).

9. BIRCHER-BENNER, M. *Nuevo libro de cocina dietética [New Dietic Cookbook]*. Madrid, Ediciones Rialp, 1980.

10. MATA, L. ET AL. Extinction of Vibrio cholerae in acidic substrata: contaminated cabbage and lettuce treated with lime juice. *Rev. Biol. Trop.*, **42**: 487-492 (1994).

11. HEANEY, R. ET AL. Absorbability of calcium from Brassica vegetables: broccoli, bok choy, and kale. *J. Food Sci.*, **58**: 1379-1380 (1993).

12. PANTOS, C.E.; MANKAKIS, P. Ascorbic acid content of artificially ripened tomatoes. *Journal of Food Science*, **38**: 550 (1973).

13. FAO Production Yearbook 1990, vol. 44. FAO/UN, Rome.

14. GAITAN, E. ET AL. Antithyroid effects in vivo and in vitro of babassu and mandioca: a staple food in goiter areas of Brazil. *Eur. J. Endocrinol.*, **131**: 138-144 (1994).

15. TENNEKOON, K.H. Effect of Momordica charantia on key hepatic enzymes. *J. Ethnopharmacol.*, **44**: 93-97 (1994).

16. BEDNAR, C.; KIES, C. Nitrate and vitamin C from fruits and vegetables: impact of intake variations on nitrate and nitrite excretions of humans. *Plant Foods Hum. Nutr.*, **45**: 71-80 (1994).

17. AWOYINKA, A.F.; ABEGUNDE, V.O.; ADEWUSI, S.R. Nutrient content of young cassava leaves and assessment of their acceptance as a green vegetable in Nigeria. *Plant Foods Hum. Nutr.*, **47**: 21-28 (1995).

18. MAGDA, R. Moringa: a health-giving, water-purifying vegetable. *Food Marketing and Technology*, **8**: 10-11 (1994).

19. SIMOPOULOS, A.P.; NORMAN, H.A.; GILLASPY, J.E. ET AL. Common purslane: a source of omega-3 fatty acids and antioxidants. *J. Am. Coll. Nutr.*, **11**: 374-382 (1992).

6. REAVEN, P. ET AL. Effect of antioxidants alone and in combination with monounsaturated fatty acid-enriched diets on lipoprotein oxidation. *Arteriosclerosis, Thrombosis and Vascular Biology*, **16**: 1465-1472 (1996).

7. BONANOME, A. ET AL. Effect of dietary monounsaturated and polyunsaturated fatty acids on the susceptibility of plasma low density lipoproteins to oxidative modification. *Arterioscler. Thromb.*, **12**: 529-533 (1992).

8. REAVEN, P.D.; GRASSE, B.J.; TRIBBLE, D.L. Effects of linoleate-enriched and oleate-enriched diets in combination with alpha-tocopherol on the susceptibility of LDL and LDL subfractions to oxidative modification in humans. *Arterioscler. Thromb.*, **14**: 557-566 (1994).

9. REAVEN P. ET AL. Effects of oleate-rich and linoleate-rich diets on the susceptibility of low density lipoprotein to oxidative modification in mildly hypercholesterolemic subjects. *J. Clin. Invest.*, **91**: 668-676 (1993).

10. REAVEN, P. ET AL. Feasibility of using an oleate-rich diet to reduce the susceptibility of low-density lipoprotein to oxidative modification in humans. *Am. J. Clin. Nutr.*, **54**: 701-706 (1991).

11. MARTIN-MORENO, J.M. ET AL. Dietary fat, olive oil intake and breast cancer risk. *Int. J. Cancer*, **58**: 774-780 (1994).

12. TRICHOPOULOU. A. ET AL. Consumption of olive oil and specific food groups in relation to breast cancer risk in Greece. *J. Natl. Cancer Inst.*, **87**: 110-116 (1995).

13. SZENDE, B.; TIMAR, F.; HARGITAI, B. Olive oil decreases liver damage in rats caused by carbon tetrachloride (CCl⁴). *Exp. Toxicol. Pathol.*, **46**: 355-359 (1994).

14. ASCN / AIN (Task force on Trans Fatty Acids). Position paper on trans fatty acids. *Am. J. Clin. Nutr.*, **63**: 663-670 (1996).

15. WILLETT, W.C.; ASCHERIO, A. Trans fatty acids: are the effects only marginal? *Am. J. Public Health*, **84**: 722-724 (1994).

16. CHISHOLM, J. ET AL. Effect on lipoprotein profile of replacing butter with margarine in a low fat diet: randomized crossover study with hypercholesteraemic subjects. *British Medical Journal*, **312**: 931-934 (1996).

17. WILLETT, W.C. ET AL. Intake of trans fatty acids and risk of coronary heart disease among women [see comments]. *The Lancet*, **341**: 581-585 (1993).

18. TYAGI, V.K.; VASISHTHA, A.K. Changes in the characteristics and composition of oils during deep-fat frying. *Journal of the American Oil Chemists' Society*, **73**: 499-506 (1996).

19. SHIELDS, P.G. ET AL. Mutagens from heated Chinese and U.S. cooking oils. *J. Natl. Cancer Inst.*, **87**: 836-841 (1995).

20. HAGEMAN, G. ET AL. Biological effects of short-term feeding to rats of repeatedly used deep-frying fats in relation to fat mutagen content. *Food Chem. Toxicol.*, **29**: 689-698 (1991).

21. KNEKT, P. ET AL. Intake of fried meat and risk of cancer: a follow-up study in Finland. *Int. J. Cancer.*, **59**: 756-760 (1994).

22. KRIS-ETHERTON, P.M. Trans fatty acids and coronary heart disease risk. *Am. J. Clin. Nutr.*, **62**: 655S-708S (1995).

23. THIEBAUD, H.P.; KNIZE, M.G.; KUZMICKY, P.A. ET AL. Airborne mutagens produced by frying beef, pork and a soy-based food. *Food Chem. Toxicol.*, **33**: 821-828 (1995).

CHAP. 8: SEAWEED

1. ENSMINGER,A. H. ET AL. *The Concise Encyclopedia of Foods and Nutrition*. Boca Raton (Florida), CRC Press, 1995, p. 587

2. STRASBURGER ET AL. *Strasburger, Lehrbuch der Botanik*, Suttgart, Gustav Fischer Verlag, 33rd ed.,1991, p. 648.

3. HERBERT, V.; DRIVAS, G. Spirulina and vitamin B₁₂. *JAMA*, **248**: 3096-3097 (1982).

CHAP. 9: MUSHROOMS

1. CHANG, R. Functional properties of edible mushrooms. *Nutr. Rev.*, **54** (11 Pt 2): S91-S93 (1996).

2. H.TAKEHARA, M.; KUIDA, K.; MORI, K. Antiviral activity of virus-like particles from Lentinus edodes (Shiitake). *Arch. Virol.*, **59**: 269-274 (1979).

3. NANBA, H.; MORI, K.; TOYOMASU, T.; KURODA. Antitumor action of shiitake (Lentinus edodes) fruit bodies orally administered to mice. *Chem. Pharm. Bull.(Tokyo)*, **35**: 2453-2458 (1987)

4. KABIR, Y.; YAMAGUCHI, M.; KIMURA, S. Effect of shiitake (Lentinus edodes) and maitake (Grifola frondosa) mushrooms on blood pressure and plasma lipids of spontaneously hypertensive rats. *J. Nutr. Sci. Vitaminol (Tokyo)* **33**: 341-346 (1987).

5. KUBO, K.; AOKI, H.; NANBA, H. Anti-diabetic activity present in the fruit body of Grifola frondosa (Maitake). *Biol. Pharm. Bull.* **17**: 1106-1110 (1994).

6. TOTH, B.; ERICKSON, J. Cancer induction in mice by feeding of the uncooked cultivated mushroom of commerce Agaricus bisporus. *Cancer Res.*, **46**: 4007-4011 (1986).

7. SHEPHARD, S.E.; GUNZ, D.; SCHLATTER, C. Genotoxicity of agaritine in the lacI transgenic mouse mutation assay: evaluation of the health risk of mushroom consumption. *Food Chem. Toxicol.*, **33**: 257-264 (1995).

CHAP. 10: HONEY, SUGAR AND CHEMICAL SWEETENERS

1. HALLFRISCH, J. Metabolic effects of dietary fructose. *FASEB J.*, **4**: 2652-2660 (1990).

2. ROLLS, B.J. Effects of intense sweeteners on hunger, food intake, and body weight: a review. *Am. J. Clin. Nutr.*, **53**: 872-878 (1991).

3. UHARI, M. ET AL. Xylitol chewing gum in prevention of acute otitis media: double blind randomised trial. *British Medical Journal*, **313**: 1180-1184 (1996).

4. UUSITUPA, M.I. Fructose in the diabetic diet. *Am. J. Clin. Nutr.*, **59** (3 Suppl): 753S-757S (1994).

5. GLINSMANN, W.H.; PARK, Y.K. Perspective on the 1986 Food and Drug Administration assessment of the safety of carbohydrate sweeteners: uniform definitions and recommendations for future assessments. *Am. J. Clin. Nutr.*, **62** (1 Suppl): 161S-168S (1995).

6. RUMESSEN, J.J. Fructose and related food carbohydrates. Sources, intake, absorption, and clinical implications. *Scand. J. Gastroenterol.*, **27**: 819-828 (1992).

7. BAR, A.; BIERMANN, C. Intake of intense sweeteners in Germany. *Z. Ernahrungswiss.*, **31**: 25-39 (1992).

8. KUBLER, W. [The consumption of sugar in the Federal Republic of Germany] *Z. Ernahrungswiss.*, **29** (Suppl. 1): 3-10 (1990).

9. WHO, Technical Report Series, 797. *Diet, Nutrition, and the Prevention of Chronic Diseases*. Report of a WHO Study Group. Geneva. 1990.

10. BIERMAN, E.L. Carbohydrates, sucrose, and human disease. *Am. J. Clin. Nutr.*, **32**: 2712-2722 (1979).

11. KONIG, K.G.; NAVIA, J.M. Nutritional role of sugars in oral health. *Am. J. Clin. Nutr.*, **62** (1 Suppl): 275S-282S (1995).

12. WOODWARD, M.; WALKER, A.R. Sugar consumption and dental caries: evidence from 90 countries. *Br. Dent. J.*, **176**: 297-302 (1994).

13. SMITH, J.B.; NIVEN, B.E.; MANN, J.I. The effect of reduced extrinsic sucrose intake on plasma triglyceride levels. *Eur. J. Clin. Nutr.*, **50**: 498-504 (1996).

14. KRUMMEL, D.A.; SELIGSON, F.H.; GUTHRIE, H.A. Hyperactivity: is candy causal? *Crit. Rev. Food Sci. Nutr.*, **36**: 31-47 (1996).

15. KANAREK, R.B. Does sucrose or aspartame cause hyperactivity in children? *Nutr. Rev.*, **52**: 173-175 (1994).

16. POLLOCK, I.; WARNER, J.O. Effect of artificial food colours on childhood behaviour. *Arch. Dis. Child.*, **65**: 74-77 (1990).

17. BREAKEY, J. The role of diet and behaviour in childhood. *J. Paediatr. Child Health*, **33**: 190-194 (1997).

18. SAILER, D. [Does sugar play a role in the development of gastroenterologic diseases (Crohn disease, gallstones, cancer)?] *Z. Ernahrungswiss.*, **29** (Suppl. 1): 39-44 (1990).

19. MOERMAN, C.J.; SMEETS, F.W.; KROMHOUT, D. Dietary risk factors for clinically diagnosed gallstones in middle-aged men. A 25-year follow-up study (the Zutphen study). *Ann. Epidemiol.*, **4**: 248-254 (1994).

20. KATSCHINSKI, B.D.; LOGAN, R.F.; EDMOND, M. ET AL. Duodenal ulcer and refined carbohydrate intake: a case-control study assessing dietary fibre and refined sugar intake [see comments]. *Gut*, **31**: 993-996 (1990).

21. CORNEE, J.; POBEL, D.; RIBOLI, E. ET AL. A case-control study of gastric cancer and nutritional factors in Marseille, France. *Eur. J. Epidemiol.*, **11**: 55-65 (1995).

22. LA VECCHIA, C.; FRANCESCHI, S.; DOLARA, P. ET AL. Refined-sugar intake and the risk of colorectal cancer in humans. *Int. J. Cancer*, **55**: 386-389 (1993).

23. BOSTICK, R.M.; POTTER, J.D.; KUSHI, L.H. ET AL. Sugar, meat, and fat intake, and non-dietary risk factors for colon cancer incidence in Iowa women (United States). *Causes Control*, **5**: 38-52 (1994).

24. LI, K.C.; ZERNICKE, R.F.; BARNARD, R.J. ET AL. Effects of a high fat-sucrose diet on cortical bone morphology and biomechanics. *Calcified Tissue International*, **47**: 308-313 (1990).

25. LENDERS, C.M.; HEDIGER, M.L.; SCHOLL, T.O. ET AL. Gestational age and infant size at birth are associated with dietary sugar intake among pregnant adolescents. *J. Nutr.*, **127**: 1113-1117 (1997).

26. LADAS, S.D.; HARITOS, D.N.; RAPTIS, S.A. Honey may have a laxative effect on normal subjects because of incomplete fructose absorption. *Am. J. Clin. Nutr.*, **62**: 1212-1215 (1995).

27. SCHNEIDER, ERNST. *La salud por la nutrición [Health through Nutrition]*. Madrid, Editorial Safeliz, 1986, p. 793.

28. DONADIEU, Yves. *Le miel [The Honey]*. Paris, Librerie Maloine S.A. éditeur, 1975, p. 23.

29. SNOWDON, J.A.; CLIVER, D.O. Microorganisms in honey. *Int. J. Food Microbiol.*, **31**: 1-26 (1996).

30. BAUER, L. ET AL. Food allergy to honey: pollen or bee products? Characterization of allergenic proteins in honey by means of immunoblotting. *Allergy Clin. Immunol.*, **97**: 65-73 (1996).

31. GROBLER, S.R.; DU TOIT, I.J.; BASSON, N.J. The effect of honey on human tooth enamel in vitro observed by electron microscopy and microhardness measurements. *Arch. Oral. Biol.*, **39**: 147-153 (1994).

32. FENICIA, L. ET AL. A case of infant botulism associated with honey feeding in Italy. *Eur. J. Epidemiol.*, **9**: 671-673 (1993).

CHAP. 11: MILK AND DAIRY PRODUCTS

1. SHERMAN, M.P.; DOCK, N.L.; EHLICH, G.D. ET AL. Evaluation of HIV type 1 western blot-indeterminate blood donors for the presence of human or bovine retroviruses. *AIDS Res. Hum. Retroviruses*, **11**: 409-411 (1992).

2. NASH, J.W.; HANSON, L.A.; ST. CYR-COATS, K. Detection of bovine immunodeficiency virus in blood and milk-derived leukocytes by use of polymerase chain reaction. *Am. J. Vet. Res.*, **56**: 445-449 (1995).

3. VENABLES, C. ET AL. Bovine immunodeficiency-like virus: inactivation in milk by pasteurisation. *Vet. Rec.*, **140**: 275-277 (1997).

4. FLEMING, D.W. ET AL. Pasteurized milk as a vehicle of infection in an outbreak of listeriosis. *N. Engl. J. Med.*, **312**: 404-407 (1985).

5. JACOBUS, C.H. Hypervitaminosis D associated with drinking milk. *N. Engl. J. Med.*, **326**: 1173-1177 (1992).

6. HOLICK, M.F.; SHAO, Q.; LIU, W.W.; CHEN, T.C. The vitamin D content of fortified milk and infant formula. *N. Engl. J. Med.*, **326**: 1178-1181 (1992).

7. HADDAD, J.G. Vitamin D-solar rays, the Milky Way, or both? *N. Engl. J. Med.*, **326**: 1213-1215 (1992).

8. SEGAL, J.J. Dietary lactose as a possible risk factor for ischaemic heart disease: review of epidemiology. *Int. J. Cardiol.* **46**: 197-207 (1994).

9. NATIONAL ACADEMY OF SCIENCES. Recommended Dietary Allowance.1989, p. 67.

10. ENSMINGER, A. H. ET AL. *The Concise Encyclopedia of Foods and Nutrition.* Boca Raton (Florida), CRC Press, 1995, p. 695.

11. SATOH, T.; GOTO, M.; IGARASHI, K. Effects of protein isolates from radish and spinach leaves on serum lipids levels in rats. *J. Nutr. Sci. Vitaminol (Tokyo)*, **39**: 627-633 (1993).

12. CROLL, K.K. Review of clinical studies on cholesterol-lowering response to soy protein. *JADA*, **91**: 820-827. (1991).

13. WEAVER, C.M. Calcium bioavailability and its relation to osteoporosis. *Proc. Soc. Exp. Biol. Med.*, **200**: 157-160 (1992).

14. WELTEN, D.C. ET AL. Longitudinal development and tracking of calcium and dairy intake from teenager to adult. *Eur. J. Clin. Nutr.*, **51**: 612-618 (1997).

15. GARREL, D.R. Milk and soy-protein ingestion: acute effect on serum uric acid concentration. *Am. J. Clin. Nutr.*, **53**: 665-669 (1991).

16. HILL, D.J.; BANNISTER, D.G.; HOSKING, C.S.; KEMP, A.S. Cow milk allergy within the spectrum of atopic disorders. *Clin. Exp. Allergy*, **24**: 1137-1143 (1994).

17. OSKI, F.A. *Don't drink your milk.* Teach services, Inc.; Brushton, New York.1995, p. 10.

18. ROSADO, J.L.; LOPEZ, P.; PALMA, M. Mala digestión e intolerancia a la lactosa en adultos mexicanos. Importancia de evaluarlas con dosis habituales de leche [Poor digestion and intolerance to lactose in Mexican adults. Importance of evaluating them with regular doses of milk]. *Rev. Invest. Clin.*, **46**: 203-208 (1994).

19. SUAREZ, F.L.; SAVAIANO, D.A.; LEVITT, M.D. A comparison of symptoms after the consumption of milk or lactose-hydrolyzed milk by people with self-reported severe lactose intolerance. *N. Engl. J. Med.*, **333**: 1-4 (1995).

20. JOHNSON, A.O. ET AL. Correlation of lactose maldigestion, lactose intolerance, and milk intolerance. *Am. J. Clin. Nutr.*, **57**: 399-401 (1993).

21. IACONO, G. ET AL. Chronic constipation as a symptom of cow milk allergy. *J. Pediatr.*, **126**: 34-39 (1995).

22. JOHNSEN, R. ET AL. Aetiology of peptic ulcer: a prospective population study in Norway. *J. Epidemiol. Community Health*, **48**: 156-160 (1994).

23. KATO, I.; NOMURA, A.M.; STEMMERMANN, G.N. ET AL. A prospective study of gastric and duodenal ulcer and its relation to smoking, alcohol and diet. *Am. J. Epidemiol.* **135**: 521-530 (1992).

24. SULLIVAN, P.B. Cow milk feeding in infancy: further observations on blood loss from the gastrointestinal tract. *J. Pediatr.*, **116**: 11-18 (1993).

25. SULLIVAN, P.B. Cow's milk induced intestinal bleeding in infancy. *Arch. Dis. Child.* **68**: 240-245 (1993).

26. SCOTT, F.W. Cow milk and insulin-dependent diabetes mellitus: is there a relationship? *Am. J. Clin. Nutr.*, **51**: 489-491 (1990).

27. GERSTEIN, H.C. Cow's milk exposure and type I diabetes mellitus. A critical overview of the clinical literature. *Diabetes Care*, **17**: 13-19 (1994).

28. DAHLQUIST, G. Non-genetic risk determinants of type 1 diabetes. *Diabetes Metab.*, **20**: 251-257 (1994).

29. NORRIS, J.M. ET AL. Lack of association between early exposure to cow's milk protein and beta-cell autoimmunity. *JAMA*, **276**: 609-614 (1996).

30. COUET, C.; JAN, P.; DEBRY, G. Lactose and cataract in humans: a review. *J. Am. Coll. Nutr.*, **10**: 79-86 (1991).

31. ARTAUD-WILD, S.M. ET AL. Differences in coronary mortality can be explained by differences in cholesterol and saturated fat intakes in 40 countries but not in France and Finland. A paradox [see comments]. *Circulation*, **88**: 2771-2779 (1993).

32. STEINMETZ, K.A. ET AL. Effect of consumption of whole milk and skim milk on blood lipid profiles in healthy men. *Am. J. Clin. Nutr.*, **59**: 612-618 (1994).

33. MALLATOU, H. Pesticide residues in milk and cheeses from Greece. *Sci. Total. Environ.*, **96**: 111-117 (1997).

34. ETHERTON, T.D.; KRIS-ETHERTON, P.M.; MILLAS, E.W. Recombinant bovine and porcine somatotropin: Safety and benefits of these biotechnologies. *J. Am. Diet. Assoc.*, **93**: 177-180 (1993).

35. URSIN, G. ET AL. Milk consumption and cancer incidence: a Norwegian prospective study. *Br. J. Cancer*, **61**: 456-459 (1990).

36. FERRER, J.F.; KENYON, S.J.; GUPTA, P. Milk of dairy cows frequently contains a leukemogenic virus. *Science*, **213**: 1014 (1981).

37. METTLIN, C.J.; PIVER, M.S. A case-control study of milk-drinking and ovarian cancer risk. *Am. J. Epidemiol.*, **132**: 871-876 (1990).

38. PAROD, P.W. Cow's milk fat components as potential anticarcinogenic agents. *Journal of Nutrition*, **127**: 1055-1060 (1997).

39. LA-VECCHIA, C. ET AL. Dairy products and the risk of prostatic cancer. *Oncology*, **48**: 406-410 (1991).

40. TAYLOR, D.M. ET AL. Absence of disease in mice receiving milk from cows with bovine spongiform encephalopathy. *Vet. Rec.*, **136**: 592 (1995).

41. GORBACH, S.L. Lactic acid bacteria and human health. *Ann. Med.*, **22**: 37-41 (1990).

42. MARTINI, M.C.; LEREBOURS, E.C.; LIN, W. ET AL. Strains and species of lactic acid bacteria in fermented milks (yogurts): effect on "in vivo" lactose digestion. *Am. J. Clin. Nutr.*, **54**: 1041-1046 (1991).

43. BOVEE-OUDENHOVEN, I. ET AL. Calcium in milk and fermentation by yoghurt bacteria increase the resistance of rats to Salmonella infection. *Gut*, **38**: 59-65 (1996).

44. SCHIFFRIN, E.J.; BRASSART, D.; SERVIN, A.L. ET AL. Immune modulation of blood leukocytes in humans by lactic acid bacteria: criteria for strain selection. *Am. J. Clin. Nutr.*, **66**: 515S-520S (1997).

45. MAJAMAA, H.; ISOLAURI, E.J. Probiotics: a novel approach in the management of food allergy. *Allergy Clin. Immunol.*, **99**: 179-185 (1997).

46. WHEELER, J.G. ET AL. Impact of dietary yogurt on immune function. *Am. J. Med. Sci.*, **313**: 120-123 (1997).

47. WHEELER, J.G. ET AL. Immune and clinical impact of Lactobacillus acidophilus on asthma. *Ann. Allergy Asthma Immunol.*, **79**: 229-233 (1997).

48. ABDELALI, H. ET AL. Antimutagenicity of components of dairy products. *Mutat. Res.*, **331**: 133-141 (1995).

49. POOL-ZOBEL, B.L. ET AL. Antigenotoxic properties of lactic acid bacteria in vivo in the gastrointestinal tract of rats. *Nutr. Cancer*, **20**: 271-281 (1993).

50. VAN'T VEER, P. Consumption of fermented milk products and breast cancer: a case-control study in the Netherlands. *Cancer Res.*, **49**: 4020-4023 (1989).

51. HITCHINS, A.D.; MCDONOUGH, F.E. Prophylactic and therapeutic aspects of fermented milk. *Am. J. Clin. Nutr.*, **49**: 675-684 (1996).

52. LINNAN ET AL. Epidemic listeriosis associated with mexican-style cheese. *New England Journal of Medicine*, **319**: 823-828 (1988).

53. FARBER, J.M.; ROSS, W.H.; HARWIG, J. Health risk assessment of Listeria monocytogenes in Canada. *Int. J. Food Microbiol.*, **30**: 145-156 (1996).

54. GOULET, V. ET AL. Listeriosis from consumption of raw-milk cheese. *The Lancet*, **345**: 1581-1582 (1995).

55. CASTELL MONSALVE, J. ET AL. Epidemic outbreak of 81 cases of brucellosis following the consumption of fresh cheese without pasteurization. *Rev. Esp. Salud Pública*, **70**: 303-311 (1996).

56. GEISS, H.K. ET AL. Food borne outbreak of a Salmonella enteritidis epidemic in a large pharmaceutical industry. *Gesundheitswesen*, **55**: 130-135 (1993).

57. O'DONELL, E.T. The incidence of Salmonella and Listeria in raw milk from farm bulk milk tanks in England and Wales. *Journal of the Society of Dairy Technology*, **48**: 25-29 (1995).

58. STAHL, V. ET AL. Prevention of Listeria monocytogenes contamination on dairy farms and in the cheese industry. *Pathol. Biol.*, **44**: 816-824, Paris (1996).

59. BIRD, N.; MACGREGOR, E.A.; WILKINSON, M.I. Ice cream headache -site, duration, and relationship to migraine. *Headache*, **32**: 35-38 (1992).

60. HENNESSY, C.W. ET AL. A national outbreak of Salmonella entiritidis infections from ice cream. *N. Eng. J. Med.*, **334**: 1281-1286 (1996).

61. TOLLIVER, B.A.; HERRERA, J.L.; DIPALMA, J.A. ET AL. Evaluation of patients who meet clinical criteria for irritable bowel syndrome. *Am. J. Gastroenterol.*, **88**: 176-178 (1994).

CHAP. 12: EGGS

1. URISU, A. ET AL. Allergenic activity of heated and ovomucoid-depleted egg white. *J. Allergy Clin. Immunol.*, **100**: 171-176 (1997).

2. DE SETA, L. ET AL. [The natural history of allergy to eggs in atopic dermatitis]. *Pediatr. Med. Chir.*, **16**: 485-487 (1994).

3. NORGAARD, A.; BINDSLEV-JENSEN, C. Egg and milk allergy in adults. Diagnosis and characterization. *Allergy*, **47**: 503-509 (1992).

4. MUHLENBERG, W. [Chicken feed contaminated with Salmonella enteritidis in a small egg-producing farm as source of a chain of infection in man problems in tracing the mode of transmission] *Gesundheitswesen*, **54**: 127-134 (1992).

5. LEVY, Y. ET AL. Consumption of eggs with meals increases the susceptibility of human plasma and low-density lipoprotein to lipid peroxidation. *Ann. Nutr. Metab.*, **40**: 243-251 (1996).

6. STEINMETZ, K.A.; POTTER, J.D. Egg consumption and cancer of the colon and rectum. *Eur. J. Cancer. Prev.*, **3**: 237-245 (1994).

7. KNELLER, R.W. ET AL. Risk factors for stomach cancer in sixty-five Chinese counties. *Cancer Epidemiol. Biomarkers Prev.*, **1**: 113-118 (1992).

8. SCHNOHR, P. ET AL. Egg consumption and high-density-lipoprotein cholesterol. *J. Intern. Med.*, **235**: 249-251 (1994).

9. ASATO, L. ET AL. Effect of egg white on serum cholesterol concentration in young women. *J. Nutr. Sci. Vitaminol. (Tokyo)*, **42**: 87-96 (1996).

10. OH, S.Y. ET AL. Eggs enriched in omega-3 fatty acids and alterations in lipid concentrations in plasma and lipoproteins and in blood pressure. *Am. J. Clin. Nutr.*, **54**: 689-695 (1991).

11. ZASTROW, K.D.; SCHONEBERG, I. [Outbreaks of food-borne infections and microbe-induced poisonings in West Germany, 1991]. *Gesundheitswesen*, **55**: 250-253 (1993).

12. LIGHTON, L.; GREENWOOD, L. Raw eggs in recipes in magazines should go. *British Medical Journal*, **308**: 595-596 (1994).

13. MISHU, B. ET AL. Salmonella enteritidis gastroenteritis transmitted by intact chicken eggs. *Ann. Intern. Med.*, **115**: 190-194 (1991).

CHAP. 13: FISH AND SHELLFISH

1. EINSMINGER, A. H. *The Concise Encyclopedia of Foods and Nutrition.* Boca Raton (Florida), CRC Press, 1995, p. 349.

2. CLARKSON, T. Environmental contaminants in the food chain. *Am. J. Clin. Nutr.*, **61**: S682-S686 (1995).

3. AHMED, F.E. ET AL. Risk assessment and management of chemical contaminants in fishery products consumed in Estados Unidos. *J. Appl. Toxicol.*, **13**: 395-410 (1993).

4. MORELL, V. Fishing for trouble. *International Wildlife*, **14**: 40-43 (1984).

5. YU, M.C.; HENDERSON, B.E. Intake of Cantonese-style salted fish as a cause of nasopharyngeal carcinoma. *IARC Sci. Publ.*, **84**: 547-549 (1987).

6. DUTIL, L.T.; COUILLARD, C.M.; BELANGER, D. A processing plant survey of external lesions of American eels (Anguilla rostrata) from Lake Ontario and the St. Lawrence River, Canada. *Prev. Vet. Med.*, **31**: 19-32 (1997).

7. FORAN, J.A.; GLENN, B.S.; SILVERMAN, W. Increased fish consumption may be risky. *JAMA*, **262**: 28 (1989).

8. SIKORSKI, Z.E.; SCOTT, D.N.; BUSSON, D.H. The role of collagen in the quality and processing of fish. *Crit. Rev. Food Sci. Nutr.*, **20**: 301-343 (1984).

9. OZONOFF, D.; LONGNECKER, M.P. Epidemiologic approaches to assessing human cancer risk from consuming aquatic food resources from chemically contaminated water. *Environ. Health. Perspect.*, **90**: 141-146 (1991).

10. ZHANG, R.F. ET AL. Role of nitrosamides in the high risk for gastric cancer in China. *IARC Sci. Publ.*, **105**: 152-157 (1991).

11. DAVIGLUS, M.L. ET AL. Fish consumption and the 30-year risk of fatal myocardial infarction. *N. Eng. J. Med.*, **336**: 1046-1053 (1997).

12. CHRISTENSEN, J.H. ET AL. Effect of fish oil on heart rate variability in survivors of myocardial infarction. *British Medical Journal*, **312**: 677-678 (1996).

13. SISCOVICK, D.S. ET AL. Dietary intake and cell membrane levels of long-chain n-3 polyunsaturated fatty acids and the risk of primary cardiac arrest. *JAMA*, **274**: 1363-1367 (1995).

14. KROMHOUT, D.; BOSSCHIETER, E.B.; COULANDER, C.L. The inverse relation between fish consumption and 20-years mortality from coronary heart disease. *N. Engl. J. Med.*, **312**: 1205-1209 (1985).

15. ASCHERIO, A.; RIMM, E.B.; STAMPFER, M.J. ET AL. Dietary intake of marine n-3 fatty acids, fish intake, and the risk of coronary disease among men. *N. Engl. J. Med.*, **332**: 977-982 (1995).

16. GLERUP, H. ET AL. A "mini epidemic" of hepatitis A after eating Russian caviar. *J. Hepatol.*, **21**: 479 (1994).

17. JONNALAGADDA, S.S. ET AL. Effects of individual fatty acids on chronic diseases. *Nutrition Today*, **31**: 90-106 (1996).

18. VALDINI, A.F. Efficacy of fish oil supplementation for treatment of moderate elevation of serum cholesterol. *J. Fam. Pract.*, **30**: 55-59 (1990).

19. HARRIS, W.S. n-3 Fatty acids and serum lipoproteins: human studies. *Am. J. Clin. Nutr.*, **65** (suppl): 1645S-1654S (1997).

20. SCHECTMAN, G. ET AL. Can the hypotriglyceridemic effect of fish oil concentrate be sustained? *Ann. Intern. Med.*, **110**: 346-352 (1989).

21. ISRAEL, D.H.; GORLIN, R.J. Fish oils in the prevention of atherosclerosis. *Am. Coll. Cardiol.*, **19**: 174-185 (1992).

22. APPEL, L.J. Does supplementation of diet with 'fish oil' reduce blood pressure? A meta-analysis of controlled clinical trials [see comments]. *Arch. Intern. Med.*, **153**: 1429-1438 (1993).

23. SACKS, F.M. The effect of fish oil on blood pressure and high-density lipoprotein-cholesterol levels in phase I of the Trials of Hypertension Prevention. *Trials of Hypertension Prevention Collaborative Research Group. J. Hypertens. Suppl.*, **12**: S23-S31 (1994).

24. OOSTHUIZEN, W. ET AL. Both fish oil and olive oil lowered plasma fibrinogen in women with high baseline fibrinogen levels. *Thromb. Haemost.*, **72**: 557-562 (1994).

25. STENSON, W.F. ET AL. Dietary supplementation with fish oil in ulcerative colitis [see comments]. *Ann. Intern. Med.*, **116**: 609-614 (1992).

26. KIM, Y.I. Can fish oil maintain Crohn's disease in remission? *Nutr. Rev.*, **54**: 248-252 (1996).

27. HAREL, Z. Supplementation with omega-3 polyunsaturated fatty acids in the management of dysmenorrhea in adolescents. *Am. J. Obstet. Gynecol.*, **174**: 1335-1338 (1996).

28. SKOLDSTAM, L. ET AL. Effect of six months of fish oil supplementation in stable rheumatoid arthritis. A double-blind, controlled study. *Scand. J. Rheumatol.*, **21**: 178-185 (1992).

29. UAUY-DAGACH, R.; VALENZUELA, A. Marine oils: the health benefits of n-3 fatty acids. *Nutrition Reviews*, **54**: S102-S108 (1996).

30. GRUBB, B.P. Hypervitaminosis A following long-term use of high-dose fish oil supplements. *Chest*, **97**: 1260 (1990).

31. BJERREGUAARD, P.; DYERBERG, J. Mortality from ischaemic heart disease and cerebrovascular disease in Greenland. *Int. J. Epidemiol.*, **17**: 514-519 (1988).

32. ALBINA, J.E.; GLADDEN, P.; WALSH, W.R. Detrimental effects of an omega-3 fatty acid-enriched diet on wound healing. *J. Parenter. Enteral Nutr.*, **17**: 519-521 (1993).

33. REUTER, W. ET AL. [Changes in parameters of lipid metabolism and anti-oxidative potentials in elderly hyperlipoproteinemic patients treated with omega-3 fatty acids]. *Z. Gerontol.*, **27**: 204-207 (1994).

34. BUDIARSO, I.T. Fish oil versus olive oil [letter; comment]. *Lancet*, **336**: 1313-1314 (1990).

35. LEVINE, D.Z. Ciguatera: current concepts. *J. Am. Osteopath. Assoc.*, **95**: 193-198 (1995).

36. MALPEZZI, E.L.; DE FREITAS, J.C.; RANTIN, F.T. Occurrence of toxins, other than paralysing type, in the skin of Tetraodontiformes fish. *Toxicon*, **35**: 57-65 (1997).

37. TAYLOR, S.L. Histamine food poisoning: toxicology and clinical aspects. *Crit. Rev. Toxicol.*, **17**: 91-128 (1986).

38. TAYLOR, S.L.; STRATTON, J.E.; NORDLEE, J.A. Histamine poisoning (scombroid fish poisoning): an allergy-like intoxication. *J. Toxicol. Clin. Toxicol.*, **27**: 225-240 (1989).

39. O'NEIL, C.; HELBING, A.A.; LEHRER, S.B. Allergic reactions to fish. *Clin. Rev. Allergy*, **11**: 183-200 (1993).

40. MATA, E. ET AL. Surimi and native codfish contain a common allergen identified as a 63-kDa protein. *Allergy*, **49**: 442-447 (1994).

41. HELBING, A. ET AL. Immunopathogenesis of fish allergy: identification of fish-allergic adults by skin test and radioallergosorbent test. *Ann. Allergy Asthma Immunol.*, **77**: 48-54 (1996).

42. DE MARTINO, M. ET AL. Fish allergy in children. *Ann. Allergy*, **71**: 159-165 (1993).

43. ADAMS, A.A.; BEEH, J.L.; WEKELL, M.M. Health risks of salmon sushi. *Lancet*, **336**: 1328 (1990).

44. SALONEN, J.T. ET AL. Intake of mercury from fish, lipid peroxidation, and the risk of myocardial infarction and coronary, cardiovascular, and any death in eastern finish men. *Circulation*, **91**: 645-655 (1995).

45. MACLEAN, J.D. ET AL. Common-source outbreak of acute infection due to the North American liver fluke Metorchis conjunctus. *Lancet*, **347**: 154-158 (1996).

46. MORENO-ANCILLO, A. ET AL. Allergic reactions to anisakis simplex parasitizing seafood. *Ann. Allergy Asthma Immunol.*, **79**: 246-250 (1997).

47. WILHELM, M. ET AL. Duplicate study on the dietary intake of some metals/metalloids by children in Germany. Arsenic and mercury. *Zentralbl. Hyg. Umweltmed.*, **197**: 345-356 (1995).

48. CASTILLO, R. ET AL. Shellfish hypersensitivity: clinical andimmunological characteristics. *Allergol. Immunopathol.*, **22**: 83-87 (1994).

49. LIPTON, J.; GILLETT, J.W. Uncertainty in ocean-dumping health risks: influence of bioconcentration, commercial fish landings and seafood consumption. *Environmental Toxicology and Chemistry*, **10**: 967-976 (1991).

50. WITTMAN, R.J.; FLICK, G.J. Microbial contamination of shellfish: Prevalence, risk to human health and control strategies. *Annu. Rev. Public Health*, **16**: 123-140 (1995).

51. WARNOCK, E.W.; MacMATH, T.L. Primary Vibrio vulnificus septicemia. *J. Emerg. Med.*, **11**: 153-156 (1993).

52. RATNER, H. Vibrio vulnificus. *Infect. Control*, **8**: 430-433 (1987).

53. GERBA, C.P. Viral disease transmission by seafoods. *Food Tech.*, **42**: 99-103 (1988).

54. WANKE, C.A.; GUERRANT, R.L. Viral hepatitis and gastroenteritis transmitted by shellfish and water. *Infect. Dis. Clin. North Am.*, **1**: 649-664 (1987).

55. O'MAHONY, M.C.; GOOCH, C.D.; SMYTH, D.A. ET AL. Epidemic hepatitis A from cockles. *Lancet*, **1**: 518-520 (1983).

56. VIVARES, C. ¿Es peligroso consumir mariscos? [Is it dangerous to eat shellfish?] *Mundo Científico*. (Spanish edition of *La Recherche*) **11**: 326-334 (1991).

57. SCOGING, A.C. Illness associated with seafood. *Can. Med. Assoc. J.*, **147**: 1344-1347 (1992).

58. MELE, A. ET AL. Risk factors for acute non-A, non-B hepatitis and their relationship to antibodies for hepatitis C virus: a case-control study. *Am. J. Public. Health*, **84**: 1640-1643 (1994).

59. ROMALDE, J.L. New molecular methods for the detection of hepatitis A and Norwalk viruses in shellfish. *Microbiología*, **12**: 547-556 (1996).

60. LE GUYADER, F. ET AL. Detection and analysis of a small round-structured virus strain in oysters implicated in an outbreak of acute gastroenteritis. *Appl. Environ. Microbiol.*, **62**: 4268-4272 (1996).

61. McDONNELL, S. ET AL. Failure of cooking to prevent shellfish-associated viral gastroenteritis. *Arch. Intern. Med.*, **157**: 111-116 (1997).

62. KIRKLAND, K.B. ET AL. Steaming oysters does not prevent Norwalk-like gastroenteritis. *Public Health Rep.*, **111**: 527-530 (1996).

63. DEL POZO, M.D. ET AL. Anisakis simplex, a relevant etiologic factor in acute urticaria. *Allergy*, **52**: 576-579 (1997).

64. CORTES-ALTAMIRANO, R.; HERNANDEZ-BECERRIL, D.U.; LUNA-SORIA, R. Red tides in Mexico: a review. *Rev. Latinoam. Microbiol.*, **37**: 343-352 (1995).

65. FENNEMA, Owen R. *Food Chemistry*. New York, Marcel Dekker, 2nd ed., 1990.

66. VAN EGMOND, H.P. ET AL. Paralytic and diarrhoeic shellfish poisons: occurrence in Europe, toxicity, analysis and regulation. *Journal of Natural Toxins*, **2**: 41-83 (1993).

67. PERL, T.; BÉDARD, L.; KOSATSKY, T. ET AL. An outbreak of toxic encephalopathy caused by eating mussels contaminated with domoic acid. *N. Engl. J. Med.*, **322**: 1775-1780 (1990).

68. TODD, E.C. Domoic acid and amnesic shellfish poisoning. A review. *J. Food Prot.*, **56**: 69-83 (1993).

69. PERL, T.M. ET AL. An outbreak of toxic encephalopathy caused by eating mussels contaminated with domoic acid. *N. Engl. J. Med.*, **322**: 1775-1780 (1990).

70. DE LA CUESTA, C.G. ET AL. Food allergy to Helix terrestre (snail). *Allergol. Immunopathol.* **17**: 337-339, Madrid (1989).

71. PIETINEN, P.; ASCHERIO, A.; KORHONEN, P. ET AL. Intake of fatty acids and risk of coronary heart disease in a cohort of Finnish men. The Alpha-Tocopherol, Beta-Carotene Cancer Prevention Study. *Am. J. Epidemiol.*, **145**: 876-887 (1997).

CHAP. 14: MEAT

1. KAEFERSTEIN, F.K.; CLUGSTON, G.A. Human health problems related to meat production and consumption. *Fleischwirtschaft*, **75**: 857-863 (1995).

2. LEWIS, S. An opinion on the global impact of meat consumption. *Am. J. Clin. Nutr.*, **59** (5 Suppl):1099S-1102S (1994).

3. MASSON, F.; TALON, R.; MONTEL, M.C. Histamine and tyramine production by bacteria from meat products. *Int. J. Food Microbiol.*, **32**: 199-207 (1996).

4. RANKEN, M.D. *Food Industries Manual*. Glasgow, Blackie & Son Ltd., 22nd ed., 1988.

5. FENNEMA, Owen R. *Food Chemistry*. New York, Marcel Dekker, 2nd ed., 1990.

6. LAUER, K. The history of nitrite in human nutrition: a contribution from German cookery books. *J. Clin. Epidemiol.*, **44**: 261-264 (1991).

7. McCUTCHEON, J.W. Nitrosamines in bacon: a case study of balancing risks. *Public Health Rep.*, **99**: 360-364 (1984).

8. RANKEN, M.D. *Food Industries Manual*. Blackie & Son Ltd. Bishopbriggs, Glasgow G64 2NZ, 22 ed.

9. GOMA, E.A. ET AL. Polycyclic aromatic hydrocarbons in smoked food products and commercial liquid smoke flavourings. *Food Addit. Contam.*, **10**: 503-521 (1993).

10. NINIVAARA, F.P.; ANTILA, P. *Der Nährwert des Fleisches* [*Nutritive Value of Meat*] Alzey, Germany, Verlag der Rheinhessischen Druckwerkstätte.

11. VAN MAANEN, J.M. ET AL. Formation of aromatic DNA adducts in white blood cells in relation to urinary excretion of 1-hydroxypyrene during consumption of grilled meat. *Carcinogenesis*, **15**: 2263-2268 (1994).

12. ADAMSON, R.H.; THORGEIRSSON, U.P. Carcinogens in foods: heterocyclic amines and cancer and heart disease. *Adv. Exp. Med. Biol.*, **369**: 211-220 (1995).

13. FELTON, J.S. ET AL. Health risks of heterocyclic amines. *Mutat. Res.*, **376**: 37-41 (1997).

14. BAKER, R. ET AL. Detection of mutagenic activity in human urine following fried meat meals. *Cancer Lett.*, **16**: 81-89 (1982).

15. BERG, I.; OVERVIK, E.; GUSTAFSSON, J.A. Effect on cooking time on mutagen formation in smoke, crust and pan residue from pan-broiled pork. *Food Chem. Toxicol.*, **28**: 421-426 (1990).

16. PROBST-HENSCH, N.M. Meat preparation and colorectal adenomas in a large sigmoidoscopy-based case-control study in California (United States). *Cancer Causes Control*, **8**: 175-183 (1997).

17. WARD, M.H. ET AL. Risk of adenocarcinoma of the stomach and esophagus with meat cooking method and doneness preference. *Int. J. Cancer*, **71**: 14-19 (1997).

18. DE STEFANI, E. ET AL. Meat intake, heterocyclic amines, and risk of breast cancer: a case-control study in Uruguay. *Cancer Epidemiol. Biomarkers Prev.*, **6**: 573-581 (1997).

19. BARRINGTON, P.J. Mutagenicity of basic fractions derived from lamb and beef cooked by common household methods. *Food Chem. Toxicol.*, **28**: 141-146 (1990).

20. NILSSON, L. ET AL. Influence of frying fat on mutagenic activity in lean pork meat. *Mutat. Res.*, **171**: 115-121 (1986).

21. LINDESKOG, P.; OVERVIK, E.; NILSSON, L. ET AL. Influence of fried meat and fiber on cytochrome P-450 mediated activity and excretion of mutagens in rats. *Mutat. Res.*, **204**: 553-563 (1988).

22. LEE, H.; LIN, M.Y.; CHAN, S.C. Formation and identification of carcinogenic heterocyclic aromatic amines in boiled pork juice. *Mutat. Res.*, **308**: 77-88 (1994).

23. TSAI, S.J.; JENG, S.N.; LEE, H. Naturally occurring dialyl disulfide inhibits the formation of carcinogenic heterocyclic aromatic amines in boiled pork juice. *Mutagenesis*, **11**: 235-240 (1996).

24. Meat –can we live without it? *World Health Forum*, **12**: 251-260; discussion 260-283 (1991).

25. DEUTSCH, Ronald M.; MORRILL, Judi S. *Realities of Nutrition*. Bull Publishing Company, Palo Alto, California (USA) 1991.

26. EINSMINGER, A. H. *The Concise Encyclopedia of Foods and Nutrition*. Boca Raton (Florida), CRC Press, 1995, p. 671.

27. AGUILAR, Miguel. *La dieta vegetariana* [*The Vegetarian Diet*]. Madrid, Ediciones Temas de Hoy, 1990.

28. Leviticus 3: 17.

29. BERGEN, W.G.; MERKEL, R.A. Body composition of animals treated with partitioning agents: implications for human health. *FASEB-J.*, **5**: 2951-2957 (1991).

30. BROWN, H.B. Diet and serum lipids: controlled studies in the Unites States. *Prev. Med.*, **12**: 103-109 (1983).

31. MOTT, G.E. ET AL. Comparison of the effects of dietary beef tallow and corn oil on pancreatic carcinogenesis in the hamster model. *Carcinogenesis*, **11**: 745-748 (1990).

32. BIRT, D.F. ET AL. Dietary cholesterol and type of fat differentially affect cholesterol metabolism and atherosclerosis in baboons. *J. Nutr.*, **122**: 1397-1406 (1992).

33. WILLETT, W.C.; STAMPFER, M.J.; COLDITZ, G.A. ET AL. Relation of meat, fat, and fiber intake to the risk of colon cancer in a prospective study among women [see comments]. *N. Engl. J. Med.*, **323**: 1664-1672 (1990).

34. RISCH, H.A. ET AL. Dietary fat intake and risk of epithelial ovarian cancer. *J. Natl. Cancer Inst.*, **86**: 1409-1415 (1994).

35. GIOVANNUCCI, E. ET AL. A prospective study of dietary fat and risk of prostate cancer [see comments]. *J. Natl. Cancer Inst.*, **85**: 1571-1579 (1993).

36. HURSTING, S.D.; THORNQUIST, M.; HENDERSON, M.M. Types of dietary fat and the incidence of cancer at five sites. *Prev. Med.*, **19**: 242-253 (1990).

37. 1 Corinthians 15: 39.

38. ROMER, ALFRED S. *The vertebrate body*. W. B. Saunders company, 4 ed., 1971.

39. OMOLOLU, A. Algunas carnes son más sanas que otras [Some meats are healthier than others]. *Foro Mundial de la Salud* [*World Health Forum*], **12**: 283-284 (1991).

40. Genesis 1: 29.

41. 2 Peter 3: 13; Isaiah 65: 25.

42. WHITE, Ellen. *Counsels on Diet and Foods*. Review and Herald Publishing Association, Hagerstown, MD 21740, p. 385.

43. KONTESSIS, P.; JONES, S.; DODDS, R. ET AL. Renal, metabolic and hormonal responses to ingestion of animal and vegetable proteins. *Kidney Int.*, **38**: 136-144 (1990).

44. ALDOORI, W.H.; GIOVANNUCCI, E.L.; RIMM, E.B. ET AL. A prospective study of diet and the risk of symptomatic diverticular disease in men. *Am. J. Clin. Nutr.*, **60**: 757-764 (1994).

45. ABELOW, B.J.; HOLFORD, T.R.; INSOGNA, K.L. Cross-cultural association between dietary animal protein and hip fracture: a hypothesis. *Calcif. Tissue Int.*, **50**: 14-18 (1992).

46. KJELDSEN-KRAGH, J.; MELLBYE, O.J.; HAUGEN, M. ET AL. Changes in laboratory variables in rheumatoid arthritis patients during a trial of

fasting and one-year vegetarian diet. *Scand. J. Rheumatol.*, **24:** 85-93 (1995).

47. SNOWDON, D.A.; PHILLIPS, R.L. Does a vegetarian diet reduce the occurrence of diabetes? *Am. J. Public. Health*, **75:** 507-512 (1985).

48. MACDONALD, K.L.; O'LEARY, M.J.; COHEN, M.L. Escherichia coli O157:H7, an emerging gastrointestinal pathogen. Results of a one-year, prospective, population-based study. *JAMA*, **259:** 3567-3570 (1988).

49. WORLD HEALTH ORGANIZATION, DIVISION OF EMERGING AND OTHER COMMUNICABLE DISEASES AND CONTROL. The medical impact of the use of antimicrobials in food animals. Report of a WHO meeting. Berlin, Germany, 13-17 October 1997.

50. ASCHERIO, A., ET AL. Dietary iron intake and risk of coronary disease among men. *Circulation*, **89:** 969-974 (1994).

51. NICKLAS, T.A.; FARRIS, R.P.; MYERS, L. ET AL. Impact of meat consumption on nutritional quality and cardiovascular risk factors in young adults: the Bogalusa Heart Study. *J. Am. Diet. Assoc.*, **95:** 887-892 (1995).

52. KAHN, H.A.; PHILLIPS, R.L.; SNOWDON, D.A. ET AL. Association between reported diet and all-cause mortality. Twenty-year follow-up on 27,530 adult Seventh-day Adventists. *Am. J. Epidem.* **119:** 775-787 (1984).

53. WHO, Technical Report Series, 797. *Diet, Nutrition, and the Prevention of Chronic Diseases*. Report of a WHO Study Group. Geneva, 1990.

54. THOROGOOD, M.; MANN, J.; APPLEBY, P. ET AL. Risk of death from cancer and ischaemic heart disease in meat and non-meat eaters [see comments]. *British Med. J.*, **308:** 1667-1670 (1994).

55. DE STEFANI, E.; OREGGIA, F.; RONCO, A. ET AL. Salted meat consumption as a risk factor for cancer of the oral cavity and pharynx: a case-control study from Uruguay. *Cancer Epidemiol. Biomarkers Prev.*, **3:** 381-385 (1994).

56. BOEING, H.; SCHLEHOFER, B.; WAHRENDORF, J.Z. Diet, obesity and risk for renal cell carcinoma: results from a case control-study in Germany. *Ernahrungswiss*, **36:** 3-11 (1997).

57. GIOVANNUCCI, E.; RIMM, E.B.; STAMPFER, M.J. ET AL. Intake of fat, meat, and fiber in relation to risk of colon cancer in men. *Cancer Res*, **54:** 2390-2397 (1994).

58. BINGHAM, S.A.; PIGNATELLI, B.; POLLOCK, J.R. ET AL. Does increased endogenous formation of N-nitroso compounds in the human colon explain the association between red meat and colon cancer? *Carcinogenesis*, **17:** 515-523 (1996).

59. GAARD, M.; TRETLI, S.; LOKEN, E.B. Dietary fat and the risk of breast cancer: a prospective study of 25,892 Norwegian women. *Int. J. Cancer*, **63:** 13-17 (1995).

60. O'DEA, KERIN ET AL. Cholesterol-lowering effect of a low-fat diet containing lean beef is reversed by the addition of beef fat. *Am. J. Clin. Nutr.*, **52:** 491-494 (1990).

61. SNOWDON, D.A.; PHILLIPS, R.L.; FRASER, G.E. Meat consumption and fatal ischemic heart disease. *Prev. Med*, **13:** 490-500 (1984).

62. WILL, R. G. ET AL. A new variant of Creutzfeldt-Jakob disease in the UK. *The Lancet*, **347:** 921-925 (1996).

63. PRUSINER, S.B. Molecular biology of prion diseases. *Science*, **252:** 1515-1522 (1991).

64. O'BRIEN, B.C.; REISER, R. Human plasma lipids responses to red meat, poultry, fish, and eggs. *Am. J. Clin. Nutr.*, **33:** 2573-2580 (1980).

65. *Eroski*, nº 193, March 1995, pp. 16-19.

66. CASTILLO-MARTINEZ, M.L. ET AL. Isolation of Campylobacter jejuni ATCC 29428 from inoculated fried pork meat and roasted chicken. *Rev. Latinoam. Microbiol.*, **35:** 15-18 (1993).

67. DI GIACOMO, R.F.; HOPKINS, S.G. Food animal and poultry retroviruses and human health. *Vet. Clin. North Am. Food Anim. Pract.*, **13:** 177-190 (1997).

68. BELL, B.P.; GOLDOFT, M.; GRIFFIN, P.M. ET AL. A multistate outbreak of Escherichia coli O157:H7-associated bloody diarrhea and hemolytic uremic syndrome from hamburgers. The Washington experience. *JAMA*, **272:** 1349-1353 (1994).

69. KNIZE, M.G.; SINHA, R.; ROTHMAN, N. ET AL. Heterocyclic amine content in fast-food meat products. *Food Chem. Toxicol.*, **33:** 545-551 (1995).

70. CHIU, B.C.; CERHAN, J.R.; FOLSOM, A.R. ET AL. Diet and risk of non-Hodgkin lymphoma in older women. *JAMA*, **275:** 1315-1321 (1996).

71. SPIKA, J.S.; DABIS, F.; HARGRETT-BEAN, N. ET AL. Shigellosis at a Caribbean resort. Hamburger and North American origin as risk factors. *Am. J. Epidemiol.* **126:** 1173-1180 (1987).

72. JACKSON, L.S.; HARGRAVES, W.A.; STROUP, W.H. ET AL. Heterocyclic aromatic amine content of selected beef flavors. *Mutat. Res*, **320:** 113-124 (1994).

73. STAVRIC, B.; MATULA, T.I.; KLASSEN, R. ET AL. Analysis of commercial bouillons for trace levels of mutagens. *Food Chem. Toxicol.*, **31:** 981-987 (1993).

74. ANDERSEN, A.; HANSEN, H.H. Cadmium and zinc in kidneys from Danish cattle. *Nord. Vet. Med.*, **34:** 340-349 (1982).

75. WHITE, ELLEN. *The Ministry of Healing*. Pacific Press Publishing Association, p. 240.

76. NANJI, A.A.; FRENCH, S.W. Relationship between porkconsumption and cirrhosis. *Lancet*, **1** (8430): 681-683 (1985).

77. BERENDS, B.R.; VAN KNAPEN, F.; SNIJDERS, J.M. Identification and quantification of risk factors regarding Salmonella spp. on pork carcasses. *Int. J. Food Microbiol*, **36:** 199-206 (1997).

78. NARAIN, J.P.; LOFGREN, J.P. Epidemic of restaurant-associated illness due to Salmonella newport. *South. Med. J.*, **82:** 837-840 (1989).

79. RODRIGUEZ, M.; NUÑEZ, F.; CORDOBA, J. ET AL. Gram-positive, catalase-positive cocci from dry cured Iberian ham and their enterotoxigenic potential. *J. Appl. Environ. Microbiol.*, **62:** 1897-1902 (1996).

80. ZANONI, B.; GARZAROLI, C.; ANSELMI, S. ET AL. Modeling the growth of Enterococcus faecium in bologna sausage. *Appl. Environ. Microbiol.*, **59:** 3411-3417 (1993).

81. LANDHEER, J.E.; MOL, H.; VINCENTIE, H.M. Staphylococcal enterotoxemia following consumption of a pork fricandeau. *Tijdschr. Diergeneeskd*, **112:** 844-846 (1987).

82. SCHRAFT, H.; KLEINLEIN, N.; UNTERMANN, F. Contamination of pig hindquarters with Staphylococcus aureus. *Int. J. Food Microbiol*, **15:** 191-194 (1992).

83. SWADDIWUDHIPONG, W.; AKARASEWI, P.; CHAYANIYAYODHIN, T. ET AL. A cholera outbreak associated with eating uncooked pork in Thailand. *J. Diarrhoeal Dis. Res*, **8:** 94-96 (1990).

84. QVIST, S.; SEHESTED, K.; ZEUTHEN, P. Growth suppression of Listeria monocytogenes in a meat product. *Int. J. Food Microbiol*, **24:** 283-293 (1994).

85. GOULET, V.; ROCOURT, J.; REBIERE, I. ET AL. Listeriosis outbreak associated with the consumption of rillettes in Francia in 1993. *J. Infect. Dis*, **177:** 155-160 (1998).

86. OSTROFF, S.M.; KAPPERUD, G.; HUTWAGNER, L.C. ET AL. Sources of sporadic Yersinia enterocolitica infections in Norway: prospective
case control study. *Epidemiol. Infect*, **112:** 133-141 (1994).

87. KAMAT, A.S.; KHARE, S.; DOCTOR, T. ET AL. Control of Yersinia enterocolitica in raw pork and pork products bygamma-irradiation. *Int. J. Food Microbiol*, **36:** 69-76 (1997).

88. SCHNEIDER, A.; MORABIA, A.; PAPENDICK, U. ET AL. Pork intake and human papillomavirus-related disease. *Nutr. Cancer*, **13:** 209-211 (1990).

89. KEEFE, M.; AL-GHAMDI, A.; COGGON, D. ET AL. Cutaneous warts in butchers. *Br. J. Dermatol.*, **130:** 9-14 (1994).

90. WORLEY, D.E.; SEESEE, F.M.; ESPINOSA, R.H. ET AL. Survival of sylvatic Trichinella spiralis isolates in frozen tissue and processed meat products. *J. Am. Vet. Med. Assoc.*, **189:** 1047-1049 (1986).

91. LANDRY, S.M.; KISER, D.; OVERBY, T. ET AL. Trichinosis: common source outbreak related to commercial pork. *South. Med. J.*, **85:** 428-429 (1992).

92. BAILEY, T.M.; SCHANTZ, P.M. Trends in the incidence and transmission patterns of trichinosis in humans in the United States comparisons of the periods 1975-1981 and 1982-1986. *Rev. Infect. Dis.*, **12:** 5-11 (1990).

93. TIBERIO, G.; RIVERO, M.; LANZAS, G. ET AL. Trichinellosis: study of 2 outbreaks in Navarre. *Enferm. Infecc. Microbiol. Clin.*, **15:** 151-153 (1997).

94. CHOI, W.Y.; NAM, H.W.; KWAK, N.H. ET AL. Foodborne outbreaks of human toxoplasmosis. *J. Infect. Dis.*, **175:** 1280-1282 (1997).

95. BUFFOLANO, W.; GILBERT, R.E.; HOLLAND, F.J. ET AL. Risk factors for recent toxoplasma infection in pregnant women in Naples. *Epidemiol. Infect*, **116:** 347-351 (1996).

96. THE CYSTICERCOSIS WORKING GROUP IN PERU. The marketing of cysticercotic pigs in the Sierra of Perú. *Bull. World Health Organ.*, **71:** 223-228 (1993).

97. Isaiah 66: 17.

98. SARASUA, S.; SAVITZ, D.A. Cured and broiled meat consumption in relation to childhood cancer: Denver, Colorado. *Cancer Causes Control*, **5:** 141-148 (1994).

99. STAVRIC, B.; MATULA, T.I.; KLASSEN, R. ET AL. Evaluation of hamburgers and hot dogs for the presence of mutagens. *Food Chem. Toxicol.*, **33:** 815-820 (1995).

100. BOEING, H.; SCHLEHOFER, B.; BLETTNER, M. Dietary carcinogens and the risk for glioma and meningioma in Germany. *Int. J. Cancer*, **53:** 561-565 (1993).

101. NANJI, A.A.; FRENCH, S.W. Hepatocellular carcinoma. Relationship to meat consumption. *Cancer*, **56:** 2711-2712 (1985).

102. JI, H.; YU, M.C.; STILLWELL, W.G. ET AL. Urinary excretion of 2-amino-3,8-dimethylimidazo-[4,5-f]quinoxaline in white, black, and Asian men in Los Angeles. *Cancer Epidemiol. Biomarkers Prev.*, **3:** 407-411 (1994).

103. MCLAUCHLIN, J.; HALL, S.M.; VELANI, S.K. ET AL. Human listeriosis and pate: a possible association. *British Med. J.*, **303:** 773-775 (1991).

104. KREDL, F.; SVOBODNIK, J. [Residues of chlorinated pesticides and polychlorinated biphenyls in pork and ham in past years and today]. *Vet. Med.*, **33:** 175-184. Praga (1988).

105. ANCELLE, T.; DUPOUY-CAMET, J.; BOUGNOUX, M.E. Two outbreaks of trichinosis caused by horsemeat in Francia in 1985. *Am. J. Epidemiol.*, **127:** 1302-1311 (1988).

106. VALTUEÑA BORQUE, ÓSCAR. *El vegetarianismo en la infancia y la adolescencia.* [Vegetarianism in infancy and adolescence]. Anales de la Real Academia de Medicina, Volume 62:2, Madrid, Spain, 1995.

107. Meat –can we live without it? *World Health Forum*, **12**: 251-260, discussion 260-283. (1991).

108. DONOVAN, U.M.; GIBSON, R.S. Iron and zinc status of young women aged 14 to 19 years consuming vegetarian and omnivorous diets. *J. Am. Coll. Nutr.*, **14**: 463-472 (1995).

109. NOBMANN, E.D. ET AL. The diet of Alaska Native adults: 1987-1988. *Am. J. Clin. Nutr.*, **55**: 1024-1032 (1992).

CHAP. 15: CONDIMENTS AND SPICES

1. Genesis 37: 25.

2. Isaiah 40: 22.

3. PAMPLONA-ROGER G. D. *Encyclopedia of Medicinal Plants*. Editorial Safeliz, Madrid, 1998, p. 193.

4. JURIM, O. ET AL. Disseminated intravascular coagulopathy caused by acetic acid ingestion. *Acta Haematol*, **89**: 204-205 (1993).

5. KAWAMATA, M. ET AL. Acetic acid intoxication by rectal administration. *J. Toxicol. Clin. Toxicol.*, **32**: 333-336 (1994).

6. LINKOSALO, E.; MARKKANEN, H. Dental erosions in relation to lactovegetarian diet. *Scand. J. Dent. Res.*, **93**: 436-441 (1985).

7. EL-MARAGHY, S.S. Effect of some spices as preservatives for storage of lentil (Lens esculenta L.) seeds. *Folia Microbiol.*, **40**: 490-492. Praga (1995).

8. CHOWDHURY, B. ET AL. *Medical Science Research*, **24**: 669-670 (1996).

9. MATA, L. ET AL. Extinction of Vibrio cholerae in acidic substrata: contaminated cabbage and lettuce treated with lime juice. *Rev. Biol. Trop. (Mars)*, **50**: 181-184 (1990).

10. MYERS, B.M.; GRAHAM, D.Y. Effect of red pepper and black pepper on the stomach. *Am. J. Gastroenterol*, **82**: 211-214 (1987).

11. NDJITOYAP-NDAM, E.C. ET AL. [Upper digestive system hemorrhages in Cameroons (apropos of 172 cases examined via endoscopy)]. *Med. Trop. (Mars)*, **50**: 487-492 (1994).

12. GRAHAM, D.Y.; SMITH, J.L.; OPEKUN, A.R. Spicy food and the stomach. Evaluation by videoendoscopy. *JAMA*, **260**: 3473-3475 (1988).

13. ODES, H.S. ET AL. Esophageal carcinoma in Indian Jews of southern Israel. An epidemiologic study. *J. Clin. Gastroenterol.*, **12**: 222-227 (1990).

14. SURH, Y.J.; LEE, S.S. Capsaicin in hot chili pepper: carcinogen, co-carcinogen or anticarcinogen? *Food Chem. Toxicol.*, **34**: 313-316 (1996).

15. SURH, Y.J.; LEE, S.S. Capsaicin, a double-edged sword: toxicity, metabolism, and chemopreventive potential. *Life Sci.*, **56**: 1845-1855 (1995).

16. URAGODA, C.G. Symptoms in spice workers. *J. Trop. Med. Hyg.*, **95**: 136-139 (1992).

17. NIINIMÄKI, A. ET AL. Spice allergy: results of skin prick tests and RAST with spice extracts. *Allergy*, **44**: 60-65 (1989).

18. NIINIMÄKI, A.; HANNUKSELA, M. Immediate skin test reactions to spices. *Allergy*, **36**: 487-493 (1981).

19. PRESCOTT, J.; STEVENSON, R.J. Effects of oral chemical irritation on tastes and flavors in frequent and infrequent users of chili. *Physiol. Behav.*, **58**: 1117-1127 (1995).

20. LOPEZ-CARRILLO, L. ET AL. Creencias sobre el consumo de chile y la salud en México DF. [Beliefs about chili intake and health in Mexico City] *Salud Publica Mex.* **37**: 339-343 (1995).

21. FUSCO, B.M.; GIACOVAZZO, M. Peppers and pain. The promise of capsaicin. *Drugs*, **53**: 909-914 (1997).

22. ANTONIOS, T.F.; MACGREGOR, G.A. Salt –more adverse effects. *Lancet*, **348**: 250-251 (1996).

CHAP. 16 NUTRITIONAL SUPPLEMENTS

1. MENARD, M.K. Vitamin and mineral supplement prior to and during pregnancy. *Obstet. Gynecol. Clin. North. Am.*, **24**: 479-498 (1997).

2. RIMM, E.B.; WILLETT, W.C.; HU, F.B. ET AL. Folate and vitamin B6 from diet and supplements in relation to risk of coronary heart disease among women. *JAMA*, **279**: 359-364 (1998).

3. HELSER, M.A.; HOTCHKISS, J.H.; ROE, D.A. Influence of fruit and vegetable juices on the endogenous formation of N-nitrosoproline and N-nitrosothiazolidine-4-carboxylic acid in humans

23. KANG, J.Y.; TENG, C.H.; WEE, A. ET AL. Effect of capsaicin and chilli on ethanol induced gastric mucosal injury in the rat. *Gut*, **36**: 664-669 (1995).

24. ELLIOTT, P.; STAMLER, J.; NICHOLS, R. ET AL. Intersalt revisited: further analyses of 24 hour sodium excretion and blood pressure within and across populations. Intersalt Cooperative Research Group [see comments] *BMJ*, **312**: 1249-1253 (1996).

25. MIDGLEY, J.P.; MATHEW, A.G.; GREENWOOD, C.M. Effect of reduced dietary sodium on blood pressure: a meta-analysis of randomized controlled trials. *JAMA*, **275**: 1590-1597 (1996).

26. XIE, J.X.; SASAKI, S.; JOOSSENS, J.V. ET AL. The relationship between urinary cations obtained from the INTERSALT study and cerebrovascular mortality. *J. Hum. Hypertens.*, **6**:17-21 (1992).

27. BRAHIMI, M.; KONDON, R.T.; TUAL, J.L. ET AL. Influence on sodium on arterial elasticity in essential hypertension. Seventh European Meeting on Hypertension. Milán, (1985).

28. DEVINE, A.; CRIDLE, A.R.; DICK, I.M. ET AL. A longitudinal study of the effect of sodium and calcium intakes on regional bone density in postmenopausal women. *Am. J. Clin. Nutr.*, **62**: 740-745 (1995).

29. TSUGANE, S.; TEI, Y.; TAKAHASHI, T. ET AL. Salty food intake and risk of Helicobacter pylori infection. *Jpn. J. Cancer Res.*, **85**: 474-478 (1994).

30. JOOSSENS, J.V.; HILL, M.J.; ELLIOTT, P. ET AL. Dietary salt, nitrate and stomach cancer mortality in 24 countries. European Cancer Prevention (ECP) and the INTERSALT Cooperative Research Group. *Int. J. Epidemiol.*, **25**: 494-504 (1996).

31. CAREY, O.J.; LOCKE, C.; COOKSON, J.B. Effect of alterations of dietary sodium on the severity of asthma in men. *Thorax*, **48**: 714-718 (1993).

32. MEDICI, T.C.; SCHMID, A.Z.; HACKI, M. ET AL. Are asthmatics salt-sensitive? A preliminary controlled study. *Chest*, **104**: 1138-1143 (1993).

33. ZOIA, M.C.; FANFULLA, F.; BRUSCHI, C. ET AL. Chronic respiratory symptoms, bronchial responsiveness and dietary sodium and potassium: a population-based study. *Monaldi Arch. Chest. Dis.*, **50**: 104-108 (1995).

34. MASSEY, L.K.; WHITING, S.J. Dietary salt, urinary calcium, and kidney stone risk. *Nutr. Rev.*, **53**: 131-139 (1995).

35. BURTIS, W.J.; GAY, L.; INSOGNA, K.L. ET AL. Dietary hypercalciuria in patients with calcium oxalate kidney stones. *Am. J. Clin. Nutr.*, **60**: 424-429 (1994).

36. JOOSSENS, J.V.; SASAKI, S.; KESTELOOT, H. Bread as a source of salt: an international comparison. *J. Am. Coll. Nutr.*, **13**: 179-183 (1994).

37. MACGREGOR, G.A.; SEVER, P.S. Salt-overwhelming evidence but still no action: can a consensus be reached with the food industry? *BMJ*,**312**: 1287-1289 (1996).

CHAP. 17: BEVERAGES

1. PETTER, L.P.; HOURIHANE, J.O.; ROLLES, C.J. Is water out of vogue? A survey of the drinking habits of 2-7 year olds. *Arch. Dis. Child.*, **72**: 137-140 (1995).

2. PAMPLONA-ROGER G. D. *Encyclopedia of Medicinal Plants*. Editorial Safeliz, Madrid, 1998, p. 752.

on controlled diets. *Carcinogenesis*, **13**: 2277-2280 (1992).

4. HATHCOCK, J.N. Vitamins and minerals: efficacy and safety. *Am. J. Clin. Nutr.*, **66**: 427-437 (1997).

5. BELTZ, S.D.; DOERING, P.L. Efficacy of nutritional supplements used by athletes. *Clin. Pharm.*, **12**: 900-908 (1993).

6. HESS, B.; ACKERMANN, D.; ESSIG, M. ET AL. Renal mass and serum calcitriol in male idiopathic calcium renal stone formers: role of protein intake. *J. Clin. Endocrinol. Metab.*, **80**: 1916-1921 (1995).

7. CLARK, L.C. ET AL. Effects of selenium supplementation for cancer prevention in patients with carcinoma of the skin. *JAMA*, **276**: 1957-1963 (1996).

8. HERTOG, M.G.; HOLLMAN, P.C.; KATAN, M.B. ET AL. Intake of potentially anticarcinogenic flavonoids and their determinants in adults in The Netherlands. *Nutr. Cancer*, **20**: 21-29 (1993).

9. FRANKEL, E.N.; KANNER, J.; GERMAN, J.B. ET AL. Inhibition of oxidation of human low-density lipoprotein by phenolic substances in red wine. *Lancet*, **341**: 454-457 (1993).

10. RAU, A.P.; HERZENBERG, A.L.; ROEDERER, C. Glutathione precursor and antioxidant activities of N-acetylcysteine and oxothiazolidine carboxylate compared in in vitro studies of HIV replication. *AIDS Res. Hum. Retrovi.*, **10**: 961 (1994).

11. KALEBIC, T.; KINTER, A. POLI, G. ET AL. Suppression in human immunodeficiency virus expression in chronically infected monocytic cells by glutathione, glutathione ester and N-acetylcysteine. *Proc. Natl. Acad. Sci. U.S.A.*, **88**: 986-990 (1991).

12. WEBER, C. ET AL. The coenzyme Q10 content of the average Danish diet. *Int. J. Vitam. Nutr. Res.*, **67**: 123-129 (1997).

13. BEMPONG, D.K.; HOUGHTON, P.J. Dissolution and absorption of caffeine from guarana. *J. Pharm. Pharmacol.*, **44**: 769-771 (1992).

14. ESPINOLA, E.B.; DIAS, R.F.; MATTEI, R. ET AL. Pharmacological activity of Guarana (Paullinia cupana Mart.) in laboratory animals. *J. Ethnopharmacol.*, **55**: 223-229 (1997).

15. BENONI, H.; DALLAKIAN, P.; TARAZ, K. Studies on the essential oil from guarana. *Z. Lebensm. Unters. Forsch.*, **203**: 95-98 (1996).

16. BYDLOWSKI, S.P.; D'AMICO, E.A.; CHAMONE, D.A. An aqueous extract of guarana (Paullinia cupana) decreases platelet thromboxane synthesis. *Braz. J. Med. Biol. Res.*, **24**: 421-424 (1991).

17. DA FONSECA, C.A.; LEAL, J.; COSTA, S.S. Genotoxic and mutagenic effects of guarana (Paullinia cupana) in prokaryotic organisms. *Mutat. Res.*, **321**: 165-173 (1994).

18. SCHWARZENBACH, F.H.; BRUNNER, K.W. Effects of a herbal yeast preparation in convalescent patients. *Schweizerische Zeitschrift fur Ganzheits Medizin*, **8**: 266-273 (1996).

19. MCKENZIE, H.; MAIN, J.; PENNINGTON, C.R.; ET AL. Antibody to selected strains of Saccharomyces cerevisiae (baker's and brewer's yeast) and Candida albicans in Crohn's disease. *Gut*, **31**: 536-538 (1990).

3. LUSSI, A.; JAEGGI, T.; JAEGGI-SCHARER, S. Prediction of the erosive potential of some beverages. *Caries Res.* **29:** 349-354 (1995).

4. WEISS, G.H.; SLUSS, P.M.; LINKE, C.A. Changes in urinary magnesium, citrate, and oxalate levels due to cola consumption. *Urology,* **39:** 331-333 (1992).

5. KERR, D.; SHERWIN, R.S.; PAVALKIS, F. ET AL. Effect of caffeine on the recognition of and responses to hypoglycemia in humans. *Ann. Intern. Med.,* **119:** 799-804 (1993).

6. SUPERKO, H.R.; MYLL, J.; DIRICCO, C. ET AL. Effects of cessation of caffeinated-coffee consumption on ambulatory and resting blood pressure in men. *Am. J. Cardiol.* **73:** 780-784 (1994).

7. VAN DUSSELDORP, M.; SMITS, P.; THIEN, T. ET AL. Effect of decaffeinated versus regular coffee on blood pressure. A 12-week, double-blind trial. *Hypertension,* **14:** 563-569 (1994).

8. PEHL, C.; PFEIFFER, A.; WENDL, B. ET AL. The effect of decaffeination of coffee on gastro-oesophageal reflux in patients with reflux disease. *Aliment. Pharmacol. Ther.,* **11:** 483-486 (1997).

9. WAHRBURG, U.; MARTIN, H.; SCHULTE, H. ET AL. Effects of two kinds of decaffeinated coffee on serum lipid profiles in healthy young adults. *Eur. J. Clin. Nutr.,* **48:** 172-179 (1994).

10. STICH, H.F. Teas and tea components as inhibitors of carcinogen formation in model systems and man. *Prev. Med.,* **21:** 377-384 (1992).

11. ISHIKAWA, T.; SUZUKAWA, M.; ITO, T. Effect of tea flavonoid supplementation on the susceptibility of low-density lipoprotein to oxidative modification. *Am. J. Clin. Nutr.,* **66:** 261-266 (1997).

12. KELI, S.O.; HERTOG, M.G.; FESKENS, E.J. ET AL. Dietary flavonoids, antioxidant vitamins, and incidence of stroke: the Zutphen study. *Arch. Intern. Med.,* **156:** 637-642 (1996).

13. HERTOG, M.; SWEETNAM, P.; FEHILY, A. ET AL. Antioxidant flavonols and ischemic heart disease in a Welsh population of men: the Caerphilly Study. *Am. J. Clin. Nutr.,* **65:** 1489-1494 (1997).

14. ENSMINGER, A. H. *The Concise Encyclopedia of Foods and Nutrition.* Boca Raton (Florida), CRC Press, 1995, p. 1011.

15. GOLDBOHM, R.A.; HERTOG, M.G.; BRANTS, H.A. ET AL. Consumption of black tea and cancer risk: a prospective cohort study. J. Natl. *Cancer Inst.,* **88:** 93-100 (1996).

16. PINTOS, J.; FRANCO, E.L.; OLIVEIRA, B.V. ET AL. Mate, coffee, and tea consumption and risk of cancers of the upper aerodigestive tract in southern Brazil. *Epidemiology,* **5:** 583-590 (1994).

17. VAN DUSSELDORP, M.; KATAN, M.B.; VAN VLIET, T. ET AL. Cholesterol-raising factor from boiled coffee does not pass a paper filter. *Arterioscler. Thromb.,* **11:** 586-593 (1991).

18. ZOCK, P.L.; KATAN, M.B.; MERKUS, M.P. ET AL. Effect of a lipid-rich fraction from boiled coffee on serum cholesterol. *Lancet,* **335:** 1235-1237 (1990).

19. BARRACLOUGH, M.S.; BEECH, J.R. Effects of caffeine on functional asymmetry in a Posner letter-recognition task. *Pharmacol. Biochem. Behav.,* **52:** 731-735 (1995).

20. BAK, A.A.; GROBBEE, D.E. Abstinence from coffee leads to a fall in blood pressure. *J. Hypertens. Suppl.,* **7:** S260-S261 (1989).

21. KAWACHI, I.; COLDITZ, G.A.; STONE, C.B. Does coffee drinking increase the risk of coronary heart disease? Results from a meta-analysis. *Br. Heart J.,* **72:** 269-275 (1994).

22. WEI, M.; MACERA, C.A.; HORNUNG, C.A. ET AL. The impact of changes in coffee consumption

on serum cholesterol. *J. Clin. Epidemiol.,* **48:** 1189-1196 (1995).

23. WENDL, B.; PFEIFFER, A.; PEHL, C. ET AL. Effect of decaffeination of coffee or tea on gastro-oesophageal reflux. *Aliment. Pharmacol. Ther.,* **8:** 283-287 (1994).

24. MOMAS, I.; DAURES, J.P.; FESTY, B. ET AL. Relative importance of risk factors in bladder carcinogenesis: some new results about Mediterranean habits. *Cancer Causes Control,* **5:** 326-332 (1994).

25. KUNZE, E.; CHANG-CLAUDE, J.; FRENTZEL-BEYME, R. Life style and occupational risk factors for bladder cancer in Germany. A case-control study. *Cancer,* **69:** 1776-1790 (1992).

26. TAVANI, A.; PREGNOLATO, A.; LA VECCHIA, C. ET AL. Coffee consumption and the risk of breast cancer. *Eur. J. Cancer Prev.,* **7:** 77-82 (1998).

27. ERNSTER, V.L.; MASON, L.; GOODSON, W.H. 3D. ET AL. Effects of caffeine-free diet on benign breast disease: a randomized trial. *Surgery,* **91:** 263-267 (1982).

28. HASLING, C.; SONDERGAARD, K.; CHARLES, P. ET AL. Calcium metabolism in postmenopausal osteoporotic women is determined by dietary calcium and coffee intake. *J. Nutr.,* **122:** 1119-1126 (1992).

29. Luke 10: 34.

30. World Health Organization, Communiqué WHO/84, November 1st, 1994.

31. DUCIMETIERE, P.; GUIZE, L.; MARCINIAK, A. Arteriographically documented coronary artery disease and alcohol consumption in French men. *The CORALI Study. Eur. Heart. J.,* **14:** 727-733 (1993).

32. CONSTANT, J. Alcohol, ischemic heart disease, and the French paradox. *Clin. Cardiol.,* **20:** 420-424 (1997).

33. YUAN, J.M.; ROSS, R.K.; GAO, Y.T. ET AL. Follow up study of moderate alcohol intake and mortality among middle aged men in Shanghai, China. *British Medical Journal,* **314:** 18-23 (1997).

34. CAMARGO, C.A.; HENNEKENS, C.H.; GAZIANO, J.M. ET AL. Prospective study of moderate alcohol consumption and mortality in United States male physicians. *Arch. Intern. Med.,* **157:** 79-85 (1997).

35. RIMM, E.B.; KLATSKY, A.; GROBBEE, D. ET AL. Review of moderate alcohol consumption and reduced risk of coronary heart disease: is the effect due to beer, wine, or spirits. *British Medical Journal,* **312:** 731-736 (1996).

36. DEMROW, H.S.; SLANE, R.; FOLTS, J.D. Administration of wine and grape juice inhibits in vivo platelet activity and thrombosis in stenosed canine coronary arteries. *Circulation,* **91:** 1182-1188 (1995).

37. FRANKEL, E.N.; KANNER, J.; GERMAN, J.B. ET AL. Inhibition of oxidation of human low-density lipoprotein by phenolic substances in red wine. *Lancet,* **341:** 454-457 (1993).

38. RENAUD, S.C.; RUF, J.C. Effects of alcohol on platelet functions. *Clin. Chim. Acta,* **246:** 77-89 (1996).

39. KLATSKY, A.L.; FRIEDMAN, G.D.; SIEGELAUB, A.B. ET AL. Alcohol consumption and blood presure: Kaiser-Permanente multiphasic health examination data. *N. Engl. J. Med.,* **296:** 1194-1200 (1977).

40. CRIQUI, M.H.; RINGEL, B.L. Does diet or alcohol explain the French paradox? *Lancet,* **344:** 1719-1723 (1994).

41. MEYER, F.; WHITE, E. Alcohol and nutrients in relation to colon cancer in middle-aged adults. *Am. J. Epidemiol.,* **138:** 225-236 (1993).

42. FERRARONI, M.; DECARLI, A.; WILLETT, W.C. ET AL. Alcohol and breast cancer risk: a case-con-

trol study from northern Italy. *Int. J. Epidemiol.,* **20:** 859-864 (1991).

43. WILLETT, W.C.; STAMPFER, M.J.; COLDITZ, G.A. ET AL. Moderate alcohol consumption and the risk of breast cancer. *N. Engl. J. Med.,* **316:** 1174-1180 (1987).

44. FALCAO, J.M.; DIAS, J.A.; MIRANDA, A.C. ET AL. Red wine consumption and gastric cancer in Portugal: a case-control study. *Eur. J. Cancer Prev.,* **3:** 269-276 (1994).

45. GRANDE, L.; MANTEROLA, C.; ROS, E. ET AL. Effects of red wine on 24-hour esophageal pH and pressures in healthy volunteers. *Dig. Dis. Sci.,* **42:** 1189-1193 (1997).

46. HERNANDEZ-AVILA, M.; COLDITZ, G.A.; STAMPFER, M.J. ET AL. Caffeine, moderate alcohol intake, and risk of fractures of the hip and forearm in middle-aged women. *Am. J. Clin. Nutr.,* **54:** 157-163 (1991).

47. KAMINSKI, M.; FRANC, M.; LEBOUVIER, M. ET AL. Moderate alcohol use and pregnancy outcome. *Neurobehav. Toxicol. Teratol.,* **3:** 173-181 (1981).

48. PAMPLONA-ROGER G. D. *Encyclopedia of Medicinal Plants.* Editorial Safeliz, Madrid, 1998, p. 158.

49. KEIL, U.; CHAMBLESS, L.E.; DORING, A. ET AL. The relation of alcohol intake to coronary heart disease and all-cause mortality in a beer-drinking population. *Epidemiology,* **8:** 150-156 (1997).

50. MESSNER, T.; PETERSSON, B. Alcohol consumption and ischemic heart disease mortality in Sweden. *Scand. J. Soc. Med.,* **24:** 107-113 (1996).

51. TRICKER, A.R.; PFUNDSTEIN, B.; THEOBALD, E. ET AL. Mean daily intake of volatile N-nitrosamines from foods and beverages in West Germany in 1989-1990. *Food Chem. Toxicol.,* **29:** 729-732 (1991).

52. RIBOLI, E.; CORNEE, J.; MACQUART-MOULIN, G. ET AL. Cancer and polyps of the colorectum and lifetime consumption of beer and other alcoholic beverages. *Am. J. Epidemiol.,* **134:** 157-166 (1991).

53. GIBSON, T.; RODGERS, A.V.; SIMMONDS, H.A. ET AL. A controlled study of diet in patients with gout. *Ann. Rheum. Dis.,* **42:** 123-127 (1983).

54. PEATFIELD, R.C. Relationships between food, wine, and beer-precipitated migrainous hea daches. *Headache,* **35:** 355-357 (1995).

CHAP. 18: THE COMPONENTS OF FOODS

1. RAUMA, A.L.; TORRONEN, R.; HANNINEN, O.; MYKKANEN, H. Vitamin B₁₂ status of long-term adherents of a strict uncooked vegan diet ("living food diet") is compromised. *J. Nutr.,* **125:** 2511-2515 (1995).

2. ENSMINGER, A. H. *The Concise Encyclopedia of Foods and Nutrition.* Boca Raton (Florida), CRC Press, 1995, p. 588.

3. HADDAD, J.G. Vitamin D–solar rays, the Milky Way, or both? *N. Engl. J. Med.,* **326:** 1213-1215 (1992).

4. IP, C.; LISK, D.J.; STOEWSAND, G.S. Mammary cancer prevention by regular garlic and selenium-enriched garlic. *Nutr. Cancer.,* **17:** 279-286 (1992).

5. CLARK, L.C. ET AL. Effects of selenium supplementation for cancer prevention in patients with carcinoma of the skin. *JAMA,* **276:** 1957-1963 (1996).

6. DIAZ-ALARCON, J.P. ET AL. Determination of selenium in cereals, legumes and dry fruits from southeastern Spain for calculation of daily dietary intake. *Sci. Total. Environ.,* **184:** 183-189 (1996).

7. OSTER, O.; PRELLWITZ, W. The daily dietary selenium intake of West German adults. *Biol. Trace Elem. Res.*, **20**: 1-14 (1989).

8. OLIVARES, M.; UAUY, R. Copper as an essential nutrient. *Am. J. Clin. Nutr.*, **63**: 791S-796S (1996).

9. RIMM, E.B.; KATAN, M.B.; ASCHERIO, A. ET AL. Relation between intake of flavonoids and risk for coronary heart disease in male health professionals. *Ann. Intern. Med.*, **125**: 384-389 (1996).

10. HERTOG, M.G.; FESKENS, E.J.; HOLLMAN, P.C. ET AL. Dietary antioxidant flavonoids and risk of coronary heart disease: the Zutphen Elderly Study. *Lancet*, **342**: 1007-1011 (1993).

11. FRANKEL, E.N.; KANNER, J.; GERMAN, J.B. ET AL. Inhibition of oxidation of human low-density lipoprotein by phenolic substances in red wine. *Lancet*, **341**: 454-457 (1993).

12. KANNER, J.; FRANKEL, E.; GRANIT, E. ET AL. Natural anti-oxidants in grapes and wines. *J. Agric. Food Chem.*, **42**: 64-69 (1994).

13. KELI, S.O.; HERTOG, M.G.; FESKENS, E.J. ET AL. Dietary flavonoids, antioxidant vitamins, and incidence of stroke: the Zutphen study. *Arch. Intern. Med.*, **156**: 637-642 (1996).

14. HERTOG, M.G.; HOLLMAN, P.C.; KATAN, M.B. ET AL. Intake of potentially anticarcinogenic flavonoids and their determinants in adults in The Netherlands. *Nutr. Cancer*, **20**: 21-29 (1993).

15. WATTENBERG, L.W. Inhibition of carcinogenesis by minor anutrient constituents of the diet. *Proc. Nutr. Soc.*, **49**: 173-183 (1990).

16. MIDDLETON, E. JR; KANDASWAMI, C.T. Potential health-promoting properties of citrus flavonoids. *Food Technology*, **48**: 115-119 (1994).

17. MULDOON, M.F.; KRITCHECSKY, S.B. Flavonoids and heart disease. *British Medical Journal*, **312**: 458-459 (1996).

18. HERTOG, M.G.; HOLLMAN, P.C. Potential health effects of the dietary flavonol quercetin. *Eur. J. Clin. Nutr.*, **50**: 63-71 (1996).

19. WONG, H. ET AL. *Journal of Agriculture and Food Chemistry*, **45**: 304-309 (1997).

20. CRAIG, W.J. Phytochemicals: Guardians of our health. *Issues on Vegetarian Dietetics*, **5** (3): 1(1996).

21. MAZZA, G. Anthocyanins in grapes and grape products. *Crit. Rev. Food Sci. Nutr.*, **35**: 341-371 (1995).

22. THOMPSON, L.U. Antioxidants and hormone-mediated health benefits of whole grains. *Crit. Rev. Food Sci. Nutr.*, **34**: 473-497 (1994).

23. HUTCHINS, A.M.; LAMPE, J.W.; MARTINI, M.C. ET AL. Vegetables, fruits, and legumes: effect on urinary isoflavonoid phytoestrogen and lignan excretion. *J. Am. Diet. Assoc.*, **95**: 769-774 (1995).

24. THOMPSON, L.U.; ROBB, P.; SERRAINO, M. ET AL. Mammalian lignan production from various foods. *Nutr. Cancer*, **16**: 43-52 (1991).

25. GORMAN, M.A.; BOWMAN, C. Position of the American Dietetic Association: health implications of dietary fiber. *J. Am. Diet. Assoc.*, **93**: 1446-1447 (1993).

26. DWYER, J.T. Dietary fiber for children: how much? *Pediatrics*, **96**: 1019-1022 (1995).